Core Topics in Critical Care Medicine

Core Topics in Critical Care Medicine

Edited by

Fang Gao Smith

Professor in Anaesthesia, Critical Care Medicine and Pain, Academic Department of Anaesthesia, Critical Care and Pain, Heart of England NHS Foundation Trust, Clinical Trials Unit, University of Warwick, UK

Associate editor

Joyce Yeung

Anaesthetic Specialist Registrar, Warwickshire Rotation, West Midlands Deanery and Research Fellow, Academic Department of Anaesthesia, Critical Care and Pain, Heart of England NHS Foundation Trust, UK

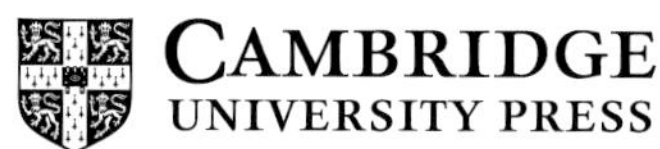

CAMBRIDGE UNIVERSITY PRESS
Cambridge, New York, Melbourne, Madrid, Cape Town, Singapore,
São Paulo, Delhi, Dubai, Tokyo

Cambridge University Press
The Edinburgh Building, Cambridge CB2 8RU, UK

Published in the United States of America by
Cambridge University Press, New York

www.cambridge.org
Information on this title: www.cambridge.org/9780521897747

First published 2010

Printed in the United Kingdom at the University Press, Cambridge

A catalogue record for this publication is available from the British Library

ISBN 978-0-521-89774-7 Hardback

Contents

Contributors

Frances Aitchison
Consultant Radiologist
Birmingham City Hospital
West Midlands Critical Care Research Network
Birmingham, UK

Prasad Bheemasenachar
Consultant Intensivist
Birmingham Heartlands Hospital
West Midlands Critical Care Research Network
Birmingham, UK

John Bleasdale
Consultant Intensivist
Birmingham City Hospital
West Midlands Critical Care Research Network
Birmingham, UK

Andrew Burtenshaw
Consultant Intensivist
Worcestershire Royal Hospital
West Midlands Critical Care Research Network
Worcester, UK

John Clift
Consultant Anaesthetist
Birmingham City Hospital
West Midlands Critical Care Research Network
Birmingham, UK

Neil Crooks
Anaesthetic Specialist Registrar
Birmingham Heartlands Hospital
West Midlands Critical Care Research Network
Birmingham, UK

Fang Gao Smith
Professor in Critical Care Medicine
Birmingham Heartlands Hospital
West Midlands Critical Care Research Network
Birmingham, UK

Nageena Hussain
Anaesthetic Specialist Registrar
University Hospital Coventry and Warwickshire
West Midlands Critical Care Research Network
Birmingham, UK

Santhana Kannan
Consultant Intensivist
Birmingham City Hospital
West Midlands Critical Care Research Network
Birmingham, UK

Zahid Khan
Consultant Intensivist
Birmingham City Hospital
West Midlands Critical Care Research Network
Birmingham, UK

Anil Kumar
Anaesthetic Specialist Registrar
University Hospital Coventry and Warwickshire
West Midlands Critical Care Research Network
Birmingham, UK

Edwin Mitchell
Consultant Intensivist
Birmingham City Hospital
West Midlands Critical Care Research Network
Birmingham, UK

Randeep Mullhi
Anaesthetic Specialist Registrar
University Hospital Birmingham
West Midlands Critical Care Research Network
Birmingham, UK

Nick Murphy
Consultant Intensivist
University Hospital Birmingham
West Midlands Critical Care Research Network
Birmingham, UK

Darshan Pandit
Consultant Intensivist
Russell Hall Hospital
West Midlands Critical Care Research Network
Dudley, UK

Mamta Patel
Consultant Intensivist
Birmingham City Hospital
West Midlands Critical Care Research Network
Birmingham, UK

Gavin Perkins
Associate Clinical Professor in Critical Care Medicine
Birmingham Heartlands Hospital
West Midlands Critical Care Research Network
Birmingham, UK

Khai Ping Ng
Medical Specialist Registrar
Birmingham Heartlands Hospital
West Midlands Critical Care Research Network
Birmingham, UK

Elinor Powell
Anaesthetic Specialist Registrar/Research Fellow
Birmingham Heartlands Hospital
West Midlands Critical Care Research Network
Birmingham, UK

George Pulikal
Medical Specialist Registrar
Derriford Hospital
Plymouth, UK

Isma Quasim
Consultant Anaesthetist
Golden Jubilee Hospital
Scotland, UK

Tara Quasim
Senior Lecturer
Glasgow Royal Infirmary
Glasgow, UK

Nick Sherwood
Consultant Intensivist
Birmingham City Hospital
West Midlands Critical Care Research Network
Birmingham, UK

Angeline Simons
Medical Specialist Registrar
Birmingham Heartlands Hospital
West Midlands Critical Care Research Network
Birmingham, UK

Harjot Singh
Consultant Anaesthetist
University Hospital Birmingham
West Midlands Critical Care Research Network
Birmingham, UK

Richard Skone
Paediatric Intensive Care Registrar
Birmingham Children's Hospital
Birmingham, UK

Catherine Snelson
Medical Specialist Registrar/Advanced Trainee in Intensive Care Medicine
Birmingham Heartlands Hospital
West Midlands Critical Care Research Network
Birmingham, UK

Roger Stedman
Consultant Intensivist
Birmingham Heartlands Hospital
West Midlands Critical Care Research Network
Birmingham, UK

David Thickett
Senior Lecturer in Respiratory Medicine
University Hospital Birmingham
West Midlands Critical Care Research Network
Birmingham, UK

Yasser Tolba
Consultant Intensivist
Birmingham Heartlands Hospital
West Midlands Critical Care Research Network
Birmingham, UK

Bill Tunnicliffe
Consultant Intensivist
University Hospital Birmingham
West Midlands Critical Care Research Network
Birmingham, UK

Sandeep Walia
Consultant Anaesthetist
University Hospital Birmingham
West Midlands Critical Care Research Network
Birmingham, UK

Tony Whitehouse
Consultant Intensivist
University Hospital Birmingham
West Midlands Critical Care Research Network
Birmingham, UK

Joyce Yeung
Anaesthetic Specialist Registrar/Research Fellow
Birmingham Heartlands Hospital
West Midlands Critical Care
Research Network
Birmingham, UK

Foreword

The range of chapter titles in this concise and focussed textbook demonstrates how far intensive care medicine has travelled along the road from the first steps of providing co-located care for patients with a single disease – respiratory paralysis from polio – to becoming a speciality caring for patients with life-threatening disease of multiple organ systems. The outcome from the polio epidemics of the 1950s was transformed by the anaesthetist Professor Bjorn Ibsen, who reduced the mortality from 90% to 40% by combining laboratory science with applied physiology to change the way care was delivered – from iron lung respirator to positive pressure ventilation via a cuffed tracheostomy tube. The 'power supply' (medical students) was soon replaced by the development of mechanical ventilators, and the scientific innovation – arterial blood gas measurement – rapidly become a standard investigation in any acutely ill patient. Although polio has virtually disappeared, intensive care was retained by hospitals convinced of its apparent utility for supporting patients with an increasingly diverse mix of diseases. In the Western world at least, we now care for patients with a substantial chronic disease burden underlying their acute illness, and intensive care has increasingly come to resemble general medical practice with its accompanying ethical issues for individuals and for society. Indeed, Professor Henry Lassen's data describing the polio epidemic (Lancet 1953) demonstrated that although the new technique of ventilatory management saved many lives, those who eventually died did so much later: intensive care has the capacity to delay, but not always prevent, death.

As a new multi-disciplinary speciality we have many challenges and opportunities ahead, from understanding the cellular mechanisms of organ dysfunction and sepsis to improving the reliability and safety of care delivered across multiple transitions in time, place and staff. The modern intensivist must combine many roles: compassionate clinician, scientist, educator and team leader amongst them. For those wishing to participate, the experience will be demanding and rewarding. This textbook provides a sound basis for that journey.

Professor Julian Bion MBBS FRCP FRCA MD
Professor of Intensive Care Medicine
University Department of Anaesthesia and Intensive Care Medicine
Royal College of Anaesthetists
Chair, Professional Standards Committee
Chair, European Board of Intensive Care Medicine

Preface

This book is primarily aimed at trainees from all specialties who are undertaking subspecialty training in critical care medicine. The book aims to provide a clear, highlighted guide, from the assessment to the management of critically ill patients. It also aims to provide comprehensive, concise and easily accessible information on all aspects of critical care medicine for trainees preparing for their specialty examinations. We have endeavoured to provide up-to-date evidence-based medicine and further reading which we encourage our readers to turn to for more detailed information. The topics in the book have been selected to complement the curriculum of SHO and SpR training by the Intercollegiate Board for training in intensive care medicine. The more advanced trainee in critical care and allied health professionals will find this book useful as a quick reference and a stimulus for further research.

Section I starts with the different practical aspects in the day-to-day work in critical care. There is an overview of the practical skills such as advanced airway management, transfer of the critically ill as well as the theory behind severity scoring systems of patients and the different uses of modern technology in critical care. Principles of the use of common drugs such as vasoactive drugs, sedation and analgesia are outlined. The often overlooked but crucial subjects of nutrition, ethics and organ donation are also discussed.

Section II covers systemic disorders and their management. This includes familiar conditions in the majority of critical care patients such as sepsis, multi-organ failure, the immunosuppressed and post-operative and post-resuscitation care. Basic theory behind acid–base disturbances, fluids and electrolyte disorders and antibiotic use is also examined here.

Section III focuses on specific organ dysfunctions and their specific management. This section expands on disorders of each organ system, including an examination of the difficult and often confusing concepts of ventilation and weaning and renal replacement therapy. There are separate chapters covering obstetric and paediatric emergencies to cover the range of scenarios encountered by the critical care trainee.

Finally, Section IV outlines higher examinations in intensive care medicine in UK and Europe. Advanced trainees in intensive care will find this a particularly useful resource and sample questions are included as reference.

Acknowledgements

We are indebted to all of the contributors of the book for all their huge efforts and also to our families and loved ones for their unyielding support.

We are grateful to Dr Seema, Dr Nick Crooks, Dr Krishsrik and Dr Ellie Powell for critically reviewing and commenting on a number of chapters.

We thank Nicola Morrow of Warwick Medical School, University of Warwick and Dawn Hill of West Midlands Critical Care Research Network, Birmingham Heartlands Hospital for their help with the abbreviation list.

Abbreviations

A&E	Accident and Emergency
ABC	Airways, Breathing, Circulation
ABCDE	airways, breathing, circulation, disability, exposure
ABGs	arterial blood gases
ABS	analgesic-based sedation
ACE	angiotensin-converting enzyme
ACE-Is	angiotensin-converting enzyme inhibitors
ACPE	acute cardiogenic pulmonary oedema
ACS	acute coronary syndrome
ACT	activated clotting time
ACTH	adrenocorticotropic hormone
ADH	antidiuretic hormone
AED	anti-epileptic drug
AEP	auditory evoked potentials
AF	atrial fibrillation
AFE	amniotic fluid embolism
AG	anion gap
AHA	American Heart Association
AHF	acute heart failure
AIDF	acute inflammatory demyelinating polyneuropathy
AIDS	acquired immunodeficiency syndrome
AIS	abbreviated injury scoring
AKI	acute kidney injury
ALERT™	Acute Life Threatening Events – Recognition and Treatment
ALF	acute liver failure
ALI	acute lung injury
ANP	atrial (A type) natriuretic peptide
AoCLD	acute on chronic liver disease
APACHE	acute physiology and chronic health evaluation
APC	activated protein C
APH	antepartum haemorrhage
APRV	airway pressure release ventilation
APTT	acitvated partial thromboplastin time
ARB	angiotensin II receptor antagonist
ARDS	acute respiratory distress syndrome
ARF	acute renal failure
ARR	absolute risk reduction
ASV	adaptive support ventilation
AT	antithrombin
ATC	automated tube compensation
ATLS	Advanced Trauma Life Support Course
ATN	acute tubular necrosis
ATP	adenosine triphosphate
ATS	American Thoracic Society
AV	atrioventricular
AVNRT	atrioventricular nodal re-entrant tachycardia
AVPU	patient is alert, responding to voice, responding to pain, unresponsive
AVRT	atrioventricular re-entrant tachycardia
BBB	bundle branch block
BIS	bispectral index
BMI	body mass index
BMR	basal metabolic rate
BNP	brain (B type) natriuretic peptide
BOOP	bronchiolitis obliterans organizing pneumonia
bpm	beats per minute
CABG	coronary artery bypass grafting
CAD	coronary artery disease
CAMP	cyclic adenosine monophosphate
CBF	cerebral blood flow
CBV	cerebral blood volume
CCK	cholecystokinin
CCO	critical care outreach
CCRISP™	Care of the Critically Ill Surgical Patient
CEMACH	confidential enquiries into maternal and child health
CI	cardiac index
CI	confidence interval
CIRCI	critical illness related corticosteroid insufficiency
CK	creatine kinase
CMV	continuous mandatory ventilation

CNS	central nervous system
CoBaTrICE	Competency Based Training in Intensive Care Medicine in Europe
COPD	chronic obstructive pulmonary disease
COX	cyclo-oxygenase
CPAP	continuous positive airway pressure
CPFA	coupled plasma filtration absorption
CPP	cerebral perfusion pressure
CPR	cardiopulmonary resuscitation
CrCU	Critical Care Unit
CRF	chronic renal failure
CSF	cerebrospinal fluid
C-spine	cervical spine
CSS	Canadian Society Classification of Angina
CT	computed tomography
CVA	cerebrovascular accident
CVP	central venous pressure
CVVH	continuous veno-venous haemofiltration
CVVHD	continuous veno-venous haemodialysis
CVVHDF	continuous veno-venous haemodiafiltration
CXR	chest X-ray
DAI	diffuse axonal injury
DI	diabetes insipidus
DIC	disseminated intravascular coagulation
DVT	deep vein thrombosis
EBV	Epstein–Barr virus
$ECCO_2R$	extracorporeal carbon dioxide removal
ECG	electrocardiograph
ECLA	extracorporeal lung assist
ECLS	extracorporeal lung support
ECMO	extracorporeal membrane oxygenation
EDH	extradural haematoma
EEG	electroencephalograph
EF	enteral feeding
EN	enteral nutrition
EPIC	evidence-based practice in infection control
ERCP	endoscopic retrograde cholangiopancreatography
ERV	expiratory reserve volume
ESC	European Society of Cardiology
$ETCO_2$	end-tidal carbon dioxide
EVLW	extravascular lung water
F/VT	frequency/tidal volume ratio
FA	flow assist
FAST	focused assessment sonography in trauma
FLAIR	fluid-attenuated inversion recovery
FRC	functional residual capacity
GABA	γ-aminobutyric acid (inhibitory neurotransmitter)
GCS	Glasgow Coma Score
GCSE	generalized convulsive status epilepticus
GEDV	global end diastolic volume
GFR	glomerular filtration rate
GIT	gastrointestinal tract
GTN	glyceryl trinitrate
GvsHD	graft versus host disease
HAART	highly active antiretrovival therapy
HBD	heart-beating donation
HBDs	heart-beating donors
HBS	hypnotic-based sedation
HCAP	healthcare-associated pneumonia
HCV	hepatitis C virus
HDU	High Dependency Unit
HE	hepatic encephalopathy
HELLP	haemolysis, elevated liver enzymes and low platelets syndrome
HepB	hepatitis B
HES	hydroxyl-ethyl starch
HFOV	high-frequency oscillatory ventilation
Hib	*Haemophilus influenzae* type B
HIT	heparin-induced thrombocytopenia
HIV	human immunodeficiency virus
HME	heat and moisture exchange unit
HPV	hypoxic pulmonary vasoconstriction
HSCT	haematopoietic stem cell transplant
HUS	haemolytic uraemic syndrome
HVHF	high-volume haemofiltration
IABP	intra-aortic balloon pump
IC	inspiratory capacity
ICD	implantable cardiovertor–defibrillator
ICF	intracellular fluid
ICH	intracranial hypertension
ICNARC	Intensive Care National Audit and Research Centre
ICP	intracranial pressure
ICS	Intensive Care Society
IHD	intermittent haemodalysis

IJV	internal jugular vein
INR	international normalized ratio
IR	infrared
IRV	inspiratory reserve volume
IRV	inverse ratio ventilation
ISP	increase pressure support
ITBV	intrathoracic blood volume
IV	intravenous
IVF	in vitro fertilization
JVP	jugular venous pressure
LBBB	left bundle branch block
LDL	low-density lipoprotein
LED	light emitting diode
LMA	left mentoanterior
LMWH	low-molecular-weight heparin
LOC	loss of consciousness
LV	liquid ventilation
LVEDP	left ventricular end diastolic pressure
LVH	left ventricular hypertrophy
MAP	mean airway pressure
MAP	mean arterial pressure
MARS	molecular absorbent recirculation system
MCQ	multiple choice questions
MDMA	methylenedioxymethamphetamine; ecstasy
MENDS	maximizing efficacy of targeted sedation and reducing neurological dysfunction
MET	medical emergency team
MI	myocardial infarction
MIC	minimum inhibitory concentration
MIP	maximum inspiratory pressure
MMDS	microcirculatory and mitochondrial distress syndrome
MODS	multiple organ dysfunction syndrome
MOF	multiple organ failure
MOST	multi-organ support therapy
MPAP	mean pulmonary artery pressure
MPM	mortality probability model
MRI	magnetic resonance imaging
MRSA	methicillin resistant *Staphylococcus aureus*
MSBT	safety of blood and tissues for transplantation
MSOF	multiple systems organ failure
MV	mechanical ventilation
MV	minute ventilation
MVV	maximal voluntary ventilation
MW	molecular weight
NAC	*N*-acetylcysteine
NAD^+	nicotinamide adenine dinucleotide
NAPQI	*N*-acetyl-*p*-benzoquinone-imine
NAVA	neurally adjusted ventilatory assistance
NCSE	non-convulsive status epilepticus
NETI	nasotracheal endotracheal intubation
NHBD	non-heart beating donor
NHS	National Health Service
NICE	National Institute for Clinical Excellence
NICO	non-invasive cardiac output
NIV	non-invasive ventilation
NKH	non-ketotic hyperglycemia
NMDA	N-methyl-D-aspartate
NO	nitric oxide
NPPV	non-invasive positive pressure ventilation
NRTI	nucleoside reverse transcriptase inhibitors
NSAID	non-steroidal anti-inflammatory drug
NTG	nitroglycerine
ODTF	organ donation taskforce
OHSS	ovarian hyperstimulation syndrome
PA	pulmonary artery
PACS	picture archiving and communication system
PACT	patient-centred acute care training
PAE	post antibiotic effect
PAFC	pulmonary artery flotation catheter
PAV	proportional assist ventilation
PAWP	pulmonary artery wedge pressure
PC	pressure control
PCA	patient-controlled analgesia
PCI	percutaneous coronary intervention
PCP	*Pneumocystis jiroveci/carinii* pneumonia
PCR	polymerase chain reaction
PCV	pressure control ventilation
PCWP	pulmonary capillary wedge pressure
PDEIs	phosphodiesterase enzyme inhibitors
PE	phenytoin, equivalents
PE	pulmonary embolus
PECLA	pumpless extracorporeal lung assist
PEEP	positive end expiratory pressure
PEG	percutaneous endoscopic gastrostomy
PF	parenteral feeding
PF4	platelet factor 4

PiCCO	pulse-induced contour cardiac output
PLEDs	periodic lateralizing epileptiform activities
PLV	partial liquid ventilation
POP	pancreatitis outcome prediction
PPH	postpartum haemorrhage
PR	per rectum
PSS	physiological scoring systems
PSV	pressure support ventilation
PTA	post-traumatic amnesia
RAP	right atrial pressure
RAS	reticular activating system
RBCs	red blood cells
RBF	renal blood flow
RCT	randomized controlled trial
RDS	respiratory distress syndrome
REM	rapid eye movement
RM	recruitment manoeuvre
ROSC	return of spontaneous circulation
RPGN	rapidly progressive glomerulonephritis
RRT	renal replacement therapy
RSBI	rapid shallow breathing index
RTA	renal tubular acidosis
RV	residual volume
rVII	recombinant activated factor VII
SAFE	saline versus albumin fluid evaluation
SAP	severe acute pancreatitis
SAPS	simplified acute physiology score
SBP	systolic blood pressure
SBT	spontaneous breathing trial
SC	subcutaneous
SCCM	Society of Critical Care Medicine
SCUF	slow continuous ultrafiltration
SDD	selective digestive decontamination
SDH	subdural haematoma
SE	status epilepticus
SIADH	syndrome of inappropriate diuretic hormone
SID	strong ion difference
SIMV	synchronized intermittent mandatory ventilation
SIRS	systemic inflammatory response syndrome
SLE	systemic lupus erythematosus
SMT	standard medical therapy
SN	sick sinus syndrome
SOFA	sequential organ failure assessment
SpO_2	spot oxygen saturation
SSI	signs and symptoms of infection
SSRIs	selective serotonin reuptake inhibitors
ST	sharp transients
SV	stroke volume
SvO_2	mixed venous saturation
SVR	systemic vascular resistance
SVT	supraventricular tachycardia
TBI	traumatic brain injury
TCAs	tricyclic antidepressants
TDS	total dissolved solids
TEDs	thromboembolic disease preventing stockings
TEG	thromboelastography
TF	tissue factor
TFPI	tissue factor pathway inhibitor
TGI	transtracheal gas insufflation
TIPS	transjugular intrahepatic portosystemic shunt
TLC	total lung capacity
TLV	total liquid ventilation
TM	thrombomodulin
TOE	transoesophageal echocardiography
TPN	total parenteral nutrition
TTP	thrombotic thrombocytopenia purpura
TV	tidal volume
URL	upper reference limit
VA	volume assist
VAD	ventricular assist device
VAP	ventilator-associated pneumonia
VC	vital capacity
VC	volume control
VCV	volume control ventilation
VF	ventricular fibrillation
VILI	ventilator-induced lung injury
V/Q	ventilation–perfusion
VRE	vancomycin resistant enterococci
VT	tidal volume
VT	ventricular tachycardia
VTE	venous thromboembolism
VZV	*Varicella zoster* virus
WBC	white blood cell
WHF	World Heart Foundation
WPW	Wolff–Parkinson–White syndrome

Section I Chapter 1

Specific features of critical care medicine
Recognition of critical illness

Edwin Mitchell

Initial assessment and resuscitation

General considerations

- Critical illness, simply defined, is a state where death is likely or imminent. All of us will experience a critical illness by definition, but the aim of intensive care is to identify patients whose critical illness pathway can be altered and steered away from a fatal outcome.
- Over the past decade, it has become clearer that intervening earlier in a patient's critical illness may lead to improved survival. Even when life-prolonging treatment is no longer in the patient's best interests, acknowledging a patient is critically ill and in the terminal phase of their illness allows appropriate palliative care to be given.
- Critical illnesses are characterized by the failure of organ systems, and it is the signs of these organ failures that the initial assessment hopes to identify. Commonly, organ systems fail in sequence over time leading to multi-organ failure, and resuscitation aims to limit this. Mortality is proportional to the number of failed organs, duration of dysfunction and severity of organ failure.
- In contrast to the treatment of many routine medical conditions, where definitive treatment is based on a thorough assessment of the patient, the assessment of the critically ill patient typically occurs simultaneously with treatment due to clinical urgency.

Assessment

- The initial assessment of the critically ill patient should begin with a brief, targeted history and an appraisal of the patient's vital signs to identify life-threatening abnormalities that merit immediate attention. Signs suggesting severe illness are listed in Table 1.1.
- Most physicians are familiar with the 'ABCDE' (Airway, Breathing, Circulation, Disability, Exposure) approach to patient assessment taught on Advanced Life Support™, Advanced Trauma Life Support™ and other nationally recognized courses. This approach is speedy, thorough and adaptable, compared to the traditional medical 'clerking'.
- The principle behind the ABCDE approach is that problems are prioritized according to the severity of threat posed. Serious physiological derangements should be dealt with at each stage before moving on to assess the next step. For example, an obstructed airway should be identified and cleared before assessing breathing and measuring blood pressure.
- In reality, information is gathered in a non-linear fashion, but it is helpful to have a clear guideline within which to work. With adequate staff training and numbers, it should be possible to deal simultaneously with multiple problems.
- Common signs of organ failure should be sought, and bedside monitoring equipment (such as pulse oximetry, automated blood pressure measurement devices and thermometers) may augment the clinical examination. Near-patient testing, using equipment such as the Haemacue™, and arterial blood gas sampling can provide useful and rapid information regarding the oxygenation of the patient and common derangements in acid–base status and haemoglobin.

Resuscitation

- The purpose of resuscitation is to restore or establish effective oxygen delivery to the tissues, in particular those of the vital organs – brain, heart,

Core Topics in Critical Care Medicine, eds. Fang Gao Smith and Joyce Yeung. Published by Cambridge University Press.

Table 1.1 Signs suggestive of critical illness

- Obstructed/threatened airway
- Respiratory rate >25 breaths/min or <8 breaths/min
- Oxygen saturations <90% on air
- Heart rate >120 bpm or <40 bpm
- Systolic blood pressure <90 mmHg
- Capillary refill >3 seconds
- Urine output <0.5 ml/kg per hour more than last 4 hours
- Glasgow coma score <15 or status epilepticus or patient not fully alert

kidneys, liver and gut. Oxygen delivery depends on adequate oxygen uptake from the lungs, an adequate cardiac output to deliver the oxygen to the tissues and an adequate haemoglobin concentration to carry the oxygen.

- These goals of resuscitation are usually achieved by the use of supplemental oxygen, fluid or red blood cell transfusion, inotropic support or antibiotics as needed. In certain circumstances, such as penetrating trauma, a surgical approach to limiting life-threatening bleeding is considered to be a part of the resuscitation process.
- Resuscitation should begin as soon as the need for it has been identified. There is now evidence showing that early intervention (within a few hours of admission) limits the degree of organ dysfunction and improves survival. Waiting until the patient reaches the intensive care unit may be too long a delay if further deterioration in the patient's condition is to be prevented.
- In some situations, such as head injury, even single episodes of hypotension or hypoxia are associated with worsened outcomes.
- Early and complete resuscitation is associated with improved outcomes.

Monitoring the progress of resuscitation

At present, there are only limited ways in which the function of individual tissue beds can be assessed. Assessing the adequacy of resuscitation is usually based on either global markers of oxygen supply and utilization (such as the normalizaton of mixed venous oxygen saturations and lactate concentration), or the clinical responses of the affected organs – urine output from the kidneys for example. Whilst resuscitation is ongoing, invasive monitors such as an arterial cannula, a central venous cannula and a urinary catheter may be placed, but these additional monitors should not detract from the clinical monitoring of the patient.

Table 1.2 Suggested goals to be achieved within 6 hours of presentation for the resuscitation of septic shock refractory to fluid therapy (after Rivers *et al.*)

- Mean arterial pressure >65 mmHg
- Central venous pressure 8–12 mmHg
- Urine output >0.5 ml/kg per hour
- Central venous oxygen saturation >70%

- Resuscitation must be tailored to the individual patient. There are now data to suggest appropriate goals or parameters for resuscitation in certain clinical states, notably sepsis (Table 1.2), acute head injury and penetrating trauma.
- Over-enthusiastic attempts at resuscitation can lead to problems with fluid overload, worsening haemorrhage through dilution of clotting factors, or rapid electrolyte shifts leading to cerebral oedema.
- The importance of early assessment by adequately trained staff, with regular review of clinical progress, cannot be over-emphasized.

Once resuscitation is under way and the patient is stabilized, it is appropriate to begin an in-depth assessment of the patient. This means taking a more complete history, making a thorough examination and ordering clinical investigations as indicated. This phase of the process aims to establish an underlying diagnosis and guide definitive treatment. If deterioration occurs over this time, the cycle of assessment and resuscitation should begin again.

Physiology monitoring systems

Physiology monitoring systems are systems that allow the integration of easily obtained and measured physiological variables into a single score or code that triggers a particular action or care pathway (see also Chapter 5: Scoring systems and outcome).

- The commonly measured physiological variables are heart rate, blood pressure, respiratory rate, temperature, urine output and consciousness level, and these can be assessed at the bedside.
- Action may be triggered by a single abnormality or by an aggregate score. Aggregate scoring systems are generally preferred as they may also allow a graded response depending on the score.
- Physiological Scoring Systems (PSS) developed from the recognition that critically ill patients, and

Table 1.3 Advantages and disadvantages of Physiological Scoring Systems

Advantages	Disadvantages
• Rapid assessment • Facilitates communication between healthcare workers • Empowers staff • Reduces time from deterioration to action	• Poor sensitivity (may not identify all critically ill patients) • Not validated in target populations • May not be appropriate for all patients (chronic health conditions, terminally ill, children, etc.) • Scores may not be calculated correctly

in particular patients who suffered cardiac arrests, often had long periods (hours) of deterioration before the 'crisis' or medical emergency occurred.

- PSS scores are often termed 'track and trigger' scores; they aim to identify and monitor patients whose clinical state is worsening over time, and then trigger an appropriate clinical response.
- The Department of Health has recognized the need for the early identification of critically ill patients and recommends the use of track and trigger systems in all acute hospitals in the UK. The current recommendation is to use PSS to assess every patient at least every 12 hours or more frequently if they are at risk of deterioration.
- PSS may have variable sensitivity and specificity for predicting hospital mortality, cardiac arrest and admission to critical care. Triggering scores may need to be set locally to maximize the benefits from these scoring systems. Typically, these scoring systems are not very sensitive but have high negative predictive power for the outcomes mentioned above. Advantages and disadvantages of PSS are summarized in Table 1.3.

Medical emergency team and outreach

It has been recognized that intensive care units will never have the capacity for all the patients that may benefit from some degree of critical care provision. The concept of 'critical care without walls' is that patients' critical care needs may be met irrespective of their geographical location within the hospital.

Medical emergency teams (METs) and critical care outreach (CCO) aim to redress the mismatch between the patient's needs when they are critically ill and the resources available on a normal ward, in terms of manpower, skills, and equipment.

- At present there is no clear consensus in the literature about the exact composition and role of these teams, nor their nomenclature.
- Currently there is emphasis in teaching critical care skills to all hospital doctors via courses such as ALERT™ (Acute Life threatening Events – Recognition and Treatment) and CCRISP™ (Care of the Critically Ill Surgical Patient).
- METs are usually understood to be physician-led. The team might typically consist of the duty medical registrar and intensive care registrar, a senior nurse and a variable number of other junior doctors.
- METs are often formed from people who do not usually work together, coming together as a team only when the clinical need dictates. The MET has an obligation to arrive quickly, to contain the necessary skill mix in its members, to document the extent of its involvement accurately, and to liaise with the team responsible for the patient's usual treatment.
- METs are summoned to critically ill patients who have been identified either by a scoring system as outlined above, because they have attracted a particular diagnosis (e.g. status epilepticus), or because of general concerns that the nursing staff have about a patient.
- METs have been shown to reduce the numbers of unexpected cardiac arrests in hospital in some observational studies, but the exact level of benefit is controversial. In some hospitals METs have replaced the traditional cardiac arrest team.

Critical care outreach (CCO) teams are typically nurse-led, and have a variety of roles compared to the MET, depending on local policy (Fig. 1.1). The nurses in CCO are typically senior nurses who have been recruited from an intensive care, coronary care or acute medical background. CCO nurses are often employed full-time in this role and may perform additional duties, such as following up patients on discharge from the intensive care unit, acute pain services, tracheostomy care and providing non-invasive ventilation advice.

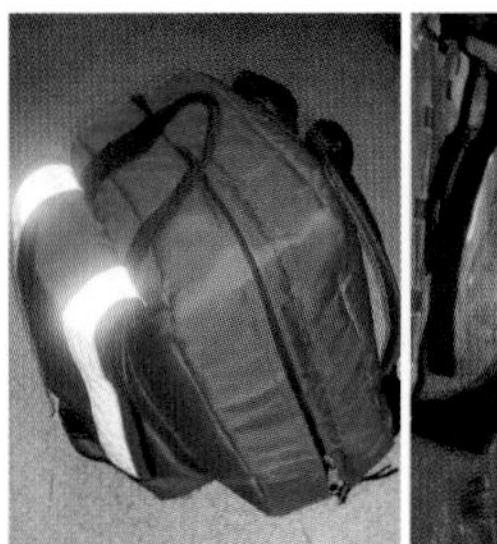
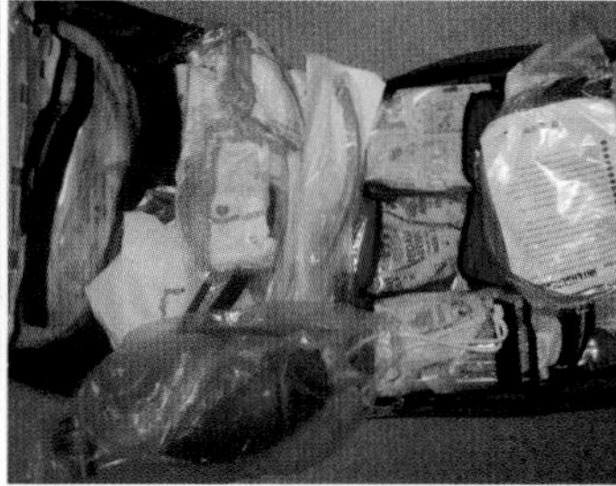

Fig. 1.1 Critical care outreach (CCO) teams often carry portable equipment to help stabilize patients in places outside of critical care areas.

- When summoned to a critically ill patient, CCO will typically make an assessment and refer directly to intensive care services, or make suggestions to the parent medical team according to the requirements of the patients.
- At present, not all CCO are staffed to provide a round-the-clock service and thus patients still often rely on junior medical staff to provide their care out of hours.

In the UK, CCO is the most frequently used model, following on from Department of Health recommendations made in the late 1990s. Their explicit purpose is to avert ITU admissions, support discharge from ITU and to share critical care skills with the rest of the hospital. Other countries, most notably Australia, have pioneered the MET model since 1990. In some hospitals both systems run side by side. Currently the systems are in a state of flux. The rapid introduction of MET/CCO systems in most hospitals has made the assessment of its impact on patient survival difficult. It is also difficult to assess how many patients at any one time need the input of a MET/CCO, and the implications that this may have for resource allocation. At the time of writing, most of the available data suggest that the MET is under-utilized.

Referral to critical care team

Critical care can offer:

- organ support technologies
- high nurse : patient ratio
- intensive/invasive monitoring
- specialist expertise in managing the critically ill

Patients who need these services should be referred to the critical care team.

Intensive care units exist to support patients whose clinical needs outstrip the resources/manpower which can be safely provided on the general wards. The patient must also generally be in a position to benefit from the treatment, rather than simply to prolong the process of dying from an underlying condition. Chronological age alone is a poor indicator of survival from a critical illness; chronic health problems and functional limitations due to these are better predictors. There should be a discussion with the patient (if possible), or their family, to explain the proposed treatment and to seek their consent for escalating management.

Most critical care facilities operate a 'closed' policy, in which the referring team temporarily devolves care to the intensive care team. The latter is led by a clinician trained in intensive care. There is evidence that this approach leads to reduced lengths of stay and increased survival rates in patients. As part of this strategy, all referrals to intensive care should be passed through the duty intensive care consultant. The referring team still has an important role to play as definitive management of a condition (e.g. surgery) is still often provided by them.

Referral to the critical care team may occur via a variety of routes. The admission may be planned well in advance in the case of elective surgery, or anticipated and discussed with the ITU consultant in the case of emergency surgery. Acute medical admissions should be referred to the ITU consultant directly from the medical consultant, but in emergencies referral may be made via the MET/CCO. The patient is usually reviewed on the ward prior to admission in order to facilitate resuscitation and safe, timely transfer to critical care.

Key points

- Early recognition and treatment of the critically ill patient may improve outcome.
- Recognition of a critically ill patient by junior or inexperienced staff may be facilitated by a scoring system.
- Physiological scoring systems are widely used, but not always well validated.
- METs and CCOs aim to provide critical care skills rapidly to critically ill patients.
- Referrals to the critical care services may happen from any level, but the final decision to admit a

patient to a critical care bed should be made by an experienced critical care physician.

Further reading

- Bickell W, Wall M, Pepe P *et al.* (1994) Immediate versus delayed fluid resuscitation for hypotensive patients with penetrating torso injuries. *N. Engl. J. Med.* **331**: 1105–9.
- Intensive Care Society (2003) *Evolution of Intensive Care.* www.ics.ac.uk/icmprof/downloads/icshistory.pdf
- Intensive Care Society (2008) *Levels of Critical Care for Adult Patients: Standards and Guidelines.* www.ics.ac.uk/downloads/Levels_of_Care_13012009.pdf
- National Institute for Clinical Excellence (2007) *Clinical Guideline CG59: Acutely Ill Patients in Hospital.* www nice.org.uk/guidance/index.jsp?action=byID&o=11810#summary
- Rivers E, Nguyen B, Havstad S *et al.* (2001) Early goal-directed therapy in the treatment of severe sepsis and septic shock. *N. Engl. J. Med.* **345**: 1368–77.

Advanced airway management

Isma Quasim

Critically ill patients may need respiratory support as part of their treatment on the intensive care unit. The provision of respiratory support is a core function of the intensive care unit; internationally around a third of patients admitted to intensive care units receive some form of mechanical ventilation for more than 12 hours. Advanced airway skills form an essential part of the intensive care clinician's armoury and are invaluable in times of emergency.

This chapter will focus mainly on the aspects of advanced airway management used most commonly in critical care: intubation and extubation, tracheostomy, cricothyroidotomy and 'mini-tracheostomy'.

Intubation

Indications for intubation (Table 2.1)

Bag–valve-mask and non-invasive ventilation are two methods of providing short-term positive pressure ventilation or intermittent airway management. However, intubation is often necessary to provide more long-term and continuous positive pressure ventilation and/or to secure and protect the airway of patients with reduced level of consciousness.

Airway assessment

Studies have suggested that difficult intubation in patients for elective operative procedures occurs approximately in 1–3% of cases, and this incidence increases up to 10% in critical care patients. In anaesthesia, there are a number of methods and parameters of airway assessment used to predict potential difficult intubation. These include the modified Mallampati score, thyromental distance, inter-incisor distance and neck mobility. In addition, difficult intubation should be anticipated in patients with certain anatomical features (protruding teeth, morbid obesity, large breasts and short necks) or pathologies such as upper airway infection (e.g. epiglottitis, laryngitis), trauma, inhalational injury, tumour, cervical spine injury, previous upper airway operations or radiotherapy.

In critical care practice, given the relative urgency for intubation in sick or non-cooperative patients, full assessments are not always possible or practical. Some vital information can still be found on an anaesthetic chart such as preoperative assessment of the airway, the grade of laryngoscopic view and techniques of airway managements. Patients should be intubated by a clinician experienced in advanced airway management with difficult airway adjuncts available.

When dealing with sick patients on the ward, conditions in the ward setting are often unfavourable due to limited equipment and lack of assistance, making intubation more difficult. Ideally patients should be transferred to a safer environment such as the critical care unit, the anaesthetic room or the operating theatre where trained assistance is available.

Rapid sequence induction

Patients who present in emergency situations are assumed to have a full stomach and in the UK, it is recommended that a rapid sequence induction (RSI) is used in intubation. This is a technique that minimizes the risks of regurgitation and subsequent aspiration of gastric contents. The principles involved are:

(1) Patient should be on a bed that can be tilted if necessary. Mandatory monitoring should be commenced including ECG, pulse oximetry, blood pressure, end-tidal CO_2 monitoring.
(2) Preparation of all essential emergency drugs before the start of procedure.

Core Topics in Critical Care Medicine, eds. Fang Gao Smith and Joyce Yeung. Published by Cambridge University Press.

(3) Equipment needed should be checked prior to the procedure including two working Macintosh laryngoscopes, endotracheal tubes, laryngeal mask airways, working suction. Airway adjuncts such as oropharyngeal airways, longer laryngoscope blades, McCoy laryngoscope or bougie that might be required in an unexpectedly difficult intubation should also be available.

(4) Trained assistance familiar with the technique should be available.

(5) Preoxygenation with high flow 100% oxygen for 3–5 minutes to maximize oxygen reserves and prevent hypoxaemia until tracheal intubation is established.

(6) A rapidly acting intravenous induction agent such as thiopentone and suxamethonium should be used to achieve rapid muscle relaxation and tracheal intubation.

(7) Sellick's manoeuvre or cricoid pressure should be applied just before patient loses consciousness.

Table 2.1 Critical care indications for intubation

Indications	Examples
Provide long-term positive pressure ventilation	Respiratory failure
Protect the airway	Glasgow Coma Scores <8
Secure the airway	Airway obstruction, inadvertent or failed extubation

This involves digital pressure against the cricoid cartilage of the larynx, pushing it backwards (Fig. 2.1). This causes compression of the oesophagus between the cricoid cartilage and the C5/C6 vertebrae posteriorly, thus minimizing passive regurgitation of gastric contents (Fig. 2.2). Force applied should be 30 N to 40 N and should be maintained until the correct placement of endotracheal tube has been confirmed by auscultation and cuff inflated. It must be released during active vomiting, to reduce the risk of oesophageal rupture.

Induction agents

Most critical care units do not have fixed protocols for the drugs used to facilitate tracheal intubation, the choice of which can vary according to the personal experience, drugs availability and the patients' pre-admission conditions or co-morbidities.

The majority of anaesthetic induction agents are vasodilators and have cardiodepressant effects. The use of these induction agents can lead to a precipitous fall in blood pressure and cardiac output in dehydrated, septic or haemodynamically unstable patients. It is good practice to monitor patients' cardio-respiratory parameters closely including invasive blood pressure monitoring prior to induction and have fluid boluses and vasopressor drugs prepared and immediately available.

It is beyond the realm of this chapter to go into the pharmacology in depth but a few of the commonly

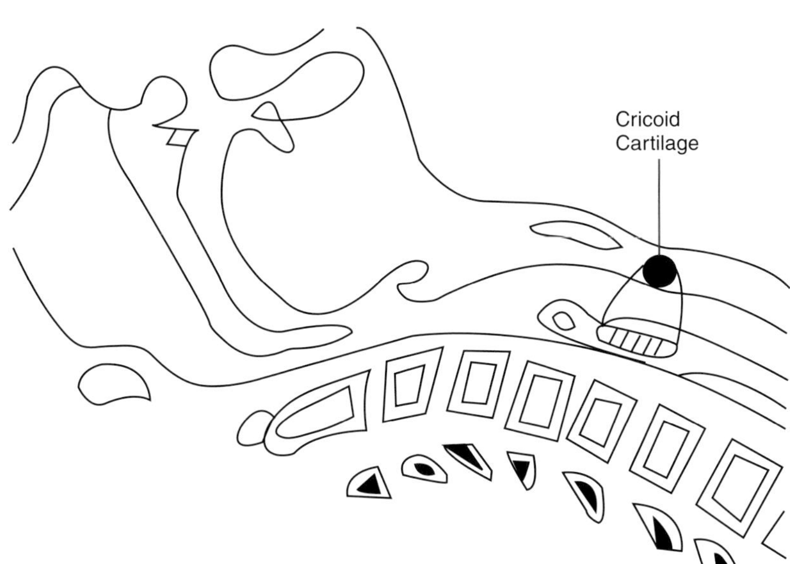

Fig. 2.1 Cricoid cartilage. (With permission of *Update in Anaesthesia*, Issue 2 (1992), Article 4: Cricoid pressure in Caesarean section.)

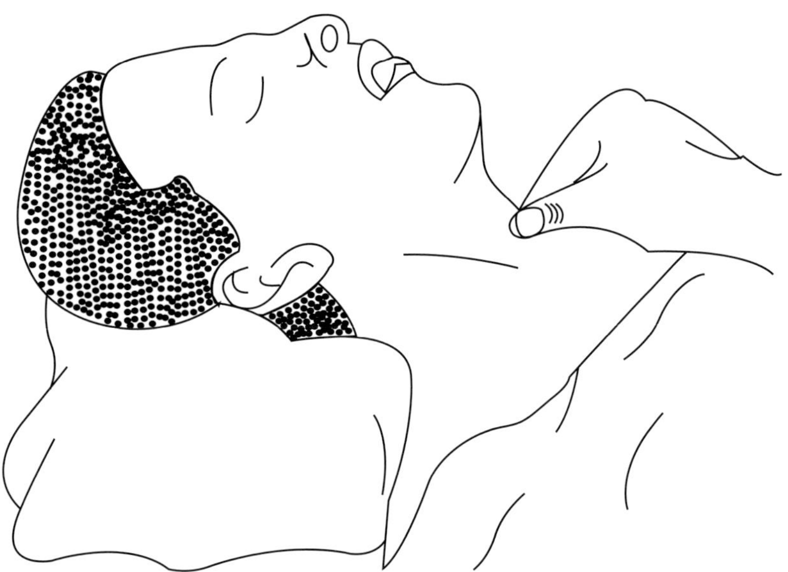

Fig. 2.2 Application of cricoid pressure. (With permission of *Update in Anaesthesia*, Issue 2 (1992), Article 4: Cricoid pressure in Caesarean section.)

used intravenous induction agents and muscle relaxants are outlined below:

Propofol – The induction dose is 1.5–2.5 mg/kg but this should be reduced in haemodynamically unstable patients as it can cause profound hypotension. It has the advantage of being able to be continued as an infusion for sedation and is a drug familiar to the majority of anaesthetists and intensivists.

Etomidate – The dose of 0.3 mg/kg causes less haemodynamic instability than propofol, and has been used as drug of choice for critically ill patients. Its use has declined as major concerns have been raised over adrenocortical suppression even when given as a single dose at induction.

Thiopentone – The classical induction agent used in RSI along with suxamethonium. It provides smooth rapid induction in a dose of 3–6 mg/kg but also produces dose-related cardiac depression. Its metabolism is slow and sedation can persist for many hours afterwards.

Muscle relaxants

In a RSI situation, only suxamethonium should be used and it is given immediately after the IV induction agent without bag-mask ventilation. In a situation in which it is safe and appropriate to use a longer-acting muscle relaxant as the primary agent, then hand ventilation must be checked prior to its administration to avoid the 'can't intubate, can't ventilate' scenario.

Suxamethonium – Suxamethonium is a depolarizing neuromuscular blocker and is the only available neuromuscular blocker with a rapid onset of effect and an ultra short duration of action of around 5 min. Given in a dose of 1–1.5 mg/kg it provides excellent intubating conditions within 60 sec but is contraindicated in conditions such as burns (>24 hours old), hyperkalaemia, malignant hyperpyrexia, myotonia and other neurological diseases. Suxamethonium is metabolized rapidly by plasma pseudocholinesterase and the duration of action is increased in patients who carry an atypical gene for this enzyme. In patients who are heterozygous for the atypical gene duration of action is increased by 50–100%; in patients who are homozygous for the atypical gene duration of action is increased to 4 hours.

Rocuronium – A dose of around 0.6 mg/kg provides good intubating conditions within 2 min; however when given in a dose of 1–1.2 mg/kg it can facilitate intubation within 60 sec and can be used in a 'modified rapid sequence induction' when suxamethonium is contraindicated. It has duration of action of around 30 min.

Atracurium – The initial dose is 0.5 mg/kg and provides intubating conditions within 2 min. It is useful in patients with renal or hepatic impairment as it is broken down by spontaneous Hoffmann degradation. It has a short duration of action of around 20–25 min and if prolonged muscle relaxation is necessary it can be given by IV infusion at 0.5 mg/kg per hour.

See Table 2.2 for a summary of induction agents and muscle relaxants.

Inhalational induction

There will be instances when an inhalational induction may be the preferred method, e.g. upper airway

Table 2.2 Commonly used induction agents and muscle relaxants

Name	Main features	Doses	Indications	Cautions
Propofol	Rapid onset; unaffected by renal or hepatic disease	1.5–2.5 mg/kg	Intravenous induction agent Given by infusion for sedation Anticonvulsant	Vasodilatory and cardio-depressant
Etomidate	Rapid onset; less cardiodepressant.	0.3 mg/kg	Induction agent	Not for use in porphyria Adrenocortical suppression even after single dose
Thiopentone	Smooth rapid onset	3–6 mg/kg	Induction agent; anticonvulsant	Avoid in porphyria. Slow hepatic metabolism
Suxamethonium	Effective within 60 sec; lasts 3–5 min	1–1.5 mg/kg	Depolarizing muscle relaxant	Not for use in malignant hyperthermia and myotonia Caution in burns, renal failure, spinal cord injuries
Atracurium	Adequate muscle relaxation within 3 min; lasts 20–25 min. Safe for use in renal and hepatic failure	0.3–0.6 mg/kg	Non-depolarizing muscle relaxant	Histamine release may cause bronchospasm and hypotension
Rocuronium	Rapid onset if dose of 1–1.5 mg/kg used. Longer duration of action of 30–40 min	0.6 mg/kg gives adequate relaxation in 2 min	Non-depolarizing muscle relaxant	Intermediate risk of anaphylaxis

obstruction, burns or status asthmaticus, and sevoflurane is one of the most commonly used agents within the UK for this technique. Inhalational induction is usually carried out by an anaesthetist and requires an anaesthetic machine and circuit.

Endotracheal intubation

Endotracheal intubation is usually via the oral route but historically nasal intubation was common practice. The oral endotracheal tube avoids the risk of sinusitis and allows a tube with a larger internal diameter to be used, reducing the work of breathing. Nasal endotracheal tubes, on the other hand, are better tolerated in awake patients and are used in some paediatric critical care units.

During intubation, the patient should be fully monitored. Equal breath sounds should be auscultated to rule out oesophageal intubation but this is not always reliable. Capnography should be used to confirm tracheal intubation as recommended by the Royal College of Anaesthetists. Lightweight portable capnography devices are available when intubation is required to be performed outside of the critical care, operating theatre or anaesthetic room environment. Chest X-rays should be performed to confirm the position of the tip of the endotracheal tube to avoid inadvertent endobronchial intubation.

Difficult and failed intubation

In an unanticipated difficult intubation situation, oxygenation should be maintained with hand ventilation until appropriate help arrives. Clinicians experienced in advanced airway management should familiarize themselves with the failed intubation drill (Fig. 2.3). The Difficult Airway Society UK website (see *Further reading*) has the following management plans:

(1) Unanticipated difficult tracheal intubation during rapid sequence induction of anaesthesia.

(2) Rescue techniques for the ‘can’t intubate, can’t ventilate’ situation.

Extubation/ weaning protocols

In 2000, a study investigated characteristics of conventional mechanical ventilation in 412 medical and surgical ICUs involving 1638 patients across North America, South America, Spain and Portugal. The study confirmed that there was similarity between countries for the primary indications for mechanical

Failed intubation, increasing hypoxaemia and difficult ventilation in the paralysed anaesthetized patient: Rescue techniques for the 'can't intubate, can't ventilate' situation

failed intubation and difficult ventilation (other than laryngospasm)

Face mask
Oxygenate and ventilate patient
Maximum head extension
Maximum jaw thrust
Assistance with mask seal
Oral ± 6 mm nasal airway
Reduce cricoid force – if necessary

failed oxygenation with face mask (e.g. SpO_2 < 90% with FiO_2 1.0)

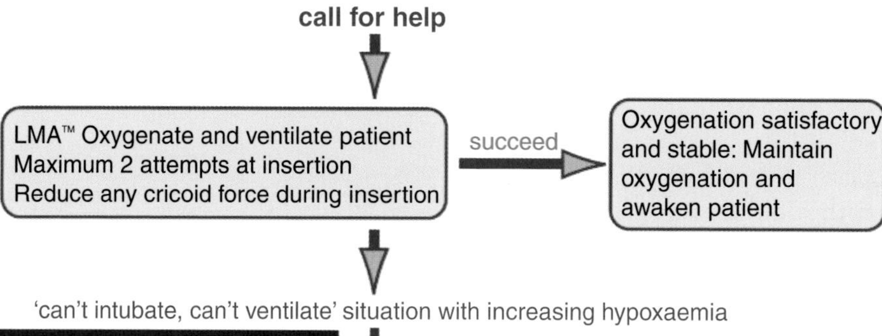
call for help
LMA™ Oxygenate and ventilate patient
Maximum 2 attempts at insertion
Reduce any cricoid force during insertion
succeed
Oxygenation satisfactory and stable: Maintain oxygenation and awaken patient

'can't intubate, can't ventilate' situation with increasing hypoxaemia

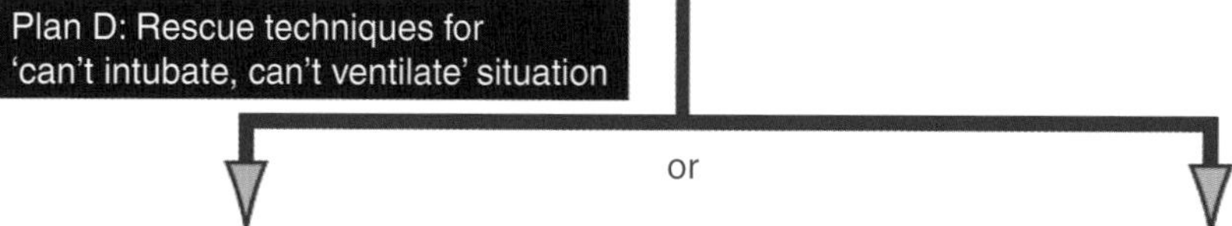
Plan D: Rescue techniques for
'can't intubate, can't ventilate' situation
or

Cannula cricothyroidotomy

Equipment: Kink-resistant cannula, e.g. Patil (Cook) or Ravussin (VBM)
High-pressure ventilation system, e.g. Manujet III (VBM)

Technique:

1. Insert cannula through cricothyroid membrane
2. Maintain position of cannula – assistant's hand
3. Confirm tracheal position by air aspiration – 20 ml syringe
4. Attach ventilation system to cannula
5. Commence cautious ventilation
6. Confirm ventilation of lungs, and exhalation through upper airway
7. If ventilation fails, or surgical emphysema or any other complication develops – convert immediately to surgical cricothyroidotomy

fail

Surgical cricothyroidotomy

Equipment: Scalpel – short and rounded (no. 20 or Minitrach scalpel)
Small (e.g. 6 or 7 mm) cuffed tracheal or tracheostomy tube

4-Step Technique:

1. Identify cricothyroid membrane
2. Stab incision through skin and membrane
   Enlarge incision with blunt dissection (e.g. scalpel handle, forceps or dilator)
3. Caudal traction on cricoid cartilage with tracheal hook
4. Insert tube and inflate cuff

Ventilate with low-pressure source
Verify tube position and pulmonary ventilation

Notes:
1. These techniques can have serious complications – use only in life-threatening situations
2. Convert to definitive airway as soon as possible
3. Postoperative management – see other difficult airway guidelines and flow-charts
4. 4 mm cannula with low-pressure ventilation may be successful in patient breathing spontaneously

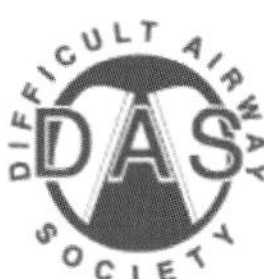
DIFFICULT AIRWAY SOCIETY
DAS

Fig. 2.3 Failed intubation algorithm. (With permission of Difficult Airway Society, UK.)

ventilation and ventilator settings, but considerable variability on the modes of ventilation or the methods of weaning.

Weaning assessment

One of the most difficult issues in critical care medicine is trying to determine which patients will be successfully extubated. There are instances where this may be easily achieved especially in patients with normal respiratory function who have been intubated for an acute event, e.g. following a drug overdose or post surgical procedure. In a significant proportion of patients however, the reduction and subsequent withdrawal from ventilatory support is more gradual and this is defined as *weaning*.

Weaning techniques

There are a number of ways in which weaning can be achieved. The mechanical ventilations may be changed from an assist-control mode to:

- Pressure support ventilation (PSV). High levels of support are gradually reduced over time as the patient increases the ability of his/her own breathing. Initially the pressure support is set to achieve a comparable tidal volume as with the assist mode and then decreased whilst the patient is monitored for weaning failure. Once the PS is at a low level (5–8 cm H_2O), they may be considered for extubation.
- Synchronized intermittent mandatory ventilation (SIMV). The initial high respiratory rate is decreased over time. Once a low level has been reached and the patient shows no signs of fatigue, then a trial of PSV/CPAP can be provided.
- Continuing full ventilation with periods of low levels of PSV (5cm H_2O)/CPAP (5 cm H_2O). This is comparable to a T-piece trial.

In 1995, the Spanish Lung Failure Collaborative Group conducted a prospective, randomized, multicentre study on comparison of four methods of weaning patients from mechanical ventilation:

(1) SIMV with an initial rate of 10 and then decreased at least twice a day. Patients were extubated once they tolerated a ventilator rate of 5 breaths/min for 2 hours with no distress.

(2) PSV initially set with pressure support around 18 cm H_2O and then reduced at least twice a day. Once the patients tolerated a pressure support of 5 cmH_2O for 2 hours with no distress they could be extubated.

(3) Intermittent trials of spontaneous breathing at least on two occasions a day on a T-piece or CPAP 5 cm H_2O. Once they could tolerate 2 hours they were extubated.

(4) Once a day spontaneous breathing trial (SBT). After 2 hours on a T-piece or CPAP 5 cmH_2O with no signs of distress the patients were extubated. If unsuccessful, full assist ventilation was continued for another 24 hours before another trial was attempted.

They found that the rate of successful weaning was significantly higher in the spontaneous breathing groups (groups 3 and 4) and that there was no significant difference in the success rate between once a day (group 4) and multiple trials of spontaneous breathing (group 3). Further work in 2002 demonstrated that spontaneous breathing trials carried out for 30 or 120 min were equivalent in recognizing those patients who would be successfully extubated.

Criteria for failed spontaneous breathing trials

Spontaneous breathing trials are the most effective way of determining whether mechanical ventilation can be discontinued. A failed SBT is said to have occurred if the patient shows signs of distress, agitation, tachypnoea (>35 breaths/min), hypoxia (SpO_2 <90%) and extremes of systolic blood pressure. The patient is then put back on full ventilatory support for the weaning process to continue at a later time.

Extubation

Critical care clinicians often use the following criteria to consider patients ready for extubation:

- Resolution of the pathology that necessitated IPPV.
- Adequate arterial oxygenation on a $FiO_2 \leq 0.5$ and PEEP $\leq$ 5 cmH_2O.
- Haemodynamic stability.
- Normal acid–base status.
- Normal fluid and electrolyte status.
- Adequate protective airway reflexes and ability to cough.
- Awake and co-operative.

There are a number of bedside tests that may be used to assess the likelihood of extubating a patient; however, they may be poor predictors of success in an individual patient.

Parameters that can be used include:

(1) PaO_2/FiO_2ratio >200 mmHg (26 kPa)

(2) Respiratory rate <35 bpm

(3) Tidal volume >5 ml/kg

(4) Maximal negative inspiratory pressure 20–30 cm H_2O

(5) Respiratory rate/tidal volume < 100 min/l

Tracheostomy

Indications for tracheostomy

Tracheostomies are commonly used in critical care units to:

- Facilitate weaning after prolonged ventilation.
- Secure and clear the airway in upper respiratory tract obstruction.
- Facilitate removal of bronchial secretions, e.g. inadequate cough.
- Protect the airway in the absence of laryngeal reflexes, e.g. bulbar palsy.
- Provide an airway in patients with injuries or surgery to the head and neck.

Contraindications for tracheostomy

The only absolute contraindication to a surgical or percutaneous tracheostomy is local severe sepsis or uncontrollable coagulopathy. Relative contraindications to a percutaneous tracheostomy are abnormal anatomy, moderate coagulopathy, children under 12 years (due to difficulty identifying anatomical landmarks) and high FiO_2 and PEEP requirements.

Timing of tracheostomy

The timing of when to perform a tracheostomy is still a clinical decision rather than one based on medical evidence. Some studies suggest that a tracheostomy performed *earlier* rather than *later* leads to improved weaning, a shorter ICU length of stay and a reduction in the incidence of nosocomial pneumonia. A systematic review performed in 2005 comparing early tracheostomy (up to 7 days after admission to ICU) with late tracheostomy (any time thereafter) suggested early tracheostomy led to a reduction in the duration of mechanical ventilation and length of ICU stay but the numbers involved in the studies were relatively small. A study investigating the effect that the timing of tracheostomy has on 30-day mortality in UK intensive care units (TrachMan trial) has been completed to compare early tracheostomy (days 1 to 4) with late tracheostomy (day 10 or after) in patients expected to require mechanical ventilation for 7 days or more. Early tracheostomy ($n = 450$) was not associated with any beneficial effect on the development of ventilator-associated pneumonia, ICU length of stay, use of sedation or 30-day mortality compared to late tracheostomy ($n = 450$). Interestingly, only 45% of the patients in the late group actually received a tracheostomy.

Techniques of percutaneous tracheostomy

The two methods of performing a tracheostomy are *surgical* or *percutaneous*. Surgical tracheostomies are best carried out by experienced surgeons and will not be discussed in any detail here. Percutaneous tracheostomy carried out using a Seldinger technique is rapidly becoming more established within the critical care setting.

At present there are at least five different techniques for carrying out a percutaneous tracheostomy, but there is no evidence that one technique is superior to another (Fig. 2.4).

(1) Classic Ciaglia technique using a guidewire over which a series of dilators are used

(2) Forceps dilational technique

(3) Retrograde translaryngeal technique

(4) Single-dilator, dilational 'Blue Rhino' technique

(5) 'PercuTwist' technique using rotational dilation with a self-cutting screw.

Complications

Complications of tracheostomy are numerous and the rates vary considerably; generally complication rates are higher for emergency tracheostomy and for airway obstruction.

Complications can be divided into:

Immediate – e.g. haemorrhage, pneumothorax, misplacement of tube.

Delayed – e.g. tube blockage by secretions, infection of stoma site, infection of

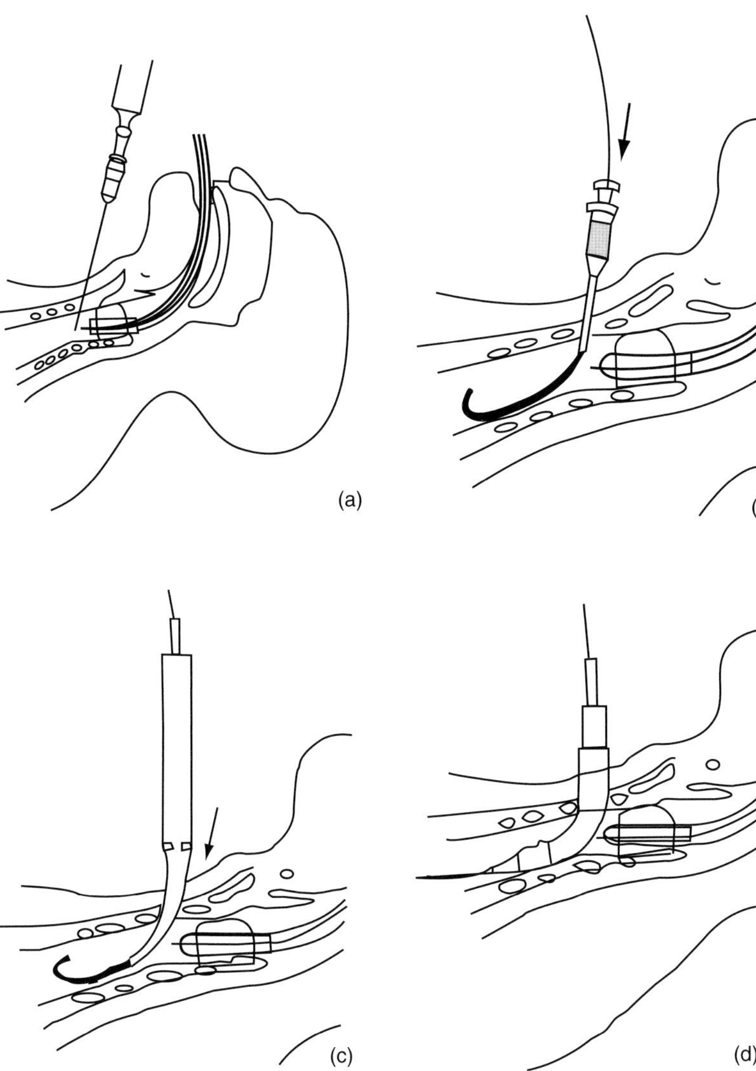

Fig. 2.4 Serial dilator percutaneous tracheostomy technique. Preparation: The patient should be positioned with neck extended and supported by pillow of a bag of fluids between the shoulders. The neck is cleansed with antiseptic solution and properly draped. The cricoid cartilage is identified, and the skin is anaesthetized with 1% lidocaine with 1: 100 000 adrenaline below the cricoid cartilage. The endotracheal tube is withdrawn so cuff is visible at the vocal cords to avoid accidental puncture. Some clinicians like to perform procedure under direct vision with fibreoptic bronchoscope. (a) A 1.5- to 2-cm transverse skin incision is made on the level of the first and second tracheal rings. A 22-gauge needle is inserted between the first and second or the second and third tracheal rings. (b) When air is aspirated into the syringe, the guidewire is introduced. (c) After the guidewire is protected, the dilators are introduced. (d) All dilators are inserted in a sequential manner from small to large diameter. The tracheostomy tube is then introduced along the dilator and guidewire. The guidewire and dilator are removed, the cuff of the tracheostomy tube is inflated, and the breathing circuit is connected. The ET tube can then be removed. (With permission from *Update in Anaesthesia* Issue 15 (2002), Article 16: Percutaneous tracheostomy.)

bronchial tree, mucosal ulceration due to cuff inflation.

Late – e.g. persistent sinus at tracheostomy site, tracheal stenosis at cuff site, scar formation requiring revision.

Tracheostomy tubes

A variety of tracheostomy tubes are available which have different properties. A patient may require many different types of tracheostomy tubes during their critical care admission.

Cuffed tracheostomy tubes – generally used for patients on positive pressure ventilation (Fig. 2.5). The cuff must be inflated to prevent air/oxygen leaking

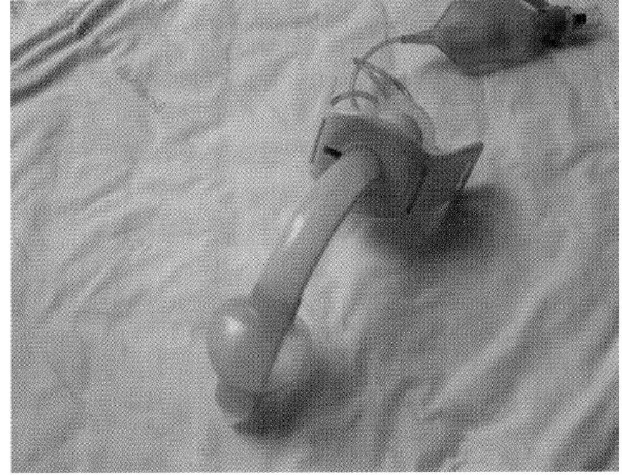

Fig. 2.5 Cuffed tracheostomy tube.

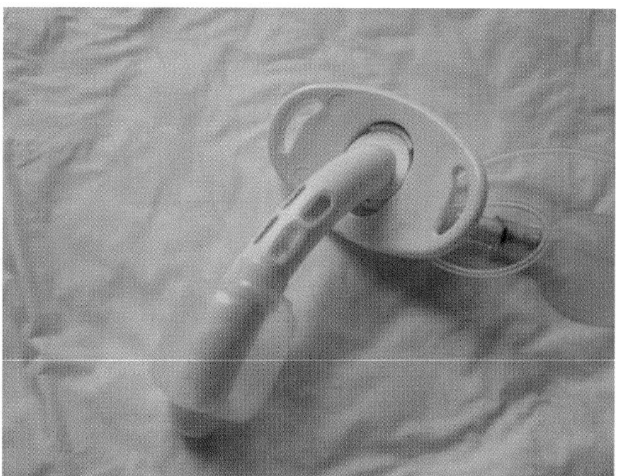

Fig. 2.6 Fenestrated tracheostomy tube.

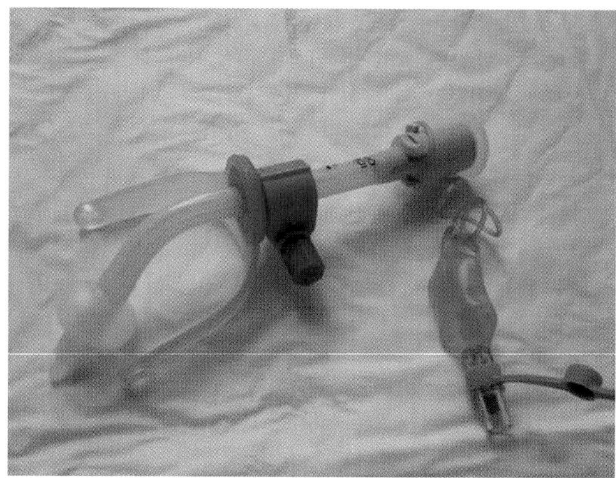

Fig. 2.7 Tracheostomy tube with adjustable flange.

backwards and reduce the chance of aspirate entering the lungs. Obstruction of a cuffed tracheostomy tube by secretions is potentially life-threatening. To minimize this risk, tracheostomy tubes should be changed frequently. Changing a tracheostomy tube carries the risk of misplacement and causes patient discomfort.

Tracheostomy tubes with an inner cannula – allows an inner cannula to be changed frequently to reduce the risk of obstruction. The main disadvantage of these tubes is the reduced inner diameter, which causes an increased work of breathing.

Fenestrated tracheostomy tubes – allow airflow to pass through the oropharynx as well as the tracheal stoma and reduce the work of breathing provided the cuff is deflated (Fig. 2.6). These should not be used if the patient is at risk of aspiration or is on positive pressure ventilation unless the fenestrations are blocked by an inner cannula.

Tracheostomy tubes with adjustable flange – useful in patients with abnormal anatomy such as obesity, neck swelling and spinal deformities (Fig. 2.7). The flanges allow the tracheostomy tube to be adjusted to a certain length.

Decannulation of tracheostomy tubes

Tracheostomy tubes should be removed as soon as possible once:

- Resolution of the primary cause of the tracheostomy has occurred.
- Patient is able to expectorate past the tube and not require regular suctioning.
- Effective swallow, gag and cough reflexes are present.
- Patient is comfortable with the cuff deflated.
- Nutritional status is adequate.
- No airway obstruction is present above the tracheostomy.

Weaning often involves increasing length of time with the cuff deflated or 'downsizing' the tube to one with a smaller diameter allowing the patient to breathe past the tracheostomy.

Speaking valves or occlusion/decannulation caps should *only* be used on non-cuffed tubes, cuffed tubes with the cuff deflated or fenestrated tubes with the cuff deflated. If the patient tolerates at least 4 hours with the occlusion cap and is able to effectively cough, then decannulation can take place.

Cricothyroidotomy and mini tracheostomy

A *cricothyroidotomy* is usually performed as an emergency procedure when a secure airway is needed and attempts at orotracheal or nasotracheal intubation have failed. The patients are likely to be profoundly hypoxic and it is important that the airway is secured quickly. This can be done either as a *needle* or as a *surgical* cricothyroidotomy.

There are several ways in which a cricothyroidotomy can be carried out. All the techniques involve an incision of the cricothyroid membrane, which is between the thyroid cartilage superiorly and cricoid cartilage inferiorly.

- A small cannula (usually inserted over a needle), which needs a high-pressure gas source such as the ManuJet system (VBM, GmbH, Sulz, Germany) to provide adequate lung inflation. The patient's airway is generally patent enough to allow exhalation, as the positive pressure within the trachea tends to open up the upper airway.

- Larger cannula (usually as a preassembled kit using a Seldinger technique, e.g. Portex, Melker), but as these are uncuffed they lead to an unprotected airway with suboptimal ventilation.
- Surgical cricothyroidotomy allows a large cuffed endotracheal tube to be placed but requires familiarity with the technique and should not be carried out by inexperienced practitioners.

Exhaled gases must be able to escape otherwise significant barotrauma can result, and in the case of an upper airway obstruction a second air outlet may be needed.

Mini tracheostomies are now available as kits which are not only used in the emergency scenario, but also in situations where sputum retention is problematic, e.g. inadequate cough, respiratory tract infection or in the post-operative period. The anatomical landmark and insertion of a mini tracheostomy are similar to performing cricothyroidotomy. Generally they are not recommended for ventilation as the airway resistance is high but recent small studies have been carried out where the combination of a mini tracheostomy plus non-invasive ventilation (NIV) has been used in patients with respiratory failure due to neuromuscular disorders. This technique avoids endotracheal intubation and IPPV and seemed to be well tolerated although patient selection may have played a role.

Key points

- Intubation of critical care patients can be difficult and the clinician should have a management plan for the unanticipated difficult airway.
- A daily assessment of ventilated patients to see whether they fit the criteria for weaning and subsequent extubation is important.
- Tracheostomies can be a useful weaning tool in certain patient groups but it is important to ensure the patients are looked after in a safe environment if they are discharged from the ICU with one in situ.
- Cricothyroidotomy is a valuable tool in securing the airway in an emergency situation. Make sure you know what equipment is available in your hospital and how to use it.

Further reading

- Esteban A, Anzueto A, Alia I *et al.* (2000) How is mechanical ventilation employed in the Intensive Care Unit? *Am. J. Respir. Crit. Care Med.* **161**: 1450–8.
- Esteban A, Frutos F, Tobin MJ *et al.* (1995) A comparison of four methods of weaning patients from mechanical ventilation: Spanish Lung Failure Collaborative Group. *N. Engl. J. Med.* **332**(6): 345–50.
- Griffiths J, Barber VS, Morgan L, Young JD (2005) Systematic review and meta-analysis of studies of the timing of tracheostomy in adult patients undergoing artificial ventilation. *Br. Med. J.* **330**: 1243.
- Henderson JJ, Popat MT Latto IP, Pearce AC (2004) Difficult Airway Society guidelines for the management of the unanticipated difficult intubation. *Anaesthesia* **57**(7): 675–94. www.das.uk.com/guidelines/downloads.html
- Perren A, Domenighetti G, Mauri S, Genini F, Vizzardi N (2002) Protocol-directed weaning from mechanical ventilation: clinical outcome in patients randomised for a 30-min or 120-min trial with pressure support ventilation. *Intens. Care Med.* **28**: 1058–63.
- Scrase I, Woollard M (2006) Needle vs. surgical cricothyroidotomy: a short cut to effective ventilation. *Anaesthesia* **61**(10): 962–74.
- Young D (2009) TracMan investigators: early and late tracheostomy on 30-day mortality. www.tracman.org.uk

Patient admission and discharge

Santhana Kannan

The critical care unit (CrCU) is one of the most resource-intensive areas of a hospital. The 233 General CrCU in England and Wales treated nearly 81 000 patients in 2003 at a cost of around £540 million, equating to approximately £1328 per day per patient. Interestingly, more recent *estimates* of costs have quoted either similar or slightly lower figures! A typical general ward patient costs £195 per day. Consider this along with the fact that the average mortality in critical care is around 30% with another 10–20% surviving less than 1 year post discharge, it is not difficult to see why the available resources have to be used in the best possible way.

In comparison to non-intensive care treatment, the incremental cost per quality adjusted life year gained of treatment in CrCU is £7010. A recent study estimated that adult intensive care represents good value for money in terms of lower cost per quality adjusted life year when compared to statin therapy.

CrCU is considered to be a 'safe haven' by most physicians, surgeons and anaesthetists leading to a persistent demand for beds. Resource crunch leads to operational levels of high bed occupancy rates in the region of 90%. Hence it is essential that robust admission and discharge procedures exist to maximize resource utilization. The increasing life expectancy, higher complexity of therapeutic interventions, higher expectations from the public and unpredictability of arrival of critically ill patients add to the challenge. This chapter will provide an outline of indications of admission to CrCU, decision to admit, a suggested admission procedure, options when the unit is full, indications for patient discharge and a suggested discharge procedure. Related issues are covered in Chapters 1, 4, 5, 6, 7, 13, 21 and 22.

Who should be admitted?

Ideally, patients who will benefit from critical care should be admitted and those who wouldn't shouldn't! The difficulty lies in the accuracy of predicting the outcome. The degree of dependency of patients in critical care is classified as follows (Table 3.1).

If a patient needs invasive ventilation (e.g. for acute severe asthma), they will be classified as level 3 even though it is only single organ support. In general, high dependency units care for level 2 patients. Patients on non-invasive ventilation alone are typically classified as level 2. This classification is used to aid nurse staffing. Some factors influencing decision to admit patient or not are outlined in Fig. 3.1.

Indications for admission to critical care

The common accepted indications of admission to critical care are given in Table 3.2.

Role of scoring systems to aid admission

Ideal scoring systems

It would be helpful if there was a simple scoring system which was 100% sensitive and 100% specific in identifying patients who will benefit from admission to critical care. To date, no such system exists. Reasons for limitations include the high number of variables that determine patient outcome and variable predictive value for data collected at the beginning of critical illness.

Potential drawbacks of scoring systems

There are *early warning scoring systems* and some lab investigations (e.g. Procalcitonin) proposed in an effort to aid early identification of critical illness. These work on the assumption that early intervention will minimize complications and improve outcome. It has been shown that early goal-directed therapy in critically ill patients can improve outcome. However,

Core Topics in Critical Care Medicine, eds. Fang Gao Smith and Joyce Yeung. Published by Cambridge University Press.

Table 3.1 Classification of levels of patient care

Level	Description	Nurse to patient ratio
Level 0	Patients whose needs can be met through normal ward care	1 : 6
Level 1	Patients whose needs are greater than what can provided by normal ward care, but may be met on acute wards with support from critical care team	1 : 4
Level 2	Patients needing support for a single failing organ system	1 : 2
Level 3	Patients needing advanced respiratory support alone, or basic respiratory support together with support of at least two organ systems	1 : 1

Table 3.2 Indications for admission to critical care

Invasive or non-invasive ventilation for acute respiratory failure
Optimization of fluid balance requiring invasive procedures
Post-operative monitoring (cardiac surgery, neurosurgery, major vascular surgery, long surgical or interventional procedures, massive blood loss, multiple co-morbidities with low systemic reserve)
Haemodynamic instability requiring inotropic support
Potential for deterioration (e.g. airway swelling, metabolic disorders, coagulopathies, hypoxaemia, hypercarbia, hypovolaemia, intracranial events, acute arrhythmias)
Interventions that cannot be performed in a general ward – continuous veno-venous haemofiltration, extra-corporeal gas exchange

it is likely that there is a window of opportunity beyond which this may lose its full benefit.

There is one other problem with the scoring systems. A 90% *probability of survival* still means that 10% of patients will die. Conversely, a 90% probability of mortality still means that 10% will survive. It is impossible to know which particular group the patient in question will fall under. However, the above statistics may aid decisions on issues such as treatment limitation and withdrawal. For example, the outcome in neutropenic sepsis requiring invasive ventilation and inotropes has a survival of around 10–15%. The majority of such patients could be in the younger age group with minimal co-morbidities. Hence, such patients are still treated in the hope that the survivor will have successful outcome with chemotherapy.

Although the correlation between *advancing age* and *mortality* in hospital patients is well known, age alone should not be a criterion for admission to critical care. An 80-year-old active patient with no known co-morbidities is likely to have a better prognosis than a 55-year-old patient with history of myocardial infarction, diabetes, renal failure and limited exercise tolerance when treated for respiratory failure due to pneumonia. It is also important that probability of survival to ward discharge is not used as a sole criterion for admission to critical care. Return to an acceptable quality of life should be aimed for. Defining this criterion has high potential for disagreement between patients, relatives and physicians. This can present difficult ethical and legal issues. It is important that all decisions and discussions with relatives are clearly documented. The decision making process should be based on evidence or accepted guidelines. The patient and relatives should be given an opportunity to clarify any doubts and also consult bodies such as Patient Advocate Liaison Service.

Some interventions including certain drugs involve *high direct costs*. In order to ensure that cost does not become a sole criterion for provision of potentially beneficial treatment, it is essential that institutional guidelines and policies are in place. These could be in the form of a checklist where a drug is authorized if certain criteria are met.

Decision to admit (Fig. 3.1)

The critical care consultant in charge should have the responsibility and be informed for all admissions, discharges and transfers. The consultant may choose to decide based on input from other members of the critical care team including Critical Care Outreach. Outreach typically consists of experienced critical care nurses. The Department of Health Comprehensive Critical Care document (2000) identified three main aims for outreach services: to avert admissions (or to ensure that admissions are timely) by identifying patients who are deteriorating; to enable discharges; and to share critical care skills.

Management of critically ill patients when unit is full

The admission criteria to the critical care unit should be based on need of the patient rather than bed availability. This means that if a patient is deemed not a

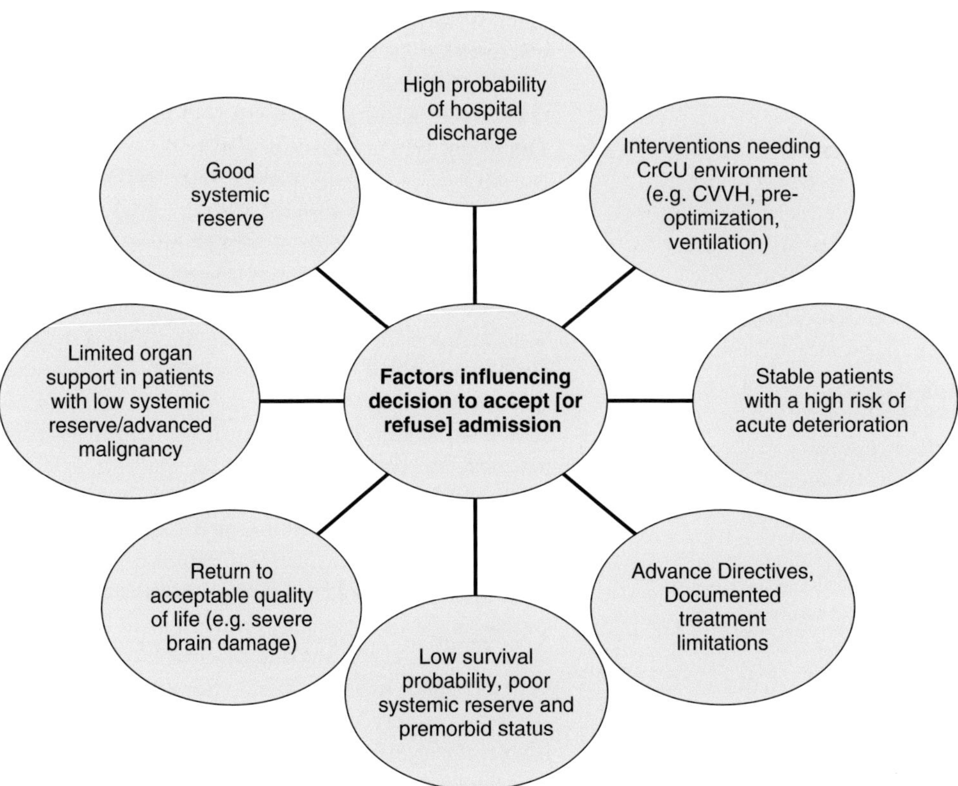

Fig. 3.1 Factors influencing decision to accept (or refuse) admission to critical care.

candidate for critical care, this should be applied even if a bed is available. Conversely, if a patient is considered a candidate for critical care, all measures should be taken to accommodate the patient in the critical care environment as early as possible.

Methods of looking after critically ill patients without CrCU beds

A number of steps could be taken if a critically ill patient presents in the absence of an available bed in the unit. The choice is often determined by the severity of illness, haemodynamic stability, ease of oxygenation, necessity of advanced interventions, time of the day and availability of medical staff.

(1) **Transfer out to another unit** – usually done in daytime hours, if the patient is haemodynamically stable and/or not too difficult to oxygenate. If definitive therapy is only available in another hospital (e.g. neurosurgery), then early transfer is essential.

(2) **Stabilization in the theatre recovery area** – after critical care nurses, the theatre recovery staff are best placed to manage a critically ill patient. Limitations include management of ventilators and limited ability to provide interventions such as continuous haemofiltration in the recovery area. This option is usually chosen out of hours or if a bed is imminently going to be available in the unit.

(3) **Earlier than planned discharge of eligible patients** – it is a common practice to discharge patients from critical care after the morning round. However, some patients may be suitable for discharge at other times. Discharge to the ward after 2200 h should be an exception rather than the rule.

(4) **Manipulation of nursing staff workload** – exceptionally, the number of nurse shift leaders could be reduced so that one of them could accommodate an additional critically ill patient. The risk and benefit of this intervention should be discussed between the nurse in charge and

consultant so that an optimum nursing skill mix is still available. Any such measures should ensure that adequate numbers of staff are available for all future shifts.

(5) **Accommodate in critical care with the aid of outreach and/or medical staff** – this option is chosen if the staff availability is likely to improve within a few hours or if the patient presents late at night when risk of transfer is deemed to be higher.

(6) **Utilize services of other monitored beds in the hospital (e.g. medical assessment unit, surgical assessment unit, coronary care unit)** – these areas have their own limitations in terms of level of monitoring and nursing skills. However, in certain circumstances, and depending upon the type of patient, their services could be used as an interim measure.

(7) **Utilize the resuscitation room in Emergency Department** – some ED nurses are trained in the management of critically ill patients. This option is least desirable since it has the potential to block ED beds.

Decision not to admit

Patients who would potentially benefit from critical care but have issued advance directives which prohibit the use of such interventions should have their views respected. These may still mean that they are admitted but have treatment limitations in place to take into account their wishes. Similarly, patients with a 'Do not resuscitate' order in place may still be admitted to critical care with treatment limitations.

Patients who are deemed to have irreversible or severe organ system damage which is likely to prevent reasonable recovery should have treatment limits in place. Some patients discharged from critical care may not be suitable for readmission to critical care in the event of deterioration (e.g. advanced lung disease with prolonged weaning). Adequate communication with the patient, relatives and other team members is essential in such situations.

Admission procedure

Adequate *communication* is vital. The priority of individual patient will vary depending upon their systemic status. For example a patient with potassium of 6.5 mmol/l unresponsive to standard measures will need urgent renal replacement therapy. However, a patient who is stable after major surgery for post-operative monitoring could wait in the recovery area for a short period before a bed is ready.

All patients who are admitted to the unit should be *handed over* to one of the critical care doctors. This should include a summary of the history, treatment received and any planned investigations, etc. The patient should then have a relevant detailed *clinical examination*. Appropriate *documentation* regarding the treatment plans should be made. Inadequate documentation and secondary errors are an important reason for weak defence in the event of litigation. It is helpful to have a 'critical care admission template' so that any relevant details are not missed. As soon as possible, *the patient and/or the relatives* should be given an explanation of current condition and plan of treatment. This will also be the ideal opportunity to address any concerns.

Discharge

A timely discharge from the CrCU is just as important as timely admission.

Risks of delayed discharge

Risks solely attributable to prolonged stay in critical care include potential cross-infection and psychological disturbances. Since a critical care bed is several times costlier than a ward bed, it is not a good use of resource if patients are kept longer than necessary. Also, with the high demand on beds, it is possible that the admission of a more deserving patient might be delayed as a result of bed blockages. Delayed discharge to wards also leads to cancellation of major elective surgery. It is essential that appropriate systems are in place to minimize delayed discharges.

Outcomes of 'premature' discharge

On the other hand, data also show that about 5% of patients are probably 'prematurely' discharged. It has been estimated that about a third of these patients have a higher mortality and might not have died if they had stayed in the critical care for 48 hours. If each patient has their bed 'held' in the ward, there will be no delay when a decision for their discharge is made. However, most hospitals in the UK and elsewhere do not have this facility due to resource issues. If the incidence of 'delayed discharges' from CrCU is low and the number of cancelled elective surgery patients due to non-availability of CrCU beds is high, it will probably be more economical to 'hold' a ward bed for

Table 3.3 Guidelines for discharge from the critical care unit to the ward

Patient not on any support or intervention (or unlikely to need them in the next 24 hours) *that cannot be provided in the ward*. This includes equipment and nurse staffing issues
Low likelihood of deterioration in the next 24 hours. For long-stay patients and those with low systemic reserve, the duration should be extended to 48 hours or more
Supplemental inspired oxygen concentration <50%
Haemodynamically stable; any fluid losses should be at a rate manageable in the ward environment
The admission aetiological factor is under control or not significant any more
Patients in whom treatment has been withdrawn and only need basic nursing care and drugs for comfort

selective CrCU patients at least for the first 24–48 hours (e.g. elective post-operative patients).

Discharge criteria

Efforts have been made to predict likelihood of a successful discharge, i.e. the patient does not deteriorate after discharge. Like any scoring system, they are not 100% sensitive or specific and hence cannot be used in a given patient. They could be applied to estimate the probability of deterioration which in turn could decide on the degree of follow up.

Discharge criteria commonly used are provided in Table 3.3.

Discharge procedure

If a *step down unit* (e.g. level 1 unit) is available, the patient could be sent there prior to transfer to a normal ward. Like admissions, the decision to discharge should be the responsibility of the consultant. The availability of outreach has certainly influenced decisions regarding discharge. The ability to follow up patients is an important part of the critical care process. Several units have *long-term follow-up clinics* which aid in the management of potentially difficult and challenging post-critical care phase of survivors.

It is desirable to have a *critical care discharge template* which has the details such as summary of critical care stay, significant events, procedures and investigations, infection risk, current medications, follow-up medications, follow-up investigations and suggestions for further management including any restrictions on readmission to critical care. It is important that a ward doctor receives a *handover* of the patient when transferred. This should ensure that the parent team is kept informed about the developments. The *patient's General Practitioner* should be informed of patient's admission and information of what to expect should be provided during the convalescence. An explanation to *the patient and relatives* also helps to alleviate anxiety about ward care.

Key points

- Critical care is a complex combination of high demand, proportionately higher mortality and higher cost. Appropriate systems should be in place so that this resource is optimally used.
- Lack of critical care beds should not delay necessary treatment.
- Advance decisions with regard to suitability for critical care and 'Do not resuscitate' orders help in minimizing communication gaps and sub-optimal care.
- Scoring systems cannot accurately predict outcome in an individual patient. They could be used to aid decisions with regard to treatment limitations and withdrawal.
- Timely discharge is as important as timely admission to critical care.

Further reading

- Bright D, Walker W, Bion J (2004) Clinical review: Outreach – a strategy for improving the care of the acutely ill hospitalized patient. *Critical Care* **8**: 33–40.
- Critical Care Stakeholders Forum and National Outreach Forum (2007) *Clinical Indicators for Critical Care Outreach Services*. London: Department of Health.
- Daly K, Beale R, Chang S (2001) Reduction in mortality after inappropriate early discharge from intensive care unit: logistic regression triage model. *Br. Med. J.* **322**: 1274.
- Department of Health (2000) *Comprehensive Critical Care*. London: Department of Health.
- Department of Health Working Group (1996) *Guidelines on Admission to and Discharge from Intensive Care and High Dependency Care Units*. London: Department of Health.
- Ridley S , Morris S (2007) Cost effectiveness of adult intensive care in the UK. *Anaesthesia* **62**: 547–54.

Chapter 4

Transfer of the critically ill

Gavin Perkins

Introduction

It is estimated that in excess of 10 000 critically ill or injured patients are transferred between hospitals each year in the UK. Special consideration to the risks and benefits of patient transfer is required. Transfers often take place out of routine working hours, with relatively junior medical staff, and are often associated with a high level of adverse/critical incidents. These factors may contribute to the increased risk of morbidity and mortality faced by patients requiring a critical care transfer.

Transfers can be divided into primary or secondary transfers. A primary transfer, from the site where a patient sustains their injury or illness, is normally undertaken by the Ambulance Service in the UK. Occasionally these transfers may be supported by doctors from the local ambulance service or pre-hospital medical care scheme (e.g. BASICS). The main involvement of anaesthetists, emergency physicians, intensivists and other acute speciality staff are in secondary transfers. These include both intra-hospital transfers (e.g. between emergency department and critical care unit or to/from a CT scanner) and inter-hospital transfers. The requirements in terms of planning and ensuring the correct equipment and personnel accompany the patient are similar whether the patient is being transferred within or between hospitals. This chapter will focus predominantly on inter-hospital transfers, but the principles are equally relevant to intra-hospital transfers.

Indications for patient transfer

The common indications for transfer of a critically ill patient are summarized in Table 4.1. Between half and three-quarters of all transfers in the UK are undertaken due to the lack of local intensive care beds or staff, followed by the need for specialist services (e.g. neurosurgery, renal replacement therapy). In 1996 the UK Department of Health published guidelines pertaining to the admission and discharge of critically ill patients from critical care units. These guidelines outline the sequence of events that should take place when considering secondary transfer of a critically ill patient due to a lack of capacity. Firstly, a review of existing critically ill patients should take place to determine if an existing patient could be safely discharged to high dependency care or ward area in order to create capacity. If this is not possible, the nearest or most appropriate empty critical care bed should be identified. This information can be obtained from a regional or national bed information service. Currently, within the UK, responsibility for secondary transfer of the critically ill patient lies with the local Critical Care Network. Within each network, individual hospitals have a pre-agreed list of hospitals to which they are able to routinely transfer patients for capacity reasons alone.

In the event that a new patient is too unstable to transfer safely, there may be the capacity to create a temporary critical care facility (e.g. emergency department, theatres, ward, etc.) until a bed becomes available. Alternatively, the secondary transfer of an existing stable critical care patient could be considered. Although part of the Department of Health guidelines, this option should be considered carefully as there are ethical and clinical implications associated with transferring a stable patient already established on intensive care. Knowing that a critical care transfer is potentially associated with increased risks, it could be difficult to justify this sort of transfer as being in the patient's best interests. If this option is considered, there must be clear communication between staff at the referring and receiving hospitals, relatives and patient (where possible) to explain the need for the transfer.

Core Topics in Critical Care Medicine, eds. Fang Gao Smith and Joyce Yeung. Published by Cambridge University Press.

Table 4.1 Indications for patient transfer

- Lack of a staffed intensive care bed at the referring hospital
- Need for specialist investigation
- Need for specialist treatment
- Repatriation

Mode of transport

The optimal mode of transport selected for a patient transfer will depend upon a number of factors. These include:

- the indication for, and urgency of, transfer
- time to organize/mobilize transport
- weather and traffic conditions
- space (particularly when additional equipment is required)
- cost.

Road transfer by ambulance – This is the commonest method used in the UK. The advantages of road transfer are relatively low costs, space, rapid mobilization (in general) and less weather dependency. The disadvantages are long journey times for transfers over long distances and unexpected delays due to traffic congestion.

Air transfer, either by helicopter or fixed-wing aircraft, can be considered for longer journeys (over 50 miles or 2 hours). The time to mobilize these resources, the reduced space available, the physiological effects of flying, the costs and the potential need (and time implications) for transferring between vehicles at the beginning and end of the transfer should be taken into account when considering this mode of transport. Some of the space considerations with helicopter transfer are illustrated in Fig. 4.1.

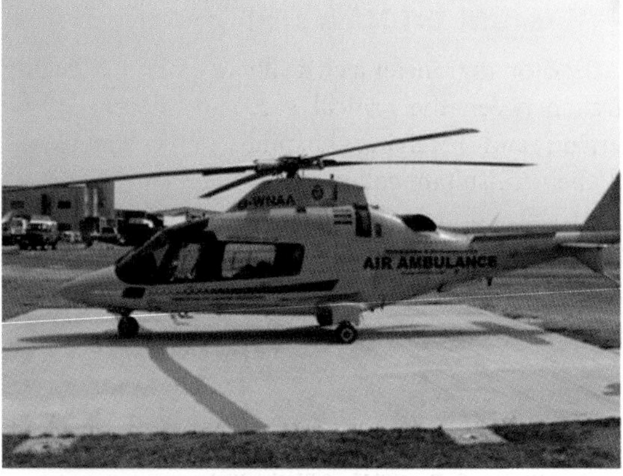

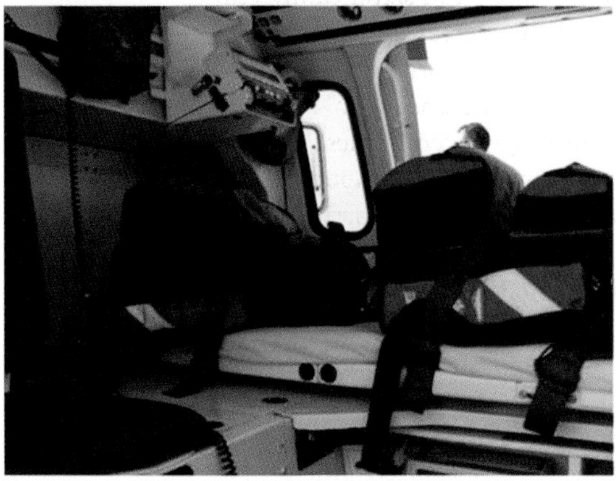

Fig. 4.1 Helicopter transfers may potentially be quicker than land-based transfers. Disadvantages of helicopter transfers includes costs, limited space, noise, time to mobilize, potential need for additional transport to/from helicopter, physiological effects related to altitude. (Pictures courtesy of Tony Bleetman, Warwickshire and Northampton Air Ambulance.)

Personnel

Current guidelines recommend that a minimum of two people accompany the transfer of a critically ill patient in addition to the staff required to operate the transport vehicle. The transfer team may be provided by the referring hospital or from a specialized retrieval service. The choice of team is usually dictated by local policy and the availability of a specialized transfer team. Observational data have shown that transfer by a specialist transfer team is associated with fewer adverse events and potentially better patient outcomes.

The personnel usually involved in a critical care transfer include a registered medical practitioner with training and experience in the transfer of critically ill patients along with a suitably experienced nurse/paramedic/technician. Rather than defining specific personnel by job title (e.g. anaesthetist, intensivist, critical care nurse, etc.), it is more important that the members of the transfer team have the relevant competencies to undertake the transfer. These have been defined in the competency-based training in intensive care medicine in Europe (CoBaTrICE) initiative which describes the knowledge, attitude and skills required for transporting a mechanically ventilated critically ill patient outside the intensive care unit (http://www.cobatrice.org/).

A clear plan for how staff will be repatriated after the transfer should be determined prior to departure and the transfer staff base institution should ensure that adequate insurance is in place to cover staff for personal injury.

Preparation prior to transfer

The decision to transfer a critically ill patient is usually shared between the critical care consultants at the referring and receiving hospitals in collaboration with their consultant colleagues in the relevant specialities. Clear communication should be established between the referring and receiving hospitals and the ambulance service. The patient (if possible) and relatives should be informed of the need for transfer at the earliest opportunity.

Patients should be stabilized prior to transfer. Time spent resuscitating and stabilizing the patient before transfer can significantly reduce complications during the actual transfer. Rare exceptions may include patients with time-critical illnesses such as ruptured aortic aneurysm or expanding intracranial haemorrhage. Even in these patients, attention to the ABC principles is paramount in order to optimize the chances of the patient arriving alive at the receiving hospital. A pre-transfer check list to assess patient suitability/stability for transfer is provided in Table 4.2.

Prior to departure, the transfer team should ensure that the full clinical details of the patient, the results and copies of relevant investigations (e.g. scans, blood results) are transported with the patient. The transfer team should contact named staff at the receiving hospital to provide an update on the patient's condition and estimated time of arrival.

Monitoring

All patients must have as a minimum continuous pulse oximetry, electrocardiographic monitoring and regular measurement of blood pressure, respiratory rate and temperature. All ventilated patients should have end-tidal carbon dioxide monitoring. In addition, the oxygen supply, inspired oxygen concentration, ventilator settings and airway pressure should ideally be monitored. Haemodynamically unstable patients (or those at risk of becoming unstable) may benefit from intra-arterial blood pressure monitoring. Intra-arterial blood pressure monitoring has the added advantage of being less sensitive to movement artefact than non-invasive techniques. Invasive cardiac output monitoring is usually impractical during transfer. In selected patients, intracranial pressure monitoring may be indicated.

Equipment

Designated lightweight, portable equipment with sufficient battery life to last the transfer should be used. The displays on portable monitors should be clear and capable of showing simultaneous ECG, SpO_2, blood pressure and $ETCO_2$ signals. All equipment should be

Table 4.2 Patient check list prior to critical care transfer

Airway

- Patients with (or at risk from) airway compromise should be intubated prior to transfer
- The tracheal tube should be secured and confirmed in correct position on a CXR
- $ETCO_2$ monitoring if intubated

C-spine

- Adequate spinal immobilization (if indicated)

Breathing

- Patient adequately sedated and paralysed if ventilated
- Ventilation established (and stable) on transport ventilator
- Adequate gas exchange on transport ventilator confirmed by arterial blood gas analysis
- Adequate oxygen supply on transfer vehicle
- Stomach decompressed by with naso- or orogastric tube
- Unclamped intercostal drain in situ if pneumothorax present (though Heimlich valve easier to manage than underwater seals)
- SpO_2 monitoring established

Circulation

- Adequate intravenous access
- Circulating volume optimized
- Haemodynamically stable
- All lines are patent and secured
- Any active bleeding controlled
- Long bone/pelvic fractures stabilized
- Adequate haemoglobin concentration
- Patient catheterized
- End-organ perfusion optimized
- ECG and blood pressure monitored

Disability

- No active seizures
- Initial treatments for raised intracranial pressure (if indicated)
- Life-threatening electrolyte disturbances corrected
- Blood glucose >4 mmol/l

Exposure

- Patient adequately covered to prevent heat loss
- Temperature monitored

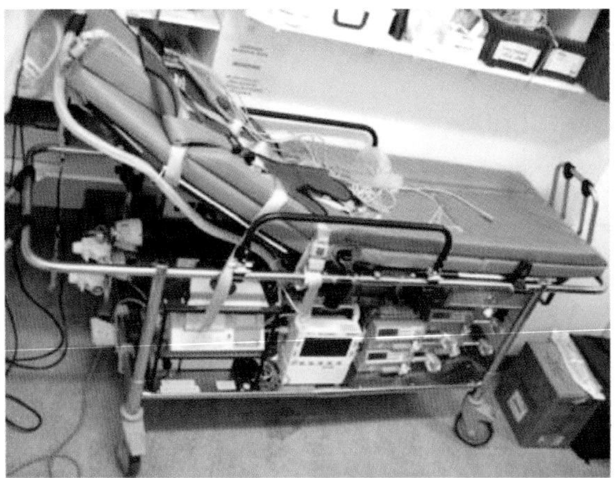

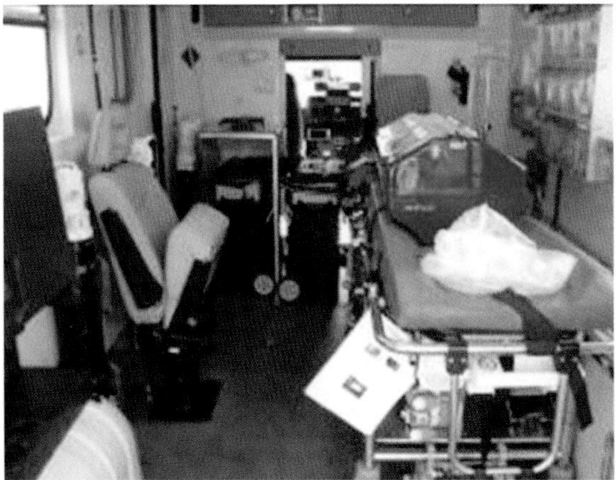

Fig. 4.2 A mobile intensive care trolley with equipment monitor, ventilator and infusion pumps which are fixed below the level of the patient. This provides a low centre of gravity and greater stability. The trolley fixes to the floor of the vehicle with a secure locking system and is not dependent on side-clamps or belt straps. (Picture courtesy of Reinout J. Mildner and Phil Wilson, Birmingham Children's Hospital NHS Foundation Trust.)

checked prior to use on a transfer. Alarm limits and volume should be checked and adjusted as necessary. Drugs and fluids should be administered by syringe/infusion pumps as gravity-fed infusions are unreliable in moving vehicles. The equipment should be left on charge until immediately prior to departure. The ambulance should carry sufficient oxygen to last the duration of the transfer, plus at least another 50% to cover unexpected delays. Enough portable oxygen to complete the journey to and from the ambulance is also required.

Equipment for advanced airway management, defibrillation and basic resuscitation drugs should be readily available. Drugs according to patient needs (e.g. sedatives, muscle relaxants, vasopressors and inotropes) and ample intravenous fluids should be carried. Detailed lists containing the minimum equipment and drug requirements for transfers are contained in the Intensive Care Society guidelines (see Further reading).

Standard ambulance trolleys are usually inadequate for patient transfer as they lack sufficient space to safely store infusions and other equipment. A bespoke transfer trolley which is compliant with the relevant regulations (British Standard 1789/2000) is recommended (Fig. 4.2). All equipment must be securely attached to the ambulance or the trolley as in the event of a crash, heavy equipment such as monitors or oxygen cylinders can cause serious injury to staff and the patient. Balancing equipment on the patient's body/between their legs is an unacceptable risk.

Patient transfer record sheet

Demographic data and clinical details about the patient's presentation and treatment should be recorded on a dedicated patient transfer record sheet. This sheet should also collect information on haemodynamics, ventilatory settings, drugs and fluids administered during the transfer. The form can also be used to record any adverse event during the transfer. A copy of the transfer record should be left with the receiving hospital and a copy returned to the referring hospital. Figure 4.3 provides an example of a critical care transfer record sheet.

Considerations during patient transfer

Continuous monitoring of the ECG, SpO_2 blood pressure and $ETCO_2$ should be maintained throughout the transfer and recorded on the patient transfer sheet. The battery life on portable monitors and infusion pumps should be monitored and batteries changed/pumps replaced if they are running low on charge. A high level of vigilance should be maintained for the common complications reported to occur during inter-hospital transfer such as line or tube displacement/disconnection, vibration artefact and equipment failure. Patients are at risk of becoming hypothermic during transfer and this is particularly true of patients who have sustained burns. Temperature should be monitored regularly during the transfer. Devices that reduce heat loss (such as insulated blankets) and portable warm air devices can be useful in maintaining the patient's temperature during the transfer.

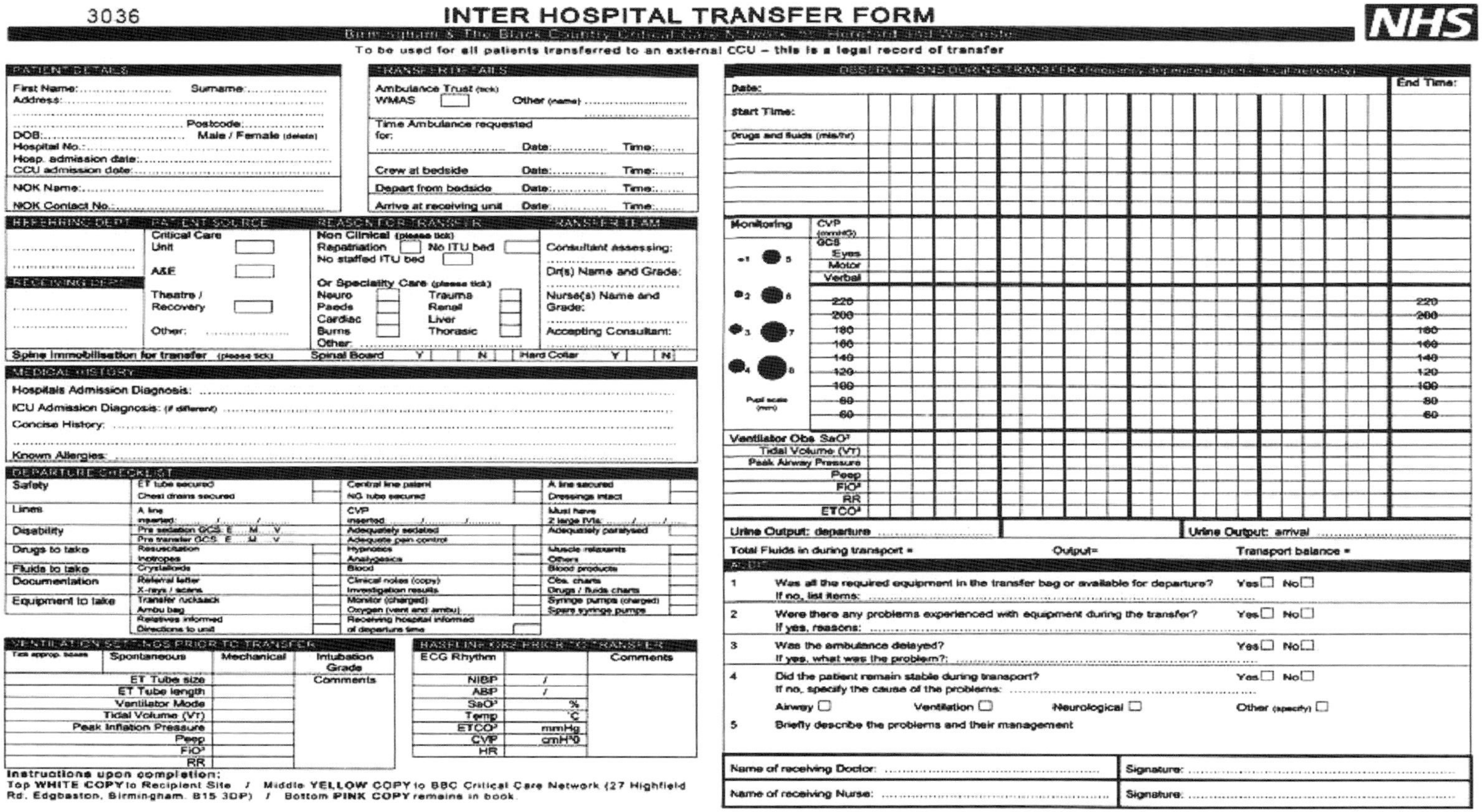

3036

INTER HOSPITAL TRANSFER FORM

NHS

Birmingham & The Black Country Critical Care Network inc Hereford and Worcester

To be used for all patients transferred to an external CCU – this is a legal record of transfer

PATIENT DETAILS

First Name: ……… Surname: ………
Address: ………
……… Postcode: ………
DOB: ……… Male / Female (delete)
Hospital No.: ………
Hosp. admission date: ………
CCU admission date: ………

NOK Name: ………
NOK Contact No.: ………

TRANSFER DETAILS

Ambulance Trust (tick)
WMAS ☐ Other (name) ………

Time Ambulance requested for:	Date:	Time:
Crew at bedside	Date:	Time:
Depart from bedside	Date:	Time:
Arrive at receiving unit	Date:	Time:

REFERRING DEPT	PATIENT SOURCE	REASON FOR TRANSFER	TRANSFER TEAM
………	Critical Care Unit ☐	Non Clinical (please tick)	Consultant assessing:
………	A&E ☐	Repatriation ☐ No ITU bed ☐	………
RECEIVING DEPT	Theatre / Recovery ☐	No staffed ITU bed ☐	Dr(s) Name and Grade:
………	Other: ………	Or Speciality Care (please tick)	Nurse(s) Name and Grade:
………		Neuro ☐ Trauma ☐	………
		Paeds ☐ Renal ☐	Accepting Consultant:
		Cardiac ☐ Liver ☐	………
		Burns ☐ Thoracic ☐	
		Other: ………	

Spine Immobilisation for transfer (please tick) Spinal Board Y ☐ N ☐ Hard Collar Y ☐ N ☐

MEDICAL HISTORY

Hospitals Admission Diagnosis: ………
ICU Admission Diagnosis: (if different) ………
Concise History: ………
Known Allergies: ………

DEPARTURE CHECKLIST

Safety	ET tube secured	☐	Central line patent	☐	A line secured	☐
	Chest drains secured	☐	NG tube secured	☐	Dressings intact	☐
Lines	A line inserted: …/…/…		CVP inserted …/…/…		Must have 2 large IVIs: …/…/…	
Disability	Pre sedation GCS E … M … V …		Adequately sedated	☐	Adequately paralysed	☐
	Pre transfer GCS E … M … V …		Adequate pain control	☐		
Drugs to take	Resuscitation	☐	Hypnotics	☐	Muscle relaxants	☐
	Inotropes	☐	Analgesics	☐	Others	☐
Fluids to take	Crystalloids	☐	Blood	☐	Blood products	☐
Documentation	Referral letter	☐	Clinical notes (copy)	☐	Obs. charts	☐
	X-rays / scans	☐	Investigation results	☐	Drugs / fluids charts	☐
Equipment to take	Transfer rucksack	☐	Monitor (charged)	☐	Syringe pumps (charged)	☐
	Ambu bag	☐	Oxygen (vent and ambu)	☐	Spare syringe pumps	☐
	Relatives informed	☐	Receiving hospital informed of departure time	☐		
	Directions to unit	☐				

VENTILATION SETTINGS PRIOR TO TRANSFER

Tick approp. boxes	Spontaneous	Mechanical	Intubation Grade
ET Tube size			Comments
ET Tube length			
Ventilator Mode			
Tidal Volume (VT)			
Peak Inflation Pressure			
Peep			
FiO_2			
RR			

BASELINE OBS PRIOR TO TRANSFER

ECG Rhythm		Comments
NIBP	/	
ABP	/	
SaO_2	%	
Temp	°C	
$ETCO_2$	mmHg	
CVP	cmH_2O	
HR		

Instructions upon completion:
Top **WHITE COPY** to Recipient Site / Middle **YELLOW COPY** to BBC Critical Care Network (27 Highfield Rd, Edgbaston, Birmingham, B15 3DP) / Bottom **PINK COPY** remains in book.

OBSERVATIONS DURING TRANSFER (frequency dependent upon clinical necessity)

Date: End Time:
Start Time:
Drugs and fluids (mls/hr)

Monitoring: CVP (mmHG); GCS: Eyes, Motor, Verbal

Pupil scale (mm): 1, 2, 3, 4, 5, 6, 7, 8

220, 200, 180, 160, 140, 120, 100, 80, 60

Ventilator Obs: SaO_2; Tidal Volume (VT); Peak Airway Pressure; Peep; FiO_2; RR; $ETCO_2$

Urine Output: departure ……… Urine Output: arrival ………
Total Fluids in during transport = Output= Transport balance =

AUDIT

1. Was all the required equipment in the transfer bag or available for departure? Yes ☐ No ☐
   If no, list items: ………
2. Were there any problems experienced with equipment during the transfer? Yes ☐ No ☐
   If yes, reasons: ………
3. Was the ambulance delayed? Yes ☐ No ☐
   If yes, what was the problem?: ………
4. Did the patient remain stable during transport? Yes ☐ No ☐
   If no, specify the cause of the problems: ………
   Airway ☐ Ventilation ☐ Neurological ☐ Other (specify) ☐
5. Briefly describe the problems and their management

Name of receiving Doctor: ……… Signature: ………
Name of receiving Nurse: ……… Signature: ………

Fig. 4.3 Critical care transfer record sheet. (Courtesy of the Birmingham and Black Country Critical Care Network.)

During a land-based ambulance transfer, staff should remain seated (with seat belts on) at all times. If the patient requires an intervention during the transfer, the vehicle should be stopped at a safe location rather than undertaking the intervention in a moving ambulance. The decision to use blue lights and sirens rests with the ambulance driver, who should be informed about the urgency of the transfer by the attending transfer team. It should be remembered that the risk of a collision greatly increases when excess speed/emergency warning devices are used.

Post transfer

Following arrival at the receiving hospital, a full handover should be provided to the admitting team. This should include leaving copies of relevant medical notes and X-rays and a copy of the inter-hospital transfer form. The transfer team should return any equipment used for the transfer and ensure that it is checked and, where applicable, is placed back on charge in readiness for future use. Most transfers are audited at a regional level and paperwork relating to the transfer should be completed and submitted in a timely manner. Any critical incidents occurring during the transfer should be reported using the appropriate mechanisms.

Conclusion

Critically ill patients frequently require secondary transfer either within or between hospitals. The decision to transfer a patient should follow a risk–benefit analysis, recognizing that the transfer of critically ill patients is associated with significant morbidity and mortality. A trained team with the requisite competencies for critical care transfers should accompany all critically ill patients during transfer. An organized and well-structured transfer system should help to minimize these risks.

Key points

- Inter- and intra-hospital transfers involving critically ill patients are relatively common. Most inter-hospital transfers result from a lack of local critical care bed capacity and usually occur within critical care networks.
- The transfer of a critically ill patient may be associated with increased risk of morbidity and mortality.
- The choice of transport modality will depend on urgency; distance to transfer; weather/road conditions; space considerations and staffing.
- Careful planning and preparation should precede all transfers and transfers should only be undertaken by appropriately trained staff.
- During transfer continuous monitoring of the ECG, SpO_2, blood pressure and $ETCO_2$ should be maintained throughout the transfer and recorded on the patient transfer sheet.

Further reading

- Advanced Life Support Group (2006) *Safe Transfer and Retrieval: The Practical Approach*, 2nd edn. Oxford: Blackwell Publishing.
- Association of Anaesthetists of Great Britain and Ireland (2006) *Recommendations for the Safe Transfer of Patients with Brain Injury*. London: The Association of Anaesthetists of Great Britain and Ireland. www.aagbi.org/publications/guidelines/docs/braininjury.pdf
- Association of Anaesthetists of Great Britain and Ireland (2009) *Interhospital Transfer*. London: The Association of Anaesthetists of Great Britain and Ireland. www.aagbi.org/publications/guidelines/docs/interhospital09.pdf
- CoBaTrICE Collaboration: Bion JF, Barrett H (2006) Development of core competencies for an international training programme in intensive care medicine. *Intens. Care Med.* **32**: 1371–83. www.cobatrice.org/
- Intensive Care Society (2002) *Guidelines for the Transport of the Critically Ill Adult*, 2nd edn. London: Intensive Care Society (UK). www.ics.ac.uk
- Warren J, Fromm RE, Orr RA, Rotello LC, Horst HM (2004) Guidelines for the inter- and intra-hospital transport of critically ill patients. *Crit. Care Med.* **32**: 256–62.

Scoring systems and outcome

Roger Stedman

Prediction is very difficult, especially about the future.
Niels Bohr, Danish physicist (1885–1962)

Introduction

Scoring systems are used widely in medicine both inside and outside the intensive care unit. They are used as an objective way of measuring and recording the severity of complex clinical conditions in order to compare patients, diseases, treatments or services. A scoring system can be specific or generic and may also be functional or anatomical. They can be designed simply as a measure of severity in order to create a 'common language' when discussing a single condition or may be a sophisticated statistical model in order to estimate probabilities of outcome or 'risk adjust' outcome data.

Types of scoring system

Specific

This type of scoring system refers to a specific condition or organ. Examples include Glasgow Coma Scale (brain injury), Ransom Score (pancreatitis) and Child–Pugh Score (liver failure).

Generic

A generic scoring system is one that can be applied to a wide range of disease conditions and uses non-specific measures of severity. For example the SOFA score (Sequential Organ Failure Assessment) grades severity of dysfunction in six organ systems according to commonly measured variables and can be used to track changes in the course of a critical illness. Other examples include APACHE I, II, III and IV (Acute Physiology and Chronic Health Evaluation), SAPS 3 (Simplified Acute Physiology Score) and MPM III (Mortality Probability Model).

Anatomical

These are typically used in trauma and include AIS (Abbreviated Injury Scoring), the more detailed ISS (Injury Severity Score) and TRISS (Trauma and Injury Severity Score). The latter is a combination of a physiological score (RTS – Revised Trauma Score) and an anatomical (ISS) and is well calibrated for evaluating outcomes of trauma care.

Functional

Also termed physiological, this group includes most of the generic scoring systems outlined above. It also includes the oldest of the widely available methods of classifying critical illness, the Therapeutic Intervention Scoring System (TISS). TISS is a detailed measure of the level of support provided for the patient. Points are assigned for various monitoring and therapeutic interventions. One of the advantages is that it does not rely on the diagnosis which is often not available at the start or even, on occasions, at the end of an intensive care period. However its long establishment has meant that it has struggled to keep up with the introduction of new monitoring and therapeutic interventions – each of which has to be weighted according to its influence on outcome.

The applications of scoring systems

Scoring systems are used for the following purposes:

- outcome probabilities
- clinical decision making and prognosis
- quality and performance assessment
- resource allocation
- pre-ICU 'at risk' and 'deteriorating patient' screening
- research.

Core Topics in Critical Care Medicine, eds. Fang Gao Smith and Joyce Yeung. Published by Cambridge University Press.

Outcome probabilities

Outcome measures

The measurement of outcome is important as considerable resources are expended in providing intensive care. It is also an intervention associated with considerable burden of treatment (pain, suffering, loss of autonomy, disability, prolonged rehabilitation and dependence) for the individual and their relatives. It is important to be able to show it is 'worth it'.

Outcome in intensive care can be measured with respect to mortality, morbidity, disability and quality of life. Death on the intensive care unit is sufficiently common and easy to measure for it to be an important outcome. Other outcomes are also important; however, they are difficult and complex to measure, and require long-term follow-up making it difficult to meaningfully inform changes in intensive care practice. This has resulted in considerably less work being done on outcomes other than death, although this is changing slowly.

There are many influences on outcome which can be broadly grouped into patient factors (age, co-morbidity), disease factors (diagnosis, severity) and intensive care factors (resources, staff, equipment, skill and timing). Generally scoring systems are used to 'adjust' measured outcomes for patient and disease factors (which can't be influenced) in order to demonstrate the effect of intensive care factors (which can be influenced).

Development of outcome probability model

The process by which a scoring system becomes an outcome probability model is through multiple logistic regression. A typical example would be the use of APACHE II scoring which gives a measure of acute physiological derangement, chronic health status and age (see Table 5.1). Data are collected on a large number of patients (development population) and each data point is weighted according to the strength of association with the outcome (death).

When the original APACHE II model was developed on a database of nearly 6000 patients it was found that each 3 point increase on the APACHE II score (0–71) was associated with a 3% increase in risk of hospital death. However, it was found that APACHE II alone was not generalizable to populations other than the development population (i.e. did not fit well when used in other settings) because the diagnosis of the acute illness had a powerful, independent influence on outcome. This led to the process of 'case mix adjustment' by which a table of possible acute diagnoses was developed and each diagnosis through the same logistic regression technique was given a weighting.

Limitations of outcome probability model

The combination of APACHE II and case mix adjustment provides a much more powerful tool for calculating outcome probabilities in intensive care. However there remain a number of limitations which arise from differences in the way the score was developed compared to the way it is applied:

(1) The population it is applied to – although the model was developed for a mixed general intensive care population its use has become widespread both in specialist intensive care units and also outside of the intensive care unit. The model is not well calibrated for these circumstances and may significantly over- or underestimate the risk of death.

(2) The timing of data collection – the model is calibrated for the collection of physiological data over the first 24 hours of the intensive care stay. In critical illness the physiological deterioration and subsequent recovery is a continuum, the data is a snapshot at a point in that continuum and may not represent the nadir of physiological deterioration. This is manifest in the phenomenon of 'lead time bias' where efficient well resourced intensive care units may pick up critically ill patients early in the natural history of the condition, stabilize them and prevent severe physiological derangement and consequently derive low APACHE scores but the severity of the acute diagnosis goes on to produce a poor outcome (i.e. the physiological nadir occurs after the initial 24-hour period). The model then underestimates probability of death.

(3) Validity, reliability and completeness of data – when developing a model, data collection will be assiduous and complete, it will be overseen by a research team who will apply consistent rules to the interpretation of the data (e.g. the scoring of GCS in sedated patients). In the application of the model data collection will be incomplete, and rules for the interpretation of data will differ between units; this can have large effects on predicted outcomes, especially if a single variable with a large impact on outcome (such as GCS) is misinterpreted.

Table 5.1 APACHE II scoring system

Physiology points	+4	+3	+2	+1	0	−1	−2	−3	−4
Rectal temperature (°C)	≥41.0	39.0 40.9		38.5 38.9	36.0 38.4	34.0 35.9	32.0 33.9	30.0 31.9	≤29.9
Mean BP (mmHg)	≥160	130–159	110–129		70–109		50–69		≤49
Heart rate (/min)	≥180	140–179	110–139		70–109		55–69	40–54	≤39
Respiration rate (/min)	≥50	35–49		25–34	12–24	10–11	6–9		≤5
Oxygenation									
$FiO_2 \geq 0.5$ A-aDO_2	66.5	46.6–66.4	26.6–46.4		<26.6				
FiO_2<0.5 PaO_2					>9.3	8.1–9.3		7.3–8.0	<7.3
Arterial pH	≥7.70	7.6–7.59		7.5–7.59	7.33–7.49		7.25–7.32	7.15–7.24	<7.15
Sodium (mmol/l)	≥180	160–179	155–159	150–154	130–149		120–129	111–119	≤110
Potassium (mmol/l)	≥7.0	6.0–6.9		5.5–5.9	3.5–5.4	3.0–3.4	2.5–2.9		<2.5
Creatinine (μmol/l)	≥300	171–299		121–170	50–120		<50		
Haematocrit (%)	≥60		50–59.9	46–49.9	30–45.9		20–29.9		<20
White cell count (10^9/l)	≥40		20–39.9	15–19.9	3–14.9		1–2.9		<1

Glasgow Coma Score – subtract GCS from 15.
Age – <45 = 0, 45–54 = 2, 55–64 = 3, 65–75 = 5, ≥75 = 6.
Chronic health points – chronic liver disease (portal hypertension, previous ALF, encephalopathy or coma), heart failure (NYHA grade 4), respiratory disease (with exercise limitation, polycythaemia or pulmonary hypertension), dialysis, immune suppression (chemo/radio therapy, high-dose steroids, leukaemia, AIDS). Additional 5 points for emergency surgery or emergency medical admission, 2 points for elective surgical admission.
Source: With permission from Knaus WA, Draper EA, Wagner DP, Zimmerman JE (1985) *Crit. Care Med.* **13**(10): 818–29.

Clinical decision making and prognosis

Clinical applications

The use of scoring systems to support clinical decision making is generally confined to specific scoring systems, for example the use of GCS to decide when to protect the airway of a brain-injured patient (or when to perform brain imaging). Another example might be the use of sedation scoring (Ramsay or RASS) to adjust the infusion of sedative drugs.

Potential drawbacks

The use of generic scoring systems to support decisions to withdraw or withhold treatment is more controversial. Although a physiological scoring system that has been well calibrated through logistic regression analysis and case mix adjustment can produce an accurate estimate of the risk of death a number of caveats have to be borne in mind when applying this to individual patients.

(1) An estimate of the risk of death is a probability (i.e. a number anywhere between 0 and 1) whereas a prediction of outcome is dichotomous (i.e. the patient will/will not survive). To convert a probability to a prediction requires a 'cut-off' to be applied to the probability – such as a risk of death of 0.9. The problem then arises if you use this to decide to withdraw care then 1/10 of the patients you withdraw on would have survived if you had continued to support them.

(2) These are statistical models that describe the population (and the results of the interventions applied to them) used to develop the model. This may be both remote in time and geography and

may not be applicable to the local circumstances. Populations and medical interventions change significantly over time and healthcare systems vary enormously in resources available to them.

(3) A statistical estimate of the risk of death will have a confidence interval. The more extreme risks will have a lower confidence (i.e. wider confidence interval) associated with them as they represent a relatively smaller proportion of the development population.

(4) Prognosis is not just survival but also disability, quality of life and the extent and burden of ongoing treatment after discharge from critical care. There have been very few if any very large studies that give reliable information of this kind following intensive care.

Quality and performance assessment

Where a scoring system has been calibrated for a clinical outcome (such as death) against a large and relevant population it can be used as a method of measuring the performance of hospitals, units or even individual clinicians.

Standardized Mortality Ratio (SMR)

An example is the Intensive Care National Audit and Research Centre (ICNARC) in the UK. ICNARC is based on APACHE II with case mix adjustment coming from a very large database of patients admitted to UK intensive care units. Units in the UK that participate in the ICNARC programme regularly submit data of their case mix, APACHE II scores and outcomes (amongst other things). ICNARC uses these data not only to add to the database but also apply the model to the submitted data in order to produce an 'expected outcome' (i.e. the number of deaths estimated by the probabilistic model); this is then used to calculate the Standardized Mortality Ratio (SMR). SMR is the ratio of expected to observed deaths. An SMR of greater than 1.0 indicates a higher than expected number of deaths following adjustment for risk of death and case mix. The SMR can then be used to compare the outcomes of intensive care units within regions or of similar units nationally. Individual units can use their SMR as a performance indicator.

Knowing that an SMR is high (or low) alone does not help improve performance as it cannot give reasons for a particular score. However it can be used to identify significant outliers within the data set. For example patients that died with a low estimated risk of death can be listed to allow case note review. The data can also be used to indentify resource issues such as high bed occupancy and turnover, high non-clinical transfer rates, early discharge and early readmission rates.

Again caution should be applied when interpreting the results of a single data set and comparing it to others. Are the units similar i.e. mixed ICU/HDU compared to ICU alone? Is the sample data set large enough that random effects aren't having a large impact on overall outcome? (For example, a small number of unexpected deaths in patients with a low estimated risk of death can have a large impact on final SMR if the sample size is small.) Does the unit have a large throughput of high-risk surgical specialties (e.g. major vascular or thoracic)?

Quality assessment and improvement is a continuous process and should take place over time. Figure 5.1 demonstrates the effects on SMR in a single unit of changing the patient population on which the model is used (Line A represents the point in time at which data began to be collected on HDU as well as ITU patients) and of a significant change in practice (Line B represents the point in time when the intensivists switched from changing daily to doing full weeks on duty).

Parsonnet score

Scoring systems can also be used to assess the performance of individual clinicians. An example is the Parsonnet score for predicting operative outcome in cardiac surgery. This is a pre-operative mortality and morbidity risk model and does not account for intra-operative events and as such can be used, in principle, to audit the performance of individual surgeons by adjusting their outcomes for pre-operative risk. The same caveats apply as for the above example.

Resource allocation

The Therapeutic Intervention Scoring System (TISS) was originally developed as a severity of illness score based on the premise that the more you have to do to a patient the more unwell they must be. The utility of TISS for this purpose was weak due to the fact that not all interventions were universally available, making comparison between sites difficult, and the introduction of new interventions necessitated recalibration of the risk model. However TISS rapidly became adopted as a useful method of identifying (particularly nursing) resource need. This enabled efficient deployment of nursing resources within a unit, and also demonstrated institutional requirements for critical care resources (i.e. number of critical care beds). By assigning points

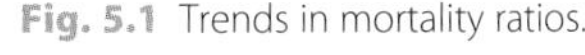

Trends in mortality ratios

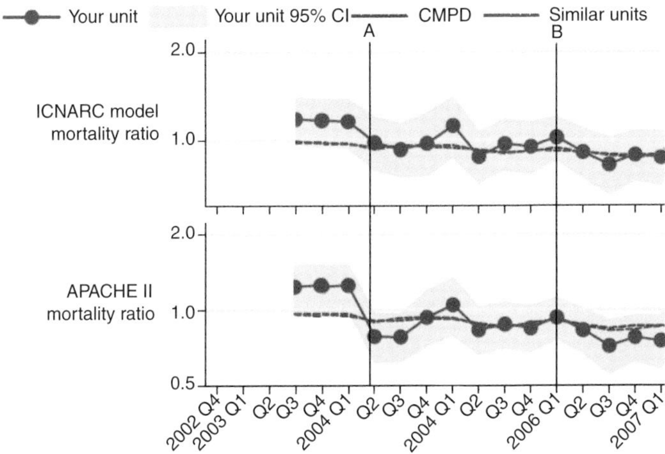

Fig. 5.1 Trends in mortality ratios.

to every intervention (from a single point for ECG monitoring or urinary catheter care up to four points for multiple vasoactive drug infusions or renal replacement therapy) a total for each patient can be summed indicating the amount of healthcare 'resource' being consumed. Patients can be stratified into four classes of dependency and the level of nursing and physician care identified for a given population.

One of the disadvantages of TISS is that the collection of information became very onerous. Points were assigned to up to 78 different nursing and medical interventions – this prompted revision and simplification of the score (down to 28 interventions) and eventually became the basis of stratification into four classes (or levels) of care.

Pre-ICU 'at risk' and 'deteriorating patient' screening

The recognition that early identification and intervention in critical illness has a large impact on outcome has resulted in the development of the critical care outreach or medical emergency team. Integral to the functioning of these teams is the use of 'early warning' scoring systems.

Features of early warning scoring systems

The essential features of an early warning scoring system are:

(1) They are based on standard ward observations (heart rate, blood pressure, oxygen saturations, respiratory rate, temperature, urine output and conscious level).

(2) They are simple to apply and calculate.

(3) They are linked to a clear escalation policy (trigger).

(4) The response to the trigger is sufficiently resourced (i.e. the outreach team are able to respond, intervene and move the patient to a higher level of care within a reasonable period of time).

(5) The application of the scoring system is universal and mandatory – no one is left out (except where a decision has been made that escalation is not appropriate, e.g. in palliative care).

Modified early warning score

A number of early warning scoring systems exist and the MEWS (Modified Early Warning Score) is typical. Table 5.2 illustrates how the score is calculated.

Early warning scores have low specificity and high sensitivity for critical illness. This means that there is a high false positive trigger rate. The setting of the trigger level is a compromise between capturing the majority of the critically ill and not overwhelming the response team.

Research

Observational studies

The small size and heterogeneous nature of the critically ill population make evaluative research through randomized controlled trials very difficult. Non-randomized and observational studies remain important and valid research methodologies in the critical care setting. However it remains important that researchers are able to describe their study populations in a way that enables clinicians to apply the findings to their own patient populations. The use of scoring systems and case mix adjustment provides a universal language for describing critical care populations and enables the fruits of research carried out in one health-care setting be applied in another.

Useful data for designing a randomized clinical trial

Scoring systems also provide a tool for researchers to stratify their study populations for risk of death and to calculate sample size of the trial when performing a randomized clinical trial.

Scoring systems in common use in critical care

There is insufficient space to cover in detail all scoring systems in common use in critical care. Here follows a list and brief description of the important ones with references for further reading at the end of the chapter.

APACHE

Now in its fourth incarnation, APACHE II remains the most commonly used. APACHE III refines the model both through the extension of the physiological data set to include laboratory data, and expands the number of co-morbid conditions. The development population was much larger than APACHE II (17 440 patients). The prognostic model is based on case mix adjustment and logistic regression as for APACHE II; however, in addition APACHE III mandates daily updates of the acute physiology score in order to incorporate a measure of 'response to therapy' and eliminate 'lead time bias'. APACHE IV is largely a recalibration of the APACHE III model based on a development population of 100 000 patients from US intensive care units admitted between 2003 and 2005.

SAPS

The Simplified Acute Physiology Score was developed as a reaction to the increasingly complicated nature of published scoring systems and the resources required to collect, process and maintain the data associated with them. The first usable version of the model developed was SAPS II and consisted of 17 easily measured physiological variables – selected from 34 analysed using logistic regression. It was an attempt to create a 'pure' physiological outcome model, the premise being that critically ill patients commonly have more than one diagnosis and determining which is the more important often impossible. The result is that SAPS models require calibrating in whichever circumstance they are used (between countries and even individual units). This limits its use as a mechanism for comparing performance between sites although its simplicity increases its utility for tracking performance over time on an individual site. Subsets of the SAPS II model have been developed for specific diagnostic groupings (for example sepsis). The SAPS III model includes limited case mix and co-morbidity adjustment.

MPM

The Mortality Probability Model is, conversely, a risk model based almost purely on diagnosis. The score is based on a list of acute and chronic diagnoses which

Table 5.2 Modified Early Warning Score

Score	3	2	1	0	1	2	3
Respiratory rate (/min)		≤8		9 – 14	15 – 20	21–29	>29
Heart rate (/min)		≤40	41–50	51–100	101–110	11–129	>129
Systolic BP (mmHg)	≤70	71–80	81–100	101–199		≥200	
Urine output (ml/kg/hr)	0	≤0.5					
Temperature (°C)		≤35	35.1–36	36.1–38	38.1–38.5	≥38.6	
Neurological				alert	responds to voice	responds to pain	unresponsive

Source: With permission from Morgan RJM, Williams F, Wright MM (1997) An early warning score for the detection of patients with impending illness. *Clin. Intens. Care* **8**: 100.

are either present or absent. Each contributes a weighted coefficient (derived by Bayesian inference) and multiplied by an age-based variable to give an overall risk score. Again the coefficients are generated from a development population which needs to be representative of the sample population for accurate probability estimation. In a similar fashion to SAPS the MPM is subject to calibration 'drift' (i.e. over time the original development population becomes less and less like the sample populations on which the model is used). MPM is currently in its third incarnation.

SOFA

Sequential Organ Failure Assessment is calculated by assigning a score of 0–4 for each of six organ systems according to objective and easily obtained measures of failure. It is performed daily, an increasing score, a high maximum and a large delta SOFA (change from admission to maximum SOFA) are associated with a high risk of mortality. SOFA is the only score (other than its similar sibling MODS – Multiple Organ Dysfunction Score) designed to provide a dynamic picture of disease severity.

Trauma scores: TRISS and ASCOT

These scores are not specific to critical care as they can be used on trauma patients in all settings. They are calculated at the time of admission to hospital. ASCOT is the most complete incorporating anatomical, physiological, age and diagnostic categories. It is well calibrated to the trauma population and is generalizable to healthcare systems outside of which it was developed. Trauma scoring systems perform better at calculating outcome probabilities than generic scoring systems (such as APACHE) when applied to trauma patients on ITU.

Key points

- Scoring systems serve many functions to support clinical decision making at the level of the individual patient right through to global healthcare policy and guideline development.
- Using scoring systems to assess critical care performance through the calculation of mortality ratios is a vital part of quality improvement.
- Using statistical models to estimate the probability of death requires recalibration due to changes in patient populations and changes in critical care practice (improvements in technology, new therapies and improved standards of care).
- Scoring systems provide a common language to describe patients with complex medical conditions.
- Scoring systems even with well-calibrated outcome models cannot predict the future.

Further reading

- Harrison DA, Parry GJ, Carpenter JR, Short A, Rowan K (2007) A new risk prediction model: the Intensive Care National Audit and Research Centre (ICNARC) model. *Crit. Care Med.* **25**(4):1091–8.
- Knaus W A, Draper EA, Wagner DP *et al.* (1991) The APACHE III prognostic system: risk prediction of hospital mortality for critically ill hospitalized adults. *Chest* **100**(6): 1619–36.
- Le Gall JR, Lemeshow S, Saulnier F (1993) A new simplified acute physiology score (SAPS II) based on a European/ North American multicentre study. *J. Am. Med. Ass.* **270**(20): 2478–86.
- Marshall JC, Cook DA, Christou NV *et al.* (1995) Multiple organ dysfunction score: a reliable descriptor of complex clinical outcome. *Crit. Care Med.* **23**(10): 1638–52.
- Rowan KM, Kerr JH, Major E *et al.* (1993) Intensive Care Society's APACHE II study in Britain and Ireland. I: Variations in case mix of adult admissions to general intensive care units and impact on outcome. II: Outcome comparisons of intensive care units after adjustment for case mix by the American APACHE II method. *Br. Med. J.* **307**: 972–81.
- Vincent J-L, de Mendonça A, Cantraine F *et al.* (1998) Use of the SOFA score to assess the incidence of organ dysfunction / failure in intensive care units: results of a multicentric, prospective study. *Crit. Care Med.* **26**(11): 1793–800.

Information management in critical care

Roger Stedman

Data is not information, information is not knowledge, knowledge is not wisdom.

Clifford Stoll (US astronomer, computer expert and author) and Gary Schubert (Associate Professor of Art & Computer Science)

Introduction

The ready availability of large amounts of information about critically ill patients is one of the defining characteristics of a critical care unit. Good information management is essential to the process of care. Having the right information in the right place at the right time is a prerequisite for the delivery of safe and effective care.

Critical care has been at the forefront of the use of technology to manage the flow of information in the clinical setting. This is undoubtedly because this technology forms the core of many of the devices used to both monitor and treat critically ill patients. The integration of bedside, ward-based and hospital-wide information systems is a considerable challenge both from the technological and the clinical points of view. It is also expensive. For this reason the majority of critical care units still remain partially if not entirely dependent on paper-based systems.

Functions of an information system

An information system in critical care has to fulfil the following functions:

(1) Bedside charting
(2) Clinical record keeping
(3) Electronic prescribing (physician order entry)
(4) Integration with other hospital systems
(5) Decision support
(6) Remote access, multi-site communication
(7) Data storage/archiving
(8) Data access for audit, research, quality and financial management
(9) Training, education and simulated environments.

Bedside charting

Paper chart

The 'ICU chart' for a long time has been the heart of information management in the critical care unit. It is often a large sheet of paper (A2 or A1) on to which is manually transcribed data from physiological monitoring, infused drugs and fluids, data from laboratory and bedside testing. It also forms part of the clinical record with a diary of events, a daily assessment of nursing needs and recording of invasive devices. It is a mechanism of communication and continuity with important clinical decisions recorded in order that all members of the multi-disciplinary team, visiting at different times, are informed. Each sheet contains 24 hours' worth of information, although much information is transcribed from preceding sheets. The creation and maintenance of the ICU chart is a time-consuming and labour-intensive task. Once created the charts often present a storage problem as they are too large to be archived with the medical record. Any information on them that is needed for audit or quality assurance has to be subsequently extracted and manually entered on to a database.

Basic requirements for an electronic chart

The replacement of these functions with electronic information gathering is logical and technically feasible. It is important to recognize that this is the 'human interface' of the information system. Although a lot of information gathering can be automated much still

Core Topics in Critical Care Management, eds. Fang Gao Smith and Joyce Yeung. Published by Cambridge University Press.

has to be entered manually. The viewing area of the screen has to be large enough to enable multiple tiled windows to be open. The input devices have to be intuitive to use, even for the technologically naive, and also compatible with infection control policies of the unit (keyboard covers and screens tolerant of cleaning chemicals). Most systems are based on adaptations of the 'spreadsheet' concept with columns representing time periods and rows representing data types. There will usually be simultaneous graphical representation of the data in an allied window (see Fig. 6.1). The interface should be customizable to enable units to determine what and how they gather their own information.

Electronic chart systems

Systems have been developed by most of the major monitoring manufacturers, which are naturally compatible with their own monitors and will claim a level of inter-compatibility with other manufacturers. However the monitor is only one of the many bedside devices to which the system has to 'talk'. A system developed by an independent manufacturer is more likely (through necessity) to have dealt with the compatibility issues of a wide range of monitors and other devices, and won't be tied to an individual monitor manufacturer for the lifetime of the information system.

Automated data capture is efficient and accurate and frees up a considerable amount of nursing time to be redeployed in direct patient care. However it is important that the data are filtered before recording. This is the process of removing factitious data (e.g. the arterial pressure during sampling from the line) before recording it. This can be achieved through the introduction of a validation step (i.e. requiring that captured data is reviewed and verified by the nurse at the bedside) or in some systems the application of rules based or fuzzy logic algorithms to clean the data. It is interesting that after the introduction of an automated data capture system many units experience an apparent increase in the severity of illness scoring for their population. The system faithfully records extremes of physiological variables that hitherto had been 'filtered out' by the nursing staff during manual transcription.

Clinical record keeping

Specific requirements

The creation and maintenance of an electronic medical record is a natural extension of the function of a bedside charting system and all systems offer this facility. The electronic clinical record, however, has a number of specific requirements that distinguish it from the bedside charting function.

(1) It is a medico-legal document. The creation, maintenance and storage of the record should meet standards that make it usable in a court of law.
(2) Access to the document must be controlled (i.e. password protected) to protect confidentiality.
(3) Entries should be date and time stamped and not modifiable or post-dated.
(4) Entries should be attributable to individual clinicians and subject to audit trails. The multidisciplinary nature of critical care means that large numbers of medical and allied healthcare professionals will need access, many of whom will not work routinely in the critical care environment.
(5) The electronic record must integrate with the main patient record. This may mean a printout to be inserted into a paper-based record or integration with a hospital electronic patient record.
(6) There must be a mechanism for archiving the record that meets medico-legal standards (for example paediatric and maternal records need to be kept for up to 25 years).
(7) A facility for producing a summary or handover document is desirable.

The electronic medical record, if carefully implemented, has distinct advantages over the traditional handwritten medical record, not least of which will be the confinement of illegible, unattributable and undated entries to history.

Electronic prescribing (physician order entry)

In principle the electronic prescribing package offers many potential benefits to safety and workflow in critical care. In practice results have been mixed, with some systems reported as virtually eliminating prescribing and administration errors, whilst others have been associated with a rise in errors and even mortality. As with electronic information systems the key is in the design and implementation of the system. The usability of the system is crucial to its acceptance by both prescribers and administrators of drugs. Many critical care information systems have a prescribing package as part of them; however, many units find

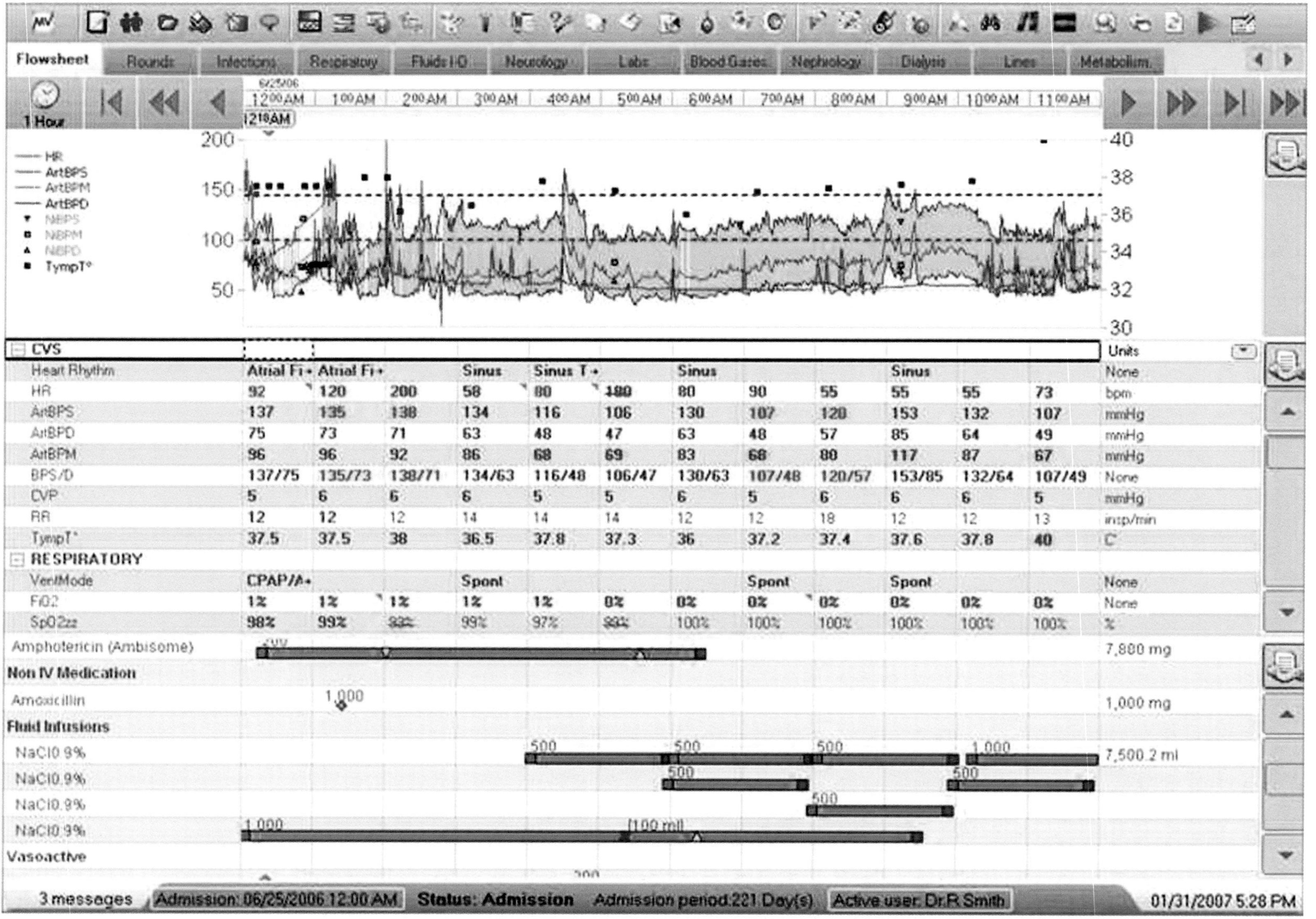

Fig. 6.1 Screen shot from the display module of an integrated critical care information system. (Courtesy of Metavision.)

themselves in institutions that have alternative systems in use already. The interoperability of different systems is vital to the usability (for example not having to log on to different systems with a different password, not having to re-enter important clinical information like allergies or renal impairment) and ultimately the safety (if it is difficult to use people will take short cuts and workarounds).

Integration with other hospital systems

No information system exists in isolation. In recent years a plethora of hospital-wide information systems have come into existence: laboratory systems, radiology systems, electronic prescribing, patient administration systems and referral and booking systems. For them to integrate and talk to each other they need a common language. The accepted common standard for communication between healthcare information systems is the HL7 (Health Level 7). This is an open standard developed since 1987 by an international community of health informatics and healthcare professionals; it is a not-for-profit organization. The HL7 as an interoperability standard has been accredited by both the American National Standards Institute (ANSI) and the International Standards Organization (ISO). It provides a framework by which different applications and systems can exchange healthcare-related information. The use of the HL7 messaging framework is an essential feature of any information system that is not to be condemned to isolation and incompatibility.

Decision support

The term decision support refers to a range of functions of a clinical information system from providing assistance in the interaction between clinician and patient at the bedside, to providing evidence for service improvement and organizational change.

At the bedside level

An information system providing decision support might offer on-screen prompts or reminders, for example, if the patient has a particular allergy, or has renal impairment and requires drug dosage adjustment. They can be used to alert a clinician to the presence of an abnormal laboratory result, even to the extent of linking to the hospital pager system. There have been attempts at developing more sophisticated decision support systems that perform a diagnostic function. An example is the integration of physiological and laboratory data to trigger a 'sepsis alert'. Information systems are an excellent way of implementing 'care bundles' and 'checklists'; not only can they remind clinicians of the elements, they can also track performance through continuous audit.

At the ward level

Decision support means the provision of timely and relevant access to protocols, guidelines and evidence-based practice. The shelves of most intensive care units are creaking with the weight of paper documents providing this type of information (and the dust gathering upon them). A paper-based guideline is generally only effective for as long as its authors and proponents maintain awareness of its existence amongst the practising clinicians. A well-indexed electronic repository of guidelines and protocols could easily be linked with the electronic patient record at the bedside with the system able to bring the relevant ones to the attention of the treating clinician.

At the organization level

Decision support means access to information on performance – both process performance (compliance with protocols, care bundles, etc.) and outcome performance (risk-adjusted outcome).

Remote access and multi-site communication

The ubiquity and robustness of modern computer networks combined with the availability of comprehensive electronic information systems means that the age of the 'virtual ICU' has arrived. It is possible to link, by electronic means, an intensive care bed to an intensive care clinician separated by many miles. Information systems can not only serve all the relevant clinical data to the clinician's desktop, they can also provide voice and video link to the bedside. This enables a single clinician to provide decision making, advice and support to a very large number of critically ill patients across a wide geographical area (Fig. 6.2).

The consolidation of healthcare organizations, for economic reasons, means that many hospitals cover multiple sites often incorporating a large central teaching or university hospital linked to a number of smaller community hospitals. Although efforts in recent decades have been made to centralize critical care resources on teaching hospital sites, there has

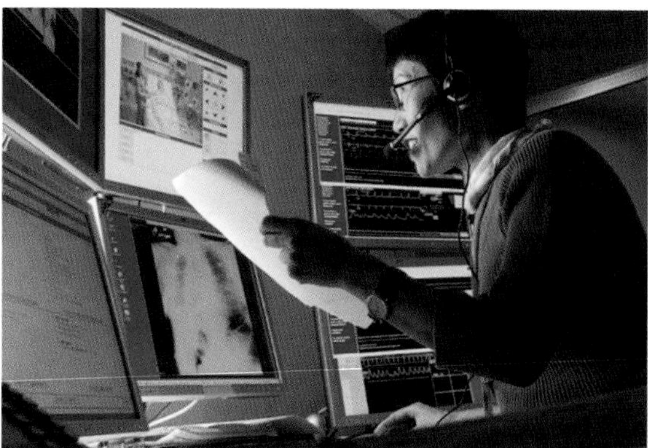

Fig. 6.2 A critical care physician on duty at an e-icu workstation.

remained a stubborn need to maintain critical care beds at smaller community hospitals. The virtual ICU provides a means of bringing the entire critical care bed stock of a multi-site healthcare organization into one 'virtual' place whilst maintaining the provision local at the point of need.

Data storage and archiving

A critical care information system generates an enormous amount of data. Attempting to keep all of it inevitably creates storage issues even in the age of the multilayer DVD and the terabyte hard drive. A good archiving system will perform a form of triage on the data that is generated based on the duration of usefulness for that data. For example, a lot of the physiological data are only useful for the duration of the patient's admission (possibly even less than that). Some data will be needed to be kept until quality and performance information is extracted from it. Research may necessitate the storage of other data. The temptation to store everything 'just in case' should be resisted as there is inevitably a trade-off between the amount of data stored and the ease and speed with which it can be accessed.

As discussed earlier there is a need to provide high-quality archive storage for information that forms the clinical record. Again the longevity of the data need to be considered. A record that needs to be accessible for 25 years will need to be written to a disk with at least that lifespan – most conventional CD ROMs have a lifespan of less than 10 years.

Data access for audit, research, quality and financial management

In order for the huge amount of data generated by a critical care information system to continue to be useful it has to be converted to a database format. This process is called 'data warehousing'. It is not a straightforward process and needs the input of specialist informatics professionals. Data need to be stored in a way that enables clinicians and managers to 'query' the database, without having specialist computer qualifications themselves. The design of the database needs to be a result of a close collaboration between the clinicians (knowing and saying what they need) and the database designers (knowing what is possible and what the best way of implementing it is). Again there is a trade-off between making every conceivable query possible and the speed and reliability of the results of those queries.

The technology of data warehousing and data mining is a huge area of endeavour within the informatics industry – not just in the healthcare arena. There are technological leaps, in the understanding and implementation of complex data structures and the software and hardware required to exploit them, occurring all of the time. These developments promise to transform the way we use and 'see' information in the morass of data available in the critical care environment.

Training, education and simulated environments

The concept of simulation has been current in critical care for some time. However the combination of the transformation of the critical care environment into an array of electronic information and the relative ease with which this can be recreated in a 'classroom' has meant that the fidelity (i.e. the realism) of simulated environments is compelling. Simulated environments are in the process of revolutionizing the way doctors and nurses are trained with enormous potential benefits for patient safety. Simulated environments not only train how to interact with the technology but also how individuals perform in stressful situations and teach vital team skills. They build understanding of how medical errors occur and self-awareness of an individual's role in preventing them.

Implementation of a critical care information system

The implementation of a critical care information system represents a major organizational change.

(1) Successful implementation requires an examination of every aspect of the workflow of a critical care unit and how the system will impact (and improve) on it. It requires a close collaboration between clinical and IT professionals, which should persist for the life of the system as requirements evolve. All stakeholders in the system need to be involved from the start. There is danger in the enthusiasts and technophiles of a department striking out on an ambitious project that leaves their more conservative (or wisely sceptical) colleagues behind.

(2) A vital aspect of the design of the system is the contingency in place if the system is down. Once dependence on an electronic information system is established then the continuous running of the system becomes 'mission critical'. Back-up servers and un-interruptible power supplies form part of this, as well as a well ordered reversion to paper-based systems in the event of a sustained catastrophe.

(3) The potential benefits need to be clearly identified and expressed as the costs are high. Costs are incurred: in the capital investment in hardware, software and structural works; for personnel for maintenance of the service; and by individuals in their personal commitment and time taken to change the way they work. However, the potential benefits of a well-designed, well-implemented and well-fitting information system in a critical care department are legion (and often unforeseeable). A step change in the quality and safety of the care delivered is possible along with a transformation of the quality of the working environment.

Key points

- The assimilation and integration of large amounts of clinical information is a defining characteristic of critical care medicine.
- Adapting this process to the electronic information age is an important challenge for the current generation of critical care practitioners.
- Critical care information systems can impact on every aspect of the workflow of a critical care department, with potential benefits in the quality and safety of the care delivered.
- There are risks if important aspects of the design of the system are not considered, including the usability of the system and the interoperability with equipment and other hospital systems.
- Costs are high: equipment, personnel and investment in organizational change.
- The benefits are a potential step change in the quality and safety of care delivered to the patient.

Further reading

- Bion JF, Heffner JE (2004) Challenges in the care of the acutely ill. *Lancet* **363**(9413): 970–7.
- Breslow MJ, Rosenfeld BA, Doerfler M *et al.* (2004) Effect of a multiple-site intensive care unit telemedicine program on clinical and economic outcomes: an alternative paradigm for intensive staffing. *Crit. Care Med.* **32**(1): 31–8.
- Fraenkel DJ, Cowie M, Daley P (2003) Quality benefits of an intensive care clinical information system. *Crit. Care Med.* **31**(1): 120–5.
- Han YY, Cacillo JA, Venkataraman ST *et al.* (2005) Unexpected increased mortality after implementation of a commercially sold computerized physician order entry system. *Pediatrics* **116**(6): 1506–12.
- Murphy JG, Torsher LC, Dunn WF (2007) Simulation medicine in intensive care and coronary care education. *J. Crit. Care* **22**: 51–5.
- Scurink CA, Lucas PJ, Hoepelman IM, Bonten MJ (2005) Computer assisted decision support for the diagnosis and treatment of infectious diseases in intensive care units. *Lancet Infect. Dis.* **5**(5): 305–12.

Chapter 7 Haemodynamics monitoring

Anil Kumar and Joyce Yeung

Essential considerations

- The purpose of the cardio-respiratory system is to ensure delivery of oxygen and nutrients to the tissues and to remove waste products. This requires an intact cardiovascular system to pump oxygenated blood with nutrients to the tissues in order to perfuse the vital organs.
- Critically ill patients may have a compromised cardiovascular system leading to impaired organ perfusion and tissue microcirculation, resulting in tissue hypoxia, which may result in multi-organ dysfunction syndrome (MODS) and has a very high mortality rate.
- It is important to monitor the physiological responses in the critically ill patients as frequent measurements of haemodynamic parameters will in turn help to detect any pathophysiological changes and gives a baseline to judge the effectiveness of any applied treatment. For example, early goal-directed therapy in severe sepsis has been shown to reduce mortality and morbidity.
- It must be remembered that no measurements can convey all aspects of the patient's condition and haemodynamic parameters need to be used in conjunction with clinical assessment.
- As the incidence of catheter-related bloodstream infection is increasing, it is imperative to ensure that all invasive procedures are done under strict aseptic conditions using barrier sterile precautions. These should include sterile gown, sterile gloves, sterile drapes and bactericidal skin preparation as recommended in the Evidence-based Practice in Infection Control (EPIC 2 guidelines, 2007).
- Haemodynamic monitoring can be broadly classified into non-invasive or invasive monitoring (Table 7.1). In this chapter we will concentrate on the invasive haemodynamic monitoring.

Invasive blood pressure monitoring

Invasive blood pressure monitoring is done by cannulating a peripheral artery and connecting it to an infusion system, transducer, recorder and display systems.

Cannulation sites

Ideally, the most peripheral artery should be chosen so that if a clot or haematoma forms, it does not threaten the circulation of the whole limb. Hence, radial and dorsalis pedis arteries are the most commonly cannulated vessels. The other arteries that can be cannulated are brachial, ulnar, femoral and posterior tibial.

Advantages of intra-arterial cannulation

- Monitor blood pressure on a beat-to-beat basis
- Repeated blood gas analysis
- Up-slope of the arterial waveform indicates myocardial contractility
- The position of the dicrotic notch on the down-slope indicates systemic vascular resistance
- Variation in arterial pressure waveform during respiratory cycle during ventilation can represent reduced preload in a patient
- The area under the systolic component of the waveform (from the beginning of upstroke to the dicrotic notch) (Fig. 7.1) is an indirect measure of stroke volume and cardiac output can be calculated by multiplying stroke volume with heart rate.

Core Topics in Critical Care Medicine, eds. Fang Gao Smith and Joyce Yeung. Published by Cambridge University Press.

Table 7.1 Classification of haemodynamic monitoring

Non-invasive monitoring	Invasive monitoring
Vital signs	Invasive blood pressure monitoring
Urine output	Central venous pressure monitoring
Electrocardiogram (ECG)	Pulmonary artery pressure monitoring
Non-invasive blood pressure monitoring	Cardiac output monitoring
Non-invasive cardiac output monitoring	
Pulse oximetry	

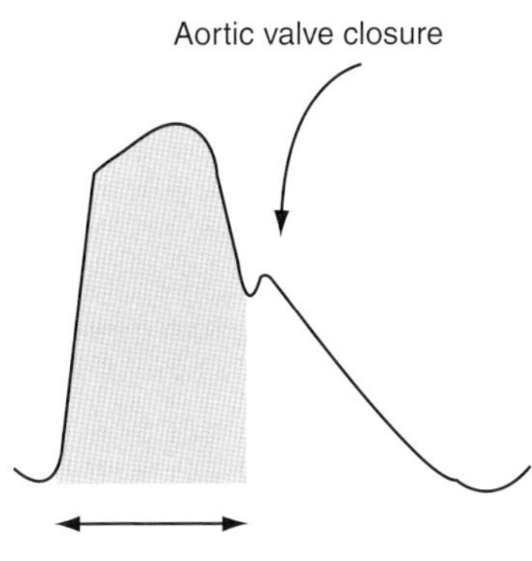

Fig. 7.1 The normal arterial pressure waveform with the shaded area representing the ejection phase.

Allen's test

Before attempting radial artery cannulation it is recommended to perform a modified Allen's test to check for collateral supply between the radial and ulnar arteries. Both the radial and ulnar arteries are compressed at the wrist and the patient is asked to clench and make a fist as tightly as possible and then unclench and open the hand. The pressure will occlude both arteries and causes blanching of the hand. With the pressure maintained over the radial artery, the pressure over the ulnar artery is released and the time taken for the colour of the palm to return to normal is noted. The test is repeated, this time with the pressure maintained over the ulnar artery. Normally colour of the palm should return to normal in less than 5–10 sec, and if it takes longer this indicates poor collateral supply between the radial and the ulnar arteries and cannulation of these arteries should be avoided.

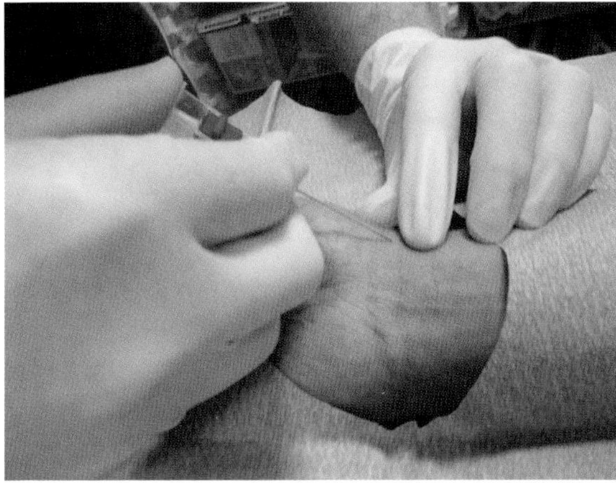

Fig. 7.2 Insertion of arterial cannula by flowswitch technique.

Techniques for radial artery cannulation

A number of arterial cannulae are commercially available which can be categorized as either catheter-over-needle technique or catheter-over-guidewire (Seldinger's) technique. An ideal arterial cannula should be short, parallel sided and made of Teflon to minimize arterial thrombosis as one of the complications from invasive arterial cannulation.

Catheter-over-needle technique

- The hand should be kept supine with wrist extended.
- Under strict aseptic conditions, radial artery is palpated and the skin over artery is infiltrated with 0.5 ml of 2% lignocaine.
- The needle is angled at 45° to the skin and inserted over the arterial pulsation and directed towards the pulsation (Fig. 7.2).
- Upon flashback, catheter is advanced by a couple of millimetres and then the needle is withdrawn and the cannula slowly withdrawn after that till flashback occurs again and then the cannula is guided in the artery (transfixation technique).
- The cannula should be sutured in place to prevent it from being dislodged.

Seldinger technique

- The hand should be kept supine with wrist extended.
- Under strict aseptic conditions, radial artery is palpated and the skin over artery is infiltrated with 0.5 ml of 2% lignocaine.
- The needle is angled at 45° to the skin and inserted over the arterial pulsation and directed towards the pulsation (Fig. 7.3).

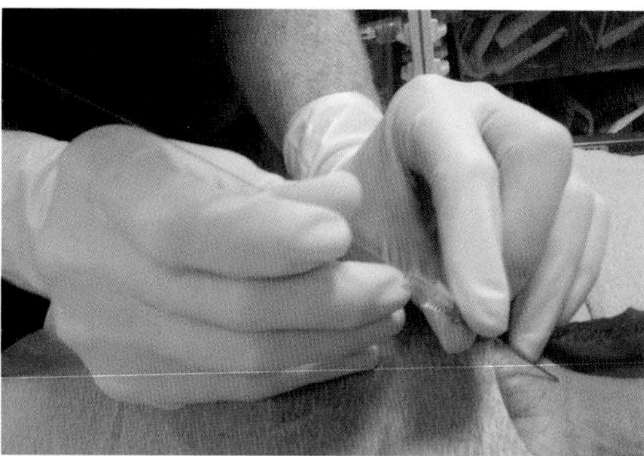

Fig. 7.3 Insertion of arterial cannula by Seldinger technique.

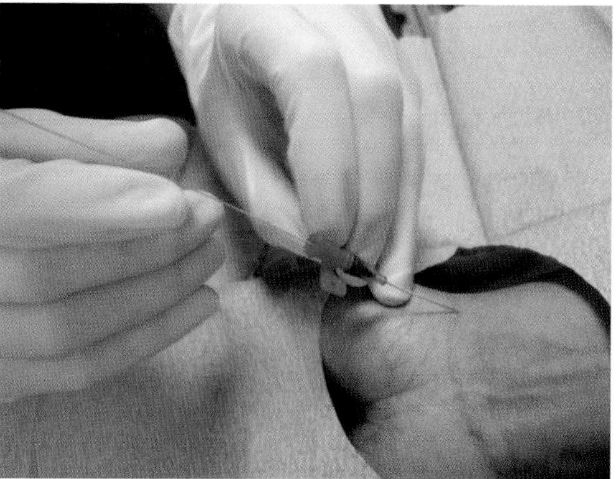

Fig. 7.4 Once flashback is seen in hub of needle, guidewire is threaded, needle removed and cannula threaded over guidewire.

- On hitting the artery, pulsatile flow of blood will be noticed; insert the guidewire through needle and remove the needle leaving the guidewire in the artery (Fig. 7.4).
- Railroad the cannula over the guidewire, and once it is in remove the guidewire, leaving the cannula in the artery.
- The cannula should be sutured in place to prevent it from being dislodged and connected to the blood pressure monitoring system.

Components of the invasive blood pressure monitoring system

Pressure tubing – a fluid-filled tubing system, connecting the cannula to the transducer. Ideally it should be short and stiff to minimize resonance.

Disposable pressure transducer – it is used to convert patient's pressure signal to electrical signal. There are four resistors connected as a Wheatstone bridge. It should be placed at the level of the right atrium at midaxillary line.

Flush device and continuous flush solution – saline is pressurized at 100 mmHg above the systolic pressure and flows at 3–4 ml/h to continuously flush the tubing and the cannula and prevent clot formation.

Monitor – has amplifier, to amplify the size of the signal to display the arterial pressure trace.

Calibration and damping

Once the artery is cannulated and the cannula is secured in place, it should be connected to the monitoring system. Once connected, the transducer system needs to be calibrated to obtain an accurate blood pressure reading. Zero calibration causes the elimination of the effect of atmospheric pressure on the measured pressure and should be done with the transducer at the level of the right atrium. At times the measured trace can be affected by damping. Damping is produced by air bubbles, clots, catheter kinking, stopcocks, and long, narrow, compliant tubing. Overdamped trace results in under-reading of systolic pressure and over-reading of diastolic pressure and underdamping causes the opposite effect. In both the situations the mean arterial pressure remains accurate (Fig. 7.5).

Complications of invasive blood pressure monitoring

- Haemorrhage and haematoma
- Thrombosis and ischaemia
- Embolism
- Infection
- Aneurysm and AV fistula
- Accidental injection of drugs.

Central venous pressure monitoring

Central venous pressure monitoring measures pressure in the great veins of the thorax usually the superior vena cava and the right atrium. It involves introducing a catheter into a vein so that the tip of the catheter lies at the junction of the superior vena cava and the right atrium. Usually it is catheterized using percutaneous technique but rarely surgical exposure 'venous cut down' may be required.

Cannulation sites

Internal jugular is the most commonly used vein. The other veins that can be cannulated are subclavian, antecubital and the femoral vein. In 2002, National Institute for Clinical Excellence (NICE) recommended the use of two-dimensional (2-D) imaging ultrasound guidance as the preferred method for insertion of central venous catheters into the internal jugular vein (IJV) in adults and children in elective situations.

Advantages of central venous catheterization

- Monitoring of central venous pressure
- Acts as a guide for fluid therapy
- Administration of drugs such as inotropes, which requires a big vein
- Total parenteral nutrition (TPN)
- Blood sampling for mixed venous saturation
- Insertion of transcutaneous pacing leads.

Changes in central venous pressure

Table 7.2 summarizes these changes

Technique for insertion of central venous catheter in internal jugular vein

There are many cannulation techniques but it is catheter-over-guidewire (Seldinger's) technique that is employed most frequently. Usually the right internal jugular vein is cannulated as it is technically easier for the right-handed operator. The thoracic duct lies on the left side and there is potential for causing chylothorax if left internal jugular is cannulated.

- Patient is usually placed supine in 15–30° Trendelenburg position to increase distension of the internal jugular vein. The head down position will also minimize risk of entraining air and causing air embolism.
- ECG, blood pressure and oxygen saturation should be continuously monitored throughout the procedure.
- Flush the central venous catheter with sterile saline solution.
- Under strict aseptic conditions, the two heads of the sternomastoid muscle and clavicle are palpated. Feel for carotid artery pulsation; internal jugular vein lies just lateral to it. Two-dimensional (2-D) imaging ultrasound should be used whenever possible to locate the artery and the vein.
- Once the vein is located, skin over it is infiltrated with 0.5 ml of 2% lignocaine.
- Under direct ultrasound guidance the needle attached to a syringe should be advanced aiming

Table 7.2 Central venous pressure can be increased or decreased as a result of various conditions

Increased by
Raised intrathoracic pressure: intermittent positive pressure ventilation, coughing
Impaired cardiac function: cardiac failure, cardiac tamponade
Circulatory overload
Superior vena caval obstruction
Decreased by
Reduced venous return: hypovolaemia

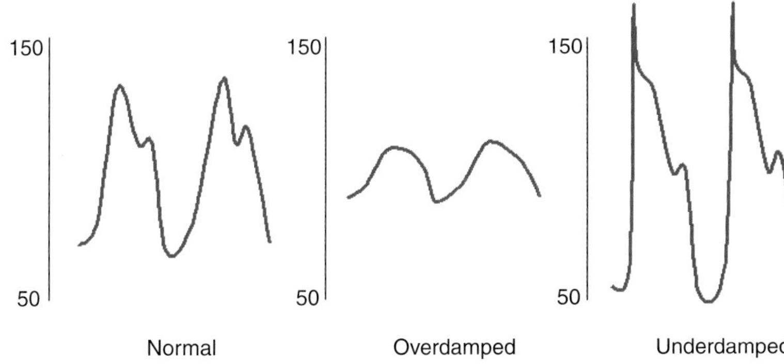

Fig. 7.5 Schematic diagram of arterial trace and effects of damping.

towards the ipsilateral nipple at an angle of 45° to the skin (Fig. 7.6).

- When in the vein, dark and non-pulsatile blood is aspirated.
- Disconnect the syringe and the insert the guidewire. It is important to monitor the ECG for cardiac arrhythmias.
- Remove the needle, leaving the guidewire in the vein.
- After dilating the insertion site a central venous catheter is railroaded over the guidewire, and ECG monitored for cardiac arrhythmias.
- The catheter should be sutured in place to prevent it from being dislodged and connected to the central venous pressure monitoring system. The components of this system are very similar to those of the invasive arterial blood pressure monitoring system.
- Correct location should be confirmed with a chest radiograph.

Complications of central venous cannulation

- Arterial cannulation
- Embolism – air or thrombus
- Pneumothorax, hydrothorax, haemothorax
- Cardiac perforation
- Cardiac tamponade
- Injury to surrounding structures – nerves and artery
- Infection.

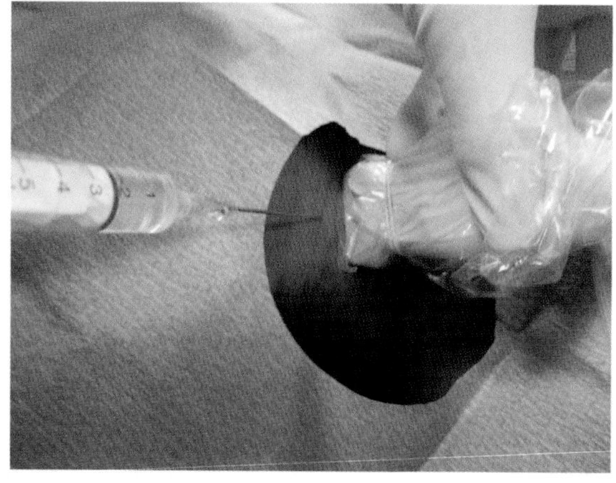

Fig. 7.6 Insertion of central venous catheter using ultrasonography.

Cardiac output monitoring

Clinical parameters may be used to determine cardiac output. Poor cerebral perfusion leads to agitation and confusion. A reduction in renal perfusion will lead to decreased urine output and subsequently to anuria. Skin perfusion is a clinically useful sign and can be determined using the capillary refill time. Progressive prolongation of the capillary refill time is seen with reduced cardiac output. As it is difficult to quantify cardiac output using the clinical parameters it is not a very objective method.

It is widely accepted that cardiac output measurement is a useful adjunct in the resuscitation of critically ill patients. There are many invasive and non-invasive methods available to monitor cardiac output. Pulmonary artery (PA) catheter is inserted via a central venous catheter sheath. The PA catheter is then 'floated' so that the tip of pulmonary artery catheter is correctly wedged in the artery by the guide of changes in pressures from right atrium, right ventricle, pulmonary artery and pulmonary capillary wedge pressure (Fig. 7.7). As this technique is invasive and can cause potential risks to the patient, other less invasive methods are gaining acceptance (Table 7.3). However, it is still widely accepted as the gold standard.

Thermodilution technique

Intermittent thermodilution technique

- 5–10 ml of cold saline is injected rapidly and smoothly through the proximal port of PA catheter

Table 7.3 Commonly used techniques for cardiac output monitoring

	Use of PA catheter	Use of CVP	Use of arterial line	Invasive
PA catheter	Yes	Yes	No	Yes
Lithium dilution	No	No	Yes	Yes
PiCCO	No	Yes	Yes	Yes
PulseCO	No	No	Yes	Yes
Trans-oesophageal Doppler	No	No	No	Yes
Trans-oesophageal echocardiography (TOE)	No	No	No	Yes
NICO (Non-invasive cardiac output)	No	No	No	No

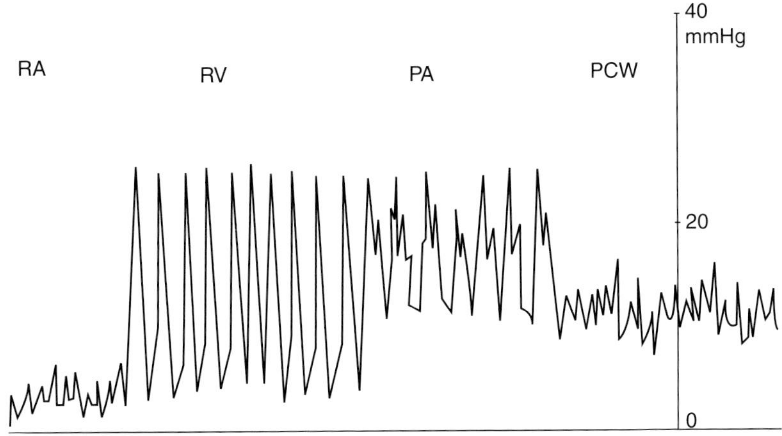

Fig. 7.7 Pressure tracing seen as the balloon of the pulmonary artery flotation catheter floats through different structures. RA, right atrium; RV, right ventricle; PA, pulmonary artery; PCW, pulmonary capillary wedge pressure.

in the right atrium and the temperature change of blood induced by the cold saline is measured with a thermistor at the catheter tip.

- The temperature change is inversely proportional to the cardiac output. Temperature drop is plotted against time and this produces thermodilution curve. Cardiac output is determined by a computer program using the area under the curve and the Stewart Hamilton equation.
- An average of at least three measurements is used.

Continuous thermodilution technique

This technique employs a different PA catheter. It has a thermal filament which heats up every 30–60 sec and adds heat to the blood and the temperature change is measured by a thermistor near the tip. Temperature change is plotted against time and this produces a thermodilution curve, and cardiac output is determined by a computer program using the area under this curve.

Causes of inaccuracies while using the thermodilution technique

- Presence of a cardiac shunt may cause differences in right and left ventricular output.
- Tricuspid or pulmonary valve regurgitation can cause underestimation of cardiac output.
- Intermittent positive pressure ventilation produces beat-to-beat variations in right ventricular stroke volume during the respiratory cycle.

Dye dilution technique

This technique is done using a PA catheter and an intra-arterial line.

- A known quantity of indocyanine green is injected in the PA and its appearance in the arterial circulation can be measured by analysing the arterial blood using a photoelectric spectrometer.
- Cardiac output is then calculated using the area under the curve and the injected dose.

Lithium dilution technique

A small dose of lithium chloride (0.15–0.3 mmol) is injected via a central or peripheral venous line.

- The resulting arterial lithium concentration–time curve is recorded by withdrawing blood past a lithium sensor attached to the patient's existing arterial line.
- Cardiac output can then be calculated using the area under the concentration–time curve.

Trans-oesophageal Doppler

Doppler ultrasound can provide a non-invasive, continuous, real-time quantification of cardiac output. The oesophagus is in close anatomical proximity to the aorta, hence signal interference from bone, soft tissue and lung is minimized.

- The Doppler probe needs to be inserted either orally or nasally into the oesophagus.
- Measurements are made with the Doppler principle: there is an increase in observed

frequency of a signal when the signal source approaches the observer and decrease when the source moves away.

- Patient's biometric data (age, sex and height) is entered and aortic cross-sectional area is estimated from nomogram.
- Changes in velocity in the descending thoracic aorta are measured. When the cross-sectional area of the aorta is known, stroke volume can be derived from the flow velocity, ejection time and aortic cross-sectional area.
- Cardiac output can be derived from the stroke volume and heart rate.
- Use is relatively contraindicated in patients with oesophageal strictures, oesophageal operations, oesophageal varices and caustic ingestion. Valvular abnormalities may give false readings.
- As measurements are made in the descending aorta, it represents only 70% of the total cardiac output.
- A real-time waveform is displayed on the monitor (Fig. 7.8). Additionally, an audible sound of the Doppler frequency shift spectrum is produced by red blood cells moving in the path of the ultrasound beam.

Fick's principle

According to Fick's principle blood flow to an organ can be calculated using a marker substance, if the amount of a marker substance taken up by the organ per unit time and the concentration of marker substance in arterial blood supplying the organ and in venous blood leaving the organ is known.

By applying the formula, the blood flow through the heart or cardiac output can be calculated:

$$CO = \frac{VO_2}{C_a - C_v}$$

where CO is cardiac output, VO_2 is amount of oxygen consumed, C_a is arterial oxygen content and C_v is venous oxygen content. This requires measurement of mixed venous and arterial blood samples.

The non-invasive cardiac output (NICO) system is a non-invasive device that applies Fick's principle to CO_2. The system uses partial CO_2 breathing to determine cardiac output non-invasively. It measures CO_2 elimination continuously. Cardiac output is proportional to the change in CO_2 elimination divided by the change in end-tidal CO_2 resulting from a short rebreathing period. The system bases its calculation on effective lung perfusion, i.e. that part of the pulmonary capillary blood flow that has passed through the ventilated parts of the lung. The effects of unknown ventilation/perfusion inequality in critical care patients may introduce inaccuracies.

Arterial pulse contour analysis

This technique combines the principles of transpulmonary thermodilution and arterial pulse contour analysis. It involves injection of a single bolus of ice-cold saline through a central venous catheter (central venous access is not required in case of PulseCO) and its modification by a special arterial cannula.

At present there are three pulse contour analytical methods available commercially:

(1) PiCCO calibrated by transpulmonary thermodilution

(2) PulseCO by lithium dilution

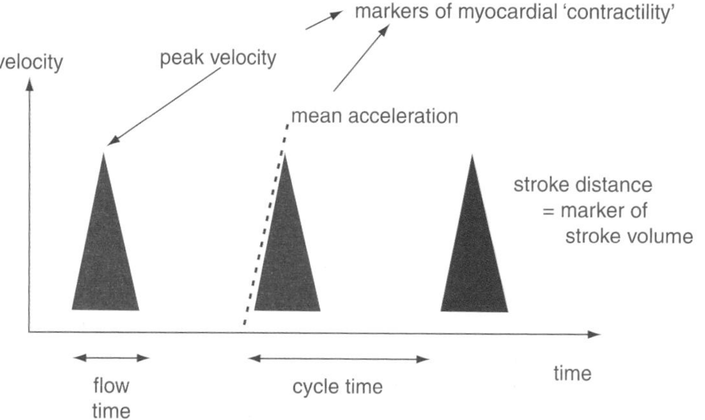

Fig. 7.8 Sample waveform from oesophageal Doppler.

(3) Modelflow by the mean of multiple conventional thermodilution measurements equally spread over the ventilatory cycle.

Pulse-induced contour cardiac output

The pulse-induced contour cardiac output (PiCCO) method uses a central venous line with a temperature sensor on the distal lumen and a thermodilution sensor arterial catheter, placed in either the femoral or brachial artery. A thermodilution curve is produced when cold saline is injected through the arterial line.

The system uses patient's height and weight and computes left ventricular stroke volume by measuring the area under the systolic part of the waveform from the end of diastole to the end of the ejection phase and dividing the area by the aortic impedance.

Formulae are then applied and give estimations of preload index such as intrathoracic blood volume and lung oedema index as extravascular lung water, and stroke volume variation as fluid responsiveness indicators (Table 7.4). Intrathoracic blood volume seems to be a good preload index but the results reported in literature are not homogeneous in all its applications.

Table 7.4 Table illustrating parameters measured by the PiCCO system

Parameter/ indices	Normal values	Notes
Intrathoracic blood volume index	850–1000 ml/m^2	<850 underfilled >1000 adequate/overfilled
Extravascular lung water index	3.0–7.0 ml/kg	>7.0 ml/kg indicates pulmonary oedema
Cardiac function index	4.5–6.5 l/min	Measured independently of preload Reflects myocardial contractile function <4.5 indicates poor myocardial contractility
Stroke volume variation	10–15%	Measured as the mean difference between the highest and lowest stroke volume over the last 30 sec Only accurately measured in ventilated patients Inaccurate in arrhythmias <10% adequate/overfilled >15% dehydrated/underfilled

Intrathoracic blood volume

Intrathoracic blood volume (ITBV) consists of the global end diastolic volume (GEDV), the volume of blood within the heart plus the pulmonary blood volume. There are three volumes within the thorax: the intrathoracic blood volume, the intrathoracic gas volume and the extravascular lung water. Due to limited expansion of the thorax, these volumes interact and change proportionally to each other. ITBV is a volumetric measurement of cardiac preload (ventricular end diastolic pressure), and is a sensitive indicator of the circulatory blood volume in mechanically ventilated patients. Studies have shown that changes in intrathoracic blood volume correlate well with changes in cardiac output and can be used as a surrogate for patient's fluid status.

Extravascular lung water

The water content in the lungs increases in left heart failure, pneumonia, sepsis and burns. Extravascular lung water (EVLW) is used to determine pulmonary function and a guide to fluid resuscitation in shock. Studies have suggested that resolution of pulmonary oedema may be more rapid when EVLW is used as a therapeutic guide. Prognosis based on EVLW has indicated a higher risk of mortality with EVLW of greater than 14 ml/kg.

Transoesophageal echocardiography

Quantifying cardiac output with transoesophageal echocardiography (TOE) involves an accurate measurement of the velocity of blood flow across a specific valve with the aid of Doppler. The area under the flow velocity curve is calculated and it represents a specific distance along which the column of blood is projected during one cardiac cycle. This measurement of the length of blood in the ascending aorta in unit time and multiplying by the cross-sectional area of the aorta can give stroke volume from which cardiac output can be derived. In addition it also allows for the assessment of ventricular function, wall motion abnormalities during myocardial ischaemia, cardiac anatomy and valve function.

In experienced hands, TOE can give valuable haemodynamic information and evaluate the ejection fraction and mechanical movement of the heart as a pump. TOE can also aid diagnosis by identifying the presence of vegetations in infective endocarditis or pericardial effusions in pericarditis.

Other methods of cardiac output monitoring

- Thoracic electrical bioimpedance
- Induction cardiography
- Electromagnetic flow measurement.

Common measured haemodynamic variables

Cardiac output (CO)	HR × SV/1000 = 4–8 l/min
Cardiac index (CI)	CO/BSA = 2.5–4 l/min/m^2
Stroke volume (SV)	CO/HR × 1000 = 60–100 ml/beat
Stroke volume index (SVI)	CI/HR × 1000 = 33–47 ml/m^2/beat
Systemic vascular resistance (SVR)	80 × (MAP–RAP)/CO = 1000–1500 dyne s/cm^3
Systemic vascular resistance index (SVRI)	80 × (MAP–RAP)/CI = 1970–2390 dyne s/cm^3/m^2
Pulmonary vascular resistance (PVR)	80 × (MPAP–PAWP)/CO = <250 dyne s/cm^3
Pulmonary vascular resistance index (PVRI)	80 × (MPAP–PAWP)/CI = 255–285 dyne s/cm^3/m^2

HR = heart rate
BSA = body surface area
RAP = right atrial pressure
PAWP= pulmonary artery wedge pressure
MPAP= mean pulmonary artery pressure

Key points

- Haemodynamic monitoring is most informative when it is used to supplement clinical judgement.
- It may be more beneficial to look at the trend of the variable being measured rather than a single value.
- One should always ensure full asepsis when inserting an invasive monitoring device into vulnerable patients.
- Good anatomical knowledge and sound technique will help in reducing some of the complications from invasive monitoring devices.

Further reading

- Allsager CM, Swanevelder J (2003) Measuring cardiac output. *Br. J. Anaesth.* **3**: 15–19.
- Association of Anaesthetists of Great Britain and Ireland (2007) *Recommendations for Standards of Monitoring during Anaesthesia and Recovery*. London: The Association of Anaesthetists of Great Britain and Ireland.
- Elliott TS, Faroqui MH, Armstrong RF (1994) Guidelines for good practice in central venous catheterization. *J. Hosp. Infect.* **28**: 163–76.
- Fletcher S (2005) Catheter-related bloodstream infection. *Contin. Educ. Anaesth. Crit. Care Pain* **5**: 49–51.
- Harvey S, Harrison DA, Singer M *et al.* (2005) Assessment of the clinical effectiveness of pulmonary artery catheters in management of patients in intensive care (PAC-Man): a randomised controlled trial. *Lancet* **366**: 472–7.
- Inweregbu K, Dave J, Pittard A (2005) Nosocomial infections. *Contin. Educ. Anaesth. Crit. Care Pain* **5**: 14–17.
- Morgan GE, Mikhail MS, Murray M (2002) Patient monitors. In *Clinical Anesthesiology*, 3rd edn. New York: McGraw Hill, pp. 86–125.
- National Institute for Clinical Excellence (2002) *Guidance on the Use of Ultrasound Locating Devices for Placing Central Venous Catheters*, Technology appraisal No. 49. London: NICE.
- Pratt RJ, Pellow CM, Wilson JA *et al.* (2007) Epic2: national evidence-based guidelines for preventing healthcare-associated infections in NHS hospitals in England. *J. Hosp. Infect.* **65**(S): S1–S64.
- Singer M, Clarke J, Bennett ED (1989) Continuous monitoring by esophageal Doppler. *Crit. Care Med.* **17**: 447–52.

Critical care imaging modalities

Frances Aitchison

All critically ill patients will have imaging tests during their time in the intensive care unit. For some patients this will be a simple procedure, such as a plain chest X-ray, however for others more complex investigations such as magnetic resonance imaging will be required.

General considerations

- It is always important that the reason for the imaging request is clearly stated on the referral form. This will allow the imaging department to ensure that the most appropriate imaging technique is used, particularly in patients with multiple pathologies where several imaging modalities may be needed. It may well be helpful to discuss the clinical problem with a radiologist. Advice is available from referral guidelines published by the UK Royal College of Radiologists 2007 (see Further reading).
- Some imaging tests are limited by considerations of patient and staff *safety* and thought must be given to the patient's clinical condition when planning investigations. For more complex examinations, such as computed tomography (CT), the imaging equipment cannot be brought to the intensive care unit and the patient will require to be moved. Up to 70% of critically ill patients undergoing intra-hospital transfer will have an unexpected adverse event (see Further reading). These adverse events include both equipment malfunction and patient instability such as hypotension, arrhythmia, increased intracranial pressure, hypocapnia and hypercapnia and significant hypoxaemia. The establishment of, and adherence to, guidelines on personnel, equipment and monitoring during intra-hospital transfer is of major importance for each critical care unit.
- Particularly in CT, it must be remembered that there are also significant risks to the critically ill patient associated with the radiation dose and the use of potentially nephrotoxic iodinated intravenous contrast.
- Most hospitals in the UK now use a picture archiving and communication system (PACS) to store X-ray, CT, magnetic resonance imaging (MRI) and ultrasound examination images directly onto the hospital computer system. PACS systems are used in conjunction with digital or computed radiography (DR or CR) equipment for plain X-rays. These have replaced the use of conventional X-ray film cassettes with an X-ray system involving reusable photo-stimulable plates. There are many advantages – the examinations should always be immediately available, are stored in chronological order and have wider latitude of exposure since the image brightness and contrast can be manipulated on the screen during viewing. This has reduced the number of repeat films and is particularly helpful for critically ill patients. However, the PACS itself and the high-resolution monitors required for viewing are expensive.

There follows a general description of each of the main imaging modalities and more detailed description of their use for particular clinical problems.

X-ray imaging

Basic principles

- All X-ray imaging involves the use of an X-ray *source* to produce a beam of radiation which is passed through the patient and a *detector* to produce an image. The detector may be a cassette

Core Topics in Critical Care Medicine, eds. Fang Gao Smith and Joyce Yeung. Published by Cambridge University Press.

placed next to the patient or may be incorporated into a CT scanner gantry which rotates around the patient.

- Modern CT scanners use a multislice helical technique, which has reduced scan times considerably. This is achieved using a row of parallel X-ray sources (numbering up to 64 in current clinical practice) with an identical number of detectors arranged on the opposite side of a large ring which rotates continuously around the patient during the scan. This allows multiple CT slices to be taken simultaneously. Computers are used to process information derived from the amount of radiation absorbed by the body at each point of the rotation and calculate the density of each of many thousand tiny squares (pixels) within the image. This forms a 2-D axial picture of the area scanned.
- A 64-slice CT scanner can image the entire chest in less than 5 sec and can produce very high quality three-dimensional reconstructions, subtracted images of vessels or 'fly through' images of hollow structures such as colon.
- Each X-ray examination involves a *radiation dose* to the patient which can be measured as the absorbed dose for each organ (in units of milliGray, mGy) or as the effective dose to the patient (in units of millisieverts, mSv). The effective dose is derived from the sum of the absorbed doses for all the organs and tissues irradiated.
- For each organ or tissue:

$$\text{equivalent dose (mSv)} = \text{absorbed dose (mGy)} \times \text{radiation weighting factor } W_R$$

- For the whole patient:

$$\text{effective dose (mSv)} = \sum \text{equivalent dose (mSv)} \times \text{tissue weighting factor } W_T \text{ for all the organs and tissues irradiated}$$

Table 8.1 shows some examples of radiation doses from commonly performed examinations.

- It should be remembered that the dose from a portable, antero-posterior (AP) X-ray is more variable and slightly higher than that from a standard, postero-anterior (PA) X-ray.

Table 8.1 Examples of radiation doses from commonly performed examinations

Diagnostic procedure	Typical effective dose (mSv)	Equivalent number of chest X-rays	Approximate equivalent period of UK natural background radiation
Postero-anterior chest	0.02	1	3 days
Lumbar spine	1.0	50	5 months
CT brain	2	100	10 months
CT abdomen	10	500	4.5 years

- Immediately after striking the patient, some of the X-rays will scatter around the patient in all directions. Hospital staff should therefore stand as far away as possible from the patient during the X-ray exposure. Staff should not remain with patients in the CT scanner during the radiation exposure.
- Dense objects such as metal wires/leads or dense bone within the scan area will alter the absorption of radiation and cause artefact. For most CT scans of chest and abdomen, patients are imaged with their arms elevated above their heads to reduce streak artefact. This is not possible in critically ill patients and consequently there may be some reduction in image quality which can be minimized by ensuring that, wherever possible, all moveable objects such as equipment leads are out of the region scanned.

Chest X-ray

The chest X-ray is the most commonly performed imaging investigation in the critical care unit and is used to assess cardiopulmonary abnormalities, the position of lines, tubes and catheters and possible complications of their insertion.

- It is not necessary for every patient to have daily chest X-rays in the critical care unit. However, all patients should have a chest X-ray on arrival in the unit, after any invasive procedures such as endotracheal intubation, central vascular catheter placement or thoracocentesis and daily chest films should always be routinely performed for ventilated patients with haemodynamic or respiratory instability.

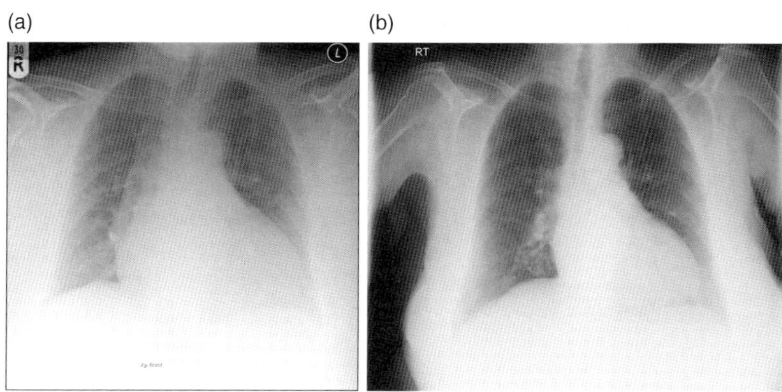

Fig. 8.1 Demonstration of (a) AP and (b) PA chest film taken on the same patient almost simultaneously.

- It is mandatory that the correct position of naso- or orogastric feeding tubes is confirmed radiologically before enteral feeding commences.

Interpretation of antero-posterior (AP) chest X-ray

The critically ill patient cannot stand erect with their anterior chest abutting the cassette and breath held in deep inspiration as required for a Postero-Anterior (PA) standard departmental film. Critical care chest X-ray films are taken as supine, AP projections with the cassette placed behind the patient and the X-ray source positioned anteriorly close to the patient. There are important consequences for interpretation of an AP chest film.

Heart and pulmonary vessels

The heart is further from the cassette than for standard projections and will appear artificially enlarged (Fig. 8.1.) In addition, the central pulmonary vessels appear larger on a supine film because of augmented venous filling.

Air or fluid in the pleural space

On a supine chest X-ray a pneumothorax or pleural effusion is much harder to see. Air in the pleural space will lie anteriorly. Only when a huge amount of air is present will the lung edge will be perceptible separate from the lateral chest wall. In a moderate sized pneumothorax a generalized reduction in density over the affected hemithorax or deepening of the ipsilateral costophrenic or cardiophrenic recess ('deep sulcus sign') will be the only abnormality visible (Fig. 8.2). Pleural fluid will accumulate in the dependent part of the chest posteriorly and when sufficient fluid

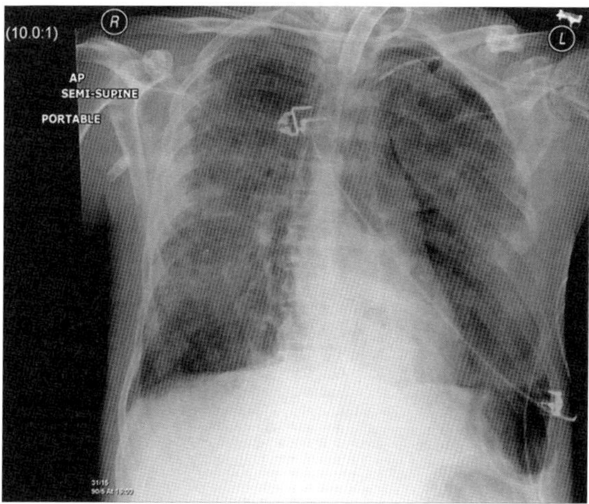

Fig. 8.2 Demonstration of pneumothorax on supine chest X-ray. The left costophrenic sulcus is deepened and of reduced density as a result of air in the pleural space. There is a tracheostomy and a left subclavian venous line (which is malpositioned, the tip being too close to the skin surface).

accumulates will cause diffuse increase in density of the hemithorax (Fig. 8.3).

Lung volume and density

When the film is not taken at full inspiration the lungs will be of smaller volume and diffusely increased density.

Assessment of tubes and catheters

Assessment of tubes and catheters should be done systematically. The following should be assessed for presence and position (Fig. 8.4):

- Endotracheal tube – lower margin should be at least 5 cm above the carina with head in neutral position.

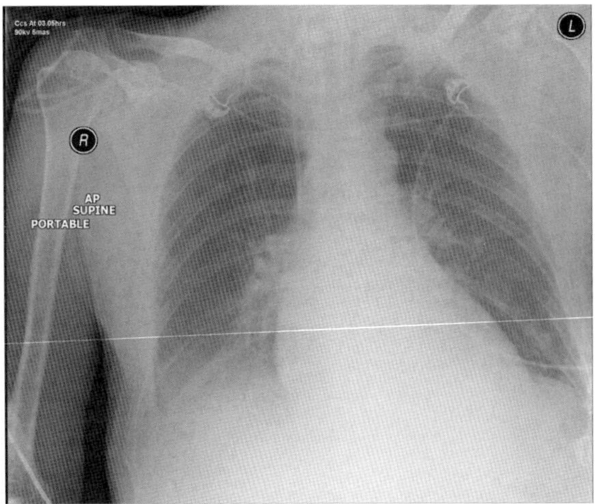

Fig. 8.3 Bilateral large pleural effusions on erect chest X-ray. There is a diffuse increase in density in the lower chest and loss of definition of the diaphragm on each side. Note the patient has a long-term tracheostomy in situ.

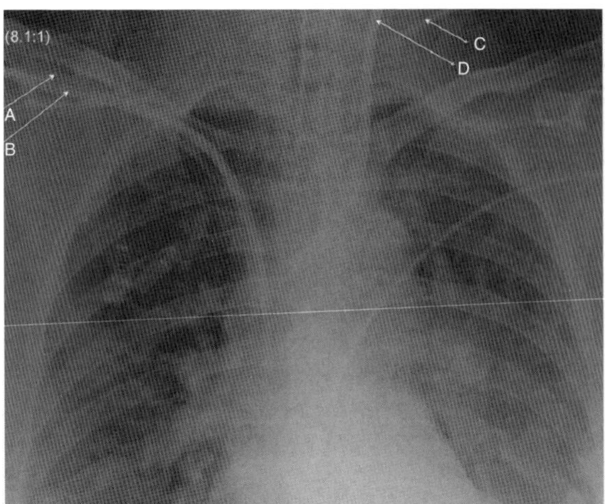

Fig. 8.5 Right subclavian and left internal jugular central venous lines (A and C) and haemofiltration lines (B and D) . All are satisfactorily positioned. There is also an endotracheal tube and nasogastric tube.

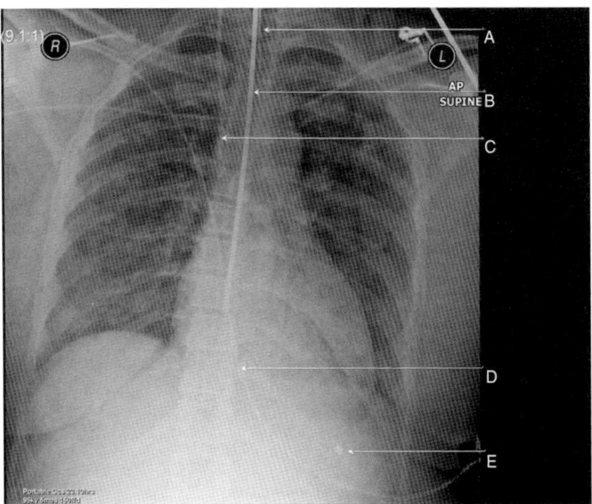

Fig. 8.4 Satisfactory positions for: A, endotracheal tube; B, oesophageal Doppler probe; C, right internal jugular venous line; D, ECG lead wire; E, tip of nasogastric tube.

- Tracheostomy tube – the T3 vertebral level defines the ideal position of the tube.
- Central venous catheters – the ideal position of the catheter tip is within the superior vena cava. Incorrect positioning of central venous catheters occurs in up to 10% of patients (see Further reading). Cannulation of the right subclavian vein is associated with the highest risk of malposition. Haemofiltration lines are of larger calibre than standard central venous lines (Fig. 8.5).
- Pulmonary artery (Swan Ganz) catheter – with an uninflated balloon, the tip of the catheter should be in the right or left pulmonary artery and within 5 cm of the midline on chest X-ray (Fig. 8.6).
- Pacing wires – chest X-rays should be checked for pneumothorax and the tip of the wire should overlie the apex of the right ventricle (Fig. 8.7).
- Chest drains – the drain should be placed postero-inferiorly for pleural fluid collections and antero-superiorly for pneumothorax. The side holes of the drain must be within the pleural space (Fig. 8.8).
- Intra-aortic balloon – the balloon should lie in the descending aorta with its tip just above the left hilum on the chest X-ray.
- Enteral tubes – the tip of nasogastric or orogastric tubes should always be below the diaphragm. Many tubes do not have a radio-opaque marker along their entire length and only the last few centimetres are visible on the X-ray.
- Oesophageal Doppler probes – tip should be in mid thorax below the level of the carina.

Appearance of lungs

The appearance of the lungs should be carefully assessed on every chest X-ray. It is particularly helpful to make a comparison with any previous chest films. Following disease progression over time will allow more accurate distinction between infection and pulmonary oedema. The presence and size of any pleural

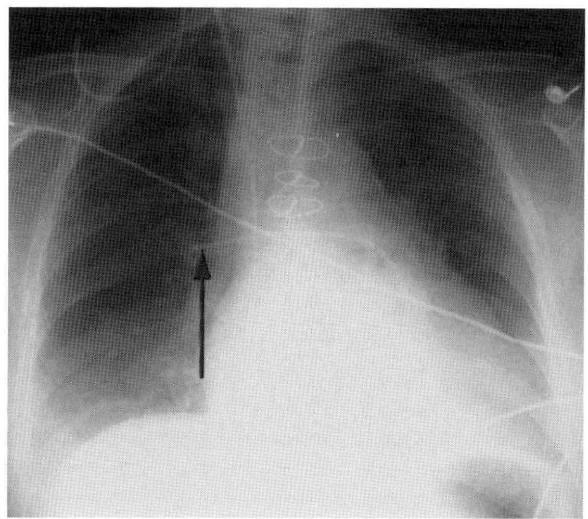

Fig. 8.6 Satisfactory position for tip of Swan Ganz catheter (arrow shows tip of catheter).

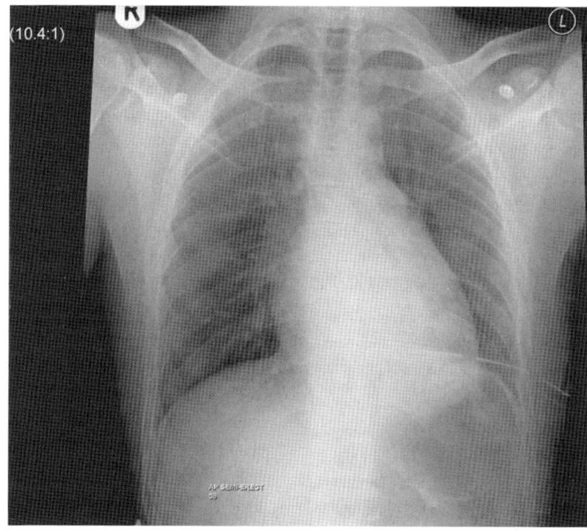

Fig. 8.8 Unsatisfactory position of left-sided chest drain with one set of side holes outside the lateral border of the ribs.

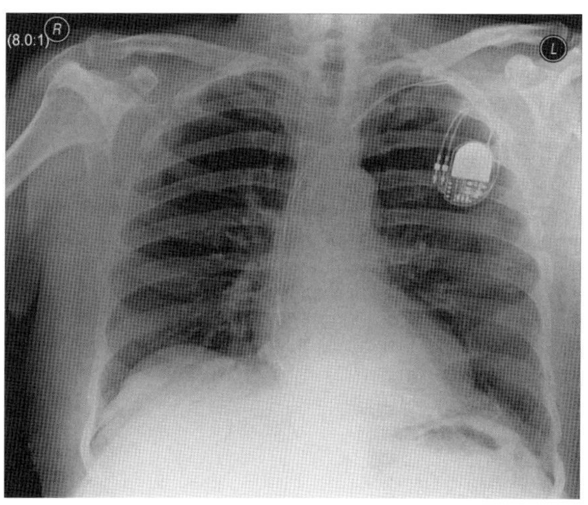

Fig. 8.7 Satisfactorily positioned dual lead permanent pacemaker with tip of the more cranial lead in right atrium and tip of more caudal lead at apex of right ventricle. Note left-sided pneumothorax as complication of insertion.

fluid collection, pneumomediastinum or pneumothorax should be documented.

Abdominal X-ray

The abdominal X-ray is useful for assessment of acute abdominal pathology. Critically ill patients are unable to have erect chest films taken; therefore if perforation of a hollow abdominal viscus is suspected evidence must be sought from abdominal X-rays. This will include the visualization of both sides of the bowel wall (Rigler's sign). Plain abdominal X-rays are used for detection of small and large bowel obstruction (Figs. 8.9 and 8.10) and are useful to demonstrate abnormal intra-abdominal opacities such as renal calculi.

CT scanning

CT scans are extremely useful in management of critically ill patients.

- Intravenous iodinated contrast is often used during CT assessment of the mediastinum, abdomen and pelvis and in CT angiography.
- Minor adverse reaction to iodinated contrast (e.g. flushing, urticaria, bronchospasm) is not uncommon. The incidence of severe reaction to modern non-ionic agents is 0.04% and very serious reaction (including death) is 0.004%. Patients most at risk are those with a history of previous contrast reaction, asthma or previous allergic reaction requiring medical treatment.
- Iodinated intravenous contrast is potentially nephrotoxic. Patients most at risk of contrast induced nephropathy are those with pre-existing renal impairment, particularly patients with GFR <30 ml/min.
- Dilute oral iodinated contrast may be used during CT of abdomen or pelvis to opacify bowel and distinguish from abnormal abdominal fluid collection or abscess. In critical care patients oral contrast may be given via a nasogastric tube.

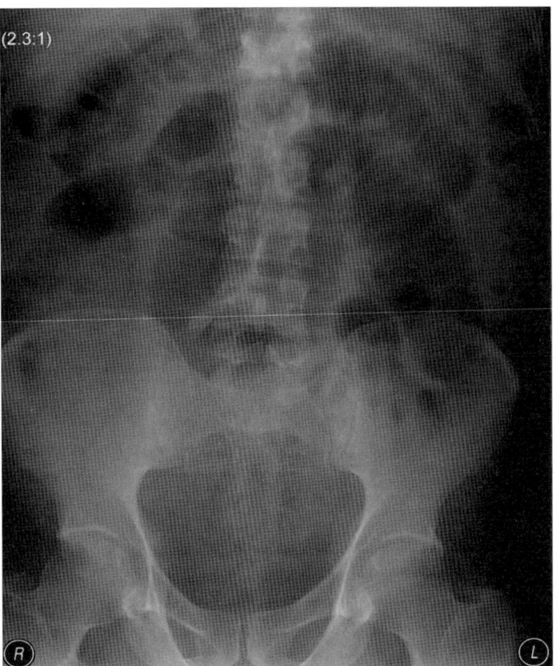

Fig. 8.9 Plain X-ray appearance of small bowel obstruction with multiple dilated loops in centre of abdomen demonstrating complete transverse mucosal folds.

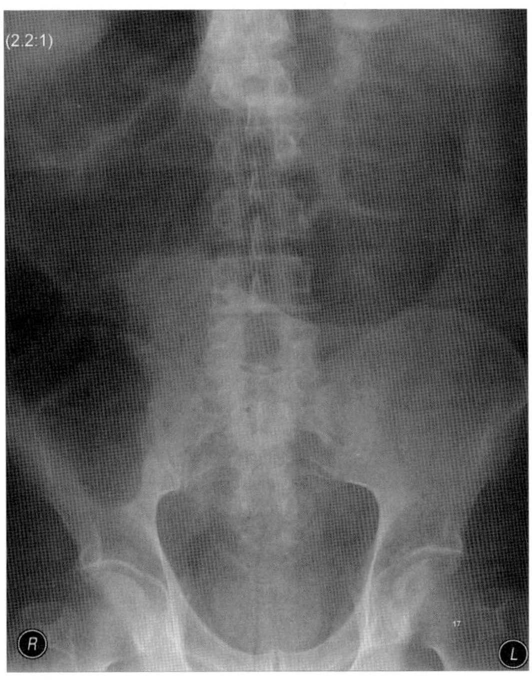

Fig. 8.10 Plain X-ray appearance of large bowel obstruction with markedly dilated loops of bowel at periphery of right and upper abdomen which have incomplete mucosal folds.

CT head

The most commonly performed CT examination in this patient group is CT head scan which is particularly useful for the detection of:

- Haemorrhage – after acute haemorrhage the area of abnormality will have the following appearance on CT relative to normal brain: 0–2 weeks, whiter (hyperdense); 2–4 weeks, same density (isodense); >4 weeks, darker (hypodense). It is important to distinguish haemorrhage with the substance of the brain itself from haemorrhage outside the brain (extra-axial bleed). Extra-axial haemorrhage can be divided into: *extradural*, egg-shaped peripheral bleed; *subdural*, more diffuse crescentic peripheral bleed (Fig. 8.11); and *subarachnoid*, widespread blood within CSF involving sulci on brain surface, basal cisterns and ventricular system (Fig. 8.12).
- Infarction: for 24–48 hours after infarction the affected brain may have normal density. Subsequently CT will demonstrate a focal area of reduced density within vascular territory affected (Fig. 8.13).
- Tumour, inflammatory disease or infection.

CT cervical spine

CT cervical spine is an increasingly commonly requested examination in trauma patients. Neck support collars and patient immobility often make plain films difficult to interpret in this group. CT cervical spine allows detailed assessment of bony structures but very limited assessment of the spinal cord itself.

Detailed guidelines on appropriate use of CT head and CT cervical spine in trauma patients can be found at www.nice.org.uk.

CT chest

CT is very useful for investigation of chest disease allowing assessment of mediastinum, lung parenchyma and chest wall. CT pulmonary angiography (CTPA) has good sensitivity and specificity for pulmonary embolic disease (Fig. 8.14).

High-resolution CT (HRCT) is performed without intravenous contrast and uses very thin slices to assess lung parenchyma. It can be used, for example, to distinguish the acute and fibrotic phases of adult respiratory distress syndrome.

CT abdomen

Critically ill patients with acute abdominal pathology are often assessed with CT for detection of bowel

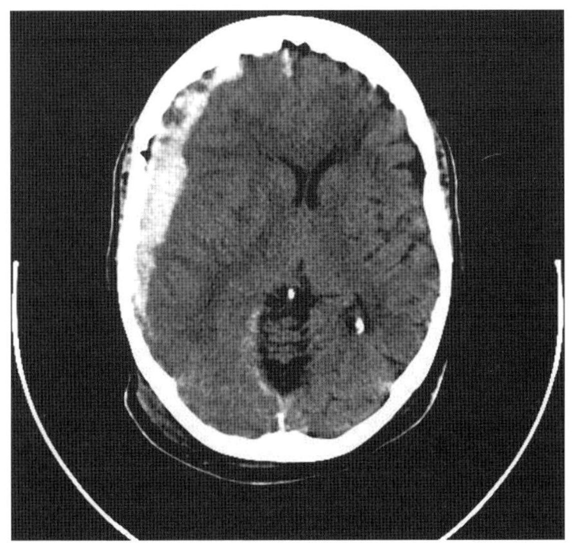

Fig. 8.11 CT demonstrating acute right-sided subdural haemorrhage.

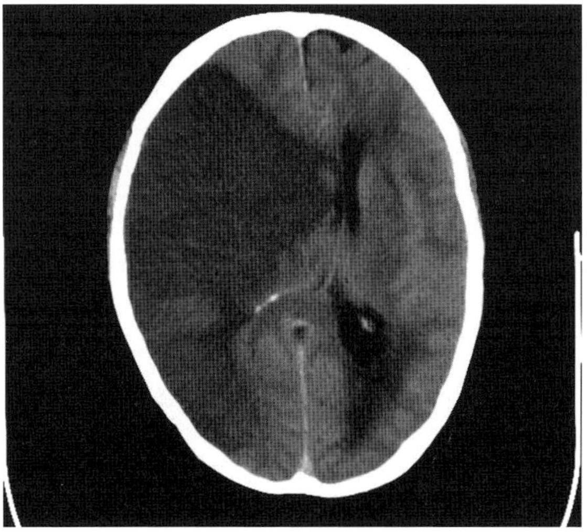

Fig. 8.13 CT demonstrating acute right middle cerebral infarct with mass effect (compression of right lateral ventricle).

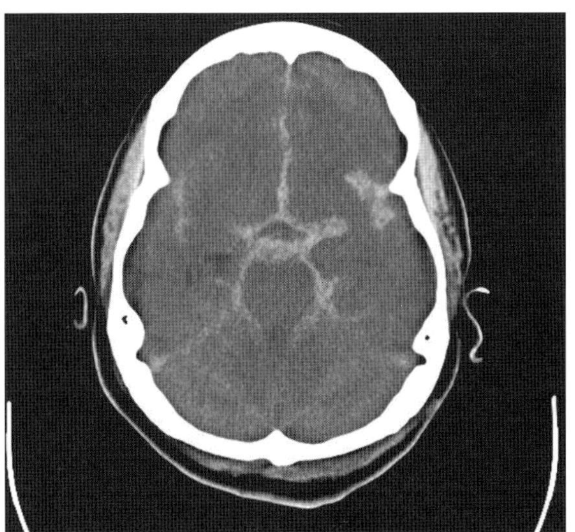

Fig. 8.12 CT demonstrating acute subarachnoid haemorrhage; hyperdense blood replaces the appearance of normal low-density CSF in the basal cisterns of the brain.

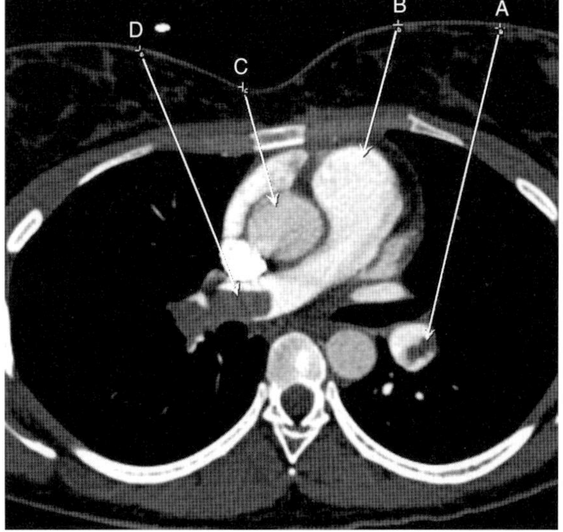

Fig. 8.14 CT pulmonary angiogram demonstrating bilateral pulmonary artery thrombus. A, clot in left main pulmonary artery; B, main pulmonary artery; C, aorta; D, clot in right main pulmonary artery.

perforation or obstruction, vascular pathology or abscess/collection.

Magnetic resonance imaging

Basic principles

Magnetic resonance imaging (MRI) uses radio waves and magnetic fields to produce extremely detailed images, particularly of soft tissues. MRI is more sensitive than CT for subtle pathology and may be the only imaging modality that can provide essential information about the posterior fossa of brain or the spinal cord (Fig. 8.15).

For the production of MRI images the patient lies in the bore of large magnet. Protons within hydrogen nuclei in the patient which would usually be spinning randomly become aligned with the magnetic field.

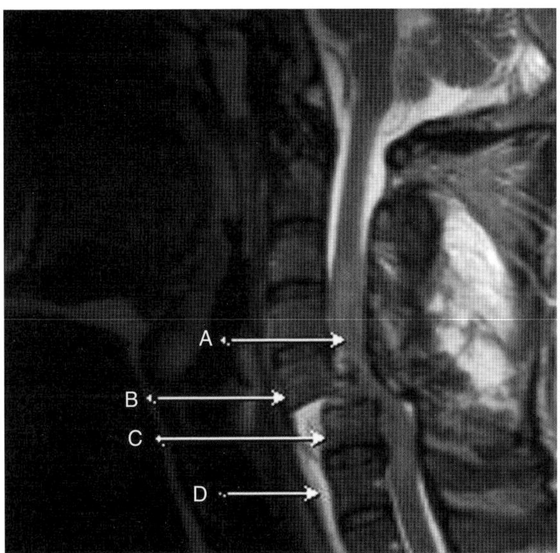

Fig. 8.15 MRI cervical spine following trauma. There is severe vertebral body malalignment and almost complete transaction of the cervical cord. A, swollen, contused cervical cord; B, C4 vertebral body; C, C5 vertebral body; D, abnormal pre-vertebral fluid collection.

A radiofrequency signal is subsequently applied which makes the protons re-align and enter a higher energy state. When the radiofrequency signal is turned off this energy is re-emitted by the protons and can be detected as a radio signal. The rate at which the energy is re-emitted varies between tissues and the information collected is used to make a map of hydrogen content and hence tissue characteristics in the area examined.

A very strong magnetic field is used to produce the image in the MRI scanner and this causes significant difficulties in performance of MRI scans in critically ill patients:

- a full history of any penetrating injury (especially to the eye), surgical procedures and implants is required before the patient can enter the scanner. The strong magnetic field in the MRI scanner can cause movement or heating of ferromagnetic objects. Any patient with a cardiac pacemaker is not allowed in the MRI scanner.
- MR compatible anaesthetic/monitoring and supportive equipment must be used. This is very expensive and available at only a limited number of hospitals.
- MRI scans take approximately 30 min; during this time the patient is in the confined area of the bore of the magnet. Patient access and monitoring is difficult, particularly in emergency situations.

Whenever possible, clinical questions should be addressed using other imaging modalities whilst the patient is critically ill.

Nuclear medicine

Basic principles

In nuclear medicine investigations, a substance is administered which is similar to a physiologically occurring compound but has an attached radioactive isotope. By taking an image of the distribution of the emitted radioactivity within the body using a gamma camera, the behaviour of the administered substance can be traced. Using different radiolabelled substances the metabolic activity and functions of the lungs, heart and bones are commonly imaged.

Nuclear medicine techniques are useful in searching for occult foci of infection by the administration of radioactive labelled white blood cells. In the past, lung scans were the most commonly requested nuclear medicine investigation in critically ill patients, but have now been replaced by CTPA.

Potential risks for the critically ill

There are some problems in arranging nuclear medicine studies for critically ill patients:

- The patient is often required to spend a long period of time in the Nuclear Medicine Department. Only a small number of hospitals have mobile gamma cameras which can be taken to the intensive care unit.
- For hours or days after the radioactive tracer has been injected there is a very small radiation dose emitted from the patient. This makes management of the patient difficult when staff are required to be close to the patient for prolonged periods of time.

Ultrasound imaging

Basic principles

Ultrasound uses sound waves of very high frequencies (above 20 kHz) which are inaudible to humans. The sound waves undergo reflection or refraction at the interface between different tissues, some being reflected back to the probe. This property is the basis of the ultrasound image.

Doppler ultrasound uses alterations in reflection of the ultrasound beam by flowing blood cells and can be used to assess either arterial or venous flow.

Use in the critically ill

- Ultrasound imaging is very well suited to the intensive care unit environment. There is no radiation dose to the patient or risk to staff and the equipment can brought to the patient's bedside. Manufacturers are now able to produce easily portable, good quality ultrasound machines even smaller than a laptop computer.
- The technology is particularly useful for the detection of fluid collections such as pleural effusion, infected collections/abscesses or free intraperitoneal fluid in cases of abdominal trauma. A skin site marking made at the time of ultrasound is useful for safe drainage of collections.
- The liver, kidneys and gall bladder are particularly well seen on ultrasound. Ultrasound will not penetrate through air and therefore bowel and lung generally cannot be assessed with ultrasound.
- Over recent years ultrasound has become increasingly used in the intensive care unit to assist in safe placement of central vascular lines.

Key points

- The reason for the imaging request should be stated on the referral form to allow the most appropriate imaging technique to be used. It may be helpful to discuss the clinical problem with a radiologist.
- Consideration should be given to patient and staff safety and the patient's clinical condition when planning investigations.
- All patients should have a chest X-ray on arrival in the unit, after any invasive procedures such as endotracheal intubation, central vascular catheter placement or thoracocentesis and insertion of naso- or orogastric feeding tubes.
- Intravenous iodinated contrast is often used during CT assessment of the mediastinum, abdomen and pelvis and in CT angiography. Risks include minor adverse reaction to iodinated contrast (e.g. flushing, urticaria, bronchospasm) and nephrotoxicity. Patients with GFR <30 ml/min are most at risk of contrast-induced nephropathy.
- MRI can produce extremely detailed images of soft tissue and is more sensitive than CT for subtle pathology, for example the posterior fossa of brain or the spinal cord.
- Ultrasound involves no radiation dose to the patient or risk to staff, and the equipment can be brought to the patient's bedside. It is used to detect fluid collections such as pleural effusion, abscesses or free intraperitoneal fluid. A skin site marking can be made for safe drainage of collections.
- Ultrasound has become increasingly used in the ICU to assist in the safe placement of central vascular lines.

Further reading

- European Society of Intensive Care Medicine (2004) *Patient Centered Acute Care Training Programme: Skills and Techniques – Clinical Imaging Module.* Brussels: ESICM.
- Papson JP, Russell KL, Taylor DM *et al.* (2007) Unexpected events during the intra-hospital transport of critically ill patients. *Acad. Emerg. Med.* **14**(6): 574–7.
- Pikwer A, Baath L, Davidson B *et al.* (2008) The incidence and risk of central venous catheter malpositioning: a prospective cohort study in 1619 patients. *Anaesth. Intens. Care* **36**(1): 30–7.
- Royal College of Radiologists (2007) *Making the Best Use of Clinical Radiology Services: Referral Guidelines*, 6 edn. London: RCR.

Vasoactive drugs

Mamta Patel

Shock is defined as the failure of the cardiovascular system to maintain adequate organ perfusion pressure. This causes inadequate oxygen delivery resulting in tissue hypoxia, lactic acidosis and end organ damage.

Causes of shock

- Cardiac or 'pump' failure – tamponade, infarction, ischaemia, cardiomyopathy
- Hypovolaemia/bleeding – haemorrhage, third space loss
- Septic shock – pancreatitis, meningitis, burns
- Obstructive – massive pulmonary embolism
- Anaphylaxis.

Oxygen delivery

The cardiovascular system comprises the heart, blood vessels and the circulating blood volume. It interacts with the lungs to maintain tissue perfusion and oxygenation.

The relationship between the respiratory and cardiovascular system (CVS) is illustrated by the oxygen delivery (DO_2) equation.

$$DO_2 = (\underbrace{SaO_2 \times Hb}_{\textbf{CVS}} \times 1.34 + \underbrace{(0.03 \times PaO_2)}_{\textbf{Lungs}}) \times \underbrace{CO}_{\textbf{CVS}}$$

where:

DO_2 = oxygen delivery (ml/min)
SaO_2 = % saturation of Hb in the blood
Hb = haemoglobin concentration (g/dl)
PaO_2 = partial pressure of oxygen in the blood (kPa)
CO = cardiac output (l/min).

CO is equated as:

$$CO = \text{stroke volume} \times \text{heart rate}$$

Thus substituting into the equation below:

$$DO_2 = (SaO_2 \times Hb \times 1.34 + (0.03 \times PaO_2)) \times \text{stroke volume} \times \text{heart rate}$$

Abnormalities in any of the above variables will result in shock and tissue hypoxia if the compensatory mechanisms of the body fail.
Stroke volume is determined by preload, afterload and contractility.

$$\text{Stroke volume} = \text{diastolic volume} - \text{end systolic volume}$$

Contractility is the ability of the heart to contract independently of preload and afterload:

- It is increased by inotropes, e.g epinephrine, dobutamine and calcium
- It is decreased by acidosis, hypoxia and hypocalcaemia.

Afterload is the force that opposes ventricular contraction.

- It is determined by the sympathetic tone, ventricular volume and pressure, the renin–angiotensin–aldosterone system and baroreceptor activity.

Preload is related to the end diastolic volume and hence central venous pressure (CVP) (Fig. 9.1).

- The Frank–Starling curve demonstrates the relationship between preload and stroke volume.
- Increasing preload will follow the curve on the diagram from A to B, augmenting stroke volume up to the peak of the curve. Beyond this, an increase in preload will not further improve stroke volume.
- Inotrope administration will increase myocardial contractility and on the diagram, this is demonstrated by a shift from A to C on the curve.

Core Topics in Critical Care Medicine, eds. Fang Gao Smith and Joyce Yeung. Published by Cambridge University Press.

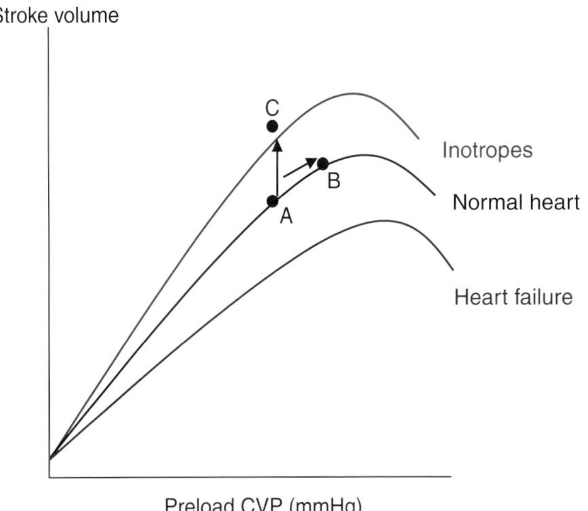

Fig. 9.1 Frank–Starling curve illustrating the relationship between stroke volume and preload in a normal heart (A and B), with inotropes (C) and in heart failure.

Vasoactive drugs

Definitions

For the purposes of the rest of the chapter the term *vasoactive drugs* refers to both inotropes and vasopressor drugs. There are very few pure inotropes or vasopressors.

- **Inotropes** affect the force of myocardial contraction. A positive inotrope will increase myocardial contractility.
- **Vasopressors** cause vasoconstriction of blood vessels (most act by α1 receptor activation) and therefore increase mean arterial blood pressure (MAP) and systemic vascular resistance (SVR).

Mechanism of action

Vasoactive drugs are used to support tissue perfusion and hence oxygenation. Vasoactive drugs act on various receptors in the body to produce their effects. Some drugs may act at more than one receptor to produce multiple effects. Some drugs have both inotropic and vasopressor activity (Table 9.1).

Alpha-1 (α1) receptors

These are present in vascular smooth muscle.

- Stimulation of α1 receptors in vascular smooth muscle activates phospholipase C via Gq proteins to increase inositol triphosphate. This increases intracellular calcium, which causes vasoconstriction.
- Examples of drugs that have α1 activity are phenylephrine and noradrenaline.

Beta (β1 and β2) receptors

Stimulation of β1 and β2 receptors via Gs proteins activates adenylate cyclase, which increases cyclic AMP (cAMP). This causes a protein kinase to phosphorylate various proteins resulting in their action, e.g. muscle relaxation, inotropy, etc.

Beta-1 (β1) receptors

These are present in the myocardium.

- Stimulation of β1 increases cAMP and subsequently intracellular calcium concentration. This increases myocardial contractility and heart rate.
- β1 receptor activation also liberates renin from the juxtaglomerular apparatus in the kidney, releasing aldosterone and increasing reabsorption of sodium and water.

Beta-2 (β2) receptors

These are present in the vascular and bronchial smooth muscle.

- β2 stimulation produces bronchial smooth muscle dilatation and vasodilatation of the blood vessels in skeletal muscle decreasing systemic vascular resistance.
- Normally the β_1:β_2 receptor ratio in the heart is 3 : 1. Excessive sympathetic drive in heart failure may cause downregulation of β1 receptors to change the ratio to 3 : 2 respectively.

Dopaminergic (D1 and D2) receptors

D1 receptors act via Gs-coupled adenylate cyclase leading to increased cAMP and cause vasodilatation in the vascular and splanchnic smooth muscle. Centrally, D1 stimulation modulates extrapyramidal activity.

D2 receptors act via Gi-coupled adenlyate cyclase leading to decreased cAMP and are located presynaptically. They have mainly modulatory functions and regulate the neurotransmission by feedback mechanisms,

Table 9.1 Action of some common vasoactive drugs

Drug	Heart rate	Mean arterial pressure	Cardiac output	Systemic vascular resistance	Bronchodilatation
Epinepherine	+++	+	+++	++	++
Norepinephrine	–	+++	+/ –	+++	0
Dopamine	++	+	++	+	0
Dobutamine	+	+	+++	–	0
Enoximone	++	– –	++	– –	0
Vasopressin	0	+++	+	+++	0
Phenylephrine	–	+++	–	+++	0

Key:

0, no effect

+, increase (mild, moderate, severe)

–, decrease (mild, moderate, severe)

+/ –, variable effect

affecting synthesis, storage and release of dopamine and norepinephrine (noradrenaline) into the synaptic cleft. Within the central nervous system, D2 receptor stimulation will lead to a reduced pituitary hormone output.

Vasopressin receptors

Please see under vasopressin.

Phosphodiesterase enzyme inhibitors (PDEI)

PDEI increase calcium by inhibiting type III phosphodiesterase enzymes in cardiac muscle.

- Type III phosphodiesterase enzymes rapidly degrade cAMP. Inhibition of PDEI causes an increase in cAMP and ionised calcium. This increases myocardial contractility.
- Phosphodiesterase inhibitors also have vasodilatatory properties. They cause vascular smooth muscle relaxation and therefore reduce afterload.
- Increased cAMP also regulates phospholamban. This increases calcium reuptake and facilitates diastolic relaxation. The combination of inotropy and diastolic relaxation is lusitropy.

Commonly used vasoactive drugs

Epinephrine (adrenaline)

Used in cardiac arrest, cardiogenic shock, low output cardiac state and anaphylaxis.

- Acts on α1, β1 and β2 receptors. It has a half-life of less than a minute.
- At low doses, the diastolic blood pressure falls due to vasodilatation and increased blood flow through skeletal muscle (β2 effect). The β2 stimulation also causes bronchodilation.
- β1 effect (predominant effect) causes tachycardia, increased contractility and cardiac output. The systolic blood pressure is increased.
- At higher doses the α1 vasoconstrictor effects predominate, causing vasoconstriction and cool extremities.
- Epinephrine stimulates glycogenolysis, lipolysis and gluconeogenesis, and causes hyperglycaemia. Insulin secretion is increased initially but then inhibited by α effects.
- Epinephrine also increases basal metabolic rate, myocardial oxygen consumption, automaticity of the heart and serum lactate.

- Na^+ reabsorption is increased by direct stimulation of tubular Na^+ transport, renin and aldosterone release. Stimulation of β2 receptors leads to increased K^+ in cells and causes hypokalaemia.
- Compared with dobutamine and norepinephrine, epinephrine worsens splanchnic perfusion.
- *Side effects* – ventricular arrhythmias, hypertension, hypokalaemia and lactic acidosis.

Norepinephrine (noradrenaline)

Norepinephrine is an endogenous catecholamine and a neurotransmitter at most of the postsynaptic adrenergic junctions in the body.

- Norepinephrine acts on both α1 and β1 receptors but has predominant α1 actions causing vasoconstriction and increased MAP.
- The increased systemic vascular resistance (α1 effect) can negate the increased cardiac output via β1 activation.
- Baroreceptor activation causes reflex bradycardia due to increased MAP.
- It is used in the treatment of septic shock and to offset vasodilatation due to spinal shock and epidurals.
- In severe sepsis norepinephrine improves splanchnic blood flow.

Studies comparing norepinephrine and dopamine to epinephrine have shown that unlike epinephrine, norepinephrine reduces serum lactate levels.

Dobutamine

Dobutamine (a derivative of isoprenaline) has β1 agonist action, which increases heart rate, stroke volume, cardiac contractility, and cardiac output.

- β2 stimulation causes dobutamine to have a vasodilatory effect reducing MAP and SVR.
- It has a half-life of 2 min.
- Its uses are mainly in cardiogenic shock and sepsis with depressed cardiac function.
- Dobutamine causes less tachycardia than epinephrine but can precipitate arrhythmias.
- Compared with dopamine, dobutamine improves gastric mucosal perfusion in patients with sepsis.
- Tachyphylaxis can occur during prolonged administration of dobutamine.

Dopamine

Dopamine is a mixed inotrope and vasoconstrictor.

- It activates dopaminergic (D1) receptors at low doses and has β and α actions with increasing doses.
- It has predominantly β1 effects at moderate dose range.
- At higher doses, the α1 effect is dominant, causing vasoconstriction. This may be due to conversion of dopamine to norepinephrine.
- Dopamine causes tachycardia, and can thus precipitate myocardial ischaemia.

There are some controversies relating to the use of dopamine.

- The 'renal protective' effect of dopamine: at low doses (<5 μg/kg per min) dopaminergic receptors in the kidneys are stimulated causing vasodilatation and increasing urinary output. This effect was initially thought to be renoprotective. However, this effect is caused by an increase in cardiac output due to increased inotropy and hence improved renal perfusion pressure. There is no evidence that low dose dopamine has any other renal protective action.
- Dopamine may interfere with pituitary and thyroid function.
- It may have an immunosuppressive effect and inhibit T cell proliferation.

Vasopressin

Vasopressin is secreted in response to increased plasma osmolality, hypovolaemia and pain.

- V1a receptors are present in smooth muscle and myocardium. Their activation causes vasoconstriction of blood vessels.
- V2 receptors are present in the collecting ducts. They are involved in water regulation.
- V3 (also known as V1b) are present in the CNS and involved in secretion of corticotrophin releasing hormone.

Vasopressin restores vascular tone in catecholamine-resistant shock by four methods:

- Activation of V1 receptors.
- Modulation of K-ATP channels.
- Modulation of nitric oxide.
- Potentiation of adrenergic and other vasoconstrictors.

Endogenous vasopressin levels are markedly reduced in adults with severe sepsis but not in children with meningococcal septic shock.

Wenzel *et al.* performed a large trial of vasopressin versus epinephrine in human cardiopulmonary arrest that had promising results, but poor neurological outcomes raised controversy in introducing vasopressin into CPR guidelines.

In severe sepsis and septic shock, current evidence suggested that although low doses of vasopressin may be effective in increasing blood pressure in patients refractory to other vasopressors, no outcome data were available and 'cautious use of vasopressin pending further studies' was recommended.

If vasopressin is used in advanced vasodilatory shock outside of clinical trials, it should be used as a supplementary vasopressor and in doses not exceeding 0.04 U/min.

Vasopressin is associated with ischaemic skin lesions in 30% of patients. Most of the skin lesions occurred on the distal limbs (68%), and 26% occurred on the tongue.

Phenylephrine

Phenylephrine is an α1 agonist with minimal β activity.

- It causes arteriolar vasoconstriction and increases SVR and MAP. It causes a reflex bradycardia due to baroreceptor activation and cardiac output is decreased as a result.
- Phenylephrine is a vasoconstrictor with minimal inotropic action. Its uses are mainly in patients with spinal shock and spinal–epidural anaesthesia.
- Phenylephrine is not routinely used as a single agent in sepsis because of its tendency to reduce cardiac output.

Phosphodiesterase enzyme inhibitors (PDEI) (e.g. milrinone/enoximone)

The two groups of phosphodiesterase inhibitors are bipyridines (amrinone) and imidazole (e.g. enoximone) derivatives.

- Phosphodiesterase inhibitors (PDEI) increase cAMP and thus intracellular calcium. This increases cardiac output. PDEIs, however, unlike β1 agonists, do not require a receptor for their action.
- PDEIs also reduce systemic and pulmonary vascular resistance.
- PDEI drugs exhibit lusitropy, i.e. they relax the heart in diastole thus increasing coronary blood flow.
- PDEIs are used in combination with other vasoactive drugs.
- Enoximone may be effective in treating right heart failure and pulmonary hypertension by causing systemic and pulmonary vasodilatation and increasing right ventricular contractility.

Levosimendan

Levosimendan is a calcium sensitizer with some PDE III inhibitory actions similar to dobutamine. It is an inodilator that exerts its effects by combining with troponin C to enhance the calcium sensitivity of the myocardium.

- A recent study in the treatment of heart failure compared levosimendan with dobutamine; levosimendan did not reduce mortality when compared with dobutamine.
- There were higher incidences of atrial fibrillation, hypokalaemia and headache in the levosimendan group.

Which vasoactive drug to use?

- Hypovolaemic shock – fluid/blood initially
- Anaphylactic shock – epinephrine
- Cardiogenic shock – consider dobutamine +/– norepinephrine and +/– epinephrine
- Septic shock – consider norepinephrine +/– dobutamine

Management of shock

When managing shock it is paramount to maintain blood pressure and tissue perfusion whilst curtailing unwanted side effects (Table 9.2). Resuscitation of a shocked patient begins with:

Table 9.2 Shock and vasoactive drugs

Type of shock	Heart rate	CVP	Cardiac output	Stroke volume	Systemic vascular resistance	Considered vasopressor/ treatment initially
Hypovolaemic	↑	↓	↓	↓	↑	Fluid/blood
Septic shock	↑	↓	↑	↓/↑	↓	Norepinephrine
Cardiogenic	↑	↑	↓	↓	↑	Dobutamine

- Optimizing airway, oxygenation and ventilation.
- Restoring the circulatory volume. This may necessitate blood transfusion for haemorrhagic shock or crystalloid/colloid for septic shock, e.g. pancreatitis.
- Supporting cardiac output. Consider vasoactive drugs, intra-aortic balloon pump, etc.
- Treating the cause of the shock, e.g. drain a cardiac tamponade.
- Treating factors that may affect cardiovascular function such as arrhythmias, hypocalcaemia, hypokalaemia, hypomagnesaemia, drug interactions and acidosis.
- Bicarbonate should only be used for severe acidosis (pH <7.15) unresponsive to adequate resuscitation. It is best to be cautious as bicarbonate can cause inadvertent intracellular acidosis by raising intracellular pCO_2.
- Institute appropriate monitoring and investigations, e.g. blood cultures and cardiac output monitoring in sepsis (see Chapter 7: Haemodynamics monitoring), echocardiogram in cardiac failure, invasive blood pressure monitoring in hypovolaemic shock.

Using vasoactive drugs

If optimization of oxygenation, ventilation and adequate fluid resuscitation fail to restore cardiac output then treatment with vasoactive drugs should be considered. When considering vasoactive drugs, the adverse effects on myocardial perfusion, oxygen demand and organ perfusion should be taken into account. End organ perfusion can be impaired further due to excessive vasoconstriction. Myocardial oxygenation requirements can increase due to increased tachycardia in an effort to maintain cardiac output. Commencing vasoactive drugs in a volume-depleted patient (absolute or relative hyporolaemia due to sepsis) can have dire consequences for the patient.

Initiating vasoactive therapy

Most vasoactive drugs have mixed vasopressor and inotropic action. At high doses, the less predominant effects become more evident. A combination of vasoactive drugs with differing pharmacological actions may be needed to provide optimal effect.

- The cause of shock should be determined, e.g. does the patient have low cardiac output state or septic shock (low SVR/MAP)?

Monitoring considerations

Appropriate parameters should be used to monitor for response and side effects e.g. ECG, ABP, CO, SV and urine output. Usually, vasoactive management is indicated to sustain a MAP greater than 60 mmHg in the fluid resuscitated patient to sustain organ perfusion.

- Patients with atherosclerosis and hypertension may need a higher MAP to maintain blood flow. 'Adequate' blood pressure is no guarantee of blood flow.
- There is no 'normal' CVP. Serial trends of CVP and its response to therapy and fluid boluses should be monitored.
- Tricuspid regurgitation, pulmonary hypertension and excessive ventilatory pressures can all give false CVP readings.
- Very high doses of some vasopressors can also cause venoconstriction. This may cause a falsely elevated CVP.

Response

Therapy may need to be started with minute-by-minute assessment of the patient's response.

The response to vasoactive drugs is often unpredictable and dependent on the cause of shock and baseline circulation. The same drug may produce different responses depending on the patient's myocardial compliance and volume status. The dosages of vasoactive agents should be reviewed frequently in the face of varying response.

For patients who are on high doses of vasoactive drugs, steroid supplementation may be considered as steroids can have a facilitatory effect on the action of inotropes. In the past, high dose steroids use was associated with higher mortality in septic patients but a recent meta-analysis by Minneci revealed a consistent and significant beneficial effect of glucocorticoids on survival and shock reversal regardless of adrenal function. The relationship between steroid dose and survival was found to be linear, characterized by benefit at low doses and increasing harm at higher doses. It is now recommended that a 5- to 7-day course of physiological hydrocortisone (150–200 mg per day in divided doses) with subsequent tapering should be given to patients with vasopressor-dependent septic shock.

Is the resuscitative therapy working?

This is assessed by collectively and serially monitoring clinical response and measured variables.

- Improved parameters, e.g. mean arterial blood pressure, stroke volume and pulse rate.
- Improved thermoregulation (e.g. cardiogenic shock patient warms up).
- Improved Urine output.
- Improved PaO_2.
- Improved base deficit.
- Reduced serum lactate.
- Return of mixed venous saturations towards normal.
- Cardiac index/output returns towards normal.

Monitoring

Serial trends and responses to monitoring are more important than isolated readings.

- ECG – to monitor for arrhythmias and signs of myocardial ischaemia.
- Arterial line – for beat-to-beat monitoring of blood pressure. A 'swing' in the blood pressure trace may indicate that the patient requires more filling. It also allows for serial sampling of arterial blood gases, base excess and lactate measurements.
- CVP – to help guide right heart 'filling' or preload. It is not very useful for monitoring individual organ perfusion. If the patient has a history of ischaemic heart disease or tricuspid regurgitation the CVP may not give any indication of left heart pressures. Its other uses include administration of vasoactive drugs and to obtain mixed venous saturation sampling if a pulmonary artery flotation catheter (PAFC) is unavailable.
- Hourly urine output.
- Echocardiogram – to determine/exclude cardiac pathology.
- Oesophageal Doppler – a non-invasive method of measuring stroke volume and cardiac output and is subject to variability.
- Pulmonary artery catheter (if indicated) – its use is not without complications and is debatable. It is an invasive method of obtaining:
  (1) an indication the left heart filling pressure and volume
  (2) measurement of cardiac output
  (3) mixed venous oxygen saturation (SvO_2) and oxygen consumption (DO_2).
- Mixed venous oxygen saturation (SvO_2) – this is determined using a blood sample obtained from the pulmonary artery. If a sample from PAFC is not available then a CVP line sample may be used. Normal SvO_2 is around 70%.
- A low SvO_2 indicates excessive extraction of oxygen from the blood or inadequate delivery.
- A high SvO_2 is difficult to interpret as it may be due to increased oxygen delivery or it may be due to the inability of the tissues to extract oxygen from the blood.
- However, care should be taken with interpretation of SvO_2. It is a very *global* measurement. If normal, it may give no indication of individual organ ischaemia.

Inotropes complications and considerations

- Excessive stimulation of α1 receptors can lead to extreme vasoconstriction and may impair tissue perfusion.
- Increased afterload may lead to impaired left ventricular function.

- Excessive stimulation of β1 receptors can lead to tachycardia and arrhythmogenicity. Tachycardia reduces diastole during which coronary perfusion occurs. This can precipitate ischaemia. Tachycardia and arrhythmias also increase myocardial oxygen demand. In susceptible patients, this can lead to myocardial ischaemia or infarction.
- Inotropes can cause vasoconstriction of the pulmonary vasculature and can worsen ventilation–perfusion mismatch and oxygen delivery.
- Central venous access is required to deliver vasoactive drugs and guide fluid resuscitation. The patient is thus exposed to the complications of CVP line insertion.
- Extravasation of vasoactive drugs can lead to tissue necrosis. The site should be washed with saline and local infiltration of 5 mg of phentolamine should be considered.
- When initiating vasoactive therapy the rate of vasoactive drug infusion should take into account the dead space in the CVP line.
- Critically ill patients are very sensitive to changes in vasoactive drug infusion syringes. 'Double pumping' where two infusion syringes, the new and the old syringe, are infused simultaneously, can minimize fluctuations in vital signs.
- Over time, a patient's response to vasoactive drugs may decrease. This may be due to adrenergic receptor downregulation and desensitization.

Key points

- Shock causes inadequate oxygen delivery resulting in tissue hypoxia, lactic acidosis and end organ damage.
- After optimizing oxygenation and circulating volume, vasoactive drugs can be used to optimize cardiac output and oxygen delivery.
- Vasoactive drugs can adversely affect myocardial perfusion, oxygen demand and organ perfusion. End organ perfusion can be impaired further due to excessive vasoconstriction. Myocardial oxygenation requirements can increase due to increased tachycardia.
- A combination of vasoactive drugs may be used to avoid side effects at high doses and provide optimal effects.
- Appropriate monitoring should be in place to assess the effects of vasoactive drugs such as invasive blood pressure monitoring, central venous pressure and hourly urine output. Other monitoring can include echocardiography, oesophageal Doppler, pulmonary artery flotation catheter and mixed venous saturation.

Further reading

- Cheryl L, Holmes A, Keith R, Walley B (2004) Vasopressin in the ICU. *Curr. Opin. Crit. Care* **10**: 442–8.
- Dellinger RP, Carlet JM, Masur H *et al.* (2008) Surviving sepsis campaign guidelines for management of severe sepsis and septic shock. *Crit. Care Med.* **36**(1): 296–327.
- Dellinger R, Phillip MD (2003) Concise definitive reviews in critical care medicine. *Crit. Care Med.* **31**(3): 946–55.
- Kellum J, Pinsky M (2002) Use of vasopressor agents in critically ill patients. *Crit. Care* **8**: 236–41.
- Levy B (2005) Bench-to-bedside review: is there a place for epinephrine in septic shock? *Crit. Care* **9**: 561–5.
- Mebazaa A, Nieminen M, Packer M *et al.* (2007) Levosimendan vs. dobutamine for patients with acute decompensated heart failure. *J. Am. Med. Ass.* **297**: 1883–91.
- Minneci PC, Deans KJ, Banks SM *et al.* (2004) Meta-analysis: The effect of steroids on survival and shock during sepsis depends on the dose. *Ann. Intern. Med.* **141**: 47–56.
- Mitchell S, Hunter JM (2007) Vasopressin and its antagonists: what are their roles in acute medical care? *Br. J. Anaesth.* **99**: 154–8.
- Wenzel V, Krismer AC, Arntz HR *et al.* (2004) A comparison of vasopressin and epinephrine for out-of-hospital cardiopulmonary resuscitation. *N. Engl. J. Med.* **350**: 105–13.

Chapter 10

Nutrition

Yasser Tolba

General considerations

The goal of nutritional support in critical care is to prevent the development of malnutrition.

Patients in critical care are at high risk of malnutrition, due to the nature of their illness and hypermetabolic catabolic state. There is loss of fat and lean body (muscle) mass: 'auto-cannibalism'. As their immune system is already compromised, they are at increased risk of infection and septicaemia.

Malnutrition in the critical care setting is an under-recognized and under-treated problem. It has been shown to be strongly linked to increased length of stay in hospital, morbidity and mortality.

Assessment of nutritional status

Nutritional status in critically ill patients can be difficult to assess.

- **Anthropometric** measurements (e.g. skinfold thickness and mid-arm circumference) are commonly used to assess populations rather than individuals.
- **Biochemical tests** also have their limitations. Albumin levels fall rapidly as part of the acute phase response. Haemoglobin is affected by haemorrhage and bone marrow suppression. Transferrin, prealbumin and lymphocyte counts can be useful; however, they are dependent on the patient being well hydrated.
- **Body mass index** (mass (kg)/height (m^2)) is used (with a BMI <18.5 classed as underweight) and has been shown to be an independent predictor of mortality in seriously ill patients. But it does not reflect the acute changes in nutritional status important in critical illness.
- **Subjective global assessment** is a widely accepted method of measuring nutritional status which is targeted history and examination. This is a structured approach to taking a *history* which includes:

  (1) Weight change (>5% of usual body weight in 3 weeks or >10% in 3 months).
  (2) Changes in food intake.
  (3) Gastrointestinal symptoms.
  (4) Functional impairment.

  This is combined with a *physical examination* looking for evidence of:

  (1) Loss of subcutaneous fat – especially in chest and triceps (body mass index <20).
  (2) Muscle wasting – especially at temporal region, deltoids and gluteals.
  (3) Oedema.
  (4) Ascites.

Despite being subjective, it has been shown to be reproducible and correlates with mortality in a variety of conditions.

Estimating nutritional requirements

A careful balance of macronutrients (protein, lipid and carbohydrate) provides the energy requirements whilst micronutrients (vitamins and minerals) are required in small amounts to maintain health but not to provide energy.

Core Topics in Critical Care Medicine, eds. Fang Gao Smith and Joyce Yeung. Published by Cambridge University Press.

Step 1: Calculate resting energy expenditure for caloric requirements

This requires sophisticated equipment so it is more often estimated using formulae. One such formula is the Harris Benedict equation, which estimates *basal metabolic rate* (BMR) in kcal/day:

$$\text{BMR for male: } 66 + (13.7 \times W) + (5 \times H) - (6.8 \times A) = \text{kcal/day.}$$

$$\text{BMR for female: } 655 + (9.6 \times W) + (1.8 \times H) - (4.7 \times A) = \text{kcal/day.}$$

Where W = body weight in kg, A = age in years, H = height in cm, 'small' calorie = 4.184 J, 'large' calorie = 1 kilocalorie (kcal).

This will usually give a result of around 25 kcal/day. The equation estimates BMR in afebrile healthy individuals. So it needs to be multiplied by the stress level:

surgery = 1.2, starvation = 0.85–1, trauma = 1.35, sepsis = 1.6, severe burn = 2.1

Fever increase BMR by 10% for each 1°C above 37°C (up to max of 40°C)

$$\text{daily energy required for maintenance} = \text{BMR} \times \text{stress factor} \times 1.25$$

(an additional 25% for hospital activity, not added if paralysed on a ventilator or heavily sedated).

$$\text{daily energy requirements for weight gain} = \text{maintenance} + 750 \text{ kcal.}$$

Step 2: Calculate protein requirements

- Normal: 0.8–1 g/kg/day protein (up to 60–70 g/day). Moderate depletion/stress: 1–1.5. Severe: 1.5–2.

Less protein is needed in patients with renal failure before dialysis and hepatic encephalopathy.

Step 3: Calculate non-protein (carbohydrates + lipids) component

- Fat calories help decrease the risk of carbohydrate overload and keep total amount of fluid down.
- Fat requirements should be less than 40% calories as fat may reduce the immune response.
- A minimum of 4% of total calories as essential fatty acids (linoleic).
- Give the remaining energy requirements as carbohydrates.

Calorie value of macronutrients (kcal/g)

Fat 9, protein 4, carbohydrates 4, IV dextrose 3.4 and 1 ml of 10% fat emulsion 1.1.

Step 4: Calculate micronutrients (vitamins, electrolytes and trace elements)

Daily requirements for vitamins

A 3300 IU, D 200 IU, E 10 IU, B1 3 mg, B2 3.6 mg, B3 40 mg, B5 15 mg, B6 4 mg, B7 60 mg, B9 0.4 mg, B12 5 mg, C 100 mg, K 2–4 mg/week.

Patients with sepsis have been shown to have large vitamin A losses.

Daily electrolyte requirements (in mmol/kg per day)

Na^+ 1.0–2.0, K^+ 0.7–1.0, Ca^{++} 0.1, M^{++} 0.1, Cl^- 1.0–2.0, PO_4^- 0.4.

Catabolism and loss of lean body mass can occur if low in K, Mg, Zn, P and S.

Daily requirements for trace elements (in micrograms)

Chromium 10–15, copper 500–1500, manganese 150–800, selenium 30–60, zinc 2500–4000.

Burns patients lose selenium, zinc and copper via their exudates and trauma patients lose selenium and zinc through their drains.

Routes of administration

Nutritional support can be given through one of two routes: *enteral feeding* (EF) (via the gastrointestinal tract) or *parenteral feeding* (PN) – intravenous (via either peripheral or central vein).

Enteral feeding (EF)

- Enteral feed involves using the gastrointestinal tract for the delivery of nutrients; this includes eating food, oral supplements and all types of tube feeding.
- If at all possible enteral is the preferred route for nutritional support. It is cheaper, more physiological, reduces the risk of peptic ulceration and minimizes mucosal atrophy.
- If the patient can eat orally then this should be encouraged. It is important to know how much the patient is eating to see whether they are receiving adequate nutrition. If not they will need supplementation either orally or enterally.

- Early enteral nutrition could lead to lower stress hormone concentrations, lower infection rates, shorter hospital stays. Better survivals have been shown in some, but not all, studies in which nutrition was started within 4–24 hours.
- Lack of enteral intake can lead to small intestinal villus atrophy, decreased villus cell count and reduced mucosal thickness. Mucosal surface patterns change from finger-like to leaf-like microvilli. Intestinal permeability is increased. These changes can be reversed with enteral feeding.
- These changes in gut integrity could cause intestinal translocation of bacteria. This can activate the gut's immune inflammatory system (Peyer's patches and hepatic Kupffer cells). The released cytokines and other mediators then exacerbate the already existing systemic inflammatory response syndrome leading to multiple organ failure. This is called the 'gut hypothesis of multiple organ failure'.
- Situations previously thought to preclude enteral nutrition, including major gastrointestinal surgery or acute pancreatitis, have now been shown to be best treated with enteral nutrition.

Requirements for enteral feeding

Patients should be haemodynamically stable with no history of massive GI bleeds, no intestinal obstruction, no severe diarrhoea, no high-output enteric fistula or abdominal distension.

Assessment of gut function

Gut output should be less than 600 ml/day. Presence of bowel sounds (does not necessarily correlate with peristalsis and passage of flatus or stool is a better marker of gut function.

Access for enteral feeding

Gastric route

The route of EF most often used in critical care is nasogastric tubes. Some patients may already have percutaneous endoscopic gastrostomy (PEG) tubes in situ, if it is known they will not be able to feed for some time after surgery.

Jejunal route

Nasojejunal tube feeding is considered ideal so as to avoid the often present gastric ileus and possibly prevent aspiration. A nasogastric tube can be passed during surgery and manually manipulated into the jejunum. In patients without surgical placement, nasogastric tubes may be placed. It is often difficult to pass such tubes from the stomach into the jejunum. Right lateral positioning and prokinetic drugs may be attempted, but often placement has to be performed under radiological or endoscopic guidance.

Jejunostomy catheter can be placed during laparotomy to start feeding within hours of bowel surgery. Complication rates are comparatively low (1.5%). The most common complications are occlusion or dislodgement of feeding catheters.

Types of feeds

Polymeric preparations

Enteral feeding solutions usually contain homogenized substrates similar to those found in normal feeds and are termed *polymeric solutions.* Elemental or semi-elemental solutions contain free amino acids or hydrolysed proteins, glucose, or oligosaccharides and medium-chain triglycerides to facilitate digestion and absorption in patients with altered digestive function. However, most patients can be fed with polymeric solutions, and these should be preferred to elemental formulae, since they are less likely to induce diarrhoea and are associated with improved nitrogen retention and improved gut trophicity, while being considerably less costly.

- Polymeric preparations contain normal proteins, fats and carbohydrates, which require digestion prior to absorption, and electrolytes, trace elements, vitamins and fibre.
- Commonly used ingredients include the protein casein (from milk), soya protein, maize and soya oils and the carbohydrate maltodextrin.
- The different preparations vary in their osmolality, calorie:nitrogen ratios and carbohydrate:lipid ratios. They provide energy between 0.5 and 2 kcal/ml although most are 1 kcal/ml.
- Standard polymeric feeds (generally 1 kcal/ml) are most often used, although there are higher-energy alternatives (1.2 or 1.5 kcal/ml) available for patients who need more calories in a shorter period of time, or who do not tolerate large volumes.

Disease-specific formulae

- Liver disease: low sodium and altered amino acid content to minimize hepatic encephalopathy.
- Renal disease: low phosphate, potassium and high energy (2 kcal/ml) to reduce volume of fluid intake.
- Respiratory disease: high fat content to reduce CO_2 production.

Elemental preparations

These preparations contain the macronutrients in a readily absorbable form, i.e. proteins as peptides or amino acids, lipids as medium-chain triglycerides and carbohydrates as mono- and disaccharides. These preparations are expensive and only indicated for patients with severe malabsorption or pancreatic insufficiency.

Parenteral nutrition (PN)

Special considerations

Intensive care clinicians should make all the efforts to improve tolerance of enteral feeding before considering parenteral nutrition. It is unclear, however, about the duration of failure in enteral feeding before PN should start, which mostly depends on pre-existing nutritional status and the disease process.

- Patients receiving less than 25% of their predicted nutrition requirements are at increased risk of sepsis. Most units believe that PN is better than no nutritional support and will start PN in patients who are expected not to tolerate adequate enteral feeding for 7 days.
- The only absolute indication for PN is gastrointestinal failure.
- PN can be used to supplement enteral nutrition, for example in short gut syndrome.
- PN can be used as the sole source of nutrition as total parenteral nutrition (TPN).

Components of parenteral nutrition

Parenteral nutrition is commonly administrated as a sterile emulsion of water, protein, lipid, carbohydrate, electrolytes, vitamins and trace elements. Components and volumes of PN are based on the recommendations discussed earlier on nutritional requirements. However, PN can be given as separate components.

Protein

Protein is given as amino acids which include essential amino acids – histidine, leucine, isoleucine, lysine, threonine, methionine, phenylalanine, tryptophan and valine and most of the non-essential amino acids.

Lipid

Lipid provides a source of essential fatty acids – linolenic acid (an omega-3 fatty acid) and linoleic acid (an omega-6 fatty acid). Lipid is also important for absorption of fat-soluble vitamins.

- Commonly given as intralipid, an emulsion made from soya with chylomicron-sized particles.
- Propofol is made of 10% intralipid and it should be included in calculation of energy requirement to avoid over-feeding.
- Intralipid can be used alone.

Carbohydrate

Commonly given as glucose. It can be given alone initially for its protein-sparing effect in starvation.

Electrolytes and micronutrients

These should usually be included in the emulsion. Otherwise, they need to be given separately.

Pharmaco/immunonutrition

This is a relatively new concept in critical care feeding for which there is a growing body of evidence reporting benefits.

Despite adequate nutritional support, nosocomial infection still remains a major problem in critically ill patients. Therefore, addition of specialized nutrients to the standard diet has been suggested in order to decrease patients' susceptibility to infection by enhancing the immune response.

The target of the so-called 'immunonutrients' can be the gastrointestinal tract (i.e. the enterocytes or the immune cells of the intestinal wall) in order to prevent or diminish the translocation of bacteria or bacterial products.

During critical illness, the amount of fuel for these rapidly renewed cells may become the rate-limiting step of an appropriate immune response. The function of circulating immune cells (mainly lymphocytes and macrophages) may also be influenced by the dietary constituents.

Data reported from several studies suggest the response of immune cells can be enhanced by immunonutrients. There is also preliminary data suggesting a beneficial effect on infection rate and length of hospital stay for some ICU patients with the use of immunonutrient-containing enteral formulae. This topic remains controversial and needs further research.

Some ICUs now have protocols for the use of immunonutrition feeds. Often where patients are admitted to the ICU for more than 24 hours they will commence on such a feed.

- *Arginine* is an amino acid shown to improve immune response to bacteria, viruses and tumour cells, promote wound healing and increase protein turnover.
- *Omega-3 fatty acids* enhance immune function by boosting neutrophil activity, and reduce inflammation.
- *Nucleotides* are essential for maintaining cellular integrity and enhancing production of repair cells.
- *Glutamine* is the most abundant amino acid in the body and becomes essential during severe stress. It is thought to promote anabolism and may be an important intestinal growth factor.

Examples of immunonutrition feeds

- *Impact* contains arginine, omega-3 fatty acids and nucleotides.
- *Oxepa* contains omega-3 and omega-6 fatty acids.
- *Stresson* contains glutamine, omega-3s and omega-6s fatty acids.
- *Recovan* contains glutamine, arginine, omega-3s and omega-6s fatty acids.

Complications of nutritional support

Refeeding syndrome

- This can happen during the first few days of nutritional support via any route in patients who are severely malnourished or starved.
- Mechanisms: starvation causes a loss of intracellular electrolytes, secondary to leakage and reduced transmembrane pumping, and intracellular stores can become severely depleted. When carbohydrate is available again there is an insulin-dependent influx of electrolytes into cells which can result in rapid and severe drops in serum levels of phosphate, magnesium, potassium and calcium.
- The clinical features include weakness, respiratory failure, cardiac failure, arrhythmias, seizures and death.
- Feeding must be introduced slowly, starting with only 25–50% of energy requirements and gradually increasing after 4 days. The recommended electrolytes should be supplemented at the same time. Thiamine and other B vitamins should also be given intravenously before starting feeding and then daily for at least three days.

Overfeeding

Deliberate overfeeding in an attempt to reverse catabolism is associated with poor outcome. It can cause uraemia, hyperglycaemia, hyperlipidaemia, fatty liver (hepatic steatosis), hypercapnia (especially with excess carbohydrates) and fluid overload. It is probable that at least some of the risks of parenteral nutrition are actually related to overfeeding and some even recommend moderate underfeeding (aiming to meet roughly 85% of requirements).

Hyperglycaemia

Hyperglycaemia can be related to overfeeding but is often not; critically ill patients become insulin resistant as part of the stress response or undiagnosed diabetes.

In 2001 Van den Berghe *et al.* reported that strict control of blood glucose (target blood glucose 4.4–6.1 mmol/l) reduced ICU mortality and morbidity in post-surgical intensive care patients compared to conventional treatment, where insulin was infused only if the blood glucose exceeded 11.9 mmol/l and was adjusted to maintain values of 10–11.1 mmol/l. Mortality was reduced by almost half (from 8.0% to 4.6%) and length of stay, ventilator days, incidence of septicaemia and requirements for both dialysis and blood transfusion were all reduced. The patients who benefited most were those who stayed on ICU for more than 5 days.

Recent studies have challenged the safety of strict glycaemic control. In 2009, the NICE-SUGAR trial, a large randomized controlled trial, randomized patients to either intensive glucose control, with a target blood glucose range of 4.5–6.0 mmol/l, or conventional glucose control, with a target of 10.0 mmol/l or less. Severe hypoglycaemia was reported in 6.8% in the intensive control group and 0.5% in the conventional control group ($P < 0.001$). No significant difference was demonstrated between the two treatment groups in the median length of stay in the ICU or hospital or the median number of days of mechanical ventilation or renal replacement therapy. The study concluded that intensive glucose control increased mortality among adults in the ICU: a blood glucose target of 10.0 mmol/l or less resulted in lower mortality than did a target of 4.5–6 mmol/l.

Electrolyte imbalances and micronutrient deficiency

Electrolyte imbalances and micronutrient deficiencies can happen particularly in those requiring prolonged periods of nutrition.

Complications of enteral nutrition

The commonest risk with enteral feeding is aspiration of feed causing pneumonia. This can be minimized by confirming tube position, feeding the patient semi-recumbent, aspirating the nasogastric tube regularly and avoiding bolus feeds to keep away from large residual gastric volumes. Prokinetics have also been shown to reduce residual gastric volumes.

Diarrhoea can also be a problem but is not an indication to stop feeds before other causes of diarrhoea have been excluded. However, if enteral feeds are the cause then a feed with more fibre can be tried.

Complications of parenteral nutrition

On intensive care, PN is commonly given via a central venous catheter. The insertion and presence of a central venous catheter has inherent risks (Chapter 7).

Overfeeding, uncontrolled hyperglycaemia and infection from parental feeding increase risk of sepsis. Bags must be sterile and discarded within 24 hours of starting. Sterile precautions must be used when changing bags and the lumen of the central venous catheter must not be used to take blood or give drugs or fluids.

Parenteral nutrition can predispose to hepatobiliary disease including fatty liver, cholestasis and acalculous cholecystitis.

Key points

- Critically ill patients are at high risk of malnutrition, due to the nature of their illness and hypermetabolic catabolic state.
- Malnutrition in critical care can lead to increased length of stay in hospital, morbidity and mortality.
- Enteral nutrition should be preferred to parenteral nutrition whenever possible, due to its trophic effects on the intestinal mucosa, lower rate of complications and lower costs.
- Guidelines for nutrition in critical care should include assessing the patient's nutritional state, the timing of nutritional support, choice of feeding route and formula, and protein–calorie requirements.
- In some patients a reduced rate of complications and length of hospital stay can result from the use of immunomodulating enteral formulae.

Further reading

- Hibbert CL, Edbrooke DL, Coates E (2001) Immunonutrition: a cost-effective approach to care? *Complete Nutri.* **1**(1): 9–13.
- Heyland DK, Dhahiwal R, Drover SW *et al.* (2003) Canadian Critical Care Clinical Practice Guidelines Committee. Canadian clinical practice guidelines for nutrition support in mechanically ventilated, critically ill adult patients. *J. of Parenteral Enteral Nutr.* **27**: 355–73.
- Heyland DK, Novak F, Drover JW *et al.* (2001) Should immunonutrition become routine in critically ill patients? A systematic review of the evidence *J. Am. Med. Ass.* **286**: 944–53.
- Jolliet P, Pichard C, Biolo G *et al.* (1998) Enteral nutrition in intensive care patients: a practical approach. *Intensi. Care Med.* **24**: 848–59.
- NICE-SUGAR Study Investigators (2009) Intensive versus conventional glucose control in critically ill patients. *N. Engl. J. Med.* **360**: 1283–97.
- Stroud M, Duncan H, Nightingale J (2003) Guidelines for enteral feeding in adult hospital patients. *Gut* **52** (Suppl. 7): vii1–vii12.
- Van den Berghe G, Wouters P, Weekers F *et al.* (2001) Intensive insulin therapy in critically ill patients. *N. Eng. J. Med.* **345**: 1359–67.
- Weitzel LB, Dhaliwal R, Drover J *et al.* (2009) Should perioperative immune modulating nutrition therapy be the standard of care? A systematic review. *Crit. Care* **13** (S1): P132
- Wellesley H (2007) *Nutrition in ICU.* London: Royal Collage of Anaesthetists. www.frca.co.uk

Chapter 11 Pain control

Edwin Mitchell

The importance of pain relief

Pain is a common finding amongst patients on the intensive care unit, and by definition is unpleasant experience. The principal reason for treating pain is humanitarian, to relieve the suffering of a fellow human being, but there are other potential benefits as well.

Effective analgesia is associated with

- improved ability to cough, clear secretions and a reduced rate of respiratory failure following major abdominal and thoracic surgery
- reduced duration of intestinal stasis following abdominal surgery
- reduced sedation requirements.
- improved compliance with physical rehabilitation, with positive outcomes on joint mobility, and lower rates of deep venous thrombosis
- minimized surgical stress response
- reduced incidence of chronic pain syndromes.

Sources of pain

Pain may be considered to originate from either the underlying pathological process, e.g. trauma, pancreatitis or myocardial infarction, or be iatrogenic from medical procedures, e.g. surgery, line insertion points and poor patient positioning.

Approximately 60% of patients on general intensive care units in the United Kingdom are suffering from surgical conditions, most of these have had an operation. Post-operative pain is common and often severe; 70–90% of patients report pain of severe/unbearable intensity following surgery.

Types and severity of pain

Most of the pain experienced on the intensive care unit is acute pain that results directly from traumatized tissue. The severity of the pain is often proportional to the amount of tissue trauma, but it must be borne in mind that patients may suffer from several painful areas at once, and it is often insufficient to treat any one painful area alone, no matter its size. The nature of surgery is often another important factor to determine the severity of acute pain. For example, thoracic open surgery brings more severe acute pain than extensive head and neck surgery.

Assessment of severity of pain

Assessing the severity of pain in intensive care patients is challenging. Patients may be sedated, or unable to communicate due to the presence of endotracheal tubes, dressings and other impediments.

Methods such as the visual analogue scale, or pain score, are frequently used to assess the severity of pain (Fig. 11.1). These are quick, easy, reproducible and sensitive to changes in the patient's condition, but can be difficult to administer in patients who have limited ability to communicate. Alternative forms of assessing pain relief that score pain behaviours (e.g. grimacing) or score physiological changes (e.g. heart rate and blood pressure changes), are available, but patients who recover from critical illness frequently recall pain of greater severity than their physiological changes have suggested.

Modalities of pain relief

Analgesia may be provided either systemically or regionally (Table 11.1). Multimodality approaches are often employed, with multiple techniques and drugs used to treat a particular pain state. This approach has the benefits of minimizing the amount of potentially toxic drugs, such as opioids, as well as providing better pain relief.

Core Topics in Critical Care Medicine, eds. Fang Gao Smith and Joyce Yeung. Published by Cambridge University Press.

Systemic analgesia

Paracetamol

A simple analgesic that is very useful for soft tissue pain and as an opioid sparing drug in more severe pain states. Paracetamol is available in an oral, rectal or intravenous preparation. Oral bioavailability is high, with absorption occurring rapidly from the duodenum. Paracetamol may cause mild derangement of liver function tests in normal doses, and caution should be exercised in patients with severe hepatic impairment. Paracetamol has anti-pyretic properties and has been associated with mild hypotension in critical care patients.

Non-steroidal anti-inflammatory drugs

Non-steroidal anti-inflammatory drugs (NSAIDs) are powerful analgesics, particularly useful for bony pain.

Table 11.1 Types of analgesia

Systemic	Regional
Paracetamol	Neuraxial blockade
NSAIDs	Peripheral nerve blocks
Tramadol	
Opioids	
Ketamine	
Inhaled – nitrous oxide	

They have an opioid sparing effect when used in combination with opioids. All NSAIDs work by the inhibition of the cyclooxygenase (COX) enzyme, and this may lead to adverse effects such as bronchospasm, renal impairment, gastric irritation, bowel perforation and platelet inhibition. The elderly are at particular risk from the adverse effects of NSAIDs. Critically ill patients who are at risk from stress ulceration and renal impairment must be carefully assessed before using NSAIDs.

Cyclooxygenase II (COX-II) inhibitors were developed in an attempt to remove the adverse side effects of traditional NSAIDs. COX-II inhibitors work by inhibiting only the induced form of cycloxygenase which is produced by tissue trauma. They have been associated with an increased risk of cardiovascular events in patients who have used these drugs for some time and their role in the critical care population is uncertain.

Tramadol

Tramadol is an atypical analgesic with antagonist actions at morphine receptors and inhibitory effects on the reuptake of serotonin and norepinephrine from the synaptic cleft. Potentiation of serotinergic neurons may be important in activating the descending pain control neuronal pathways. It is useful for moderate pain and may be administered orally or by intravenous injection. Oral bioavailability is high, approaching 100% with repeated dosing. The major adverse reaction is nausea and vomiting, but it is also associated with sedation, confusion and hallucinations, particularly in the elderly.

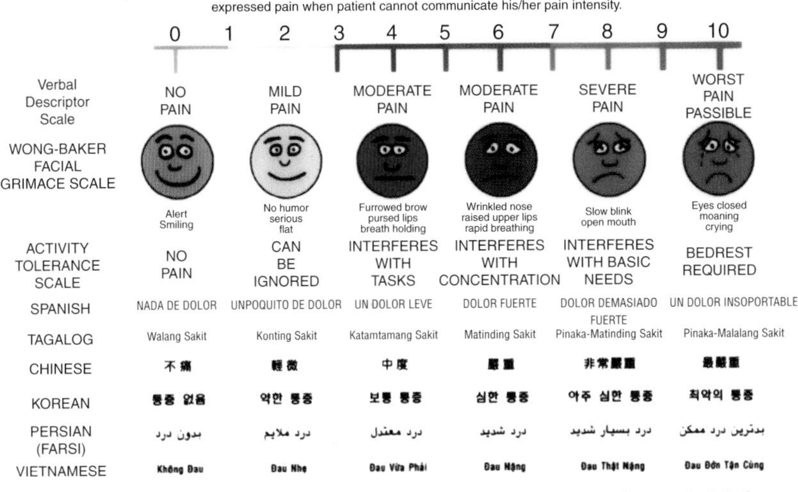

Fig. 11.1 An example of a pain assessment tool.

Opioids

Opioids are the most potent analgesics widely available and form the basis of most critical care pain management treatments.

All opioids act via opioid receptors, which are found centrally, in the spinal cord and peripherally. Opioids mimic endogenous neuropeptides, such as endorphins, which have analgesic properties. Activation of the morphine receptor causes inhibition of adenyl cyclase, hyperpolarization of the neuron, and a reduction in signal transmission.

Opioids have a similar range of effects through their actions at the morphine receptors:

- analgesia
- sedation
- respiratory depression
- miosis
- nausea and vomiting
- reduced intestinal motility
- tolerance and dependence.

The first two of these properties make opioids popular choices in sedation regimes in the critically ill. The different drugs may have differing pharmacokinetic properties, however (Table 11.2).

Morphine

Morphine may be administered orally, subcutaneously, intramuscularly, intravenously, epidurally or intrathecally. Its oral bioavailability is only 50%. Morphine is widely used due to the versatility in route of administration and low cost. Morphine undergoes conjugation in the liver to a number of metabolites, including morphine-6-glucuronide, a molecule which retains opioid agonist activity, and may accumulate in renal failure.

Table 11.2 Pharmacokinetic properties of opioids

Drug	Vd (l/kg)	Clearance (l/min)	$t_{½}$ (h)
Alfentanil	0.8	6	1.6
Fentanyl	4.0	13	3.5
Morphine	3.5	15	3
Remifentanil	0.4	40	0.1
Tramadol	2.9	6	7

Diamorphine

Diamorphine is a diacylated morphine pro-drug. It has no intrinsic analgesic activity, but is rapidly deacetylated into morphine in vivo. Diamorphine hydrochloride is more soluble than morphine sulfphate, and this allows it to be prepared in smaller volumes, an advantage when preparing small-volume syringe drivers.

Fentanyl

A synthetic opioid with a very high lipid solubility, fentanyl has a shorter half-life in the plasma than morphine following bolus administration, principally due to redistribution. Following multiple boluses or infusions redistribution may become slower and elimination half life then becomes important. Fentanyl depends on hepatic clearance. It is often used in epidural analgesic regimes at very low concentrations.

Alfentanil

A synthetic opioid similar to fentanyl, but with a lower potency due to lower lipid solubility. More alfentanil is present in the unionized state in plasma compared to fentanyl, and this means it has a more rapid onset of action than fentanyl. Compared to fentanyl and morphine, alfentanil has a shorter terminal half-life, meaning recovery is more rapid following infusions. Alfentanil is metabolized in the liver, and its clearance is relatively unaffected by renal failure.

Remifentanil

Remifentanil is an ester that is rapidly hydrolysed in the plasma to a virtually inactive compound. The half-life in plasma of remifentanil is less than 10 mins, resulting in a rapid recovery from its effects. Analgesia provided by infusion with remifentanil may be suitable where the painful stimulus is not expected to be long lasting, and in patients with renal failure.

Codeine

Codeine is a weak opioid. Approximately 10% of an orally administered dose is *O*-demethylated to morphine which accounts for the analgesic action. This depends on cytochrome CYP2D6 enzyme activity in the liver (10% of the UK population lack this enzyme). Codeine is much less efficacious for pain relief in these patients. Codeine has higher bioavailability than morphine when administered orally.

Ketamine

Ketamine is a NMDA antagonist with potent analgesic and sedative effects. In larger doses (>1–2 mg/kg) it is an anaesthetic agent. Ketamine causes activation of the sympathetic system and is associated with a rise in blood pressure and a mild tachycardia. It is widely used for short-lived, repeated procedures, such as dressing changes in burns patients. Typically given intravenously, ketamine may also be administered intrathecally or orally. The major adverse effect of ketamine is psychotomimetic reactions which may take the form of hallucinations or nightmares. These may persist for some time, although their incidence may be reduced with the concomitant use of benzodiazepines.

Nitrous oxide

Nitrous oxide is a colourless, odourless gas with analgesic properties. It is typically presented in a 50:50 combination with oxygen (Entonox™). Usually administered via a patient-activated inhalational device, it may be used for short-lived painful procedures, such as reducing fractures and changing dressings.

Regional analgesia

Regional anaesthesia is commonly provided in conditions where the pain intensity is expected to resolve over time, as its major limitation is the duration over which it may be administered safely. This is typically no more than 3–4 days. It is most widely used in the context of post-operative pain control, and the major benefits may be seen in the reduction of opioid use, with the associated complications. In certain other circumstances, such as following rib fractures, regional anaesthesia may minimize respiratory complications and speed recovery.

Regional analgesia can be divided into neuraxial or peripheral techniques.

Neuraxial blockade

Neuraxial techniques involve the administration of local anaesthetics or other drugs to the spinal cord or nerve roots. The two most commonly used techniques are spinal or epidural analgesia.

Spinal analgesia

Spinal anaesthesia is the administration of an analgesic drug into the cerebrospinal fluid, usually via a needle introduced between the third and fourth lumbar vertebrae. It is typically a 'single-shot' technique; continuous infusions have been used but are associated with nerve damage and toxicity. Local anaesthetics administered intrathecally have a short duration of action, typically only a few hours. Morphine has a longer duration of action and may provide analgesia for up to 24 hours. This technique is used following major abdominal or thoracic surgery, giving good analgesia with minimal cardiovascular complications. Unfortunately there is a higher incidence of respiratory insufficiency compared to other techniques.

Epidural analgesia

The epidural space is a potential space extending from the base of the skull to the coccyx containing fat, loose connective tissue, blood vessels and the nerve roots emerging from the spinal cord. Epidural analgesia is the administration of an analgesic drug into the epidural space, usually via a catheter introduced by the specially designed Tuohy needle.

The catheter may be placed anywhere along the vertebral column depending on the site of the pain, and will provide dermatomal anaesthesia. Local anaesthetic preparations are most commonly infused into the epidural space, the rate of infusion governing the degree of spread and area of anaesthesia. Opioids may be added to the infusion mixture. These reduce the amount of local anaesthetic required to produce a given area of analgesia, and minimize unwanted side effects associated with sympathetic blockade. Opioids infused into the epidural space diffuse into the cerebrospinal fluid and bloodstream and may cause systemic side effects (Table 11.3).

Table 11.3 Complications related to epidural insertion

Related to insertion of epidural	Related to administered drugs
• Failure of placement • Localized backache • Misplacement of catheter (blood vessel/CSF) • Post dural puncture headache (1:100) • Nerve damage (1:10 000) • Epidural abscess (1:2–10 000) • Epidural haematoma (1:10 000)	Local anaesthetic • Numbness • Hypotension • Bradycardia • Systemic local anaesthetic toxicity Opioids • Nausea and vomiting • Itch • Hallucinations

The benefits of epidural analgesia compared to systemic opioids are:

- The abolition of the surgical stress response.
- Reduced incidence of deep venous thrombosis.
- Faster return of gastrointestinal motility following abdominal surgery.
- Reduced rate of respiratory failure.

It has been difficult to demonstrate a reduction in post-operative mortality, however.

The complications associated with epidural analgesia are related either to the insertion of the epidural, or the drugs used in the epidural. The more serious complications of epidural abscess and epidural haematoma are rare, but are neurosurgical emergencies, requiring the drainage of the pus or blood within a few hours before pressure builds up within the epidural space causing infarction of the spinal cord or nerve roots. Epidural abscesses or haematomas may present with a new fever, pain in the back or weakness in the legs, and these signs may be masked in a patient who is having difficulty with communication on the intensive care unit. The difficulties in assessing the function, toxicity and potential side effects of epidural analgesia have to be weighed carefully against the theoretical benefits of a reduced surgical stress response in sedated patients.

Peripheral nerve blocks

Instillation of local anaesthetic solutions around nerve can be used to provide analgesia to localized areas of the body, most frequently the limbs. Catheters can be placed alongside nerves or nerve plexuses and infusions of local anaesthetics used to maintain anaesthesia for several days.

Using a regional technique may avoid the systemic side effects of opioids and the unwanted hypotension associated with epidural analgesia, but no benefits over these techniques in terms of patient outcome or satisfaction have been shown.

The complications of regional anaesthesia are similar to those of epidural analgesia, with trauma to the nerve on insertion, or subsequent haematoma formation being the most feared complications.

Adjuncts to acute pain management

Anxiolysis is an important part of pain management, and it is important to keep the patient fully informed of their progress and to address any concerns that they may have. Judicious pharmacological interventions to aid sleep or reduce anxiety may be of benefit. In some patients complementary therapies such as massage or aromatherapy may help.

Chronic pain management

Many patients suffer from chronic pain conditions, and these are often overlooked unless they are the direct reason for admission to the intensive care unit. Advice should be sought from physicians experienced in the management of chronic pain states.

Key points

- Pain is a common finding amongst critical care patients.
- Assessing the degree of pain a patient is in can be difficult.
- Multimodal approach to pain relief allows better pain control with minimization of adverse effects.
- Opioids should be prescribed according to their need and pharmacokinetic properties.
- Regional anaesthesia has theoretical benefits, but the associated risks may be unjustified in patients who are heavily sedated.

Further reading

- Bromley L (2005) Opioids and codeine. In *Core Topics in Pain*, eds. Holdcroft A and Jaggar S. Cambridge: Cambridge University Press, pp. 269–76.
- Payen JF, Bossen JL, Chanques G *et al.* (2009) Pain assessment is associated with decreased duration of mechanical ventilation in the intensive care unit: a post-hoc analysis of the DOCOREA study. *Anesthesiology,* **111**: 1308–16.
- Rigg J, Jamrozik K, Myles P *et al.* (2002) Epidural anaesthesia and analgesia and outcome of major surgery. *Lancet* **359**: 1276–82.
- Schulz-Stubner S, Boezaart A, Hata J (2005) Regional analgesia in the critically ill. *Crit. Care Med.* **33**: 1400–7.

Chapter 12

Sedation

Joyce Yeung

Introduction

For many patients, the critical care environment can be a frightening and stressful environment and analgesics and sedatives are used to improve the comfort and safety of critically ill patients. Agitation is believed to be present in at least 71% of patients on intensive care. The majority of critically ill patients cannot communicate easily the way they feel or what they need. Procedures such as tracheal intubation, ventilation, suction and physiotherapy cannot be tolerated without adequate level of sedation. However, continuous administration of sedatives can prolong the time on mechanical ventilation and ICU stay. The correct management of sedation is one of the most important and often difficult goals to achieve in critical care.

Although the mainstay of therapy will be pharmacological, other approaches are just as important and should not be neglected. Good communication and regular assurance from nursing staff can help alleviate anxiety of patients in unfamiliar surroundings. Environmental control such as temperature, noise and lighting can provide a restful environment. The management of thirst, constipation and full bladder can help with the general comfort and well-being of patients.

Aims

The American College of Critical Care has recommended that the use of analgesics, sedatives and neuroleptics for treatment of pain, anxiety or psychiatric disturbance in the intensive care unit should be used as 'agents to mitigate the need for restraining method and not overused as a method of chemical restraint'. The main goals should be:

(1) Patients should be comfortable and provided with adequate analgesia. Studies have shown that 70% of patients in ICU remembered being in pain despite their healthcare providers believing them to be pain free. Adequate analgesia can often reduce the need for deep sedation.

(2) Anxiety should be minimized as it can reduce efficiency of ventilatory support and agitated patients have higher metabolic rate and higher oxygen consumption.

(3) Patients should be able to tolerate procedures and organ system support.

(4) Patients should be calm, co-operative and able to sleep when undisturbed.

(5) Patients should not be paralysed and awake.

Levels of sedation

The required level of sedation will vary according to the patient being cared for. Deep sedation will be required for status epilepticus but the modern ventilator can work with patients who are lightly sedated and spontaneously breathing. The desired level of sedation should be documented and once sedation is started, the level of sedation should be regularly assessed. Oversedation will lead to increase time on mechanical ventilation, increased risk of nosocomial pneumonia and unnecessarily prolonged ICU stay. It may also increase the need for frequent neurological assessments such as CT scans and increase the incidence of long-term cognitive and psychological problems in patients. Undersedation, on the other hand, can cause hypercatabolism, immunosuppression, hypercoagulability and increased sympathetic activity.

Many scoring systems have been devised to provide an assessment of levels of sedation. Vital signs, such as blood pressure and heart rate, are not specific or sensitive markers of sedation and not useful in assessing sedation. A reliable and practical objective method of assessment is still being developed.

Core Topics in Critical Care Medicine, eds. Fang Gao Smith and Joyce Yeung. Published by Cambridge University Press.

Assessment tools

Clinical scoring systems

There are many clinical scoring systems and commonly used ones include Ramsay (Table 12.1) and Bloomsbury scales (Table 12.2). These are designed to give a quantitative score which can be done regularly by nursing staff and documented on observation charts. Their limitations include interpreter variability and the lack of discrimination between deeper levels of sedation.

Electroencephalograms

Electroencephalograms (EEG) can provide a measure of cerebral activity. This technique is complex and requires trained personnel. It is more suitable for the assessment of depth of anaesthesia and can be difficult to interpret in the encephalopathic patient.

Table 12.1 Ramsay Scale

	Level	Response
Awake	1	Patient anxious and agitated or restless or both
	2	Patient co-operative, orientated and tranquil
	3	Patient responds to commands only
Asleep	4	Brisk response to a light glabellar tap or loud auditory stimulus
	5	Sluggish response to a light glabellar tap or loud auditory stimulus
	6	No response to a light glabellar tap or loud auditory stimulus

Table 12.2 Bloomsbury Scale

Sedation score	
3	Agitated and restless
2	Awake and comfortable
1	Aware but calm
0	Roused by voice
−1	Roused by touch
−2	Roused by painful stimuli
−3	Unrousable
A	Natural sleep
P	Paralysed

Bispectral index

The bispectral index (BIS) has been used successfully to monitor the depth of anaesthesia in the operating theatre environment (Fig. 12.1). The monitor gives a quantitative value between 0 to 99, with value of 0 representing EEG silence and 100 representing a fully awake patient. Some studies have shown good correlation between Ramsay Score of 1–5 and BIS in critical care settings but correlation is more variable when Ramsay Score is 6.

Auditory evoked potentials

Evoked potential monitors measure electrical activity in certain areas of the brain in response to stimulation of specific sensory nerve pathways. Auditory evoked potentials (AEP) monitoring technique isolates the neurophysiological signal generated during stimulation of cranial nerve VIII using a repetitive auditory stimulus (Figs. 12.2 and 12.3). The repeated sampling allows the signal to be extracted from the background EEG noise. Studies have suggested that long latency auditory evoked potentials can provide an objective electrophysiological analogue to the clinical assessment of sedation independent of the sedation regime used.

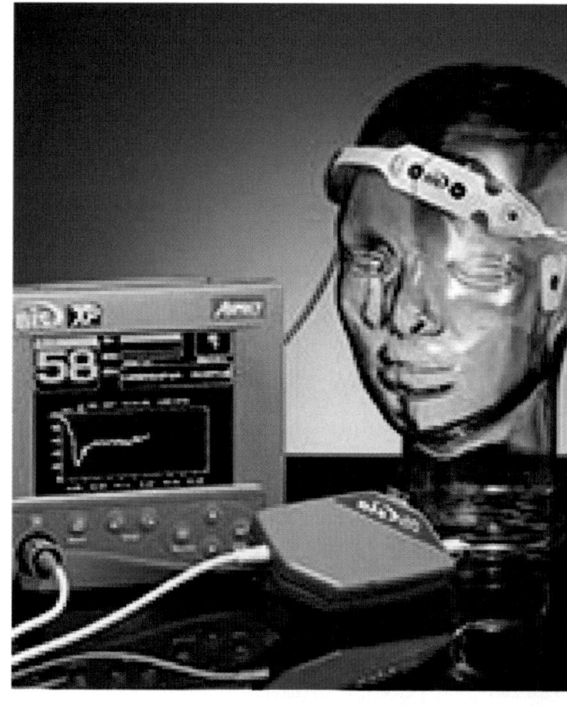

Fig. 12.1 A bispectral index (BIS) monitor displaying BIS value with BIS sensor strips for attachment. (Photo courtesy of Aspect Medical Systems.)

Pharmacological management

Loading dose

It takes four half-lives of a drug given by intravenous infusion to achieve steady state. It is therefore necessary to start with a loading dose to minimize delays to achieve adequate sedation. However, the initial high infusion rates for a loading dose are often not required to be continued once the steady state is achieved. Any increase in infusion rates should be by small increments as high infusion rates will encourage tolerance to sedatives.

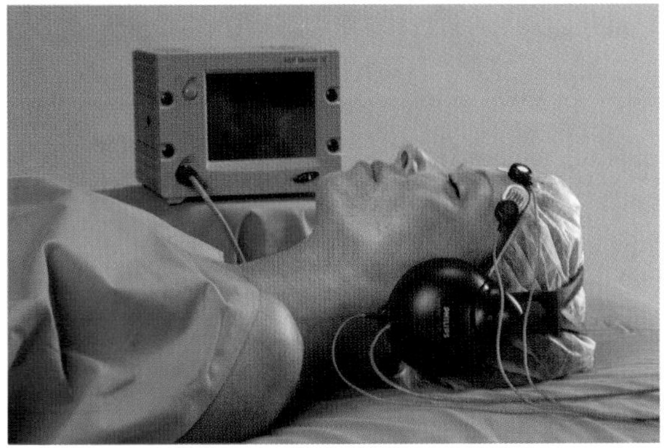

Fig. 12.2 AEP monitor attached to surface electrodes on patient's head and headphones providing the auditory stimulus. (Photo courtesy of Aspect Medical Systems.)

Side effects of sedatives

Currently there is no ideal sedative agent available and pharmacological agents will all share the same side effects:

- Accumulation with prolonged infusion leading to delay in weaning from organ support and prolonged ICU stay.
- Adverse effects on circulation and blood pressure resulting in inotropic support.
- Adverse effects on pulmonary vasculature, increasing V/Q mismatch leading to increased ventilatory support and risk of nosocomial pneumonia.
- Tolerance with continued use.
- Withdrawal symptoms when sedation is stopped.
- Sedative agents do not provide rapid eye movement (REM) sleep needed for rest. REM sleep deprivation is an important cause of ICU psychosis.
- Reduced intestinal motility interfering with the absorption of enteral feed and drugs.

Ideal properties of sedatives

The ideal properties of sedatives are summarized in Table 12.3.

Commonly used sedatives

Choice of sedative will vary according to local guidelines and cost effectiveness. Combinations of sedatives

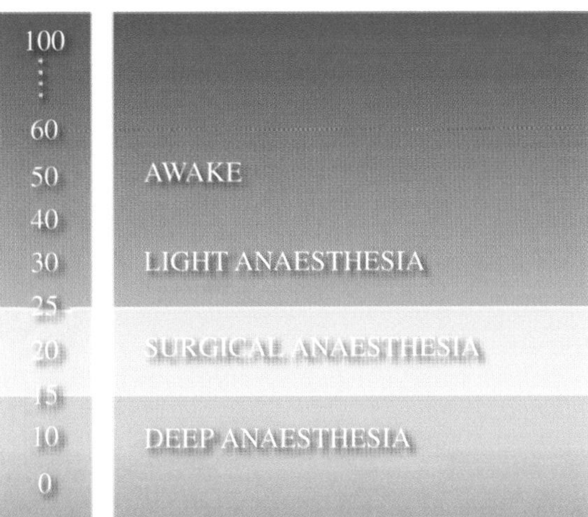

Fig. 12.3 Diagram illustrating AEP monitor displaying index number of 21. For this particular monitor, an index of below 25 indicates adequate anaesthesia. (Photos and illustration courtesy of Danmeter, Denmark.)

that act via different mechanisms are more effective than single agents at high dose (Table 12.4).

Pharmacokinetc considerations

The choice of sedative agents in critically ill patients is difficult as their pharmacokinetics will be affected by the following factors:

- patient's volume status
- capillary leak affecting the volume of distribution
- serum protein levels affecting protein binding
- renal function
- hepatic function
- hepatic blood flow
- combination of drugs competing for carrier molecules and metabolic pathways.

Table 12.3 Properties of the ideal sedative

Hypnosis/sleep
Anxiolysis
Amnesia
Anti-convulsant
Non-accumulative
Non-toxic
Titratable effect
Independent of renal or hepatic metabolic pathways
Minimal cardio-respiratory effects
Rapid onset and offset time
No prolonged effect on memory
No long-term psychological effects
No interactions with other drugs
Cheap
Water soluble
Long shelf-life

Intravenous anaesthetic agents

Propofol

Propofol is one of the most commonly used anaesthetic agents in intensive care. It is fast-acting, effective, titratable and has a rapid offset of action. Some studies have demonstrated that the use of propofol is associated with a reduced time on mechanical ventilation compared to benzodiazpine sedation; but it has not been shown to reduce ICU stay. Propofol can cause myocardial depression, reduced systemic vascular resistance and hypotension especially in susceptible patients who are hypovolaemic. Propofol infusion is also lipid-rich and has a caloric value of 0.9 calorie/ml. Prolonged infusion can cause metabolic acidosis and muscle necrosis due to impairment of oxidation of fatty acid chains and inhibition of oxidative phosphorylation in mitochodria. The use of propofol has been associated with increased mortality in children and is currently not licensed for use in children less than 3 years old.

Thiopentone

The use of thiopentone on ICU is now reserved only for specific indications such as status epilepticus and to treat uncontrolled raised intracranial pressure. Its use as a sedative agent is limited by its poor titratability and low clearance and long half-life due to zero order kinetics.

Ketamine

Ketamine is a phencyclidine derivative. It produces dissociative anaesthesia, analgesia and amnesia by

Table 12.4 Pharmacology of commonly used sedatives on intensive care

Agent	Onset	Half-life	Metabolic pathway	Active metabolite	Unique side effect	Infusion range
Propofol	1–2 min	26–32 hr	Oxidation	None	↑triglycerides, pain on injection	5–8 μg/kg/min
Midazolam	2–5 min	3–11 hr	Oxidation	Yes		0.04–0.2 mg/kg/hr
Lorazepam	5–20 min	8–15 hr	Glucuronation	None	Solvent-related acidosis/ renal failure in high doses	0.01–0.1 mg/kg/hr
Remifentanil	<1.5 min	3–10 min	Plasma esterases	None	Rebound analgesia	0.6–15 μg/kg/min
Clonidine		8.5 hr		None	Hypotension, bradycardia, rebound hypertension	0.014 μg/kg/min
Haloperidol	3–20 min	18–54 hr	Oxidation	Yes	↑QT interval	0.04–0.15 mg/kg/hr

antagonizing the excitatory neurotransmitter glutamate at NMDA receptors. Its use on the intensive care as a sedative is limited by emergence phenomena and sympathetic stimulation causing tachycardia, systemic and pulmonary hypertension and raised intracranial pressure. Its analgesic effect gives ketamine a role in the management of severe burns and its bronchodilator effect makes ketamine a useful adjunct in the management of status asthmaticus.

Etomidate

Despite a favourable haemodynamic profile, the use of etomidate has been associated with increased mortality on intensive care units and it is no longer used for sedation. Even a single bolus can cause significant adrenocortical suppression via inhibition of 11β-hydroxylase.

Volatile anaesthetic agents

Volatile anaesthetic agents are not routinely used on intensive care because of the more complex set-up and cost of administering the agents. Isoflurane has been used to treat status asthmaticus due to its bronchodilatory effects.

Benzodiazepines

Benzodiazepines are widely used on critical care units for their hypnotic, amnesic and anxiolytic effects. It is important to remember they do not provide analgesia. In fact, benzodiazepines are commonly used synergistically with opioids for their analgesic, respiratory and cough suppressive effects, allowing for lower dosages to be used. Benzodiazepines depress the excitability of the limbic system via reversible binding at the GABA–benzodiazepine receptor complex, resulting in intracellular influx of chloride ions when activated.

Benzodiazepines are commonly administered as continuous or intermittent infusion titirated to effect. Their clinical effects will be affected by the patient's age and physiological reserve, prior exposure to benzodiazepines or alcohol, concurrent therapy and any renal or hepatic dysfunction. After long-term administration, dose of benzodiazepines should be reduced gradually to avoid withdrawal symptoms.

Midazolam

Midazolam is one of the most popular sedatives used in intensive care. It is a water-soluble molecule at acidic pH, but once injected, it becomes fat soluble at physiological pH, resulting in rapid transit across the blood–brain barrier. It has a rapid onset of action and a short elimination half-life. It is 94–98% bound to plasma protein and has a volume of distribution of 1.7 l/kg. It is extensively metabolized by cytochrome P450 to 1-hydroxymidazolam glucuronide (1-OHMG) which has active sedative properties and is excreted in the urine.

Lorazepam

Lorazepam is a unique agent as its elimination depends primarily on non-cytochrome-mediated glucuronide conjugation in the liver. It is ideal for patients with hepatocellular dysfunction. However, as the conjugates are renally excreted, it can still accumulate in patients with renal failure.

Opioids

Although opioids are used primarily for their analgesic effects in critical care, they do possess varying degrees of anxiolytic and sedative properties. All opioids share the same side effect profile including nausea and vomiting, respiratory depression, histamine release causing urticaria, rash, hypotension and bradycardia.

Remifentanil and analgesic-based sedation

Remifentanil has been used as sole agent to provide analgesic-based sedation. It acts as a pure μ agonist and is metabolized by non-specific blood and tissue esterases. It has a context-sensitive half-life of 3–10 min irrespective of the duration of infusion. A large randomized, double-blind controlled trial has found that remifentanil provided effective and rapid sedation without the need for propofol in most patients. Analgesic-based sedation has also been shown to shorten the duration of mechanical ventilation compared with traditional hypnotic based sedation by up to 10 days. However, the use of remifentanil can be associated with problems of withdrawal symptoms and inadequate analgesia after cessation of infusion. Longer-acting opioids should be commenced and allowed to take effect before remifentanil infusion is stopped.

Alpha-2 receptor agonists

Clonidine

Clonidine is an imidazoline derivative and acts as sedative by stimulating alpha-2 (α2) receptors in lateral reticular nucleus of medulla, reducing sympathetic outflow, resulting in sedation and analgesia. It also causes haemodynamic changes by first causing hypertension but subsequently reducing sympathetic tone causing hypotension and bradycardia in prolonged infusion. Clonidine has an elimination half-life of 8.5 hours and is metabolized in the liver and excreted in urine. It should be used with caution in patients with hepatic or renal failure.

Dexmedetomidine

Dexmedetomidine is a highly selective α2 receptor agonist and has been used as a sole agent for sedation and analgesia in intensive care. It has a shorter elimination half-life of 2 hours compared to clonidine. The Maximizing Efficacy of Targeted Sedation and Reducing Neurological Dysfunction (MENDS) Trial was a randomized double-blind study which showed a reduction in delirium and coma and a trend of reduced ICU stays and more ventilator-free days.

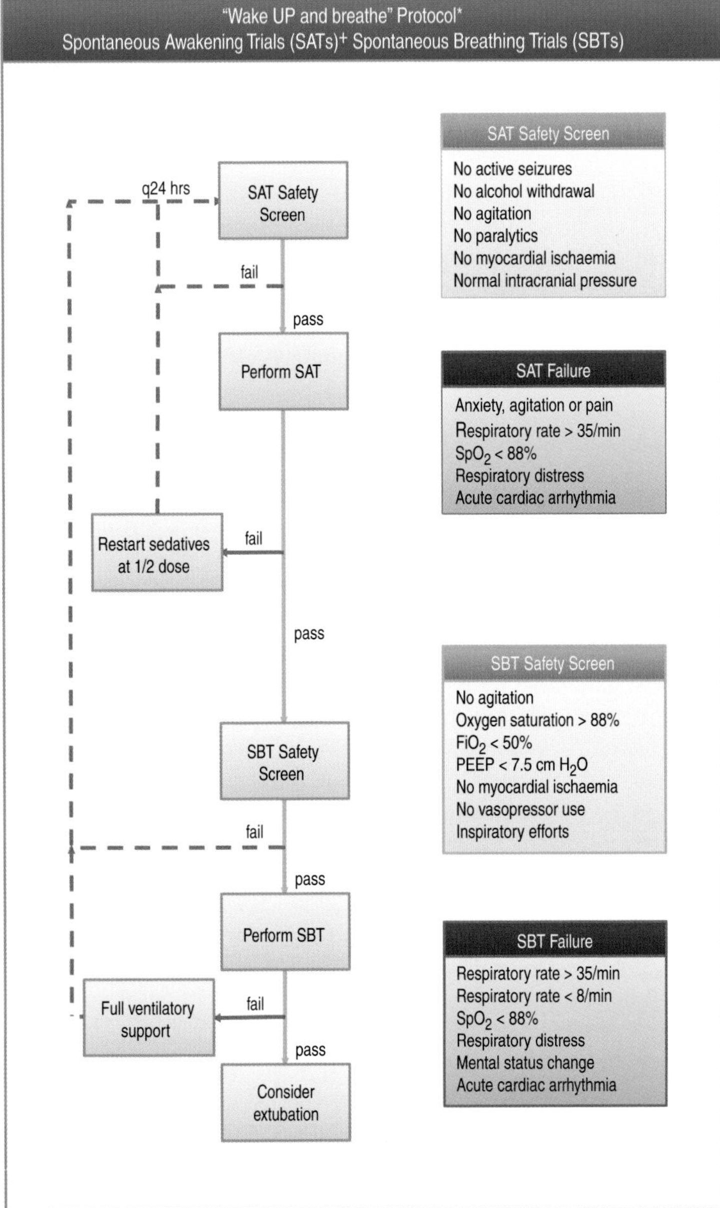

Fig. 12.4 'Wake up and breathe' protocol: spontaneous awakening trials (SATs) + spontaneous breathing trials (SBTs). (Adapted from Girard TD *et al.* (2008) *Lancet* **371**: 126–34.)

Neuroleptic agents

Haloperidol and chlorpromazine are useful agents for treating post-operative psychosis and delirium in critical care. They act via a range of receptors including dopaminergic, α-adrenergic, histamine, serotonin and cholinergic receptors. The desired effects of neurolepsis are reduced motor activity, anxiolysis, reduced aggression and indifference to external environment. Their effects on different receptors also give rise to a wide range of side effects including extrapyramidal effects, anticholinergic affects, arrhythmias, hypotension and neuroleptic malignant syndrome.

Neuromuscular blockade

It is important to remember that neuromuscular blocking agents do not have sedative properties. Their use should be limited to patients who remain difficult to oxygenate despite optimum ventilation strategies and are on alternative ventilation strategies such as inverse ratios, or high-frequency oscillatory ventilation. Patients who receive neuromuscular blocking agents must be adequately sedated and should have regular assessments for continued need of paralysis. Prolonged use is associated with chronic muscle weakness and critical care myopathy.

Use of protocols and sedation breaks

The inability to assess a patient's mental state during the course of critical illness is a major drawback of deep sedation. A protocol-driven approach with daily interruptions of sedation will provide a time when depth of sedation can be evaluated and adjusted according to the individual patient's needs. It will minimize the effect of accumulation of drugs in fat stores and redistribution back to the circulation can take place by stopping sedation. The ICU team should be aware that not all patients will wake appropriately with sedation breaks. Excessive agitation should lead to cessation of the waking attempt to avoid incidents such as self-extubation.

The recent Awakening and Breathing Control (ABC) Trial suggested that a 'wake up and breathe' protocol (Fig. 12.4) which pairs daily spontaneous awakening trials with daily spontaneous breathing trials results in better outcomes for mechanically ventilated patients in intensive care. Results from the group with daily sedation break had earlier extubation and more ventilator-free days. Previous studies have demonstrated that daily sedation breaks were associated with lower incidence of complications of critical illness such as ventilator-associated pneumonia, venous thromboembolism and bacteraemia. Interestingly, the same group of researchers also found that no patient from the sedation break group reported post-traumatic stress disorder compared with one-third of those who did not have daily sedation breaks.

Future developments

Traditionally, the most common approach is hypnotic-based sedation (HBS), where midazolam and propofol are used with opioid as an analgesic. However, the advent of remifentanil has allowed for greater use of analgesic-based sedation (ABS) where the relief of pain is the main objective. Many critical care units have adapted and developed their own sedation strategy and protocol. The goal is to provide a comfortable and stress-free environment for the patients by using a balanced approach to analgesia and sedation. In the future, the focus will be on how best to deliver and monitor sedation in critically ill patients, with more sensitive and easy to use monitoring equipment becoming more widely available.

Key points

- Agitation is very common in critical care patients.
- Analgesics and sedatives are used to improve the comfort and safety of critically ill patients.
- Oversedation can lead to prolonged mechanical ventilation and ICU stay, and an increased risk of nosocomial infection.
- Required level of sedation should be assessed regularly for each patient and scoring systems used to provide monitoring of patient's level of sedation.
- There is currently no ideal sedative available and each agent should be used with caution as to its potential side effects.
- Neuromuscular blockade should be avoided.
- The recent Awakening and Breathing Control (ABC) trial suggested that a 'wake up and breathe' protocol that pairs daily spontaneous awakening trials with daily spontaneous breathing trials results in better outcomes for mechanically ventilated patients in intensive care.

Further reading

- Girard TP (2008) Efficacy and safety of a paired sedation and ventilator weaning protocol for mechanically ventilated patients in intensive care (Awakening and Breathing Controlled trial): a randomised controlled trial. *Lancet* **371**(9607): 126–34.
- Guttormson JL, Chlan L, Weinert C *et al.* (2009) Factors influencing nurse sedation practices with mechanically ventilated patients: a US national survey. *Intens. Crit. Care Nurs.* Nov. 27 (Epub ahead of print).
- Jacobi J (2002) Clinical practice guidelines for the sustained use of sedatives and analgesics in the critically ill adult. *Crit. Care Med.* **30**(1): 119–36.
- Kress JP (2000) Daily interruption of sedative infusions in critically ill patients undergoing mechanical ventilation. *N. Engl. J. Med.* **322**(20): 1471–7.
- Muellejans B (2004) Remifentanil versus fentanyl for analgesia based sedation to provide patient comfort in the intensive care unit: a randomized, double-blind controlled trial. *Crit. Care* **8**: R1–R11.

Chapter 13

Ethics

John Bleasdale

Doctors have an ethical obligation to show respect for human life; protect the health of their patients; and to make their patients' best interests their primary concern. This means offering those treatments where the possible benefits outweigh any burdens or risks associated with the treatment, and avoiding those treatments where there is no net benefit to the patient.

Introduction

Ordinarily, when discussing treatment options with a patient, doctors manage to fulfil this ethical obligation by ensuring that the patient's treatment choices are accommodated as far as possible. For a variety of reasons this is not always possible in critical care.

The particular nature of critical care does not mean that we can forgo our ethical obligations when providing care, for even in the apparently impersonal and technical critical care environment clinical decision making is essentially an encounter between two human beings and, as such, is rooted in a moral context.

The purpose of this chapter is to provide a starting point for understanding the ethical framework of critical care; some ethical theories will briefly be considered before suggesting an approach to decision making. The problems of consent in critical care will be reviewed and finally a consideration of end-of-life decision making.

Ethical framework of critical care

Ethical theories

Though an ethical judgement is a decision of the moment, pertinent to the circumstances of the individual case, philosophers and ethicists believe that there are basic theories that we can use when faced with such problems. There are many different ethical theories but three have become the most influential in medical ethics. Two of these theories are best thought of as a concept for trying to define what the good is in making a decision. For the deontologist the good is doing your duty, for the utilitarian it is maximizing happiness. Unfortunately these theories often conflict when a clinician is faced with a difficult decision.

Deontology – the ethics of absolutes. Based on the work of Immanuel Kant (1724–1804) who considered that the ethical duty lay in the action itself, irrespective of the outcome. The fundamental rule and the basic good for Kantian ethics is that you must never act in any way that cannot be universally applied. Therefore 'bending' the rules to achieve a desired outcome in an individual case is not sustainable. If this were universally applied and the rules were 'bent' in all cases it would render rules pointless. Therefore 'It is always wrong to lie' and 'It is always wrong to bring about the death of another human being' (whatever the circumstances) are Kantian absolutes.

Utilitarianism – the greatest good for the greatest number. Utilitarianism is based on the work of Jeremy Bentham (1748–1832) and John Mill (1806–1873). Utilitarians considered that an action is right if it produces consequences that are of net social benefit, the balance of happiness against unhappiness is maximized over society. The correct act is that which, in the individual case, produces the greatest happiness for the greatest number.

These two theories consider clinical decision making from opposite approaches. A utilitarian considers the consequences of the act to be the basis for ethical decision making whereas for the deontologist the origin or will of the act is the significant factor. Some argue that utilitarianism is a morally superior approach as it generates more happiness for more parties. However it also permits the interests of the majority to trample on the rights of the minority.

Principlism – is an alternative approach, drawing its ideals from many different ethical theories, including

Core Topics in Critical Care Medicine, eds. Fang Gao Smith and Joyce Yeung. Published by Cambridge University Press.

deontology and utilitarianism. Rather than considering the value of an individual act (or medical decision) principlism considers that for any act there are a set of values that need to be balanced before an act can be viewed as ethical. Using this system any ethical decision is reached after considering four key ethical principles:

(1) Beneficence – acting for the benefit of patients.
(2) Non-maleficence – an obligation not to inflict harm on patients.
(3) Respect for autonomy – ensuring patients remain in control of their own lives.
(4) Justice – ensuring treatment is fair, equitable and appropriate.

Unfortunately, as with deontology and utilitarianism, some of these principles conflict (e.g. should I do what the patient wants or should I do what I think is best for this patient?). But there is no natural ranking order leading to potential conflict between clinicians and with patients.

To actually understand what beneficence, non-maleficence, autonomy and justice mean you must start with a set of presuppositions about the meaning of good, bad, free will and fairness. These are ultimately rooted in your own, and your patient's, ideology, leading to personal interpretations which may conflict. This may lead to a form of social/cultural relativism when applying them to clinical decision making. In a multi-faith, pluralist society such as ours, there will generally be no consensus on the ranking or appropriateness of the principles. Thus in any two individual cases given the same clinical scenario there may develop different treatment decisions. This is not a failing of principlism but one of its strengths.

The principles are essentially those of Western culture and relying on them exclusively may cause conflict with other cultural groups. Some ethicists, and some cultural groups, would suggest that other principles, such as love, sacrifice for others and interdependence, have at least equal priority. And patients may introduce these when discussing treatment options.

A practical approach to decision making

In critical care prompt decisions are often required and we may not have the luxury of approaching a complex decision by considering each of the ethical theories and principles outlined above. (There are, of course, other ethical theories and approaches we could also consider – see Further reading list). What we need is a reproducible approach for identifying the ethical problems of a case that can be applied in all circumstances. The system of Jonsen, Siegler and Winslade described in *Clinical Ethics: A Practical Approach to Ethical Decisions in Clinical Medicine* is a clear and systematic four-step approach that can be used for every medical encounter.

For every decision on each case, especially those raising an ethical problem, consideration should be given to the medical indications, patient preferences, quality of life and contextual features of the decision. By considering each of these steps in turn the ethical problems can be identified and placed into the context of the clinical problem.

The four steps provide a system for considering the clinical encounter in the context of ethical principlism.

Medical indications – beneficence and non-maleficence

What are the benefits for this patient from my proposed treatment and what is the likely outcome? After considering the history, diagnosis and prognosis, consider the goals of treatment. Is it curable or not? What is the best outcome treatment can offer and what are the probabilities of success? It is also imperative to review what could be done in the event of treatment failure.

Patient preferences – autonomy

Has everything been done to ensure that the patient's right to choose has been respected? Are they competent (see consent issues below)? Establish their wishes for treatment and whether they have previously expressed any limitations (e.g. Jehovah's Witnesses).

Quality of life – beneficence, non-maleficence and autonomy

Could there be a change in the patient's quality of life if treatment succeeds? Is that your judgement or theirs? Would that be acceptable to them? Ensure that treatment failure is considered and palliative care is considered (see withdrawal of care below).

Social, economic, legal and administrative context – justice

What are the family/cultural/religious issues and do they affect treatment decisions? Is there a problem of resource allocation that may affect the treatment plan? Consideration will also have to be given to legal issues and whether there is any conflict of interest on the part of the doctors or the hospital.

The significance and implication of the ethical principles and any conflicts they provide can only be truly appreciated when considered within the context of the whole case. Once this system has been applied and the facts of the case are made clear the relevant issues will become clear and an appraisal of the principles will reveal which one is the priority. Only then can an honest discussion take place between the patient and the doctor, and by trying to understand each other's arguments, can a reasoned treatment plan be devised.

Consent

One of the cornerstones of good medical practice is that before providing treatment or involving a patient in teaching, or research, you must be satisfied that you have a valid authority. Usually this requires the patient to consent to the proposed treatment.

However, in any situation where treatment is immediately necessary to save life or avoid significant deterioration and consent cannot be obtained, you may provide such treatment. This is the necessity principle; you cannot 'use' this principle to perform procedures that are not essential for the patient's survival and any treatment given must not be more extensive than is necessary. Even so if the patient has made an advanced refusal, that you are made aware of, you must respect it.

Beyond the necessity principle, obtaining consent may not be particularly straightforward. For consent to be valid all the relevant information must be provided to patients in an easily understandable form. They must take part in the decision making process and freely submit to treatment. However, the complexities of treatment options and severity of the patient's illness make it difficult to establish whether they can offer a truly valid consent. Patients who are considered unable to offer a valid consent are said to lack capacity or be incompetent.

Capacity

When it is unclear whether a patient possesses or lacks capacity we need guidance. Direction on the validity of consent, due to the capacity of an individual, has previously been obtained from common law. Unfortunately the guidance available from these rulings is unclear. This changed in 2007 with the enactment of the Mental Capacity Act 2005 (England and Wales).

Mental Capacity Act 2005 – Section 1 states that it must be assumed all persons have capacity. It also makes clear that all practicable steps have to be taken to help them make a decision and that merely because a decision is unwise does not indicate incapacity.

The Act then goes on to establish, in civil law, a description of what renders a person incapacitated (Section 2):

People who lack capacity

(1) *For the purposes of this Act, a person lacks capacity in relation to a matter if at the material time he is unable to make a decision for himself in relation to the matter because of an impairment of, or a disturbance in the functioning of, the mind or brain.*

(2) *It does not matter whether the impairment or disturbance is permanent or temporary.*

(3) *A lack of capacity cannot be established merely by reference to –*
   - (a) *a person's age or appearance, or*
   - (b) *a condition of his, or an aspect of his behaviour, which might lead others to make unjustified assumptions about his capacity*

It would appear that, because of their medical condition, many critical care patients could be considered incompetent. The Act makes it clear that the extent of the patient's condition and complexity of the treatment do not automatically preclude the patient from providing a valid consent. As each consent issue has to be viewed as an independent event, 'at the material time', we must make an assessment of a patient's capacity for each decision. Though incompetent to consent on one treatment a patient may be more than capable of consenting, or refusing their consent, for another.

The Act then goes on to provide guidance on assessing a person's inability to make decisions (Section 3):

Inability to make decisions

(1) *For the purposes of section 2, a person is unable to make a decision for himself if he is unable –*
   - (a) *to understand the information relevant to the decision,*
   - (b) *to retain the information,*
   - (c) *to use or weigh that information as part of the process of making the decision, or*
   - (d) *to communicate his decision (whether by talking, using sign language or any other means)*

The Act has provided us with a legal definition of capacity and some tests we must apply before deciding that a patient lacks capacity. For a patient to be capable of offering a valid consent all the relevant information must be provided in an easily understandable form, they must then demonstrate that they can understand and retain the information then communicate this decision to us.

Best interests

If we establish that a patient lacks capacity how then are we to provide treatment that is not necessarily life saving?

Doctors are allowed to provide care in this situation by considering the patient's best interests. The Act (Section 5.1) allows a doctor (D) to act in connection with the care of a patient (P) lacking capacity if:

(b) *when doing the act, D reasonably believes –*
  - (i) *that P lacks capacity in relation to the matter, and*
  - (ii) *that it will be in P's best interests for the act to be done.*

Though the Act outlines who should be consulted (anyone named, caring for or interested in the patient's welfare) and what to consider when determining a patient's best interests (wishes, feelings and belief values of the patient), there is no definition of best interest proposed.

For guidance we must turn to established interpretations of best interests. In the past, best interests were exclusively medical, giving rise to the prolongation of life at almost any cost. However, with the ability of modern critical care to prolong life beyond the irreversible loss of awareness, the wider best interests (e. g. wishes, values and family life) of the patient are acquiring equal importance. If we restrict ourselves to medical best interests we have a common law test for guidance. Best interests are judged by what other doctors consider as being reasonable, so long as this belief is logical. If we expand best interests to include the wider interests of the patient then it is not clear if doctors are necessarily best placed to make these decisions and this test may be inappropriate.

End-of-life care

Society has developed an unrealistic belief that we can prolong life indefinitely and that death is no longer an inevitability but a failure of medicine. Though we may be able to prolong life far beyond what was previously possible we must not forget that the primary goal of medicine is the reinstatement of a patient's health as far as possible. For the majority the prolongation of life, sometimes without a return to prior levels of health, is an appropriate goal. However, the prolongation of life at all costs, without regard to the quality of that life or the burdens imposed by treatment, may not always be desirable.

In critical care the hardest decisions are those concerning when to withhold or withdraw treatment. Despite this the majority of patients who die in critical care departments do so after a decision to withhold or withdraw life-prolonging care.

Withholding and withdrawing life-prolonging care

It may seem that withholding a treatment and withdrawing a treatment that has already started are very different decisions. This is not the case, for just as a doctor cannot offer a treatment that is non-beneficial neither can a treatment continue if it is no longer providing any benefit. Once it is clear that a treatment cannot provide the desired benefit then the justification for its use, or continued use, is removed.

The benefit derived from a treatment can be viewed on two levels. Firstly if the benefit is the restoration of physiological targets, and a treatment is either unable to achieve these targets, or once started is failing to achieve them, then this is clearly a medical decision and the decision to withhold or withdraw it is medical. Though this should be communicated to the patient (and/or their family) consultation with them is not necessary to make such a decision. Secondly if a treatment can provide a medical benefit we must consider whether it can provide a broader benefit, to include the balance of physiological outcome and the burdens of treatment. This is a decision based on the best interests of the patient and will require a discussion with the patient or their family before it can be considered valid.

During discussions with patients and their families the term 'futility' has been applied to these two types of decision. This is best avoided as it causes confusion between the two types of decision and is often too inflammatory a term to be using with patients and families at this stage in their illness.

Refusing life-prolonging care

Whenever life-prolonging treatment is being considered some competent patients decide that there is a stage in their illness beyond which they do not wish such treatment to be continued. They make this known to the medical team and, as with all other medical decisions, their wishes must be respected. Other patients feel that during a serious or life-threatening illness there may not be the time for these discussions to take place and, if they lose their capacity to be involved, continued life-prolonging treatment would result in a quality of life they would find unacceptable. In these circumstances they may express their views in an advance decision or appoint a welfare attorney to act on their behalf.

Advance decision

An advance decision can cover a range of circumstances (e.g. birth plan, Jehovah's Witnesses' refusal of blood transfusions) but most commonly applies to life-prolonging treatment. An advanced decision must be expressed at a time when the patient is competent, acting free of pressure and has been offered accurate information. It will only apply when they lose capacity. An advance decision may be presented as a formal written document, but it is not necessary for the refusal to be in writing for it to be valid. If, during a discussion about treatment, a patient clearly indicates their wishes this will have the same status as a written advance directive. Any decision in an advance decision is binding, but can be reversed by the patient if they are judged to be competent at the time of reversal.

Welfare attorney

The Mental Capacity Act makes provision for the appointment of persons with lasting power of attorney. This transfers the authority to make personal (property and affairs) and welfare (health) decisions from the patient to a specified spokesperson in the event of a loss of capacity. This person is responsible for ensuring that decisions are made in accordance with the Act and in the best interests of the patient. This is the only circumstance where one adult can consent on behalf of another. Consent must be sought from the welfare attorney before all non-necessary treatment can start but the authority of the welfare attorney only extends to life-prolonging treatment if specified.

In the event of a disagreement between medical staff and a welfare attorney regarding life-prolonging treatment the Court of Protection may be approached for a declaration.

In the UK the majority of patients admitted to critical care do not have an advance decision recorded or welfare attorney appointed. If these patients lose their capacity to be involved in decision making then treatment may be provided, withheld or withdrawn only if the doctor is satisfied that such treatment is in the patient's best interest. The assessment of best interests in these circumstances is exactly the same as for any medical decision where a patient lacks capacity. As the family are best placed to consider the broader best interests of the patient their input is crucial.

If a patient lacking an advance decision or welfare attorney does not have any close relatives or friends to help in these deliberations then an Independent Mental Capacity Advocate (IMCA) must be consulted. An IMCA cannot consent on behalf of such a patient but their views must be taken into account when assessing the best interests of the patient.

Whether there are relatives or an IMCA, in the absence of an advance decision or appointed welfare attorney, the treatment decision rests with the doctor.

Key points

- Good ethical decision making is the cornerstone of critical care medicine.
- By being aware of a few ethical theories and the particular problems surrounding consent, then considering the case as a whole rather than as individual ethical vignettes, better treatment decisions will be made.
- The Mental Capacity Act provides a test for considering capacity that we must use whenever we are considering treatment as well as providing a structure for establishing decisions for those who lack capacity.
- When considering end-of-life issues good communication with patients and their relatives is essential for establishing priorities and ensuring that the wishes of the patient are paramount.

Further reading

- Adults with Incapacity (Scotland) www.opsi.gov.uk/legislation/scotland/acts2000/20000004.htm
- Beauchamp TL, Childress JF (2001) *Principles of Biomedical Ethics*, 5th edn. New York: Oxford University Press.

- British Medical Association (2007) *Withholding and Withdrawing Life-Prolonging Medical Treatment*, 3rd edn. London: BMJ Books.
- General Medical Council (2002) *Withholding and Withdrawing Life-Prolonging Treatments: Good Practice in Decision Making*. Manchester, UK: General Medical Council. www.gmc-uk.org/guidance/current/library/witholding_lifeprolonging_guidance.asp
- Intensive Care Society (2007) *Ethical Issues in Intensive Care*, Critical Care Focus No. 13. London: Intensive Care Society.
- Jonsen AR, Siegler M, Winslade WJ (2006) *Clinical Ethics: A Practical Approach to Ethical Decisions in Clinical Medicine*, 6th edn. New York: McGraw Hill.
- Mental Capacity Act 2005 www.opsi.gov.uk/acts/acts2005/20050009.htm
- Neuberger J (2004) *Caring for Dying People of Different Faiths*, 3rd edn. Abingdon, UK: Radcliffe Medical Press.
- Walton DN (1987) *Ethics of Withdrawal of Life-Support Systems*. New York: Praeger.

Chapter

14 Organ donation

Angeline Simons and Joyce Yeung

Introduction

Organ and tissue transplantation is one of the major medical success stories of our time. The first reported corneal graft dated back to 1905 in the Czech Republic and in 1954, Dr Joseph Murray performed the first successful kidney transplant between two identical twins in USA. Since then, over a million people worldwide have had their lives saved or their quality of life improved by an organ transplant.

Results of organ transplantation continue to improve and 1-year survival post transplant is now as high as 90%. This success has led to the current situation where the demand for organs outstrips supply. The NHS can only continue to meet the need for organs and tissues for transplantation if the public is educated about organ donation. Critical care staff have to continue to identify all potential donors and co-ordinate with transplant professionals who will retrieve high quality organs and tissues.

The Department of Health's policy for the development of transplant services in England is set out in *Saving Lives, Valuing Donors: A Transplant Framework for England*. This aims to increase organ donation and transplant rates by investing in programmes aimed at maximizing both living and cadaveric organ donation.

Epidemiology

In the UK there are currently 26 adult NHS renal transplant units, seven liver transplant units and seven cardiothoracic transplant units. In addition, other surgeons perform well over 10 000 surgical procedures involving tissue transplants. Despite their efforts, the UK has one of lowest rates of organ donation in the Western world.

During the year 2007–2008, there was a 5% increase in solid organ transplant mainly due to an increase in the number of living organ donors. The majority of organ donations were from deceased donors and 80% of these were on the organ donation register. Only 30% of renal transplants in the UK were from living donors compared to 80% in some Nordic countries.

Every year, many patients die whilst waiting for a transplant. The need for transplanted organs is always increasing due to the changing demographics of the population. In 2009 the active transplant list stands at around 8000; however, this underestimates the true need as patients who do not fulfil set criteria are not added to the transplant list even if they are in need of one.

People from South Asian backgrounds are four times more likely than those from European backgrounds to require a renal transplant. This is due to increased prevalence of diseases such as diabetes and hypertension; however, this population group is much less likely to be on the organ donation register. Ethnic minorities are under-represented on the organ donation register and there has been a strong drive to encourage ethnic minorities to join the register.

Types of organ donation

There are four types of organ donation: living donation, xeno-transplantation, non-heart-beating donation (NHBD) and heart-beating donation (HBD). The latter two are both forms of cadaveric donation and are most relevant in the critical care setting.

Heart-beating donation

All patients who have confirmed brainstem death can be heart-beating donors (HBD). Further consideration will then take into account their past medical history, past surgical history and the events during hospital admission.

The number of HBDs is declining and this is likely to continue for two reasons. Fewer young people are

Core Topics in Critical Care Medicine, eds. Fang Gao Smith and Joyce Yeung. Published by Cambridge University Press.

dying as a result of severe injury or catastrophic cerebrovascular events. This together with changes in diagnosis and management of severe brain injuries means that fewer patients will fulfil the brainstem testing criteria. At present, death is increasingly likely to follow withdrawal of active treatment and so in the future, NHBDs are likely to become more important in maintaining the organ transplant programmes.

Brainstem death

In the UK, the term of brainstem death was accepted in 1976. Brainstem death produces a state of irreversible loss of consciousness associated with the loss of central respiratory function. It is accepted as being equivalent to somatic death as it represents a state when 'the body as an integrated whole has ceased to function'.

Brainstem death is diagnosed in three stages:

(1) It must be established that the patient has suffered an event of known aetiology resulting in irreversible brain damage with apnoeic coma.
(2) Reversible causes of coma must be excluded.
(3) Bedside brainstem tests are undertaken to confirm the diagnosis of brainstem death.

Preconditions to brainstem death testing

There are three important preconditions that must be met prior to testing:

(1) The patient's condition is due to irreversible brain damage of known aetiology. This may be obvious such as a severe head injury or intracranial haemorrhage. However, when a patient has suffered primarily from cardiac arrest, hypoxia or severe circulatory insufficiency with cerebral hypoxia, it may take longer to establish the diagnosis. It is generally recommended therefore that if brainstem death is secondary to generalized cerebral hypoxia from cardiac arrest the tests should not be performed until a minimum of 24 hours have elapsed.
(2) The patient is in unresponsive coma. Coma is due to cerebral damage of known aetiology and reversible causes of coma have been excluded.
(3) The patient is apnoeic and mechanically ventilated.

Reversible causes of coma

Potentially reversible causes of coma must be excluded and include:

(1) Sedative drugs: sedatives may have prolonged action, particularly in the presence of hypothermia, renal or hepatic failure. In order to exclude the effects of sedative drugs, it may involve prediction according to pharmacokinetic principles, the measurement of drug concentrations or the use of antagonists in the case of opioids or benzodiazepines. If the patient is thought to be brainstem dead, it is advisable to wait to perform the tests when the effect of sedatives can be excluded.
(2) Neuromuscular blocking agents: the effect of neuromuscular relaxants must be excluded as the cause of coma or respiratory failure by eliciting adequate neuromuscular function with a peripheral nerve stimulator.
(3) Hypothermia: the core temperature must be >34° C.
(4) Circulatory, metabolic or endocrine disturbances: circulatory, metabolic and endocrine disturbances can occur as a result of the physiological consequences of brainstem compression and death; these should not preclude certification of death by brainstem testing. However, the correction of these physiological abnormalities is advisable before brainstem testing if the severity of the disturbance is profound enough to cause depression of consciousness (e.g. severe hypernatraemia or profound hypotension).

Confirmation of brainstem death

These tests must be performed by two experienced clinicians, who have been registered with GMC for more than 5 years, on two separate occasions. They should be competent in critical care and in the certification of brainstem death. One clinician must be of a consultant level and neither can be members of the transplant team.

This relies on testing the cranial nerves whose nuclei are in the brainstem and testing spontaneous respiration.

The tests are as follows:

- Pupillary light reflex (cranial nerves II and III) – a light is shone into both pupils and reaction is noted. Trauma and drugs affecting pupillary reaction would have been excluded.
- Corneal reflex (cranial nerves V and VII) – the cornea is stimulated with cotton wool to look for blink response.

- Gag reflex (cranial nerve IX) – a suction catheter is applied down the endotracheal tube to stimulate the gag reflex.
- Oculovestibular reflex (cranial nerves VI and VII) – before testing patient's ears should be examined with otoscope to ensure that tympanic membranes can be directly visualized. 50 ml of cold water is then irrigated into the external auditory meatus over 1 min and patient's eyes are examined to look for absence of movement or nystagmus.
- No motor response to central stimulation.
- No motor response within the cranial nerve or somatic distribution in response to supraorbital pressure.
- Apnoea test. Before the test, the patient should be pre-oxygenated with 100% oxygen for 15 min. An arterial blood gas should be taken to confirm a $PaCO_2 > 5$. If this is not achieved the patient can be ventilated with 95% oxygen and 5% carbon dioxide. Once the $PaCO_2 > 5$, the patient should be disconnected from the ventilator and given oxygen of 100% via a suction catheter down the endotracheal tube. Serial arterial blood gases are done to monitor the $PaCO_2$. If $PaCO_2$ reaches 6.65 and there is no evidence of spontaneous respiration, persistent apnoea has been confirmed and the patient is reconnected to the ventilator.

Non-heart-beating donation

This should be considered in any patient who is:

- >60 years of age
- has an irreversible condition so that after withdrawing treatment death is inevitable.

Criteria to be fulfilled for non-heart-beating donation (NHBD):

- no abnormal liver or renal biochemistry
- BMI < 30
- no long-standing untreated hypertension
- no long-standing diabetes mellitus
- no high dose inotropic requirements
- no history of ischaemic heart disease prior to admission
- no untreated sepsis or treated but unresponsive sepsis.

Once the criteria for non-heart-beating donation have been fulfilled and the decision to withdraw treatment has been made independent of the transplant team there are strict time constraints from the time of treatment withdrawal to death of the patient. This is to ensure that the organs have not suffered from hypoxic damage or haemodynamic compromise. Unfortunately this leaves a very short time for the family to say goodbye before the patient is taken to theatre for organ retrieval (Fig. 14.1).

Contraindications to tissue donation

The Advisory Committee on the Microbiological Safety of Blood and Tissues for Transplantation (MSBT) provides national guidance on donor evaluation and testing. This guidance is updated regularly on their website and the donor transplant co-ordinator will be aware of the latest advice and guidance. Essentially, the guidance sets out criteria for screening potential donors so as to identify the risk of transmission of disease from donor to recipient (Table 14.1).

Other clinical conditions may affect the eligibility of organ donation. Please refer to the MSBT website for most up to date information. Some examples of contraindications are given below:

- Active TB/encephalitis/meningitis.
- Previous organ transplant.
- Growth hormone therapy.
- Malignancies of blood and bone marrow, leukaemia, myeloma, lymphoma.
- High-risk behaviour predisposing to HIV, hepatitis B and C.
- Disorders of the CNS where no clear diagnosis has been identified.
- Colonization with MRSA.

Further exclusion criteria

- Patient must pass away within 3 hours of withdrawal of treatment.
- If saturations are <80% for more than 30 min.
- If systolic BP <50 mmHg for more than 30 min.

Organs that can be donated

- Kidneys
- Liver

Table 14.1 Requirements for microbiological testing of all donors

Infection	Test	Organs	Tissues	Cells
HIV1 and 2	HIV1 and 2 antibody	X	X	X
Hepatitis B	HBsAg	X Consider only in life-saving situations (after discussion of implications with recipients) or in patients already infected or immune to hepatitis B	X	X Except autologous transplants and related where chemoprophylaxis and immunization may be acceptable
Hepatitis C	HCV antibody	X Consider only in life-saving situations (as above) or in those already infected	X	X Except autologous transplants and cord blood donation where mother is infected
Syphilis	Treponemal specific antibody	Acceptable	Acceptable for cornea and sclera	Acceptable

X denotes contraindicated.

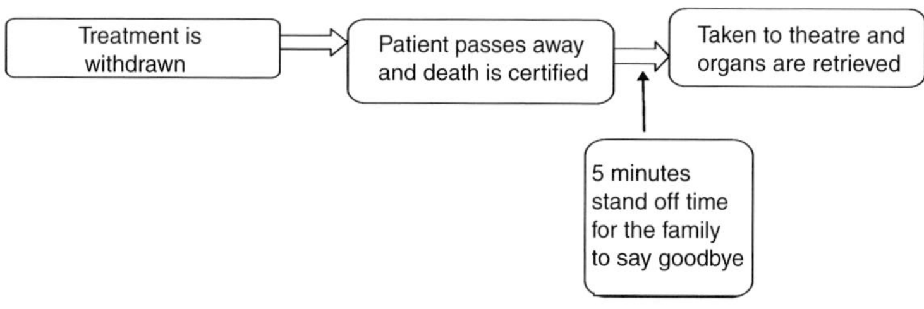

Fig. 14.1 Schematic diagram illustrating the process for non-heart-beating organ donation.

- Cornea
- Pancreas
- Heart
- Lungs
- Skin
- Bone
- Cartilage

Corneal donation

The criteria for corneal donation are not as strict. Corneas have been harvested up to 24 hours after asystole. The main contraindications for corneal donation are diseases affecting the eye such as:

- Leukaemias, myelomas, lymphomas.
- Scarring corneal ulcers.
- Malignant ocular tumours.

Role of the donor transplant co-ordinator

Within the Transplant Framework, the donor transplant co-ordinator has an important educational and supportive role for healthcare professionals and for the families of potential organ and tissue donors (Figs. 14.2 and 14.3).

It is essential that the donor transplant co-ordinator is informed of all potential donors as early as possible so that any retrieval can be expedited. The co-ordinator can ascertain the suitability of potential donors and provide advice to staff on donor identification and clinical management. However, the relatives of HBDs should not be formally approached until after the first set of brainstem tests has been performed unless the topic of organ donation has already been raised by the relatives during discussions about the patient's prognosis. Early referral will also ensure that the donor transplant co-ordinator is able to attend

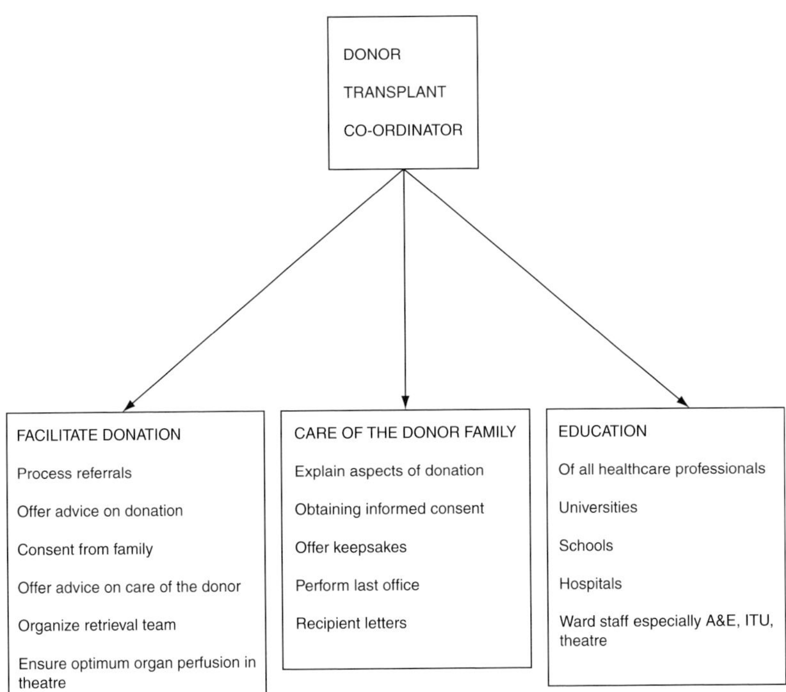

Fig. 14.2 Role of the donor transplant co-ordinator.

the referring unit at an early stage to facilitate the organ donation process.

Management of the potential donor

The process of donation can take time and it is vital that a potential HBD receives full physiological support so that organs remain in optimal condition. Whilst ethically this may not be in the best interest of the patient, it will be in the best interest of the recipient of the organs. An organ that has been retrieved and transplanted in a suboptimal condition is a major cause of graft failure. Physiological parameters should be kept as close to normal as possible until organ transplantation takes place:

- The donor should remain intubated and ventilated to maintain adequate oxygenation.
- Inotropes may need to be commenced or continued to maintain adequate perfusion pressure to all the major organs.
- Hypoglycaemia and hyperglycaemia should be avoided by the use of insulin sliding scale.
- Electrolyte imbalance should be corrected and hydration maintained by intravenous maintenance fluids.

The donor operation takes place in an operating theatre at the referring hospital and is performed by surgeons from the retrieving hospital. Retrieval teams normally bring all the equipment and staff they need although at present this may not routinely include an anaesthetist. An anaesthetist or intensivist from the referring hospital provides valuable liaison between visiting teams and operating theatre staff and assistance during the operation.

Ethics and consent

The public is very supportive of organ donation in principle, with 15 million already on the NHS Organ Donor Register. However, the actual donation rate remains poor, partly due to 40% of relatives refusing to give consent. The removal, storage and use of organs or part organs from a deceased person for the purpose of transplantation are governed by the Human Tissue Act 2004. The Act makes it lawful for donation from the deceased to take place provided that consent was given by the person prior to their death. In the absence of their wishes, consent can be obtained from the person nominated to act on their behalf, from a family member or a person close to the patient. Although legally if a patient has been registered on the Organ Donor Register, their consent has been obtained and transplantation can take

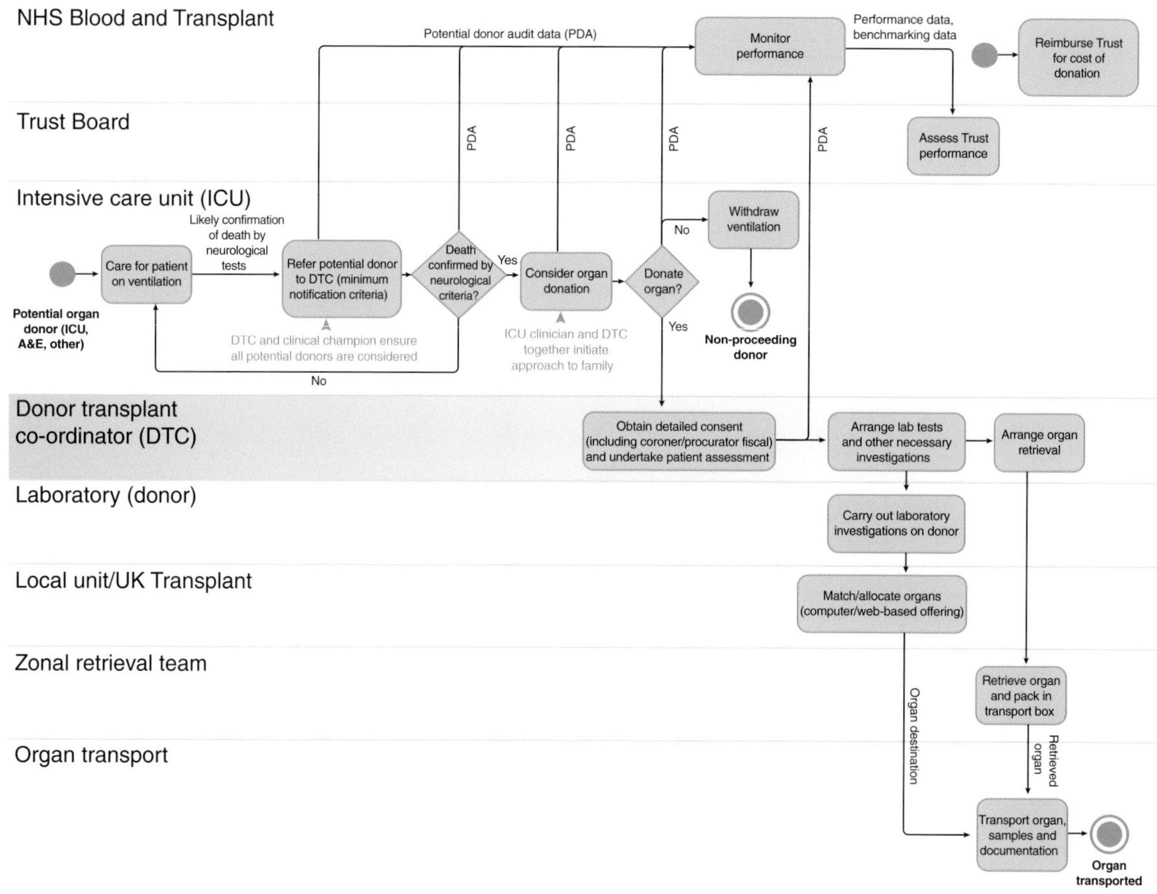

Fig. 14.3 The Transplant Framework in UK. (Courtesy of NHS Blood and Transplant.)

place legally, the wishes of their next of kin are respected and if consent is withdrawn then transplantation will not take place.

Although discussing organ donation at a time of great loss for the family may seem insensitive, it has been shown to provide some solace for them to know that they have given the gift of life to others. It is important that the staff caring for the patient and the family have a sound knowledge of different areas such as brainstem testing, and the need for continued invasive monitoring so they can provide explanation to the family. The donor transplant co-ordinator can be of support for both the critical care staff and the family. The approach to the family should be sensitive and the best time to discuss organ donation is found to be at the time of discussing the outcome of brainstem tests. It should be done in a quiet, private place where there will be no disturbances. It must be ensured that the family understand the outcome of the tests and that time is allowed for any questions. All aspects of organ donation should be discussed and time given for the family to ask questions.

The Organ Donation Taskforce

In 2006, the UK government set up the Organ Donation Taskforce (ODTF) to identify barriers to organ donation and draw up actions needed to increase organ donation. The ODFT is made up of medical professionals, NHS managers, patients and patient representatives and ethicists. The Taskforce has forecasted that a 50% increase in organ donation is 'possible and achievable in the UK within 5 years'.

The first report by the Taskforce in January 2008 has made some recommendations to unify the service into a nationwide Organ Donation Organization. The report also identified the need for the NHS to embrace organ donation as a usual event and to educate and promote organ donation to the general public.

In November 2008, the ODTF published a second report outlining an opt-out or presumed consent organ donation system and its potential impact in UK. The Taskforce concluded that whilst an opt-out system would have potential benefits, the challenges it would present may not be necessary to deliver the desired increase in organ donation rates and it should not be introduced at the present time.

Key points

- Organ transplantation is life-saving and the results continue to improve. However, demand greatly outstrips supply.
- Health inequality exists in that while the South Asian population is more likely to require organ transplantation, they remain under-represented in the Organ Donor Register.
- Critical care staff are most likely to be involved in the care of heart-beating donors (HBDs) and non-heart-beating donors (NHBDs).
- In HBD, brainstem death needs to be ascertained by brainstem testing. Brainstem death produces a state of irreversible loss of consciousness associated with the loss of central respiratory function and is accepted as being equivalent to somatic death.
- For patients whose condition is irreversible and death is imminent once treatment is withdrawn, then NHBD should be considered.
- The process of donation can take time and it is vital that a potential HBD receives full physiological support so that organs remain in optimal condition. An organ that has been retrieved and transplanted in a suboptimal condition is a major cause of graft failure.
- The removal, storage and use of organs or part organs from a deceased person for the purpose of transplantation are governed by the Human Tissue Act 2004. Although it is legal for organ donation to take place if patient is on the Organ Donor Register, if consent is withdrawn by next of kin, this is respected and transplantation will not take place.

Further reading

- Academy of Medical Royal Colleges (2008) *A Code of Practice for the Diagnosis of Brain Stem Death*. London: AC.
- Conference of Medical Royal Colleges and their Faculties in the United Kingdom (1996) Diagnosis of brainstem death. *Lancet* **ii**: 1069–70.
- Council of Europe (2001) *Meeting the Organ Shortage: Transplant Newsletter*. Madrid: Fundación Renal.
- Council of Europe (2003) *Guide to Safety and Quality Assurance for Organs, Tissues and Cells*. Brussels: Council of Europe.
- Department of Health (2000) *Guidance on the Microbiological Safety of Human Organs, Tissues and Cells Used for Transplantation*. London: Department of Health.
- Department of Health (2003) *Saving Lives, Valuing Donors: A Transplant Framework for England*. London: Department of Health.
- Institute of Medicine 2000 *Non-Heartbeating Organ Transplantation: Practice and Protocols*. Washington, DC: National Academy Press.
- Nicholson M (2002) *Kidney Transplantation from Non-Heartbeating Donors*. Peterborough, UK: National Kidney Research Fund.

Useful websites

- www.organdonation.nhs.uk NHS Blood and Transplant
- www.dh.gov.uk/en/Healthcare/Secondarycare/Transplantation/index.htm Department of Health website dedicated to organ donation and transplantation
- www.advisorybodies.doh.gov.uk/acmsbtt/index.htm. Website of Advisory Committee on the Microbiological Safety of Blood, Tissues & Organs for Transplantation

Section II Chapter

15 Systemic disorders and management

Sepsis

Yasser Tolba and David Thickett

Background and definitions

In 1992, the American College of Chest Physicians (ACCP)/Society of Critical Care Medicine (SCCM) introduced into common parlance the systemic inflammatory response syndrome (SIRS) and defined sepsis, severe sepsis and septic shock.

In 2001, ACCP/SCCM/ATS (American Thoracic Society)/SIS (Surgical Infection Society) revisited the definitions for sepsis and related conditions, which remained essentially unchanged (Table 15.1):

- Sepsis is the systemic response to infection.
- Infection: a pathological process induced by a micro-organism.
- Bacteraemia: the presence of viable bacteria in the blood.

The 1992 statement first introduced the concept *systemic inflammatory response syndrome* (SIRS). SIRS can be triggered by localized or generalized infection, trauma, thermal injury or sterile inflammatory processes, e.g. acute pancreatitis (Fig. 15.1). SIRS is therefore too non-specific to be of use in diagnosing cause for sepsis or in identifying a distinct pattern of host response.

The 2001 statement recommended the term of *signs and symptoms of infection* (SSI) to improve the limitations of SIRS criteria.

Sepsis is the clinical syndrome defined by the presence of both a SIRS and documented or suspected new infection. However, findings indicative of *early organ dysfunction* such as haemodynamic instability, arterial hypoxaemia, oliguria, lactic acidosis, coagulopathy, thrombocytopenia or altered liver function tests may be the first symptoms noted by clinicians at the bedside. Therefore, 2001 International Sepsis Definitions Conference suggests these criteria can be used to establish the diagnosis of sepsis.

Severe sepsis refers to sepsis complicated by organ dysfunction that can be defined by the Sequential Organ Failure Assessment (SOFA) scores ≥3 (see Table 15.2). Nevertheless, findings indicative of early organ dysfunction as described above are recommended for evaluation for severe sepsis screening tools to implement severe sepsis care bundles in Surviving Sepsis Campaign (SSC).

Septic shock in adults refers to a state of acute circulatory failure characterized by persistent arterial hypotension despite adequate volume resuscitation. Sepsis induced hypotension is defined by a systolic blood pressure <90 mmHg, a MAP <60, or a reduction of >40 mmHg from baseline, in the absence of other causes for hypotension. Patients who are receiving inotropic or vasopressor agents may not be hypotensive at the time that the perfusion abnormalities are measured. This is a subset of severe sepsis.

In neonates, post-operative patients and patients with trauma, burns, pancreatitis and neutropenia or organ transplantation, the diagnosis of infection may be unreliable using the SIRS criteria. Consequently, a number of laboratory markers have been evaluated as more specific indicators of sepsis, such as procalcitonin (PCT) or C-reactive protein (CRP), which could help in differentiating infectious from non-infectious causes of SIRS.

Pathophysiology

Opinions on the causes and potential therapies for sepsis have evolved significantly over the last 20 years. Mounting evidence suggests that beside well-established factors, such as virulence of pathogens or site of infection, individual differences in disease manifestation are a result of the genetic predisposition of the patient with sepsis. In this section we have concentrated upon the basic mechanisms of the septic process that are particularly relevant to clinical management.

Core Topics in Critical Care Medicine, eds. Fang Gao Smith and Joyce Yeung. Published by Cambridge University Press.

Table 15.1 Diagnostic criteria for sepsis from 2001 International Sepsis Definitions

Infection – a pathological process caused by the invasion of normally sterile tissue or fluid or body cavity by pathogenic or potentially pathogenic micro-organisms.

Signs and symptoms of infection (SSI) requires any two of following signs and symptoms both present and new to the patient:

temperature >38.3°C or <36.0°C
heart rate >90 beats per min (bpm)
respiratory rate >20 breaths per min
acutely altered mental status
leucocytosis – WBC >12 000/μl
leukopenia – WBC <4000/μl
hyperglycaemia (plasma glucose >7.7 mmol/l) in absence of diabetes
plasma C-reactive protein >2 SD above the normal value.

Sepsis is the clinical syndrome defined by the presence of both signs and symptoms of infection as described above and documented or suspected new infection.

Severe sepsis refers to sepsis complicated by one organ dysfunction that can be defined by the Sequential Organ Failure Assessment (SOFA) score.

Multi-organ failure: two or more organ dysfunction.
PaO_2/FiO_2 ≤26.7 kPa
Noradrenaline/adrenaline ≥0.1 μg/kg per min
Creatinine ≥330 μmol/l
Platelets ≤50 × 103/l
Bilirubin ≥102 μmol/l
Glasgow Coma Score <9

Septic shock in adults applies to a state of acute circulatory failure unexplained by other causes, defined as persistent arterial hypotension (a systolic blood pressure (SBP) <90, MAP <60, or a reduction in SBP 40 mmHg from baseline despite adequate volume resuscitation).

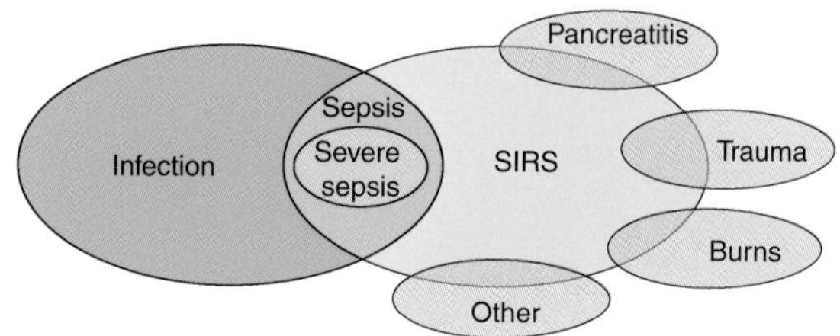

Fig. 15.1 Sepsis and SIRS. (Adapted from Bone RC *et al.* (1992) Definitions for sepsis and organ failure and guidelines for the use of innovative therapies in sepsis. *Chest* **101**: 1644–55.)

Cytokine cascade: too much of a good thing?

The inflammatory response is a central component of sepsis as it drives the physiological alterations that are recognized as SIRS. A successful inflammatory response eliminates the invading micro-organisms without causing lasting damage.

Sepsis develops when the initial, appropriate host response to an infection becomes amplified, and then excessive. Bacterial cell wall components such as lipopolysaccharide act as ligands for specific toll receptors and trigger monocytes, neutrophils, and endothelial cells (EC) to initiate an inflammatory cascade (Fig. 15.2).

Many believe that sepsis develops as a result of exuberant production of proinflammatory molecules such as TNF-α and IL-1, IL-6, lysosomal enzymes, superoxide-derived free radicals, vasoactive substances, such as platelet-activating factor (PAF), tissue factor (TF) and plasminogen activator inhibitor-1 (PAI-1).

Pro-inflammatory mediator release occurs in conjunction with increases in the expression of inducible nitric oxide (NO) synthase and NO release with resultant coagulopathy, endothelial dysfunction and vascular instability, and eventually leads to apoptosis (i.e. programmed cell death) and multi-organ failure.

Unfortunately, despite clinical trials of agents blocking single mediators, for example TNF-α and IL-1, results have been disappointing.

Cytokine cascade: too little of a good thing?

In contrast to the hypothesis of exuberant inflammatory response in sepsis is the finding that septic patients may have a relative anti-inflammatory environment. Thus, TNF : IL-10 ratios may be reduced, producing the equivalent of a blunted inflammatory response.

Defective mediator production in response to stimuli has been seen in both monocytes and T lymphocytes from sepsis patients. The blunted monocyte response seen in sepsis has been successfully reversed with interferon γ and this proved effective in a small series of sepsis patients. However, a larger trial of trauma patients showed that although interferon γ did reduce deaths due to infections, it did not reduce overall mortality.

A role for endothelial apoptosis in sepsis?

Cellular death may be a key factor in sepsis and its related mortality. Cells that are destined to die can do so by two mechanisms: apoptosis (programmed cell death) and necrosis:

- The role of endothelial cell apoptosis in sepsis remains inconclusive due to the challenges involved in study of endothelial cell death in vivo.

Table 15.2 Sequential Organ Failure Assessment (SOFA) scores

SOFA scores	1	2	3	4
Respiratory: PaO_2/FiO_2 (kPa)/(mmHg)	<53.2/400	<39.9/300	<26.6/200	<13.3/100
Coagulation: Platelets (× 10^9/l)	<150	<100	<50	<20
Liver: Bilirubin (μmol/l)	20–32	33–101	102–204	>204
Cardiovascular (mmHg) (μg/kg/min)	MAP <70	Dopamine <5 and/or dobutamine (any dose)	Dopamine 5.1–15 or Adrenaline <0.1 or Noradrenaline <0.1	Dopamine ≥15 or Adrenaline >0.1 or Noradrenaline >0.1
CNS: Glasgow Coma Score	13–14	10–12	6–9	<6
Renal: Creatinine (μmol/l) or urine output/24hr (ml)	110–170	171–299	300–440	>440
			<500	<200

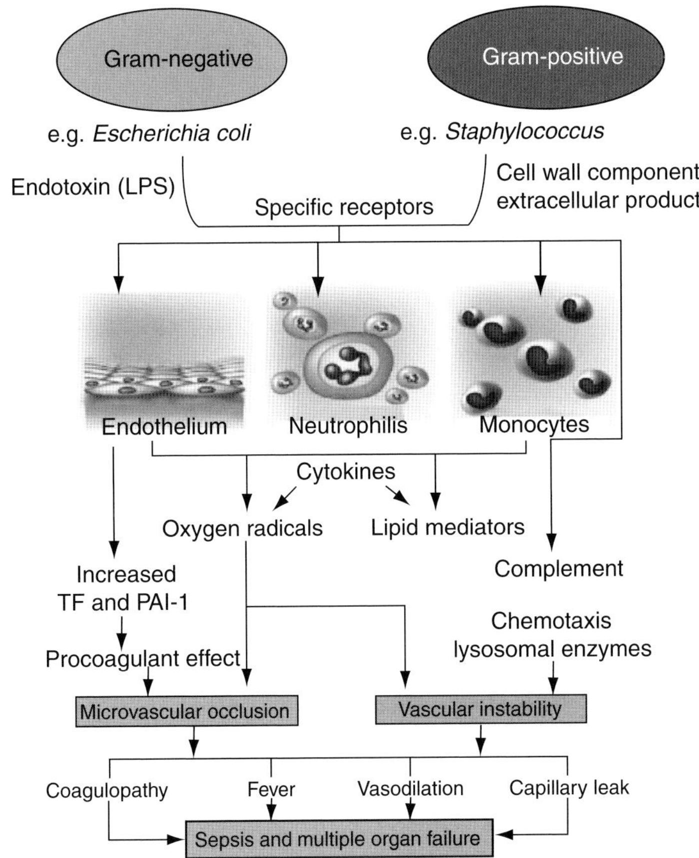

Fig. 15.2 Pathophysiology of sepsis and multi-organ failure. (Adapted from Cohen J (2002) *Nature*, with permission.)

- Soluble Fas ligand (a pro-apoptotic mediator) levels are elevated in patients with multi-organ failure and levels fall during recovery.
- Circulating levels of nuclear matrix protein, a general cell death index, are also elevated in sepsis-related multi-organ dysfunction patients and correlate with severity.
- Finally, circulating endothelial cells have been detected in the blood of patients with sepsis supporting a role of endothelial cell death in early sepsis.

Sepsis-induced coagulopathy

In sepsis, cytokine-induced coagulopathy triggers increased activity of TF and PAI-1 and decreased levels of the natural anticoagulant protein C on mononuclear and endothelial cells (Fig. 15.3). TF in turn activates a series of proteolytic cascades, converting prothrombin to thrombin, with subsequent generation of fibrin from fibrinogen. Simultaneously, PAI-1 prevents the conversion of plasminogen to plasmin, which results in impaired fibrinolysis.

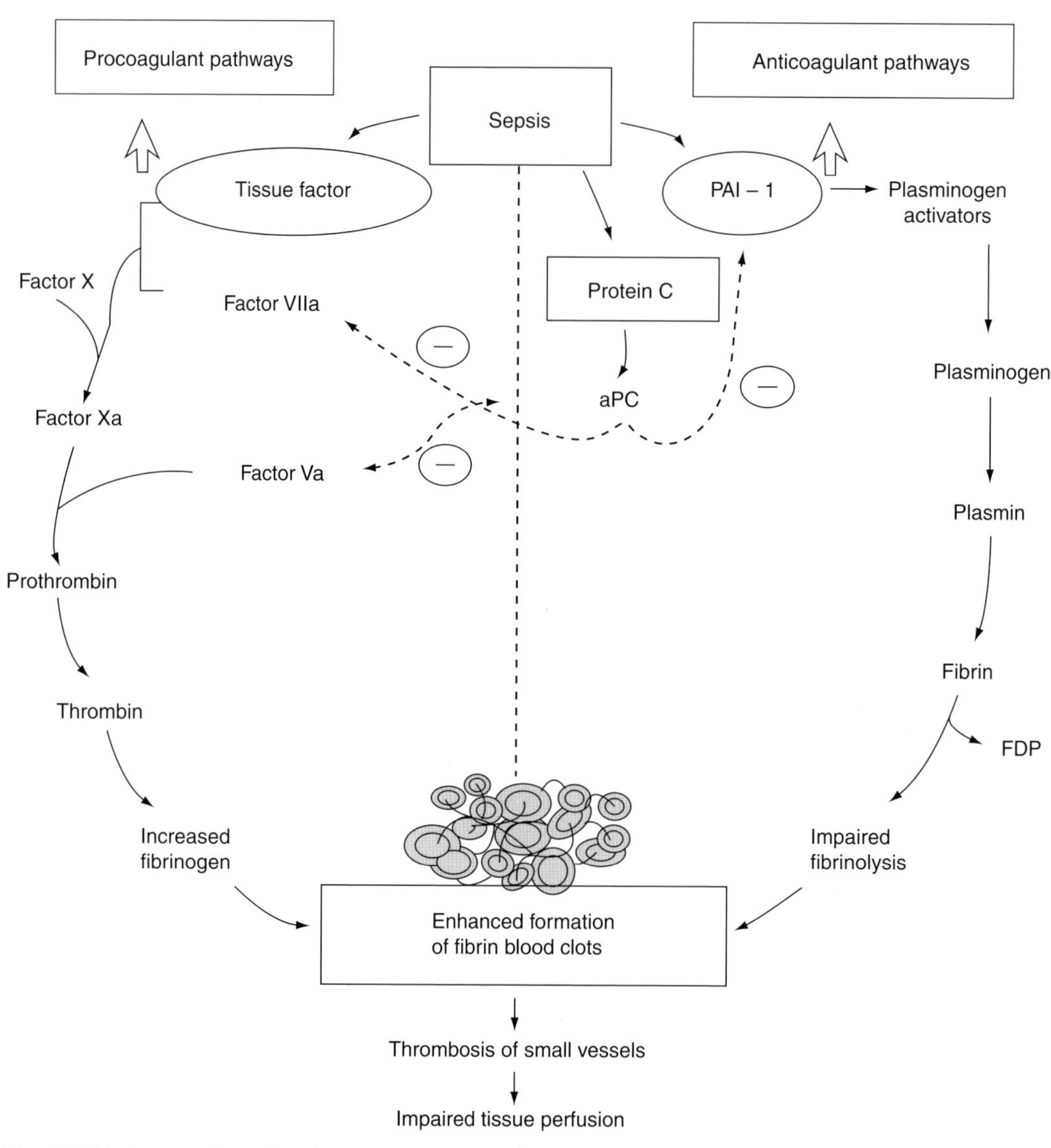

Fig. 15.3 Mechanisms of coagulopathy in sepsis. (Adapted from Cohen J (2002) *Nature*, with permission.)

The activated form of protein C, aPC, formed when thrombin links with thrombomodulin (TM), inactivates factors Va and VIIa, and inhibits PAI-1 activity; hence, protein C deficiency results in further procoagulant effect. The net result is enhanced formation of fibrin clots in the microvasculature, leading to microvascular occlusion, impaired tissue perfusion, and then multi-organ failure.

Recombinant activated protein C (drotrecogin alfa, rhAPC) is currently the only pharmacological intervention available with antithrombotic and profibrinolytic properties to treat severe sepsis but its use remains controversial.

Vascular damage in sepsis

The endothelium is involved in the control of vascular tone, vascular permeability and coagulation, and a number of changes in it follow exposure of endothelial cells (EC) to relevant proinflammatory mediators.

- Widespread endothelial damage and death is believed to occur during human sepsis and leads to organ dysfunction and failure: the multi-organ dysfunction syndrome (MODS).
- Pan-endothelial damage is particularly important within the pulmonary circulation and results in high permeability pulmonary oedema that is clinically recognized as acute respiratory distress syndrome (ARDS) and necessitates mechanical ventilation.

Circulatory and metabolic pathophysiology of septic shock

The predominant haemodynamic feature of septic shock is arterial vasodilatation. Diminished peripheral arterial vascular tone causes dependency of blood pressure on cardiac output which may result in hypotension and shock if insufficiently compensated by a rise in cardiac output.

Early in septic shock, the rise in cardiac output often is limited by hypovolaemia and a fall in preload because of low cardiac filling pressures. When intravascular volume is augmented, the cardiac output usually is elevated (the hyperdynamic phase).

Even though the cardiac output is elevated, the performance of the heart, reflected by stroke work as calculated from stroke volume and blood pressure, usually is depressed.

The myocardial depression seen in sepsis is multifactorial but appears related to myocardial depressant substances, coronary blood flow abnormalities, pulmonary hypertension, various cytokines, nitric oxide and β-receptor downregulation.

Management

Despite technological advances in medicine and our increased understanding of the pathophysiology of infection, sepsis remains a global health problem with mortality remaining high.

- The resuscitation of a patient with severe sepsis should begin as soon as the syndrome is recognized and should not be delayed pending ICU admission. Early goal-directed therapy (Fig. 15.4) has been recommended to guide fluid management outside intensive care area.
- Treatment of severe sepsis is best guided by protocols /care bundles: *resuscitation bundle* and *management bundles* in patients with severe sepsis. Compliance with the sepsis treatment bundles has been associated with a reduction in hospital mortality.

The sepsis resuscitation bundle

The following tasks should be accomplished as soon as possible during the first 6 hours of resuscitation:

(1) Measure serum lactate level.

(2) Obtain blood cultures before antibiotic administration.

(3) From the time of presentation, administer broad-spectrum antibiotics within 3 hours for emergency department admissions and within 1 hour for non-emergency department ICU admissions.

(4) In the event of hypotension and/or lactate level greater than 4 mmol/l, administrate an initial minimum of 20 ml/kg of crystalloid (or colloid equivalent); use vasopressors for hypotension not responding to initial fluid resuscitation to maintain mean arterial pressure of 65 mmHg or greater and urine output of 0.5 ml/kg per hour or greater.

(5) In the event of persistent hypotension despite fluid resuscitation (septic shock) and/or lactate level greater than 4 mmol/l, achieve central venous pressure of 8 mmHg or greater and achieve central venous oxygen saturation of 70% or greater or a mixed venous oxygen saturation of 65% or greater.

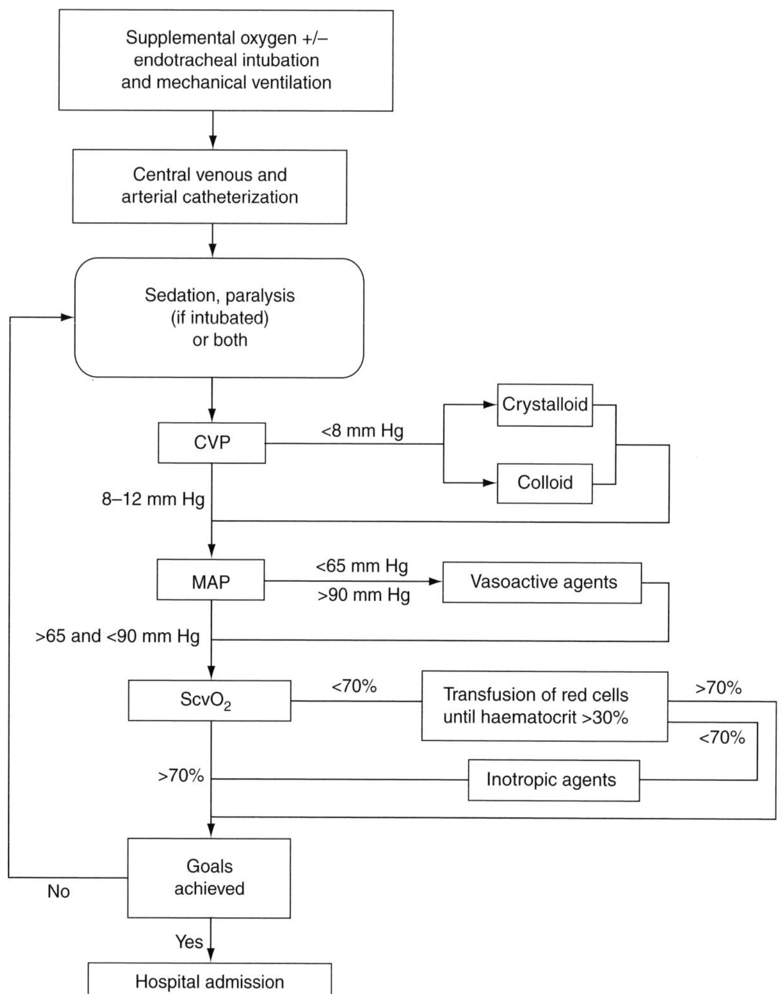

Fig. 15.4 Protocol for early goal-directed therapy. CVP, central venous pressure; MAP, mean arterial pressure; $ScvO_2$, venous oxygen saturation. (With permission from: Rivers E, Nguyen B, Havstad S *et al.* (2001) Early goal-directed therapy in the treatment of severe sepsis and septic shock. *N. Engl. J. Med.* **345**: 1368–77.)

The sepsis management bundle

The following tasks should be accomplished as soon as possible during the first 24 hours:

(1) Low-dose steroids for severe septic shock, following a standardized ICU protocol.

(2) Activated drotrecogin alfa should be administered in severe sepsis following a standardized ICU protocol.

(3) Glucose control should maintain glucose level at or above the lower limit of normal, but less than 150 mg/dl (8.3 mmol/l) using a validated protocol for insulin dose adjustment.

(4) For mechanically ventilated patients, inspiratory plateau pressures should be maintained at less than 30 cm H_2O.

Inotropic and vasopressor therapy (see Chapter 9: Vasoactive drugs)

There is little evidence to support the use of a particular inotrope in sepsis.

- In the face of the vasodilatation and reduced systemic vascular resistance that characterizes 'warm sepsis', most clinicians would opt for noradrenaline (norepinephrine).
- High dose dopamine is still used as a vasopressor in continental Europe.
- As sepsis can depress myocardial function, dobutamine is often introduced to provide inotropy and chronotropy.
- Adrenaline (epinephrine) is not a commonly used agent because of lack of selective α or β effects and lactic acidosis.

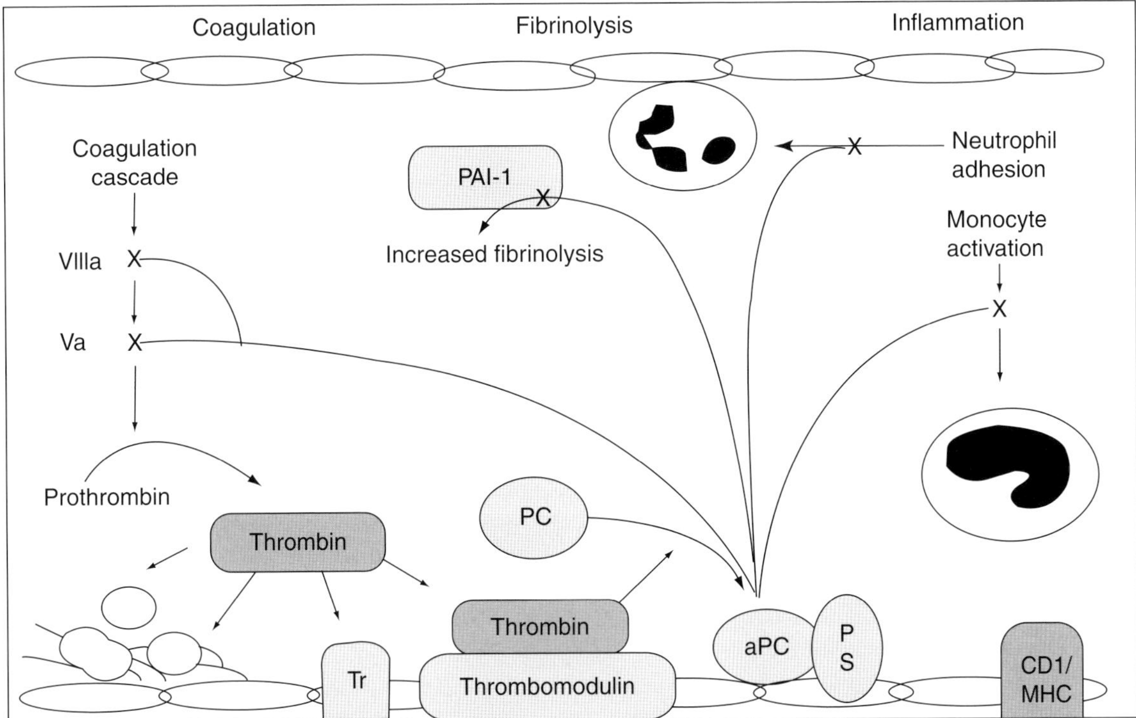

Fig. 15.5 Role of activated protein C in the pathophysiology of severe sepsis and its relationship with mediators of inflammation, coagulation, and fibrinolysis. aPC indicates activated protein C; CD1/MHC, major histocompatibility complex; PAI-1, plasminogen activator inhibitor-1; PC, protein C; PS, protein S; Tr, thrombin receptor; Va, activated factor V; VIIIa, activated factor VIII. (With permission from Bench S (2003) *American Journal of Critical Care* **11**(6): 537–42.)

The use of vasopressin

Previous studies have shown that patients with septic shock demonstrate a state of 'relative vasopressin deficiency', with circulating levels significantly lower than expected for the degree of hypotension.

Vasopressin cannot be recommended for routine use in septic shock, but in selected patients it can be used safely and may improve blood pressure and reduce the infusion requirements of other traditional vasopressors.

As with many areas of critical care, individual patient management must be considered when choosing vasopressor agents and their combinations. This should be guided by cardiac output monitoring.

Activated protein C in sepsis

The main physiological effect of protein C is reducing the production of thrombin, by inactivating factors Va and VIII. Thrombin is proinflammatory, procoagulant and antifibrinolytic. In addition, protein C inhibits the influence of tissue factor on the clotting system, reduces the production of IL-1, IL-6 and TNF-α by monocytes, and has profibrinolytic properties by inactivating PAI-1 (Fig. 15.5).

- In patients with sepsis, levels of protein C are depleted and the ability to produce endogenous activated protein C is impaired, shifting the balance towards greater systemic inflammation, intravascular coagulation and organ failure.
- Recombinant activated protein C (drotrecogin alfa, rhAPC) is an endogenous protein that enhances fibrinolysis, inhibits thrombosis and has anti-inflammatory properties.
- rhAPC is recommended for use in adult patients who have severe sepsis that has resulted in multiple organ failure and who are being provided with optimum intensive care support.
- Activated protein C is indicated in severe sepsis with Acute Physiology and Chronic Health Evaluation (APACHE) II score >25 (USA) or in patients with two or more acute organ failures caused by sepsis (Europe).

- The drug should be ideally administrated within 24 hours of meeting the criteria. The recommended standard treatment regimen for is to infuse 24 mg/kg body weight per hour for 96 hours.
- The primary risk of rhAPC is associated with its increased risk of bleeding. Therefore, its contraindications include:
  (1) Patients with a pre-existing coagulopathy (except for acute coagulopathy secondary to sepsis)
  (2) Severe thrombocytopenia of platelets $<30 \times 10^9$/l
  (3) Active bleeding
  (4) Gastrointestinal bleed within the last 6 weeks
  (5) Recent administration of thrombolytic therapy (within 3 days) or warfarin
  (6) Recent surgery (less than 12 hours after major surgery)
  (7) Severe head injury, intracranial or spinal surgery, or haemorrhagic or ischaemic stroke within the previous 3 months or in patients with CNS lesion (mass, cerebral aneurysm, etc.)
  (8) Within 6 hours from removal of an epidural catheter
  (9) Pregnancy or breastfeeding.

Steroid therapy of septic shock

Critical illness related corticosteroid insufficiency (CIRCI) is defined as inadequate cellular steroid activity for the severity of the patient's illness.

- CIRCI occurs as a result of either a decrease in adrenal steroid production (adrenal insufficiency) or tissue resistance to glucocorticoids (with or without adrenal insufficiency).
- Clinical assessment rather than the ACTH (corticotrophin) stimulation test is used to identify patients with septic shock who should receive steroid therapy for CIRCI. For example, intravenous hydrocortisone should be given to septic shock patients only if their blood pressure is poorly responsive to fluid resuscitation and vasopressor therapy.
- Hydrocortisone can be given in a dose of 200 mg/day in four divided doses for 7 days.
- Fludrocortisone (50 μg orally once a day) may be included as an alternative to hydrocortisone as it lacks significant mineralocorticoid activity.
- Steroid therapy may be weaned by reducing doses once vasopressors are no longer required.
- Reinstitution of treatment should be considered with recurrence of signs of septic shock.

Glycaemic control and nutritional support

In patients with severe sepsis, a strategy of glycaemic control using intravenous insulin should include a nutritional protocol with preferential use of the enteral route (see Chapter 10: Nutrition).

- Initiating glycaemic control without adequate provision of calories and carbohydrates will increase the risk of hypoglycaemia. This strategy of strict glycaemic control should be carefully coordinated with the level of nutritional support and metabolic status, which changes frequently in septic patients.
- Blood glucose should be monitored every 1–2 hours (4 hours when stable) in patients receiving intravenous insulin.

Key points

- The definitions of infection, sepsis, severe sepsis and septic shock have remained essentially unchanged since 1992. However, the 2001 statement recommended the term *signs and symptoms of infection* (SSI) to improve the limitations of SIRS criteria.
- Sepsis results in excessive production of cytokines, lysosomal enzymes, vasoactive substances and decreases in physiological concentration of NO leading to coagulopathy, endothelial dysfunction and vascular instability and eventually to apoptosis (i.e. programmed cell death) and multi-organ failure.
- Surviving Sepsis Campaign documents provide international guidelines for management of severe sepsis and septic shock.

Further reading

- American College of Chest Physicians/Society of Critical Care Medicine Consensus Conference (1992) Definitions for sepsis and organ failure and guidelines for the use of innovative therapies in sepsis. *Crit. Care Med.* **20**: 864–74.

- Dellinger RP, Levy MM, Carlet JM *et al.* (2008) Surviving Sepsis Campaign: international guidelines for management of severe sepsis and septic shock. *Intens. Care Med.* **34**: 17–60 and *Crit. Care Med.* **36**(1): 296–327.
- Ferreira FL, Bota DP, Bross A *et al.* (2002) Serial evaluation of the SOFA scores to predict outcome in critical care ill patients. *J. Am. Med. Ass.* **286**: 1754–8.
- Gao F, Linhartova L, Johnson AMcD, Thickett DR (2008) Statins and sepsis. *Br. J. Anaesth.* **100**: 288–98.
- Levy MM, Fink MP, Marshall JC *et al.* (2001) SCCM/ESICM/ACCP/ATS/SIS International Sepsis Definitions Conference. *Crit. Care Med.* **31**: 1250–6.
- Rivers E, Nguyen B, Havstad S *et al.* (2001) Early goal-directed therapy in the treatment of severe sepsis and septic shock. *N. Engl. J. Med.* **345**: 1368–77.

Multiple organ failure

Zahid Khan

Definitions

Multiple organ failure (MOF)

This is the commonest cause of death in intensive care unit patients. There is little consensus over definitions and criteria used to describe the condition and causes despite being first described in surgical patients more than 30 years ago.

MOF can affect any organ and systems not thought of as organs such as endocrine, immune, haematological and therefore it has also been called multiple systems organ failure (MSOF). It is not an all-or-none phenomenon and the clinical course is variable.

Multiple organ dysfunction syndrome (MODS)

Because dysfunction precedes failure with progression over time and can often be restored to normal in survivors, multiple organ dysfunction syndrome (MODS) has recently become a more appropriate and commonly used term.

MODS can be defined as the potentially reversible failure of two or more organ systems following a severe physiological insult in an acutely ill patient such that intervention is required to maintain homeostasis.

Secondary multiple organ dysfunction syndrome (MODS)

It has been understood for some time that critically ill patients rarely die from a single organ failure that led to their admission but from the cumulative effect of progressive failure of multiple interdependent organ systems caused by activation of uncontrolled host inflammatory response.

This is known as secondary MODS to differentiate from multiple organ dysfunctions directly attributable to the initiating insult such as multiple trauma which is known as primary MODS.

Primary MODS can however progress to secondary MODS.

Pathophysiology

When multiple organ failure was first described within an intensive care unit in 1977, in 69% of the cases the significant aetiology was bacterial infection. Over the last 30 years, infection and sepsis remain the most common aetiology for MOF (see Chapter 15: Sepsis), and in some series 90% of cases of MODS are attributed to sepsis. (Table 15.1 in Chapter 15 describes the definitions of infections, sepsis and severe sepsis.)

It is not clear why only certain individuals with sepsis or SIRS develop MODS, but genetic predisposition plays a role by upregulation of inflammatory mediators expression. In Chapter 15 (Sepsis), pathophysiological alterations during the process of sepsis are described in detail and summarized in Figs. 15.2 and 15.3. The initial changes that occur due to inflammation may be adaptive and possibly protective.

However, it is believed that the inflammatory mediators disrupt communication pathways between the multiple cell populations and cell signalling pathways involved in this complex condition. If the inflammatory response is severe in SIRS or sepsis, self-sustaining and progressive MODS is likely to follow.

The release of TNF-α has positive feedback and causes further increase in cytokine levels, platelet activating factor and eicosanoids. The complement and coagulation systems are activated with prothrombotic pathways such as tissue factor, with development of microthrombi. Fibrinolytic pathways are downregulated with decreased levels of activated protein C,

Core Topics in Critical Care Medicine, eds. Fang Gao Smith and Joyce Yeung. Published by Cambridge University Press.

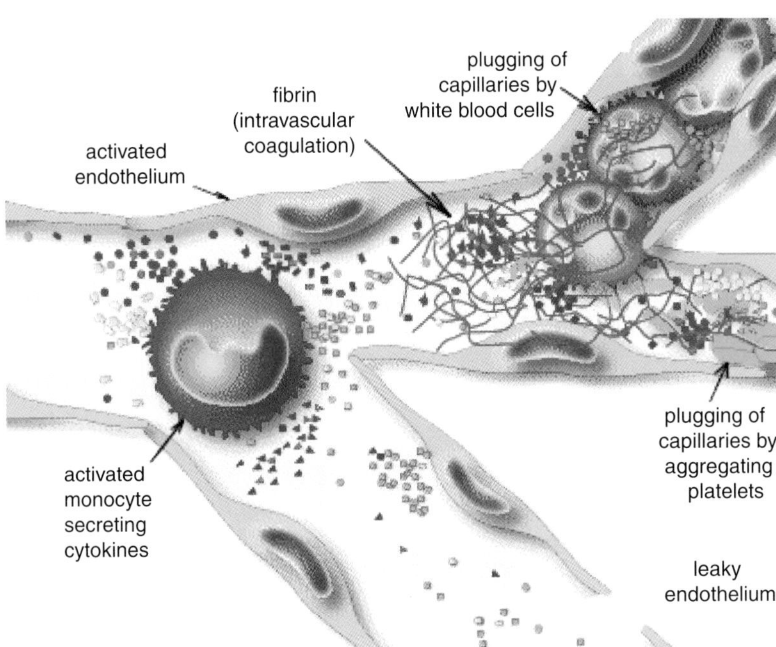

Fig. 16.1 Diagram illustrating effects of inflammatory mediators and cytokines.

antithrombin III and tissue factor pathway inhibitor leading to microvascular thrombosis (Fig. 16.1).

There is also activation of polymorphonuclear leucocytes, macrophages and lymphocytes. Activated leucocytes migrate from blood vessels to the interstitial space. These processes all cause end organ damage.

Hypotension, low cardiac output and hypoxia result in tissue hypoxia and organ hypoperfusion leading to further organ damage, cytokine release and immune suppression with an imbalance of proinflammatory mediators and anti-inflammatory mediators.

The gastrointestinal tract (GIT) has been proposed as both the initiator and the propagator of multiple organ failure following a remote insult. The upper GIT is often colonized with bacteria. Mucosal injury due to gut ischaemia following reduced intestinal perfusion can lead to bacterial translocation across a permeable intestinal luminal mucosa into the splanchnic circulation (Fig. 16.2). This may trigger or further propagate the inflammatory cascade.

The lungs receive all blood supply; they are also a rich source of inflammatory markers and cytokine release.

- *Hypoxic hypoxia* occurs when the ability to extract oxygen at a tissue level is reduced by a microcirculatory dysfunction and mitochondrial depression.
- *Microcirculatory dysfunction* – there is increased endothelial permeability which leads to widespread tissue oedema. Plugging of capillary lumen by red blood cells, intrinsic and extrinsic compression of capillaries leads to a decrease in the number of functional capillaries.
- *Mitochondrial depression* – oxygen is consumed by cell mitochondria to produce adenosine triphosphate (ATP) by oxidative phosphorylation. Nitric oxide and cytokines deplete cellular stores of nicotinamide adenine dinucleotide (NAD^+) which inhibits mitochondrial electron transport and therefore impairs oxygen utilization.
- *Cytopathic hypoxia* refers to oxygen utilization deficiency rather than failure of oxygen delivery. Cytopathic hypoxia is a major pathophysiological feature of septic shock, as demonstrated in patients with elevated levels of skeletal muscle tissue oxygen but with reduced levels of ATP. This condition is correlated with increased severity of MOF and mortality.
- The term *microcirculatory and mitochondrial distress syndrome* (MMDS) has been used to encapsulate both failure of oxygen delivery and impairment in oxygen utilization. MMDS causes a further cascade of biochemical and physical changes as a final pathway to MODS.
- Apoptosis (i.e. programmed cell death) of lymphocytes is responsible for an immune anergy which facilitates the development of secondary infection. Apoptosis of activated macrophages and

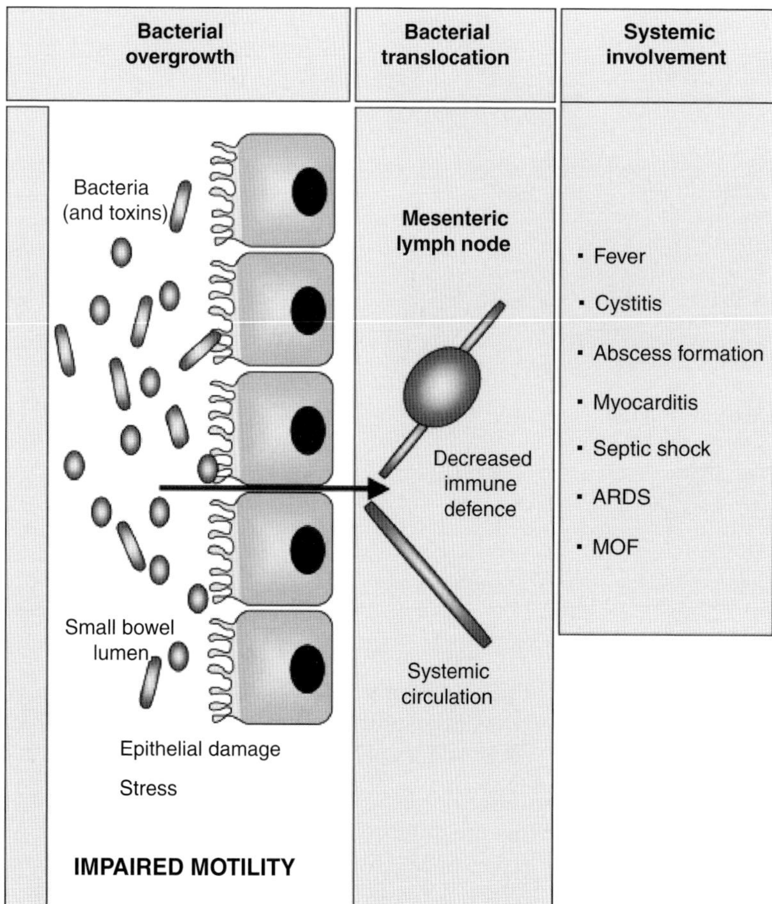

Fig. 16.2 Bacterial translocation in gut ischaemia.

neutrophils leads to accelerated death of gut epithelium. The intensity of immunoparalysis predicts poor prognosis.

- Organ functions are interdependent and coupled to each other by neurological and hormonal communication pathways. Sepsis disrupts these pathways contributing further to the development of MODS.
- Histology of organs involved in MODS shows evidence of oedema, inflammation, ischaemia with tissue necrosis and fibrosis but the pathophysiology of MODS does not consistently lead to histopathological comparisons.
- In MOF further pathophysiological alterations can be associated with supportive treatments we have provided. Resuscitation of hypoperfused organs can lead to reperfusion injury from release of free radicals.

Clinical presentation and outcome

Possible predictors of poor outcomes

MODS is described by the number of organ systems that have failed or the interventions required to support the organ dysfunctions.

- Patients with MODS make up 10–15% of the intensive care unit population and typically have two to three organ system dysfunctions at time of diagnosis; hypoxia, shock and oliguria are the most common combination.
- The risk of death increases as the number of organ failures or the severity of dysfunction increases and the longer dysfunction persists. Each new organ dysfunction adds 15% to the baseline risk of death.
- The Sequential Organ Failure Assessment score (SOFA) is the most widely applied of the organ

failure scores (see Chapter 15, Table 15.2). Daily SOFA scores can track the critical patient's physiological status; worse scores are associated with increased mortality. Patients with two organ system failure have mortality between 50% and 70%; those with four organ failures on admission have a mortality of 90%.

- A third of deaths occur early within 2 days, with nearly 80% occurring within 14 days.
- Poor prognostic factors include high severity of illness score and low pH, elderly patients, infection with resistant organisms, impaired immune response and existing poor functional status. This is seen in a number of descriptive scales which have numerically quantified organ dysfunction and its association with mortality. They have all used the respiratory, cardiovascular, renal, hepatic, neurological and haematological organ systems to characterize multiple organ failure.
- Improved survival from renal failure and acute respiratory distress syndrome (ARDS) have recently been reported, but with patient populations more elderly and increases in co-morbidities it is difficult to predict outcome from epidemiological data. Survival depends on physiological reserve of individual patients and the restoration of the balance between inflammation and immunoparalysis. The kidneys are the only organ to show residual damage following recovery in the medium to long term, but only 10% of patients will require long-term dialysis.
- The hospital mortality for MODS is 30–45% and even survivors will have utilized considerable resources. Those who survive initial insults will require prolonged intensive care support and rehabilitation and after 6 months only 50% have returned to their usual activity level. Because of the high mortality considerable psychological and emotional support for patients, relatives and carers is required.

Clinical presentations

MODS has been described in two distinct presentations.

(1) The most common form of MODS has lung injury as the predominant symptom, and this often remains the predominant organ failure in the process. Patients present with a primary lung disorder such as pneumonia, aspiration or exacerbation of chronic obstructive lung disease. The primary pulmonary disorder progresses to ARDS with accompanying encephalopathy and/or mild coagulopathy and persists for 2–3 weeks. Recovery then ensues but if the patient progresses to develop major multiple organ failure, a poor outcome is likely.

(2) The other form of MODS has a source of sepsis or a trigger of inflammation in organs other than the lungs, commonly intra-abdominal sepsis or pancreatitis. Lung injury or ARDS develops early with early development of multiple organ failure, e.g. hepatic, haematological, cardiovascular and renal. Patients remain with organ dysfunction for 2 weeks with subsequent recovery or deterioration and death.

Management

Possible causes for each organ failure should be sought with a multi-displinary team approach.

- The key management for MOF is supportive treatment for each failed organ guided by the international, national or local clinical guidelines or protocols.
- Frequent clinical reassessment, invasive or non-invasive monitoring with appropriate interpretations of the values may help timely adequate management.

Mechanisms and managements of MODS

Cardiovascular system

Cardiovascular dysfunction can be a consequence of MODS as well as a cause because cardiovascular dysfunction impairs oxygen delivery and contributes to failure of other organs. Cardiovascular impairment results from generalized peripheral vasodilatation due to local release of endothelial nitric oxide with reduced cardiac filling and a relative reduction in cardiac output. Impaired secretion of vasopressin may be responsible for some of the vasodilatation.

- The reduction in systemic vascular resistance can increase cardiac output because of the reduction in afterload, although the overall effect is dependent on intravascular volume status and the patient's pre-existing cardiac status. Ventricular dilatation occurs with ejection fraction reduced to less than

30% even with increased cardiac output. Low cardiac output may be the main feature as the disease progresses and along with diastolic dysfunction correlates with a worse outcome.

- Increased capillary permeability occurs with increased peripheral oedema and hypovolaemia. In the lungs the increased permeability results in pulmonary oedema and impaired gas exchange.
- Myocardial depression with predominantly right heart failure resulting from direct myocardial depressant effects of some cytokines is demonstrated in 44% of patients with severe sepsis. Reduced myocardial perfusion occurs because of reduced diastolic blood pressure. Oliguria and confusion are often present due to reduced cardiac output.
- Tachycardia is common in response to inflammatory mediators and the increase in sympathetic drive. An increase in pressure-adjusted heart rate is the product of the heart rate and the ratio of central venous pressure and the mean arterial pressure.
- Signs of inadequate oxygen delivery and tissue hypoxia include worsening metabolic acidosis and increasing blood lactate. Patients who survive usually recover myocardial function.
- MMDS alters regional blood flow to certain organs via arteriovenous shunting resulting from microvasculature occlusion by abnormal erythrocytes and leucocytes, reduction in the number of functional capillaries and microvascular plugging. Microcirculation imaging techniques such as orthogonal polarization spectral (OPS) and sublingual sidestream darkfield (SDF) techniques have demonstrated the redistribution of capillary blood flow in the clinical setting of sepsis preceding global cardiovascular dysfunction.
- Chapters 24, 25 and 26 highlight management for specific cardiac conditions including acute coronary syndrome, cardiac arrhythmias, acute heart failure and cardiogenic shock.
- Supportive management for cardiovascular failure are briefed in this book. Chapters 9 and 18 outline the use of inotropes and antibiotics, Chapters 10, 19 and 20 highlight the general managements for nutrition, fluid, electrolytes and acid–base balance. Chapter 7 provides you with essential knowledge on haemodynamics monitoring which can be informative and critical for the bedside management.
- Attempts to increase oxygen delivery to supranormal values in all critically ill patients have not been shown to be beneficial. However, well-timed resuscitation and achievement of normal haemodynamics is crucial. Central venous oxygen saturation and lactate measurements are routinely used in identifying and correcting oxygen debt. Resuscitation with fluids plus inotropes and blood is necessary in the first 6 hours of severe sepsis and septic shock and significantly reduces organ failure and mortality. Early goal-directed therapy protocols are available.
- Currently a number of minimally invasive devices for cardiovascular monitoring are used in critical care units; these include oesophageal Doppler, bioimpedance, pulse contour and lithium dilution cardiac output monitors with little evidence of efficacy. The use of the pulmonary artery catheters has decreased, whilst the use of echocardiography has increased.

Respiratory system

Respiratory failure is the most common organ dysfunction and is an important and an acute feature of MODS. Direct aetiology includes pneumonia, gastric contents aspiration, smoke/toxin inhalation, thoracic trauma or near-drowning. Indirect aetiology is associated with sepsis, cardiopulmonary bypass, pancreatitis, non-thoracic trauma or increased work of breathing and diaphragmatic dysfunction.

- Chapters 27, 28 and 29 highlight the classifications, causes and pathophysiological mechanisms of respiratory failure, ventilator associated pneumonia, acute lung injury and ARDS.
- Chapters 27, 29, 30, 31 and 32 stress the detailed respiratory management using appropriate modes of mechanical ventilation, fluid management for patients with ARDS, weaning from mechanical ventilation and respiration, unusual strategies including rotation, oscillation, proning, liquid and extracorporeal membrane oxygenation (ECMO).
- In those patients that develop acute lung injury or ARDS and are mechanically ventilated mortality benefit from volume limited tidal volumes of 6 ml/kg and plateau pressures limited to 30 cm H_2O has been demonstrated. The strategy may

minimize barotraumas, volutrauma and biotrauma. The use of high positive end expiratory pressures, prone positioning, surfactant, steroids and nitric oxide have not demonstrated mortality benefits. High-frequency oscillation, β_2-agonist infusions and liquid ventilation trials are awaited.

Renal system

Acute renal dysfunction is a common component of MODS with multifactorial aetiology. It is an independent risk factor for mortality, which ranges from 45–70% when associated with sepsis. Combined renal and respiratory failures have a significant increase in mortality compared with other combinations of MODS.

- Chapter 37 underlines classifications, causes, diagnosis, proganosis and management of different types of renal failure.
- Acute renal failure is not reversed by renal dose dopamine or by the use of frusemide. Any nephrotoxins should be stopped and be avoided.
- Chapter 38 emphasizes the principles, indications and various modes of renal replacement therapy.
- It has been shown that continuous or intermittent daily veno-venous haemofiltration is better than alternate-day renal replacement therapy. The use of high-dose haemofiltration therapy has not demonstrated a mortality benefit. The rationale for multiple organ support therapies (MOST) would require a more complex extracorporeal system in terms of hardware and software than currently available.

Gastrointestinal system

Gastrointestinal failure results from reduced regional blood flow, impaired motility and alterations in microbial flora. The gut plays a key role in the development of nosocomial pneumonia. Increases in gut permeability due to nitrosylation of gut epithelial cytoskeleton correlate with increase in MODS.

- Patients become intolerant of enteral feeding and often develop diarrhoea.
- The use of stress ulcer prophylaxis, early diagnosis of infection and improved resuscitation has reduced the incidence of upper gastrointestinal haemorrhage secondary to stress ulceration.
- Gastric tonometry can be used as a monitor of splanchnic perfusion.
- H_2 blockers, e.g. ranitidine, are routinely used for stress ulcer prophylaxis in mucosa vulnerable to ischaemia and have reduced incidence of gastrointestinal bleeding to 2%. The use of H_2 blockers is controversial as they lead to colonization with bacteria and increased incidence of nosocomial pneumonia. Sucralfate reduces the incidence of pneumonia as it does not reduce acid but acts as a barrier.
- Enteral nutrition is recommended, but if there is gastric stasis use prokinetic drugs e.g. erythromycin, nasojejunal feeding tubes and feeding jejunostomies. There is a lack of benefit from parenteral nutrition compared to not feeding patients up to 10 days. Parenteral feeding has an increased infection rate and increased gut permeability due to gut atrophy and lack of nutrition in gut lumen.

Hepatic system

Because the liver has a lavish blood supply from the hepatic portal vein and artery it may have a critical role in the development of MODS. Critically ill patients often have non-specific derangement of liver function tests.

- Acute hepatic dysfunction is seen mainly with cholestasis and increased bilirubin levels rather than hepatocellular dysfunction. Liver transaminases can significantly increase following ischaemia and the hepatocyte reduction–oxidation potential is reduced. Levels of acute phase response proteins such as protein C initially increase. Alpha-1 anti-trypsin levels are elevated and albumin levels depressed.

Neurological system

Most common neurological problems are an altered level of consciousness due to hypoxia and hypotension with a reduction in the Glasgow Coma Score. Depression of consciousness levels includes non-specific encephalopathy, metabolic alterations, cerebral oedema, reduced cerebral perfusion pressure and micro-abscesses in the brain. Chapter 40 describes common conditions of abnormal levels of consciousness and draws attention to clinical features, diagnosis and management of these conditions.

- The use of sedatives and analgesics makes assessment difficult. 70% of patients ventilated for more than 5 days may have abnormal EEG. Encephalopathy-induced coma correlates with mortality.

- Critical illness polyneuropathy and myopathies (subtle or profound) with peripheral demyelination and axonal damage are not uncommon. Muscle wasting and necrosis also occurs. Causes of neuromuscular injury include use of non-depolarizing muscle relaxants, microvascular occlusion and immune effects.
- Apoptosis mediated by nitric oxide in neurons and glial cells of cardiovascular centres of the autonomic nervous system play a role in cardiovascular dysfunction.

Haematology

Leucocytosis in response to acute stress is common as is mild anaemia due to bone marrow suppression and blood taking. Restrictive transfusion policy if haemoglobin greater than 7g/dl is generally accepted practice in intensive care units.

Thrombocytopenia is a marker of organ failure and has a number of causes including heparin induced thrombocytopenia, intravascular consumption and reduced production due to bone marrow suppression.

- Chapter 23 highlights management of coagulopathy and thrombocytopenia.
- Disseminated intravascular coagulation (DIC) is a severe form of haematological failure with an incidence of 10–15%. In DIC there is prolonged clotting, low platelets, low fibrinogen, low protein C resulting in bleeding and anaemia. DIC-induced microvascular coagulation contributes to tissue hypoxia and end organ damage. Chapter 23 describes the detailed management for DIC.
- The routine use of deep vein thrombosis prophylaxis is recommended.
- Activated protein C modulates coagulation, inflammation and endothelial function. The use of recombinant activated protein C is not universally accepted despite showing mortality benefit when used early in severe sepsis with high risk of death.

Immunology

Immunological dysfunction is exhibited as impaired delayed type hypersensitivity responsiveness, altered production of antibodies or abnormalities in lymphocyte response. This dysfunction can result in a virulent organism causing infection.

- The early use of the right antibiotics can improve mortality in severe sepsis.
- Selective decontamination of the digestive tract (SDD) with non-absorbable antibiotics reduces the colonization of the upper GIT with bacteria and decreases the incidence of ventilator associated pneumonia due to aspiration of pharyngeal secretions.

Endocrinology and metabolism

There is disruption of the four main neuroendocrine axes:

(1) Cytokines affect the *hypothalamic–pituitary–adrenal axis* with resultant increase in plasma cortisol levels. Cortisol levels may be inadequate; there is often a relative adrenal insufficiency. Cortisol levels are associated with the degree of shock and prognosis. However, the use of low-dose corticosteroids is only recommended in septic shock not responding to vasopressors.

(2) *The glucose–insulin axis* – hyperglycaemia is common due to relative insulin resistance caused by proinflammatory cytokines IL-1 and TNF-α, and an increase secretion of hyperglycaemic hormones. Hyperglycaemia increases TNF-α synthesis so is self-sustaining. The use of tight glycaemic control of 4.4–6.1 mmol/l remains controversial despite showing a reduction in MOF with proven sepsis; a less strict glucose control of 8 mmol/l is recommended.

(3) There is a relative *vasopressin* deficiency in septic shock.

(4) Disruption of the *hypothalamic–thyroid axis* leads to sick euthyroid syndrome; falls in T_4 correlate with increased mortality.

The causes of hyperlactaemia are multifactorial, but monitoring of blood lactate as a marker of critical illness is recommended. The relationship of lactic acidosis, organ failure and poor outcome is well established.

Prevention of multiple organ failure

No single treatment for MODS can be recommended because it is a maladaptive response to acute severe inflammation and therefore a complication to be prevented rather than a syndrome to treat.

It is crucial to identify patients at risk of developing MODS and those with evolving multiple organ dysfunction. This is best achieved by close monitoring of physiological parameters of at-risk patients. These patients may have a suitable underlying cause, signs of inflammation with or without evidence of infection and progressive deteriorating organ function.

- Patients with impaired host defence mechanisms are at greatly increased risks of developing sepsis and MODS. These include patients on chemotherapy, the elderly, those with burns, severe trauma, diabetes mellitus, chronic renal or hepatic failure, and those on ventilator support and with invasive catheters.
- Once identified the patient needs prompt treatment of the underlying cause and appropriate resuscitation with referral to the ICU for organ support. Sepsis requires urgent antibiotics and source control with or without surgery.

Key points

- Multiple organ failure complicating sepsis or SIRS is the commonest of death in ICU.
- Tissue hypoxia resulting from microvascular and cellular abnormalities causes organ dysfunction.
- Susceptibility to the effects of inflammation is determined genetically and better understanding may improve therapies in the future.
- Early detection of organ dysfunction and management with proven strategies may improve survival.

Further reading

- Blanco J, Muriel-Bombín A, Sagredo V *et al.* (2008) Incidence, organ dysfunction and mortality in severe sepsis: a Spanish multicentre study. *Crit. Care* **12**(6): R158.
- Fink MP, Evans TW (2002) Mechanisms of organ dysfunction in critical illness: report from round table conference held in Brussels. *Intens. Care Med.* **28**: 369–75.
- Harrois A, Huet O, Duranteau J (2009) Alterations of mitochondrial function in sepsis and critical illness. *Curr. Opin. Anaesthesiol.* **22**(2): 143–9.
- Marsh R, Nadel ES, Brown DF (2005) Multisystem organ failure. *J. Emerg. Med.* **29**(3): 331–4.
- Marshall JC, Cook DJ, Christou NV *et al.* (1995) Multiple organ dysfunction score: a reliable descriptor of a complex clinical outcome. *Criti. Care Med.* **23**: 1638–52.
- Martin CM, Priestap F, Fisher H *et al.* (2009) A prospective, observational registry of patients with severe sepsis: the Canadian Sepsis Treatment and Response Registry. *Crit. Care. Med.* **37**(1): 81–8.
- Pinsky MR, Matuschak GM (1989) Multiple systems organ failure: failure of host defence homeostasis. *Crit. Care Med.* **5**(2): 199–220.

Chapter 17

Immunosuppressed patients

Tara Quasim

The immune system is a highly complex physiological cascade that protects the body from 'foreign' pathogens. A defect at any point in this system can lead to both an increase in the incidence and an increase in the severity of infections. An immunosuppressed patient is unable to mount the normal, co-ordinated immune response to trauma and infection. The aetiology of the immune defects can be divided into primary (congenital) or secondary (acquired) disorders (Fig. 17.1).

Improvements in the treatment of immune disorders have increased the number of referrals and admissions to the ICU. Patients may present because of their primary illness or a new pathology which is complicated by their immunosuppressant therapy, for example a perforated viscus.

Whilst chronic illnesses such as diabetes mellitus can predispose to a degree of immunosuppression, the groups that will be discussed in this chapter include:

- Patients with cancer or haematological malignancies.
- Recipients of solid organ transplants.
- Patients with HIV/AIDS.
- Patients with asplenia or functional hyposplenism.

General considerations

Infection

(1) Respiratory failure or sepsis are the commonest reasons for immunosuppressed patients to require ICU admission. The exceptions to this are patients post solid organ transplant.

(2) Whilst there is no specific therapy for the immunosuppressed patient, the principles outlined in the surviving sepsis guidelines (www.survivingsepsis.org) should be followed.

(3) Immunosuppressed patients may be critically ill yet display little in the way of signs or symptoms. This key point means a detailed history, together with a high index of clinical suspicion, is vital. Knowing the aetiology of the immunosuppression can provide invaluable clues as to the likely pathogen causing the infection. For example, neutropenia confers susceptibility to bacteraemia whilst long-term steroids (>15–20 mg/day) increase host susceptibility to viruses, fungi and parasites as well as bacteria.

(4) The infections they sustain are often of greater severity and may have a rapid progression. The prior use of prophylactic and therapeutic antibiotics may mean that the potential for resistant organisms is increased. Microbiological diagnosis should be pursued and early liaison with microbiology is vital to ensure broad spectrum cover.

(5) Invasive procedures such as CT-guided needle biopsy, broncho-alveolar lavage and transbronchial biopsy may be required to obtain a sample of sputum or tissue when a respiratory source is suspected. These investigations can lead to further complications, especially if patients are requiring high inspired concentrations of oxygen and high positive end expiratory pressure (PEEP) levels. When infection is suspected, a reduction in the dose of immunosuppressant therapy may be equally as important as commencing antibiotics to allow an adequate host response.

(6) Particular risk factors for developing infection include:

- Neutropenia – an absolute neutrophil count below 0.5×10^9/l or those in whom the neutrophil count is falling rapidly.

Core Topics in Critical Care Medicine, eds. Fang Gao Smith and Joyce Yeung. Published by Cambridge University Press.

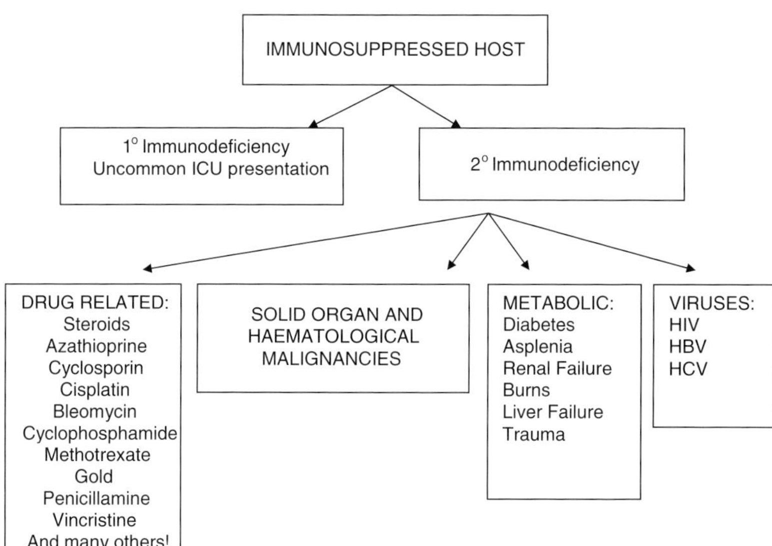

Fig. 17.1 Common causes of immunosuppression in patients presenting to the ICU.

- New leukaemia or lymphoma.
- Recent haematopoietic stem cell transplant (HSCT) recipients and allogenic HSCT recipients with significant degrees of graft versus host disease (GvsHD).
- Recent infections especially due to cytomegalovirus (CMV), or with known colonization with fungi or resistant bacteria.
- Co-morbid illnesses requiring hospitalization.
- The use of peripheral and central venous catheters and urinary catheters.

See Table 17.1 for a summary of patterns of infection.

Respiratory failure

Respiratory failure can result from multiple simultaneous pulmonary processes, both infectious and non-infectious. Non-infectious complications include thromboembolism, tumour, radiation pneumonitis, atelectasis, pulmonary oedema, drug allergy or toxicity and pulmonary haemorrhage.

In addition to the usual 'common' pathogens, these patients are at increased risk of opportunistic infections and reactivation of latent infections such as toxoplasmosis, herpes viral infections or tuberculosis.

The common pathogens include:

- Bacteria: *Streptococcus pneumoniae, Haemophilus influenzae, Mycoplasma, Legionella*
- Viruses: CMV is the most common virus of concern, especially in transplant recipients, and is often difficult to distinguish from non-invasive viral infection. Its incidence is related to the intensity of the immunosuppressant therapy and usually occurs in the first few months post transplant. In patients not receiving prophylaxis *Pneumocystis jiroveci/carinii* (PCP) is associated with CMV infection.
- Fungi: *Cryptococcus neoformans, Aspergillus* (invasive aspergillosis is increasing in incidence and is associated with a high mortality), *Pneumocystis jiroveci/carinii* (not uncommon in patients receiving steroids as part of a chemotherapeutic or maintenance regimen).

Special considerations

Patients with cancer and haematological malignancies

As a consequence of both the primary illness and its treatment, patients with malignancies are prone to episodes of neutropenia. The presence of a fever in a neutropenic patient is to be taken seriously. It is often the only sign of a bacteraemia. Factors contributing to the pathogenesis of infection include the direct effects of chemotherapy on mucosal barriers and the immune deficits related to the underlying malignancy.

Table 17.1 Predominant causes of infection in immunocompromised patients

Condition	Predominant causes of infection
Cancer	
Neutropenia ≤10 days	PUO Gram-positive organisms, gram-negative organisms, respiratory viruses or herpes viruses
Neutropenia >10 days: a wider range of infections are seen in these patients, and fungal and viral infections are more common with longer durations of neutropenia	PUO Gram-positive organisms including coagulase-negative *Staphylococcus* spp., *Streptococcus* spp./ group A *Streptococcus* spp., *Enterococcus* spp., *Staphylococcus aureus* Gram-negative organisms including *Escherichia coli, Pseudomonas aeruginosa* Respiratory syncytial virus, cytomegalovirus or herpes simplex virus; parainfluenza virus and adenoviruses found in profoundly neutropenic patients *Candida, Cryptococcus, Trichosporon, Fusarium, Phaeohyphomycosis* *Aspergillus* spores, *Pneumocystis carinii* or *Toxoplasma*
Transplantation	
Bone marrow: pattern of infection is influenced by time since transplantation and type of procedure (i.e. autologous or allogeneic)	
Early: patients are at risk from a similar range of pathogens to high-risk cancer patients, having received high-dose chemotherapy	Patients who receive bone marrow transplants are initially at high risk of infection from a wide range of pathogens Gram-positive or gram-negative aerobes or anaerobes at sites of mixed infection *Candida, Cryptococcus, Trichosporon, Fusarium, Phaeohyphomycosis* *Aspergillus* spores *Pneumocystis carinii* or *Toxoplasma* Respiratory syncytial virus, parainfluenza virus, adenoviruses, herpes simplex virus or cytomegalovirus
Late: (more than 100 days after transplantation)	*Streptococcus pneumoniae* and latent viruses including herpes simplex virus and CMV
Solid organ: the pattern of infection is influenced by time since transplantation and type of transplant	Transplant patients are at lifelong risk from *Cryptococcus* infection The single most important pathogen in solid organ transplantation is cytomegalovirus (CMV)
Early (up to 1 month post transplantation)	Kidney: Enterococci (including vancomycin-resistant enterococci), *Pseudomonas aeruginosa*, herpesvirus, polyomavirus Liver: Enterococci (including vancomycin-resistant enterococci), human herpesvirus, hepatitis C, *Candida* Heart/lung: Gram-positive and gram-negative bacteria, hepatitis B and C viruses
Late (2–6 months post transplantation)	CMV, Epstein–Barr virus, *Candida, Aspergillus, Cryptococcus* CMV, Epstein–Barr virus, adenovirus *Aspergillus, Toxoplasma*, CMV, Epstein–Barr virus
Splenectomy	Primarily encapsulated bacteria, especially *Streptococcus pneumoniae* (the most common organism), *Neisseria meningitidis, Haemophilus influenzae, Escherichia coli* or *Capnocytophaga canimorsus* Parasites: babesia, malaria
HIV/AIDS: infection type depends to a large extent on CD4+ levels Viral and fungal infections tend to occur after longer periods of immunosuppression	Incidence of *Streptococcus pneumoniae* has increased in adults; other encapsulated bacteria, *Salmonella*, enteric bacteria, *Pseudomonas*; mycobacteria, especially *Mycobacterium avium* complex and *Mycobacterium tuberculosis* (an early AIDS-defining illness) Herpes simplex virus, cytomegalovirus, herpes zoster virus, Epstein–Barr virus or respiratory viruses (especially respiratory syncytial virus, adenovirus, parainfluenza virus, measles virus)

Table 17.1 (cont.)

Condition	Predominant causes of infection
	Candida (can be invasive in patients with urinary catheters), *Cryptococcus, Aspergillus* (uncommon), *Histoplasma, Coccidioides, Penicillium marneffei* (depending on location), *Pneumocystis carinii, Toxoplasma, Cryptosporidia* or *Microsporidia*
Diabetes: hyperglycaemia increases risk of infection due to the negative influence on neutrophil function. Areas of vascular insufficiency are prone to infection following local trauma	Oral and vaginal candidiasis are common Foot infections are a major problem: infected ulcers, cellulitis, osteomyelitis and a combination of chronic osteomyelitis and soft tissue infection known as a fetid foot
Corticosteroid treatment: clinical signs of infection may be suppressed. Patients often carry steroid cards.	Chickenpox may be severe Measles is also a risk Septicaemia and tuberculosis in particular may be difficult to detect in their early stages Ocular fungal and viral infections are also a risk
Rheumatoid arthritis: immunosuppression may result from the disease itself or from treatments such as methotrexate, corticosteroids (see above) and anti-TNF therapies	Possible increased risk of pulmonary infections and septic arthritis

Source: Adapted from: Pizzo PA (1999) Fever in immunocompromised patients. *New England Journal of Medicine* **341**(12): 873–900.

The likelihood of there being an underlying bacterial cause is greatest when the neutrophil count is $<1 \times 10^9$/l. The high mortality associated with gram-negative organisms has led to the use of prophylactic antibiotics; however, gram-positive organisms are now common isolates, especially in patients with long-term vascular access catheters.

Validated regimens that are commonly used include antipseudomonal penicillin and aminoglycoside or a single-agent regimen such as a third-generation cephalosporin or a penem. As these agents give relatively poor gram-positive cover consideration should be given to introducing vancomycin.

After 5 days, if the patient has continued fever but is clinically stable and has resolving neutropenia, the initial antibiotic regimen can be continued. However, if there is evidence of progressive disease then consideration should be given to changing or adding further antibiotics. Treatment should continue for at least 1 week and ideally until the neutrophil count is $>0.5 \times 10^9$/l or 14 days have elapsed.

A high, swinging pyrexia in the absence of a readily identifiable focus should raise the possibility of a deep fungal infection. Fungi are common pathogens and the risk of a fungaemia increases with the duration and severity of neutropenia, prolonged antibiotic use and the number of chemotherapy cycles. Consideration should be given to adding an antifungal agent if there is a persistent temperature after 72 hours.

Unique considerations post haematopoietic stem cell transplant

Haematopoietic stem cell transplat (HSTC) can be either autologous (derived from the patient) or allogenic (from a donor). Despite advances, the success of HSCT remains limited by severe complications that are related to the toxicity of the conditioning regimen required prior to allogenic HSCT, immunosuppression and GvsHD. Complications usually occur in the first 100 days post HSCT. The presence of more than one organ failure, regardless of organ type, increases the mortality in this patient population. Mortality rates of 75–85% have been quoted in patients requiring mechanical ventilation.

HSCT recipients are prone to unique pulmonary complications.

- **Engraftment syndrome** – occurs within 96 hours of engraftment and can arise in autologous and allogenic recipients. It can cause fever, erythematous rash, diarrhoea, renal impairment and multi-organ failure. The syndrome coincides with neutrophil recovery and the treatment is supportive.
- **Diffuse alveolar haemorrhage** – injury to the endothelial cells of small blood vessels and thrombotic microangiopathy due to high dose chemotherapy can cause this condition. Symptoms include progressive dyspnoea, cough, fever and

hypoxia. The treatment is supportive; however, the prognosis is poor with most patients dying of sepsis and multi-organ failure rather than respiratory failure.

- **Idiopathic pneumonia syndrome** is a syndrome of diffuse lung injury that develops post HSCT where an infectious cause is not found.
- **Bronchiolitis obliterans organizing pneumonia (BOOP)** is related to GvsHD and usually responds to steroids. It has a good prognosis and doesn't usually require critical care services.

Infection and complications in solid organ transplant recipients

Despite rigorous screening, transmission of infection from the donor organ can occur. Some donors may have active infection at the time of procurement.

- Fever, bacteraemia or even mycotic aneurysms at anastomotic sites can occur in the recipients. Proof of adequate treatment of such infections must be established prior to organ donation. Other infections may not be apparent, or be accelerated in the recipient, after commencing immunosuppressant therapy.
- Viral infections, especially CMV and Epstein–Barr virus (EBV), can cause particular problems in the transplant recipient. The greatest risk is seen in the sero-negative recipient and sero-positive donor.
- Late, latent infections, including TB, can also activate many years after transplantation.
- Not surprisingly, lung transplant patients have a higher risk of developing pulmonary infection than other solid organ transplant recipients. Reasons for this include:
    - An extended intubation period leading to colonization of the lower respiratory tract
    - Trauma sustained by the lung during transplantation.
    - Mechanical factors such as decreased ciliary action and reduced cough reflex.

Complications post organ transplant can be divided into three timelines:

(1) Up to 6 weeks post transplant
Infections can be derived from the donor or recipient; in addition there is the potential for the usual post-operative infectious complications and hospital acquired infections. In these patients the effects of immunosuppression are not often evident unless they have been receiving immunosuppressant therapy pre-operatively.

(2) 1–6 months post transplant
It is in this time period that patients are at most risk of developing opportunistic infections, although problems from the perioperative period can persist. The major infections due to opportunistic pathogens include PCP, latent infections, viral pathogens and TB. Viruses can also cause direct clinical effects such as fever and neutropenia (CMV), pneumonitis (respiratory viruses), hepatitis (HBV, HCV), etc.
Graft rejection is thought to be mediated by proinflammatory cytokine release and may require an increase in immunosuppressant therapy leading to an increased risk of opportunistic infection.

(3) After 6 months
At this time most patients are receiving stable and reduced levels of immunosuppression and are prone to the usual community acquired pathogens.

Common immunosuppressant drugs

- **Steroids** limit cytokine and chemokine synthesis, induce apoptosis and limit acquired immune responses predominantly by attenuating T cell actions. The risk of infection is dose and time related. The highest risk occurs with doses >0.5 mg/kg per day of prednisolone or equivalent agents, or a cumulative total dose of >700 mg. The risk of sepsis is related to diminished phagocytosis and killing of bacterial and fungal pathogens. Long-term therapy can cause defects in cell mediated immunity and cause opportunistic infections.
- **Cytoreductive agents** induce dose-related reductions in rapidly dividing cell lines and cause neutropenia and mucositis. When used in lower doses as an immune modulator, methotrexate has been associated with opportunistic infections.
- **Immunophilin binding agents** are used primarily in transplantation, limiting cytotoxic T lymphocyte expansion and graft rejection. This is achieved by attenuating the signalling system for IL-2 production by calcineurin inhibition (cyclosporine and tacrolimus) or inhibition of lymphocyte mRNA transplantation and IL-2 synthesis (sirolimus or rapamycin). As they

primarily affect T cells the risk of bacterial and fungal infection is quite low.

- **Mycophenolate** specifically inhibits the de novo pathway of purine synthesis in B and T cells. There is specific inhibition of lymphocyte clonal expansion on exposure to appropriate antigens. The risk of sepsis is reduced but its use has been associated with opportunistic, intracellular viral infections, specifically CMV disease and EBV associated with lymphoproliferative disorder.
- **Anti-TNF agents** inhibit the host innate and acquired immune responses to microbial pathogens. Anti-TNF treatment (infliximab, etanercept) is used in severe rheumatoid arthritis and Crohn's disease and has been associated with severe, disseminated infection.

HIV and AIDS

With the advent of highly active antiretroviral therapy (HAART), the prognosis of patients with HIV and AIDS has improved enormously. Compared with other ICU groups with similar severity of illness, HIV patients no longer have a worse outcome. Patients are increasingly admitted to the ICU with HIV as a co-morbid disease rather than as the primary admission reason.

HIV and its therapy can cause multisystem problems:

- **Respiratory failure** still remains the commonest cause for ICU admission. This can be due to varied pathologies including PCP, TB or other mycobacterial disease. Patients with PCP and a pneumothorax requiring mechanical ventilation still have a mortality approaching 100%.
- **Cardiac disease** can occur in these patients as HAART is associated with atherogenesis and metabolic complications such insulin resistance and diabetes. It is also known that HIV patients who undergo percutaneous coronary intervention have higher restenosis rates than those who do not.
- **End-stage liver disease** secondary to viral hepatitis can cause significant morbidity and mortality. Patients receiving concurrent HIV and HBV treatment should ideally continue both therapies as severe relapses of hepatitis B may occur if it is stopped.
- **Renal impairment** is a frequent cause of mortality and morbidity. Treatment options include renal replacement therapy transplantation. The HIV infection itself appears to be the cause of HIV associated nephropathy and in this clinical scenario HAART can slow disease progression.
- **Immunological reconstitution** can occur when established HAART therapy reduces the viral load and causes a general increase in proinflammatory mediators and effects. A number of disorders are related to this and are collectively termed the immune reconstitution inflammatory syndrome (IRIS). With the addition of steroids HAART can often be continued in this situation.
- **Co-infection** of HIV and HCV has major mortality effects. HCV-related deaths are more common after improved HIV treatment with HAART. It appears that impaired cellular immunity from HIV leads to accelerated HCV reproduction. Conversely HCV has also accelerated the progression of HIV disease.

Antiretroviral therapy in ICU

HAART generally consists of two nucleoside reverse transcriptase inhibitors (NRTIs) and either one non-nucleoside reverse transcriptase inhibitor (NNRTI) or one or two protease inhibitors (PIs) (Table 17.2).

General principles for deciding on whether to commence HAART in the ICU are as follows.

- If the patient is not on treatment but admitted with an AIDS-related illness, consider commencing antiretrovirals.

Table 17.2 Components of highly active antiretroviral therapy (HAART)

Nucleoside reverse transcriptase inhibitor	Protease inhibitor	Non-nucleoside reverse transcriptase inhibitor
Zidovudine	Amprenavir	Efavirenz
Abacavir	Fosamprenavir	Nevirapine
Didanosine	Indinavir	
Emitricitabine	Lopinavir	
Lamivudine	Nelfinavir	
Stavudine	Ritonavir	
Tenofovir	Saquinavir	
Zalcitabin		

- If not admitted with an AIDS related illness this decision can probably be deferred. If the CD4 count is less than 200/mm^3 and the patient is having a prolonged ICU stay consider treatment, as this increases risk of an opportunistic infection.

The main problems encountered with HAART in the ICU are as follows.

Continuation of drug therapy

Achieving adequate plasma levels in those patients that cannot swallow may be problematic. If an oral solution is not available, tablets or capsules have to be crushed. If the enteral route cannot be utilized, few drugs have an intravenous formulation. Potential problems therefore include sub-therapeutic drug levels and drug resistance, or supra-therapeutic drug levels and adverse effects. In addition, discontinuing HAART in the ICU is undesirable, as it may also lead to the selection of a drug resistant virus.

Pharmacokinetics and pharmacodynamics

Commonly used ICU interventions such as enteral feeding, proton pump and H_2 antagonists can affect the pharmacokinetics and pharmacodynamics of antiretrovirals.

Renal insufficiency decreases the clearance of most NRTIs, therefore these patients cannot use most of the fixed dose NRTI combinations. Hepatic impairment will also decrease the metabolism of many protease inhibitors and NNRTIs.

Drug interactions

There are many interactions between antiretrovirals and common ICU drugs; protease inhibitors are particularly vulnerable as they are metabolized by the cytochrome P450 system. Commonly used drugs that can interact with HAART include:

- Midazolam: interacts with most PIs and NNTRIs leading to increased sedative effects.
- Amiodarone, Diltiazem and Nifedipine: interact with some PIs to cause increased cardiac effects.

Toxicity

HAART has decreased the incidence of AIDS-related illnesses; however, it has been implicated in rare life-threatening conditions such as Stevens–Johnson syndrome. Other toxic side effects include pancreatitis, lipodystrophy, insulin resistance and hyperlipidaemia. NNRTIs can cause a fatal lactic acidosis by disrupting mitochondrial DNA replication by selective inhibition of DNA polymerase-γ. This can cause hepatic steatosis, lactic acidosis or mitochondrial myopathy. Treatment involves stopping the drug.

Asplenia

Splenic macrophages have an important filtering and phagocytic role in removing bacteria and parasitized red cells from the circulation. Life-threatening infection is a major long-term risk post splenectomy. Most serious infections are due to encapsulated bacteria.

With the advent of vaccinations, this risk can be minimized and national guidelines are in place to offer prophylaxis to all patients who have either undergone a surgical splenectomy or have functional hyposplenism (sickle cell, thalassaemia major, lymphoproliferative disorders, bone marrow transplant).

Vaccines against pneumococcus, meningococcus and *Haemophilus influenzae* B should be administered 2 weeks prior to an elective splenectomy or as soon as possible after surgery and certainly prior to hospital discharge. These patients are also offered the flu vaccine on a yearly basis.

Lifelong antibiotics should be offered to all patients; however, the first 2 years post splenectomy appear especially important. The antibiotic prophylaxis of choice is oral phenoxymethylpenicillin 250–500 mg twice daily or erythromycin if the patient is penicillin allergic.

Key points

- Immunosuppressed patients may be critically unwell, yet display minimal clinical signs and symptoms.
- In addition to the usual pathogenic organisms, these patients are prone to opportunistic infections and reactivation of latent infections. Knowing the aetiology of the immunosuppression can help target therapy.
- Early liaison with microbiologists is vital to ensure patients are given appropriate broad-spectrum cover.
- Patients with HIV and those post HSCT can have their own unique clinical syndromes.

Further reading

- Gea-Banacloche JC, Opal SM, Jorgensen J *et al.* (2004) Sepsis associated with immunosuppressive medications: an evidence based review. *Crit. Care Med.* **32**(11): S578–S590.
- Huang L, Quartin A, Jones D, Havlir DV (2006) Intensive care of patients with HIV infection. *N. Engl. J.Med.* **355**(2): 173–81.
- Morris A, Masur H, Huang L (2006) Current issues in the critical care of the human immunodeficiency virus-infected patient. *Crit. Care Med.* **34**(1): 42–9.
- Rosen MJ, Narasimhan M (2006) Critical care of immunocompromised patients: human immunodeficiency virus. *Crit. Care Med.* **34**(9): S245–S250.
- Soubani AO (2006) Critical care considerations of haematopoietic stem cell transplantation. *Crit. Care Med.* **34**(9): S251–S267.
- Warrell DA, Cox TM, Firth JD, Benz EJ (2003) *Oxford Textbook of Medicine*. Oxford: Oxford University Press.

Chapter 18

Principles of antibiotics use

Edwin Mitchell

Introduction

The development of antibiotics and synthetic antimicrobial agents in the twentieth century revolutionized the treatment of infectious disease, reducing the mortality of many common infections dramatically. Hand in hand with vaccination programmes and improved public health, death from infectious disease early in life has become unusual in developed countries.

Despite these advances, infection is still the world's largest killer, and remains a major problem on intensive care units. Crude death rates from sepsis have remained relatively constant at around 40% for the past decade. The emergence of drug resistant strains of organisms has made several antibiotics almost obsolete. New infections have emerged such as human immunodeficiency viruses (HIVs) and severe acute respiratory syndrome (SARS), and previously rare infections have become common as a result of healthcare practices, e.g. *Clostridium difficile* diarrhoea.

Principles of rational antibiotic testing

Culturing or otherwise identifying the organism responsible for an infection is a cornerstone of rational antibiotic practice (see Table 18.1). Infected patients who do not have an organism identified have a worse prognosis than those in whom antibiotic therapy is active against the causative microbe.

- Antibiotics should only be administered after microbiological specimens are taken, except in emergencies.
- Bacteraemia typically results in a spike in fever 30–90 min afterwards, so it is important to take blood cultures as soon as a change in temperature has been noted.
- In the emergency situation, antibiotics should be given on a 'best guess' basis, depending on the clinical picture and knowledge of local bacterial patterns. This is often the case on critical care units.
- Once an organism has been identified, it is further cultured to allow sensitivity testing to a range of antibiotics to which it may be susceptible. When these results are known, the spectrum of antibiotic therapy should be narrowed to cover only the identified organism. This strategy may help reduce the incidence of unwanted side effects, reduce the probability of developing *C. difficile* diarrhoea and prevent the emergence of resistant organisms.
- Although in vitro activity does not guarantee in vivo clinical success, drugs with no in vitro activity are unlikely to lead to successful treatment.
- Knowledge of the causative organism allows a correct duration of therapy to be selected. Typically 5–7 days of intravenous antibiotics are all that is required, although some infections, particularly those in areas with poor antibiotic penetration (such as infective endocarditis) may require considerably longer courses.
- Close liaison with the local microbiological team is essential in deciding length of therapy.
- For some antibiotics (e.g. vancomycin, gentamicin), serum levels may be measured to ensure that the concentration of drug in the blood remains above the minimum inhibitory concentration required to inhibit bacterial growth or cause bacterial killing, yet below levels known to be toxic to the body.

Core Topics in Critical Care Medicine, eds. Fang Gao Smith and Joyce Yeung. Published by Cambridge University Press.

Table 18.1 Principles of rational antibiotic therapy

- Minimize infective load – surgical drainage/debridement/ removal of infected device
- Drug chosen with activity against causative organism
- Drug penetrates to site of infection
- Spectrum narrowed according to sensitivity testing
- Appropriate duration of treatment
- Clinical/laboratory assessment of progress
- Avoidance of drugs with high incidence of side effects
- 'Best guess' drug treatments based on local microbiological patterns
- Minimize cost of treatment

Pharmacokinetics

Prescribing in renal failure

Most antibiotics are removed from the body via the kidneys. Renal failure may cause the accumulation of a drug, or its metabolites. This is a particular problem with glycopeptides and aminoglycosides where toxic levels are associated with severe and permanent side effects such as ototoxicity and renal impairment.

- Accumulation of β-lactams or quinolones in renal failure may result in seizures.
- These problems may be minimized by measuring drug levels in the blood and adjusting doses, or by dose reduction according to estimations of the glomerular filtration rate.
- Where levels are employed, usually pre-dose (trough level) and immediately post-dose (peak level) measurements are taken. Trough levels are manipulated by changing the dosage interval, peak levels may be changed by altering the dose administered.
- Patients being treated on the intensive care unit for severe infections are often being treated concurrently with continuous renal replacement therapy.
- Drug clearance whilst a patient is receiving haemofiltration depends on a number of factors including protein binding, charge, volume of distribution, pump pressures, porosity of the membrane and the degree of residual renal function.
- Limited data are available to support the choice of dose regime in a given patient, and advice should be sought from the pharmacological service in combination with the clinical microbiology team.

Post antibiotic effect

Post antibiotic effect (PAE) refers to the ability of some antibiotics to continue killing bacteria despite the concentration of the drug falling below the minimum inhibitory concentration (MIC). This is particularly marked with aminoglycosides and virtually absent with many beta lactams.

Other aspects of antimicrobial prescribing

In vitro testing of antibiotics reveals that some drugs kill bacteria (bacteriocidal), whilst others inhibit their replication (bacteriostatic). In theory it is desirable to have bacteriocidal antibiotics in conditions where there may be a high bacterial load, or where the patient is immunosuppressed, but in practice it has been difficult to demonstrate marked differences in success rates. Antibiotics that inhibit protein synthesis (e.g. clindamycin) may prevent toxin release from some organisms.

Multi-resistant organisms

Micro-organisms may have intrinsic resistance to some antimicrobials (e.g. *Pseudomonas* spp., *Acinetobacter* spp.), or they may acquire resistance via natural selection or plasmid transfer from other microbes.

Organisms resistant to multiple antibiotics such as methicillin-resistant *Staphylococcus aureus* (MRSA) and vancomycin-resistant enterococci (VRE) have emerged in healthcare environments and have proved difficult to control in many countries.

- Intensive care units typically have more resistant organisms than general hospital wards, with 60% of new *S. aureus* infections being MRSA in one European study.
- Infection with a resistant organism is associated with increased mortality, morbidity, length of hospital stay and cost of healthcare – even when treated with an antibiotic to which the organism is sensitive.
- There is little doubt that person–person transmission of resistant organisms is the most important route of spread, and the importance of basic hygiene measures such as handwashing and wearing protective gloves cannot be over-emphasized.
- Advice from the clinical microbiology team regarding choice and duration of antibiotic therapy is essential.

Table 18.2 Strategies to reduce impact of multi-resistant organisms

- Basic hygiene measures to prevent cross-infection
- Appropriate use of disinfectants
- Avoidance of antibiotics known to be associated with high rates of resistant organisms (e.g. third-generation cephalosporins, fluoroquinolones)
- Restriction in antibiotic availability without specialist advice
- Rotation of antibiotic availability within an institution
- Avoidance of combination therapy where possible

- Strategies being used to try and reduce the impact of multi-resistant organisms are given in Table 18.2.

Prophylaxis

Prophylaxis is recommended where a bacteraemia is expected, and the resultant infection may result in significant morbidity or mortality (Table 18.3). It is particularly useful where:

- A high inoculum of normal commensal bacteria may be introduced into the blood (e.g. large bowel surgery) and/or
- The patient is at high risk of developing an infection (e.g. immunocompromised) and/or
- The presence of prosthetic material may lead to a persistent infection (e.g. mechanical heart valve).

The prophylactic regime chosen must be active against the likely bacteria that will be introduced, for example gram-negative and anaerobic cover for bowel surgery, gram-positive cover where the skin is breached (often with specific anti-staphylococcal activity). Fungal prophylaxis is indicated in select patient groups, usually those with severe immunosuppression.

Commonly used antibiotics on intensive care unit

The most commonly used antibiotics in intensive care are:

beta-lactams
carbapenems
aminoglycosides
glycopeptides
quinolones
macrolides
rifampicin
oxazolidinone
nitroimidazoles.

Table 18.3 Example of antibiotic prophylaxis protocol for general and vascular surgery

- Antibiotic prophylaxis should be administered immediately before or during a procedure (Evidence Grade A)
- Additional doses of prophylaxis not indicated unless blood loss >1500 ml or haemodilution up to 15 ml/kg (Evidence Grade B)
- Patients with a history of anaphylaxis/urticaria/rash after penicillin administration should not receive prophylaxis with a β-lactam antibiotic (Evidence Grade B)

Upper gastrointestinal surgery

- Oesophageal surgery (Evidence Grade C) Recommended
- Gastroduodenal surgery (Evidence Grade A) Recommended
- Endoscopic gastrostomy (Evidence Grade A) Recommended
- Small bowel surgery (Evidence Grade C) Recommended
- Open biliary surgery (Evidence Grade A) Recommended
- Laparoscopic cholecystectomy (Evidence Grade C) NOT recommended
- First choice: single dose co-amoxiclav 1.2g IV at induction
- Penicillin allergic patients: single dose gentamicin 160 mg IV plus metronidazole 500 mg IV

Lower gastrointestinal surgery

- Colorectal surgery (Evidence Grade A) Highly recommended
- First Choice: single dose co-amoxiclav 1.2 g IV on induction.
- Penicillin allergic patients: gentamicin 160 mg IV plus metronidazole 500 mg IV
- Appendicectomy (Evidence Grade A) Recommended
- Single dose co-amoxiclav 1.2 g IV or metronidazole 1 g PR at induction
- If there is evidence of perforation or peritonitis, antibiotics should be continued as per a therapeutic regime (refer to treatment guidelines)
- Penicillin allergic patients: gentamicin 160 mg IV plus metronidazole 500mg IV

Hernia surgery

- Antibiotic prophylaxis is not required for routine hernia repair

Vascular surgery

- Lower limb amputations (Evidence Grade A) Recommended
- Abdominal and lower limb (Evidence Grade A) Recommended
- First Choice: Single dose co-amoxiclav 1.2 g IV at induction
- Penicillin allergic patients: gentamicin 160 mg IV plus metronidazole 500 mg IV at induction

MRSA colonized patients/redo vascular surgery

- Teicoplanin 400 mg IV at induction

These are described in detail in the following sections.

Beta-lactams (penicillins, cephalosporins)

- The first antibiotics containing a β-lactam ring (benzylpenicillin) typically had efficacy against gram-positive infections, but little activity against many gram-negative organisms.
- Newer generations of these drugs have extended gram-negative cover (cefuroxime) and/or anti-pseudomonal activity (ticarcillin, ceftazidime).

- Resistance to the earlier penicillins is mediated by a bacterial penicillinase, and newer penicillins have been developed that are not sensitive to bacterial penicillinase.
- An alternative approach has been to prepare the penicillin with a penicillinase inactivator such as tazobactam or clavulinic acid.
- Extended spectrum β-lactamase-producing bacteria that are resistant to extended spectrum drugs such as piperacillin are becoming more common.
- Beta-lactams exhibit time-dependent killing of bacteria, and tissue penetration is relatively poor. There is little post antibiotic effect.

Carbapenems (imipenem, meropenem)

- These antibiotics are a subset of β-lactams, differing in the substitution of a sulphur atom for a carbon atom within the β-lactam ring. This confers resistance to many bacterial penicillinases.
- They have the widest spectrum of all antibiotics, covering most gram-positive, aerobic and gram-negative organisms, including *Pseudomonas aeruginosa*.
- They are well distributed throughout the body.
- Imipenem is broken down on the brush border of renal tubules, and is given in combination with cilastatin, a competitive inhibitor of this process. Meropenem does not require cilastatin.
- Carbapenems are most useful for serious infections where the organism has not been identified, mixed infections, or where the organism is resistant to conventional β-lactams.

Aminoglycosides (gentamicin, amikacin)

- Gentamicin is the archetypical aminoglycoside, and is a mixture of three very closely related molecules.
- It has activity against gram-negative organisms.
- High peak concentrations of gentamicin are required for optimal bacterial killing. The peak concentrations achieved are often ten times the minimum inhibitory concentration.
- There is a significant post antibiotic effect, and this means that gentamycin may be best given in a once daily large dose.
- Aminoglycosides are renal and ototoxic, and the doses must be adjusted according to renal function. Normograms are available for once-daily dosing of gentamicin.
- Resistance is well described, usually through modification of the side chains of gentamicin.
- Amikacin may still be useful in gentamicin-resistant infections.

Glycopeptides (vancomycin, teicoplanin)

These are very large molecules which are not absorbed from the gut. They have marked activity against gram-positive organisms, including *Staphylococcus aureus* and MRSA.

- Glycopeptides exhibit time-dependent killing, and may be best given by continuous infusion, although, unlike penicillins, they have a post antibiotic effect and are commonly given by twice daily dosing.
- Vancomycin is ototoxic and may cause 'red man syndrome' (erythema caused by generalized mast cell degranulation and IgE release) on rapid infusion.
- Levels must be carefully monitored, especially in renal failure.
- Tissue penetration is poor, with frequent treatment failures in pneumonias and infective endocarditis.
- Currently, vancomycin is one of the only antibiotics active against MRSA, and its general use should be restricted.
- Vancomycin-resistant enterococci (VRE) have been described, and these infections can be very difficult to control, especially once they become endemic in an intensive care unit.

Quinolones (ciprofloxacin, levofloxacin)

- Quinolones are DNA gyrase inhibitors, with a wide spectrum of action.
- They are most often employed in the treatment of gram-negative sepsis. Fluoroquinolones may be used in the treatment of *Pseudomonas* infections.
- Excreted principally in the urine, quinolones have been used extensively for urinary tract infections.
- Quinolones kill bacteria best in a concentration-dependent fashion, although toxicity (seizures) occurs at high serum concentrations limiting the

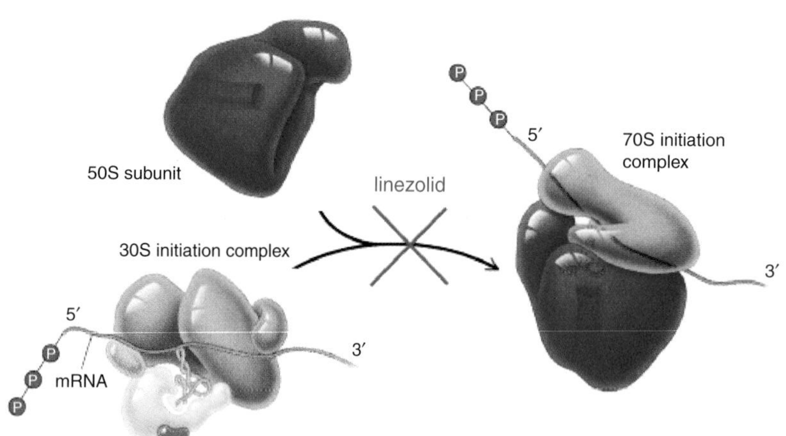

Fig. 18.1 Linezolid – mechanism of action. Linezolid binds to the 50S subunit of ribosomes, stopping the initiation of bacterial translation.

utility of a once-daily dose. Quinolones have a high oral bioavailability.

- Resistance to quinolones is an increasing problem, due to indiscriminate use and the secretion of the drug onto the skin which may allow the overgrowth of resistant bacteria.

Macrolides (erythromycin, clarithromycin)

The macrolides are bacterial protein synthesis inhibitors with activity against a diverse range of bacteria. They are most used in patients with streptococcal infections who are penicillin allergic, and in the treatment of community acquired pneumonia where 'atypical' organisms such as mycoplasma may be responsible.

- Erythromycin is irritant to veins and is not widely used on many ITUs, except as a prokinetic agent in intestinal stasis.
- Resistance is common, plasmid transferred, and often confers resistance to clindamycin which has a similar mode of action to the macrolides.

Rifampicin

Principally used for the treatment of mycobacterial infections – brucellosis, legionnaire's disease, endocarditis, tuberculosis and leprosy – rifampicin also has marked anti-staphylococcal properties and may be used in the treatment of MRSA.

- Resistance is common and frequently develops during treatment.
- It is widely distributed throughout the body.
- Rifampicin is orange-red and may colour the urine, sweat and tears.

Oxazolidinones (linezolid)

One of the most recently introduced antimicrobials, linezolid is a completely synthetic molecule developed from research into monoamine oxidase inhibitors (Fig. 18.1). It inhibits the binding of ribosomes, preventing the synthesis of mRNA.

- Linezolid has anti-gram-positive activity, with only minimal anti-gram-negative activity.
- It has good tissue penetration and may be used in the treatment of MRSA.
- Oral bioavailability is 100%, although an intravenous form is more commonly used.
- Resistance has been described. There have been occasional reports of myelosuppression and seizures associated with linezolid usage.

Nitroimidazoles (metronidazole)

- Metronidazole is active against anaerobic bacteria and some parasitic infections, e.g. *Giardia*.
- It damages the target cells' DNA.
- Resistance is uncommon, and it is well distributed throughout the body.
- The most serious side effect is neurotoxicity, although this is rare.

Antifungals

Fungi are important pathogens on the intensive care unit. Most infections are caused in debilitated immunosuppressed hosts, or those with prosthetic material in situ.

- Fungal infections can be difficult to identify, as colonization without infection is common, and blood cultures lack sensitivity. Novel methods of identification such as polymerase chain reaction (PCR) and antigen testing may help.

- There are three major classes of anti-fungal drug used for the treatment of invasive fungal disease:
  (1) Azoles (fluconazole, voriconazole)
  (2) Polyenes (amphotericin B)
  (3) Echinocandins (caspofungin).

All three target the cell wall. Azoles target ergosterol synthesis in the cytoplasmic membrane. Polyenes, of which the only current clinical example is amphotericin, bind ergosterol. Echinocandins inhibit synthesis of glucan, a molecule important in the construction of the cell wall.

- The most important fungal infections encountered on the ITU are usually due to *Candida* spp. Fluconazole is often used to treat candidaemias, with amphotericin B used for treatment failure.
- Caspofungin is indicated for either infections unresponsive to or patients intolerant of amphotericin.
- Echinocandins are likely to have a greater role in the treatment of severe fungal infections in future; evidence is accruing of equal or greater efficacy with lower toxicity compared to other antifungals.

Key points

- Successful treatment of severe infections depends on prompt removal of the infected material where possible, and speedy administration of antibiotics covering the likely pathogen.
- Stopping antimicrobial therapy when no longer indicated and narrowing the spectrum of antimicrobial cover once the infectious agent is known may help prevent the emergence of resistance.
- Close liaison with the microbiology service and knowledge of local patterns of infection is invaluable.

Further reading

- Bochud P-Y, Bonten M, Marchetti O, Calandra T (2004) Anitmicrobial therapy for patients with severe sepsis and septic shock: an evidence-based review. *Crit. Care Med.* **32**: S495–S512.
- Niederman M (2003) Appropriate use of antimicrobial agents: challenges and strategies for improvement. *Crit. Care Med.* **31**: 608–16.
- Roberts JA, Lipman J (2009) Pharmacokinetic issues for antibiotics in the critically ill patient. *Crit. Care Med.* **37**: 840–51.
- Salgado C, O'Grady N, Farr B (2005) Prevention and control of antimicrobial-resistant infections in intensive care patients. *Crit. Care Med.* **33**: 2372–82.
- Trotman R, Williamson J, Shoemaker M, Salzer W (2005) Antibiotic dosing in critically ill adult patients receiving continuous renal replacement therapy. *Clin. Infect. Diseases* **41**: 1159–66.

Fluid and electrolyte disorders

Prasad Bheemasenachar

General points

Fluid and electrolyte balance is an important everyday practice on the intensive care unit. It is an integral part of everyday care of the patient. It is governed by many processes and is difficult at times to manage.

There are a plethora of measurements available to make an assessment of the fluid balance in the critically ill. Some of these measurements are based on static filling pressures of the right and left chambers of the heart, some are based on dynamic changes to left ventricular output due to respiratory variations in venous return and some are based on achieving optimal oxygen delivery to the tissue.

Types of fluid (Table 19.1)

Crystalloids

This is the term commonly used to refer to solutions in water of inorganic ions and small organic molecules used for intravenous therapy.

- They are either glucose or sodium chloride (saline) based and may be isotonic, hypotonic or hypertonic.
- In addition, potassium, calcium and lactate are common constituents added to make the composition of the intravenous fluid closer to that of plasma.
- A 1-litre infusion of isotonic crystalloid is thought to result in less than 250 ml expansion of the circulating volume and a significant expansion of the extracellular volume.

Hartmann's solution

- It contains potassium and calcium in concentrations that approximate the free (ionized) concentrations in plasma.
- The addition of these cations requires a reduction in sodium concentration for electrical neutrality, so Hartmann's has a lower sodium concentration than either isotonic saline or plasma.
- The addition of lactate (28 mEq/l) similarly requires a reduction in chloride concentration, and the resultant chloride concentration in lactated Ringer's solution (109 mEq/l) is a close approximation of the plasma chloride concentration (103 mEq/l).

Normal (isotonic) saline

- It is a solution of 0.9% sodium chloride in water, it contains equal quantities of sodium and chloride (154 mEq/l).
- It has a much higher concentration of chloride compared to plasma and infusion of large volumes of isotonic saline can produce a metabolic acidosis.

Dextrose

In the days before the introduction of enteral and parenteral nutrition, dextrose was added to intravenous fluids to provide calories. However, with the advent of effective enteral and parenteral nutrition regimens, the popularity of dextrose infusion fluids is no longer justified.

- Severe stress hyperglycaemia has several deleterious effects in critically ill patients, including immune suppression, increased risk of infection, aggravation of ischaemic brain injury and an increased mortality.
- In head injury only fluid with the same concentration of sodium as plasma should be used. When dextrose-containing solutions are given, the dextrose is metabolized into water and reduces the

Core Topics in Critical Care Medicine, eds. Fang Gao Smith and Joyce Yeung. Published by Cambridge University Press.

concentration of sodium in the plasma. The water then crosses the blood–brain barrier by osmosis where the concentration of sodium is higher. This worsens brain swelling and raises intracranial pressure. Dextrose-containing solutions should not be given to patients with head injury.

Colloids

Colloids can be either natural (primarily human albumin) or artificial, for example, hydroxyethyl starch (HES) or gelatin solutions.

- Artificial colloids are cheaper than human albumin but may be associated with a risk of anaphylactic reactions and other undesired effects.
- Colloid fluids are more effective than crystalloid fluids for expanding the plasma volume because they contain large, poorly diffusible, solute molecules that create an osmotic pressure to keep water in the vascular space. Colloid fluids are about three times more effective than crystalloid fluids for increasing plasma volume.
- Individual colloid fluids differ in their ability to augment the plasma volume, and this difference is a function of the colloid osmotic pressure of each fluid.

Albumin

Albumin is a versatile and abundant protein that is synthesized almost continuously by the liver (an average of 10 g is produced daily).

The average-sized adult has about 120 g of albumin in plasma and another 160 g in the interstitial fluid. Thus albumin is located primarily in the interstitial fluid, which is perplexing in light of the important role played by albumin in the plasma.

- Albumin is the principal transport protein in blood and is also responsible for 75% of the colloid osmotic pressure in plasma.
- It also acts as a buffer and has significant antioxidant activity.
- Following acute infusions of 25% albumin, plasma volume increases by 3 to 4 times the infusate volume.
- The effect is produced by fluid shifts from the interstitial space, so interstitial fluid volume is expected to decrease by equivalent amounts.
- About 70% of the infusate volume remains in the plasma for the first few hours post-infusion, but the increment in plasma volume dissipates rapidly thereafter, and the effect can be lost after just 12 hours.

Starch

Hydroxyethyl starch (hetastarch) is a chemically modified starch polymer that is available as a 6% solution in isotonic saline or buffered Ringer's solution.

- There are three types of hetastarch solution based on the average molecular weight (MW) of the starch molecules: high MW (450 000 Da), medium MW (200 000 Da) and low MW (70 000 Da).
- There is some evidence to suggest that use of high MW starches could possibly result in a higher incidence of renal failure.
- The performance of 6% hetastarch as a plasma volume expander is very similar to 5% albumin. The oncotic pressure (30 mmHg) is higher than 5% albumin (20 mmHg), and the increment in plasma volume can be slightly higher as well. The effect on plasma volume usually is lost by 24 hours.

Gelatins

Gelatins are polydispersed polypeptides produced by degradation of bovine collagen.

- Three types of modified gelatin products are now available: cross-linked or oxypolygelatins (e.g. Gelofundiol), urea-cross-linked (e.g. Haemacel), and succinylated or modified fluid gelatins (e.g. Gelofusine).
- Molecular weight (MW) ranges from 5000 to 50 000 Da with an average MW of 30–35 000 Da. The various gelatin solutions have comparable volume-expanding power, and all are said to be safe with regard to coagulation and organ function (including kidney function).

Table 19.1 Components of crystalloids and colloids

Solution	pH	Na^+ (mmol/l)	Cl^- (mmol/l)	K^+ (mmol/l)	Ca^{2+} (mmol/l)	Lactate (mmol/l)	Glucose (g/l)	Osmolality (mosm/l)	Other
0.9% normal saline	5.0	154	154	0	0	0	0	308	0
Hartmann's solution	6.5	130	109	4	3	28	0	275	0
5% dextrose in water	4.0	0	0	0	0	0	50	252	0
0.45% normal saline with dextrose	4.5	77	77	0	0	0	50	406	0
Albumin (5%)	6.4–7.4	130–160	130–160	<1	0	0	0	309	50 g/l albumin
Albumin (25%)	6.4–7.4	130–160	130–160	<1	0	0	0	312	250 g/l albumin
Hetastarch 6%	5.5	154	154	0	0	0	0	310	60 g/l starch
Pentastarch 10%	5.0	154	154	0	0	0	0	326	100 g/l starch
Dextran-40 (10% solution)	3.5–7.0	154	154	0	0	0	0	311	100 g/l dextran
Dextran-70 (6% solution)	3.0–7.0	154	154	0	0	0	0	310	60 g/l dextran
Haemaccel 3.5%	7.4	145	145	5	6.25	0	0	293	35 g/l gelatin
Gelofusine	7.4	154	125	0	0	0	0	308	40 g/l gelatin

Colloid vs. crystalloids

Although many studies have been performed, methodological flaws (e.g. underpowered, not blinded) limit interpretation of their findings, and two meta-analyses have yielded different conclusions.

Investigators in Australia and New Zealand conducted the randomized double-blind SAFE (Saline versus Albumin Fluid Evaluation) study to test the hypothesis that rates of death from any cause within 28 days do not differ, whether patients are treated with 4% albumin or normal saline. Nearly 7000 patients in 16 intensive care units who required fluid resuscitation received either 4% albumin or normal saline. Patients received other aspects of standard care. The absolute difference in rates of death from any cause within 28 days between the two groups was 0.2%; the relative risk for death in the albumin group was 0.99. Mean length of stay in the ICU and in the hospital, and number of days of mechanical ventilation, did not differ between the two groups.

The SAFE study identified six predefined subgroups: patients with and without trauma, with and without severe sepsis, and with and without acute respiratory distress syndrome (ARDS). Within the predefined subgroups there was limited evidence of a treatment effect favouring saline in patients with trauma, and favouring albumin in patients with severe sepsis. The detrimental effect of albumin in patients with trauma was limited to patients with evidence of traumatic brain injury (Glasgow Coma Score <14 prior to sedation and evidence of brain injury on CT scan). However, the investigators cautioned readers that such subgroup differences frequently occur by chance.

There is too much discussion about which type of resuscitation fluid (colloid or crystalloid) is most appropriate in critically ill patients because it is unlikely that one type of fluid is best for all patients.

Sodium balance

Main points

(1) Disorders of sodium concentration are nearly always caused by excess free water (hyponatraemia) or free water loss (hypernatraemia).

(2) Severe or symptomatic acute hyponatraemia should be corrected at steady rate (2 mEq/l per hour) but only partially, generally using hypertonic saline.

(3) Severe hypernatraemia should be corrected only slowly, since rapid correction risks cerebral swelling.

Hyponatraemia

Hyponatraemia is of concern because of increasing evidence that it is a cause of significant morbidity and mortality in the hospital population. Hyponatraemia can occur in glucocorticoid deficiency, primary adrenal failure, or secondary pituitary ACTH deficiency.

- Hyponatraemia (serum sodium less than 135 mEq/l) has been reported in 50% of hospitalized patients with neurological disorders, 5% of hospitalized elderly patients and 1% of post-operative patients.
- Between 1% and 2% of patients present with levels below 125 mEq/l; whilst these levels are well tolerated in chronic situations, patients manifest neurological symptoms in acute situations. Early symptoms, such as weakness, nausea, vomiting, and headache, are non-specific. The level at which neurological symptoms appears is variable, often depending on the rapidity with which the hyponatraemia has developed. In acute hyponatraemia, fits can occur when plasma sodium levels are 123 mmol/l or less, but patients with chronic hyponatraemia appear to tolerate levels that are much lower than this, although brain damage may occur.
- The iatrogenic contribution to its development is significant. Patients may be receiving drugs such as thiazide diuretics, selective serotonin antagonists and proton pump inhibitors which are associated with hyponatraemia.
- Excessive beer drinking and excessive water drinking associated with Ecstasy may be a cause in young people.

Pseudohyponatraemia

Plasma is 93% water by volume, and sodium is restricted to this aqueous phase of plasma. The traditional method of measuring the sodium concentration in plasma (flame photometry) uses the entire volume of the sample, which includes both the aqueous and non-aqueous phases of plasma. Sodium is present only in the aqueous phase of plasma, so the measured sodium concentration in plasma will be lower than the actual sodium concentration.

- Plasma is normally 93% water by volume, so the difference in measured and actual plasma sodium is negligible in normal subjects.
- Extreme elevations in plasma lipids or proteins will increase the volume of the non-aqueous phase of plasma. In this situation, the measured plasma sodium concentration can be significantly lower than the actual (aqueous phase) sodium concentration. This condition is called *pseudohyponatraemia*.
- Many clinical laboratories now have ion-specific electrodes that measure sodium activity in water only.

True hyponatraemia

True hyponatraemia represents an increase in free water relative to sodium in the extracellular fluids. It does not necessarily represent an increase in the volume of extracellular fluids. The extracellular volume can be low, normal or high in patients with hyponatraemia. The diagnostic approach to hyponatraemia can begin with an assessment of the fluid balance.

Hypovolaemic hyponatraemia

This condition is characterized by fluid losses combined with volume replacement using a fluid that is hypotonic to the lost fluid (e.g. diuresis replaced by drinking tap water). The result is a net loss of sodium relative to free water, which decreases both the extracellular volume and the extracellular sodium concentration.

Causes: renal sodium losses would be seen in diuretic overuse, adrenal insufficiency and in cerebral salt-wasting syndrome, whereas extrarenal sodium losses can occur with diarrhoea and persistent vomiting.

Isovolaemic hyponatraemia

Isovolemic hyponatraemia is characterized by a small gain in free water, but not enough to be detected clinically. In this situation, the major disorders to consider are inappropriate release of antidiuretic hormone (ADH) and acute water intoxication (psychogenic polydipsia). The urine sodium and urine osmolality will help distinguish between these two disorders.

The inappropriate (non-osmotic) release of ADH is characterized by an inappropriately concentrated urine (urine osmolality above 100 mOsm/kg H_2O) in the face of a hypotonic plasma (plasma tonicity below 290 mOsm/kg H_2O). This condition can be seen in certain groups of 'stressed' patients, such as patients who have undergone recent surgery. It can also be produced by a variety of tumours and infections. This latter condition is known as the syndrome of inappropriate ADH (SIADH), and it can be accompanied by severe hyponatraemia (plasma sodium below 120 mEq/l).

Hypervolaemic hyponatraemia

Hypervolaemic hyponatraemia represents an excess of sodium and water, with the water gain exceeding the sodium gain. In this situation, the urine sodium can sometimes help identify the source of the problem.

Common causes	Urine sodium
Heart failure	>20 mEq/l
Renal failure	<20 mEq/l
Hepatic failure	>20 mEq/l

The urine sodium can be misleading if the patient is also receiving diuretics (which are commonly used in these conditions). The clinical picture is usually helpful, although these conditions can co-exist in critically ill patients.

Hyponatraemic encephalopathy

The most feared complication of hyponatraemia is a life-threatening metabolic encephalopathy that is often associated with cerebral oedema, increased intracranial pressure and seizures, and can be accompanied by ARDS. Correction of the hyponatraemia can also be associated with an encephalopathy that is characterized by demyelinating lesions, pituitary damage and oculomotor nerve palsies.

This is usually seen when the sodium concentration is corrected too rapidly. A specific demyelinating disorder known as central pontine myelinolysis has also been attributed to rapid correction of hyponatremia.

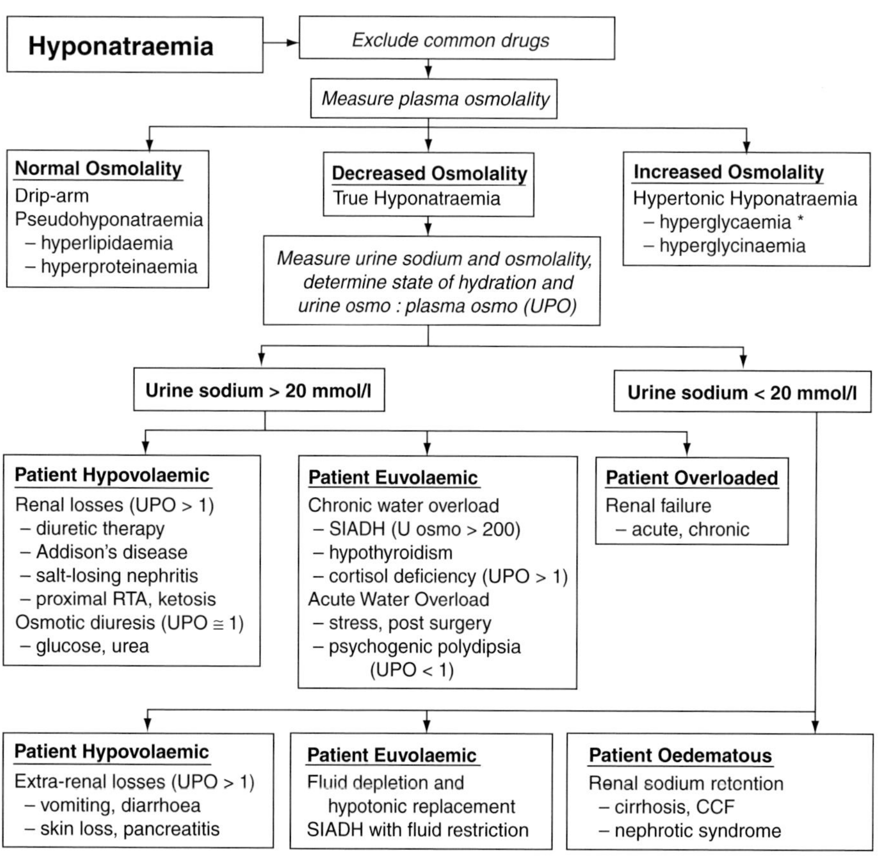

Fig. 19.1 Treatment algorithm of hyponatraemia.

Management strategies

The management of hyponatraemia is determined by the state of the extracellular volume (i.e. low, normal or high) and by the presence or absence of neurological symptoms (see Fig. 19.1).

- In many mild cases, an underlying illness may simply require treatment, whilst water intake should be restricted when appropriate.
- Symptomatic hyponatraemia requires more aggressive corrective therapy than asymptomatic hyponatraemia. However, to limit the risk of a demyelinating encephalopathy, the rate of rise in plasma sodium should not exceed 0.5 mEq/l per hour and the final plasma sodium concentration should not exceed 130 mEq/l.

The general management strategies based on the fluid balance are as follows:

- Hypovolaemic – infuse hypertonic saline (3% NaCl) in symptomatic patients, and isotonic saline in asymptomatic patients.
- Euvolaemic – combine frusemide diuresis with infusion of hypertonic saline in symptomatic patients, or isotonic saline in asymptomatic patients.
- Hypervolaemic – use frusemide-induced diuresis in asymptomatic patients. In symptomatic patients, combine frusemide diuresis with judicious use of hypertonic saline.

Sodium replacement

When corrective therapy requires the infusion of isotonic saline or hypertonic saline, the replacement therapy can be guided by the calculated sodium deficit. This is determined as follows (using a plasma sodium of 130 mEq/l as the desired end-point of replacement therapy).

The normal total body water (in litres) is 60% of the lean body weight (in kg) in men, and 50% of the lean body weight in women. Thus, for a 60-kg woman with a plasma sodium of 120 mEq/l, the sodium deficit will be $0.5 \times 60 \times (130 - 120) = 300$ mEq. Because 3% sodium chloride contains 513 mEq of sodium per litre, the volume of hypertonic saline needed to correct a sodium deficit of 300 mEq will be 300/513 = 585 ml. Using a maximum rate of rise of 0.5 mEq/l per hour for the plasma sodium (to limit the risk of a demyelinating encephalopathy), the sodium concentration deficit of 10 mEq/l in the previous example should be corrected over at least 20 hours. Thus, the maximum rate of hypertonic fluid administration will be 585/20 = 29 ml/hour. If isotonic saline is used for sodium replacement, the replacement volume will be 3.3 times the replacement volume of the hypertonic 3% saline solution.

Hypernatraemia

The normal plasma (serum) sodium concentration is 135 to 145 mEq/l. Therefore, hypernatraemia (i.e. a serum sodium concentration above 145 mEq/l) can be the result of loss of fluid that has a sodium concentration below 135 mEq/l (hypotonic fluid loss) or gain of fluid that has a sodium concentration above 145 mEq/l (hypertonic fluid gain).

Hypotonic hypernatraemia

Hypotonic hypernatraemia indicates loss of hypotonic fluids. Common causes are excessive diuresis, vomiting and diarrhoea. The two consequences of hypotonic fluid loss are hypovolaemia and hypertonicity. The most immediate concern in hypovolaemic hypernatraemia is to replace volume deficits and maintain the cardiac output. Volume replacement can be guided by the cardiac filling pressures, cardiac output, urine output, etc. When hypovolaemia has been corrected, the next step is to calculate and replace the free water deficit. The hypertonicity of the extracellular fluids predisposes to cellular dehydration. The most serious consequence of hypertonic hypernatraemia is a metabolic encephalopathy. Hypernatraemic encephalopathy has an associated mortality of up to 50%, but management should proceed slowly.

The management strategy is to replace the sodium deficit quickly (to maintain plasma volume) and to replace the free water deficit slowly (to prevent intracellular overhydration). The brain cells initially shrink in response to a hypertonic extracellular fluid, but cell volume is restored within hours. This restoration of cell volume is attributed to the generation of osmotically active substances called idiogenic osmoles. Once the brain cell volume is restored to normal, the aggressive replacement of free water can predispose to cerebral oedema and seizures. To limit the risk of cerebral oedema, free water deficits should be replaced slowly so that serum sodium decreases no faster than 0.5 mEq/l per hour.

Isotonic hypernatraemia

Isotonic hypernatraemia indicates a net loss of free water. This can be seen in diabetes insipidus, or when loss of hypotonic fluids (e.g. diuresis) is treated by replacement with isotonic saline in a 1:1 volume-to-volume ratio. The management strategy is to replace the free water deficit slowly (to prevent intracellular over hydration).

Diabetes insipidus

The most noted cause for hypernatraemia without apparent volume deficits is diabetes insipidus (DI), which is a condition of impaired renal water conservation. This condition results in excessive loss of urine that is almost pure water (devoid of solute). The underlying problem in DI is related to ADH, a hormone secreted by the posterior pituitary gland that promotes water reabsorption in the distal tubule. Two defects related to ADH can occur in DI:

(1) Central DI is caused by failure of ADH release from the posterior pituitary. Common causes of central DI in critically ill patients include traumatic brain injury, anoxic encephalopathy, meningitis and brain death. The onset is heralded by polyuria that usually is evident within 24 hours of the inciting event.

(2) Nephrogenic DI is caused by defective end-organ responsiveness to ADH. Possible causes of nephrogenic DI in critically ill patients include amphotericin, dopamine, lithium, radiocontrast dyes, hypokalaemia, aminoglycosides and the polyuric phase of acute tubular necrosis. The defect in urine concentrating ability in nephrogenic DI is not as severe as it is in central DI.

Diagnosis

The hallmark of DI is dilute urine in the face of hypertonic plasma. In central DI, the urine osmolarity is often below 200 mOsm/l, whereas in nephrogenic DI the urine osmolarity is usually between 200 and 500 mOsm/l. The diagnosis of DI is confirmed by noting the urinary response to fluid restriction.

Management

The fluid loss in DI is almost pure water, so the replacement strategy is aimed at replacing free water deficits only. The free water deficit is corrected slowly (over 2 to 3 days) to limit the risk of cerebral oedema. In central DI, vasopressin administration is also required to prevent ongoing free water losses. The usual dose is 2 to 5 units of aqueous vasopressin subcutaneously every 4 to 6 hours. The serum sodium must be monitored carefully during vasopressin therapy because water intoxication and hyponatraemia can occur if the central DI begins to resolve.

Non-ketotic hyperglycaemia

The formula for plasma tonicity predicts that hyperglycaemia will be accompanied by a hypertonic extracellular fluid. When progressive hyperglycaemia does not result in ketosis, the major clinical consequence is a hypertonic encephalopathy.

Clinical manifestations

Patients with non-ketotic hyperglycaemia (NKH) usually have an altered mental status and may show signs of hypovolaemia. The altered mental status can progress to frank coma when the plasma tonicity rises above 330 mOsm/kg H_2O. Advanced cases of encephalopathy can be accompanied by generalized seizures and focal neurological deficits, as described for hypernatraemic encephalopathy.

Fluid management

Volume deficits tend to be more profound in NKH because of the osmotic diuresis that accompanies the glycosuria. Therefore, rapid correction of the plasma volume may be necessary.

Free water deficit

Once the plasma volume is restored, free water deficits are estimated and replaced slowly. However when calculating the free water deficit that accompanies hyperglycaemia, it is necessary to correct the plasma sodium for the increase in plasma glucose. The restoration of brain cell volume can occur rapidly in hypertonic states due to hyperglycaemia. Therefore, the free water replacement should be particularly judicious in NKH.

Insulin therapy

Because insulin drives both glucose and water into cells, insulin therapy can aggravate hypovolaemia. Therefore, in patients who are hypovolaemic, insulin should be withheld until the vascular volume is restored. Once this is accomplished, insulin therapy can be given as advised for diabetic ketoacidosis. The insulin requirement will diminish as the hypertonic condition is corrected, so plasma glucose concentrations should be monitored hourly during intravenous insulin therapy in NKH.

Hypertonic hypernatraemia

Hypertonic hypernatraemia indicates a gain of hypertonic fluids. This is seen with aggressive use of

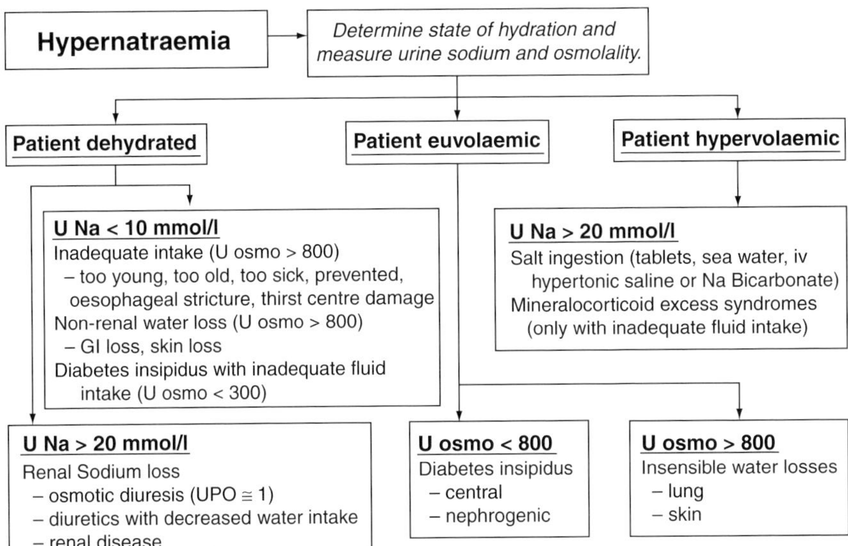

Fig. 19.2 Treatment algorithm of hypernatraemia.

hypertonic saline or sodium bicarbonate solutions. The management strategy is to induce sodium loss in the urine with diuresis and to replace the urine volume loss with fluids that are hypotonic to the urine. Hypernatraemia from hypertonic fluid gain is uncommon. Possible causes are hypertonic saline resuscitation, sodium bicarbonate infusions for metabolic acidosis, and ingestion of excessive amounts of table salt.

Management

In patients with normal renal function, excess sodium and water are excreted rapidly. When renal sodium excretion is impaired, it might be necessary to increase renal sodium excretion with a diuretic (e.g. frusemide). Because the sodium concentration in urine during frusemide diuresis is approximately 75 mEq/l, excessive urine output will aggravate the hypernatraemia (because the urine is hypotonic to plasma). Therefore, urine volume losses must be partially replaced with a fluid that is hypotonic to the urine (see Fig. 19.2).

Potassium balance

Main points

(1) Potassium is mainly an intracellular cation; only 2% of the potassium is outside cells. Serum potassium concentration is not an accurate reflection of total body potassium stores.

(2) The ratio between intracellular and extracellular potassium concentrations strongly influences cell membrane polarization, which in turn influences important cell processes, such as the conduction of nerve impulses and muscle (including myocardial) cell contraction.

(3) Hypokalaemia associated with diuretic therapy is often the result of magnesium depletion, and potassium replacement will not correct the problem unless magnesium is also replaced.

(4) While hypokalaemia is often well tolerated, hyperkalaemia (serum K^+ greater than 5.5 mEq/l) can be a serious and life-threatening condition.

(5) If hypokalaemia is really due to potassium depletion, don't expect an extra 40 mEq of potassium to correct the problem because for each 0.5 mEq/l decrease in serum K^+, you will have to replace about 175 mEq of potassium to replenish total body K^+ stores.

The total body potassium content in healthy adults is approximately 50 mEq/kg, so a 70-kg adult will have 3500 mEq of total body potassium. However, only 70 mEq (2% of the total amount) is found in the extracellular fluids. Because the plasma accounts for approximately 20% of the extracellular fluid volume, the potassium content of plasma will be about 15 mEq, which is about 0.4% of the total amount of potassium in the body. This suggests that the plasma potassium will be an insensitive marker of changes in total body potassium stores.

Hypokalaemia

Hypokalaemia is a serum potassium concentration below 3.5 mEq/l. Hypokalaemia can be caused by an intracellular shift of potassium (transcellular shift) or can be due to loss of potassium. Loss of potassium from the body is either due to loss from the kidneys or from loss from extrarenal deficits like diarrhoea or vomiting.

Causes

Hypokalaemia can be caused by decreased intake of potassium but is usually caused by excessive losses of potassium in the urine or from the GI tract.

GI tract losses

Abnormal GI potassium losses occur in chronic diarrhoea and include losses due to chronic laxative abuse or bowel diversion. Other causes include vomiting, and gastric suction (which removes HCl, causing the kidneys to excrete potassium). GI potassium losses may be compounded by concomitant renal potassium losses due to metabolic alkalosis and stimulation of aldosterone due to volume.

Renal losses

The leading cause of renal potassium wasting is diuretic therapy. Other causes likely to be seen in the ICU include nasogastric drainage leading to alkalosis, and magnesium depletion. Magnesium depletion impairs potassium reabsorption across the renal tubules and may play a very important role in promoting and sustaining potassium depletion in critically ill patients, particularly those receiving diuretics. Excretion can increase in adrenal steroid excess due to direct mineralocorticoid effects on potassium secretion by the distal nephron. The urinary chloride is low (less than 15 mEq/l) when nasogastric drainage or alkalosis is involved, and it is high (greater than 25 mEq/l) when magnesium depletion or diuretics are responsible. Renal potassium wasting can also be caused by numerous congenital and acquired renal tubular diseases.

Intracellular shift

The transcellular shift of potassium into cells also causes hypokalaemia. Stimulation of the sympathetic nervous system, particularly with β_2-agonists, may increase cellular potassium uptake. This can also occur in glycogenesis during total parenteral nutrition (TPN) or enteral hyperalimentation or after administration of insulin. Similarly, severe hypokalaemia occasionally occurs in thyrotoxic patients from excessive β-sympathetic stimulation (hypokalaemic thyrotoxic periodic paralysis). Familial periodic paralysis is a rare autosomal dominant disease characterized by transient episodes of profound hypokalaemia thought to be due to sudden abnormal shifts of K into cells.

Clinical manifestations

Mild hypokalaemia (plasma K 2.5–3.5 mEq/l) rarely causes symptoms. Severe hypokalaemia with plasma potassium levels <2.5 mEq/l generally produces muscle weakness and may lead to paralysis and respiratory failure.

Cardiac effects of hypokalaemia are usually minimal until plasma K levels are <3 mEq/l. Hypokalaemia produces sagging of the ST segment, depression of the T wave, and elevation of the U wave. With marked hypokalaemia, the T wave becomes progressively smaller and the U wave becomes increasingly larger. Sometimes, a flat or positive T wave merges with a positive U wave, which may be confused with QT prolongation. Hypokalaemia may produce premature ventricular and atrial contractions, ventricular and atrial tachyarrhythmias, and 2nd- or 3rd-degree atrioventricular block. Such arrhythmias become more severe with increasingly severe hypokalaemia; eventually, ventricular fibrillation may occur. Patients with

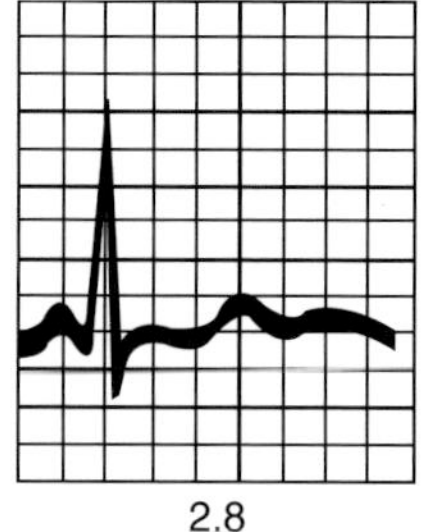

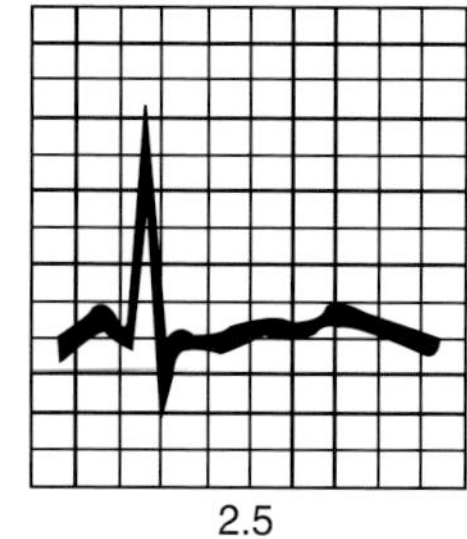

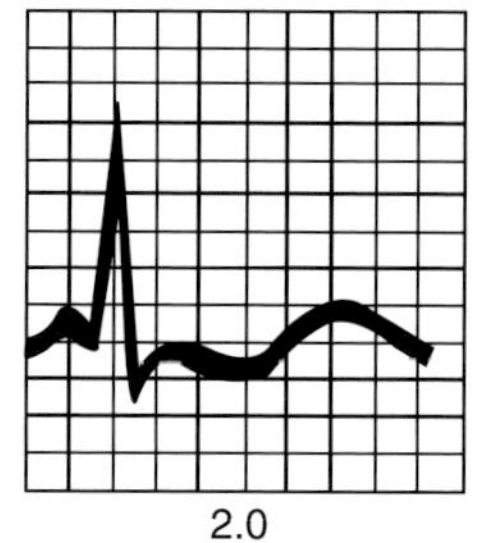

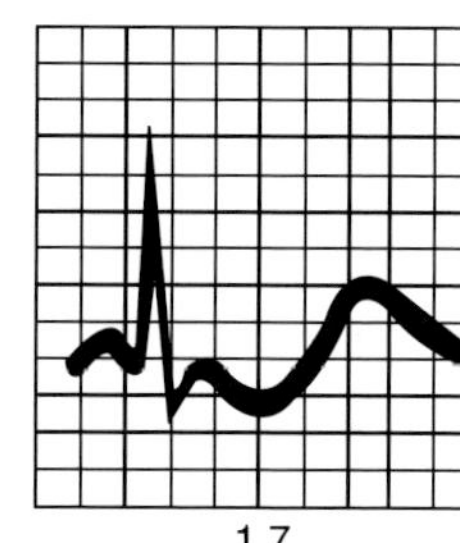

Fig. 19.3 Some ECG features of hypokalaemia.

significant pre-existing heart disease and/or those receiving digoxin are at risk of cardiac conduction abnormalities even from mild hypokalaemia (see Fig. 19.3). Some of these changes could be the result of other accompanying electrolyte abnormalities, e.g. hypocalcaemia and hypomagnesaemia.

Potassium replacement

In mild cases of hypokalaemia the oral route is used to top up potassium. When hypokalaemia is severe, is unresponsive to oral therapy or occurs in hospitalized patients with active disease, potassium must be replaced parenterally. Because potassium solutions can irritate peripheral veins, the concentration should not exceed 40 mEq/l. The rate of correction of hypokalaemia is limited because of the lag in potassium movement into cells. Routine infusion rates should not exceed 10 mEq/hour. In hypokalaemia-induced arrhythmia, IV potassium must be given more rapidly, usually through a central vein or using multiple peripheral veins simultaneously. Infusion of 40 mEq KCl/hour can be undertaken but only with continuous cardiac monitoring and hourly plasma potassium determinations. If the hypokalaemia is due to potassium depletion, a potassium deficit of 10% of the total body potassium stores is expected for every 1 mEq/l decrease in the serum potassium.

In potassium deficit with high plasma potassium concentration, as in diabetic ketoacidosis, IV potassium is deferred until the plasma potassium starts to fall. When hypokalaemia occurs with hypomagnesaemia, both the potassium and magnesium deficiencies must be corrected to stop ongoing renal potassium wasting.

Hyperkalaemia

Hyperkalaemia is serum K concentration >5.5 mEq/l resulting from excess total body K stores or abnormal movement of K out of cells. The usual cause is impairment of renal excretion; it can also occur by trans cellular shifts.

Pseudohyperkalaemia

Potassium release from traumatic haemolysis during the venipuncture can produce a spurious elevation in serum potassium. This is more common than suspected, and has been reported in 1 in 5 of blood samples with an elevated serum potassium. Potassium release from cells during clot formation in the specimen tube can also produce pseudohyperkalaemia when severe leucocytosis (white blood cell count greater than 50 000/mm^3) or thrombocytosis (platelet count greater than 1 million/mm^3) is present. When this condition is suspected, the serum potassium should be measured in an unclotted blood sample.

Causes of hyperkalaemia

Transcellular shift

Hyperkalaemia may be caused by transcellular movement of potassium out of cells in metabolic acidosis as in diabetic ketoacidosis and moderately heavy exercise. Drugs that can promote hyperkalaemia via transcellular potassium shifts include β-receptor antagonists and digitalis. Serious hyperkalaemia (i.e. serum potassium above 7 mEq/l) is possible only with digitalis toxicity.

Impaired renal excretion

Hyperkalaemia from total body potassium excess is particularly common in oliguric states (especially acute renal failure) and with rhabdomyolysis, burns, bleeding into soft tissue or the GI tract, and adrenal insufficiency. In chronic renal failure, hyperkalaemia is uncommon until the glomerular filtration rate (GFR) falls to <10–15 ml/min. Other potential causes of hyperkalaemia in chronic renal failure are hyporeninaemic hypoaldosteronism (type 4 renal tubular acidosis), angiotensin-converting enzyme (ACE) inhibitors, K-sparing diuretics, fasting (suppression of insulin secretion), β-blockers and NSAIDs. Other drugs that may limit renal potassium output, thereby producing hyperkalaemia, include cyclosporine, lithium, heparin and trimethoprim.

Urine potassium

Hyperkalaemia can be caused by potassium release from cells (transcellular shift) or by impaired renal potassium excretion. If the source of the hyperkalaemia is unclear, the urinary potassium concentration can be helpful. A high urine potassium (greater than 30 mEq/l) suggests a transcellular shift, and a low urine potassium (less than 30 mEq/l) indicates impaired renal excretion.

Clinical manifestations

The most serious consequence of hyperkalaemia is the slowing of electrical conduction in the heart (Fig. 19.4).

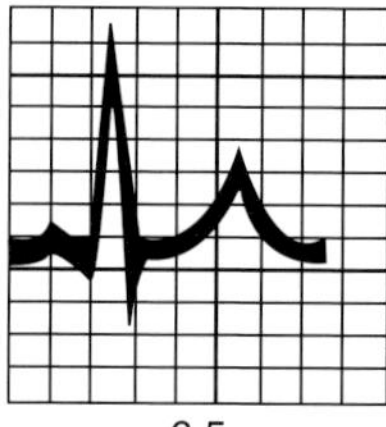

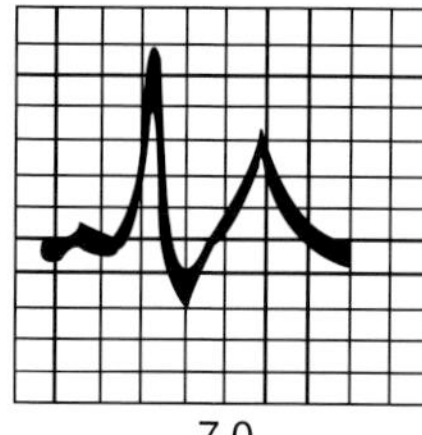

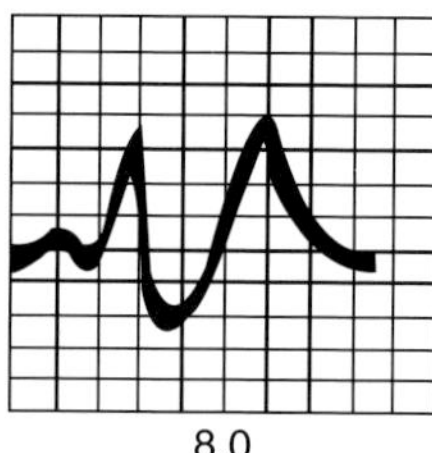

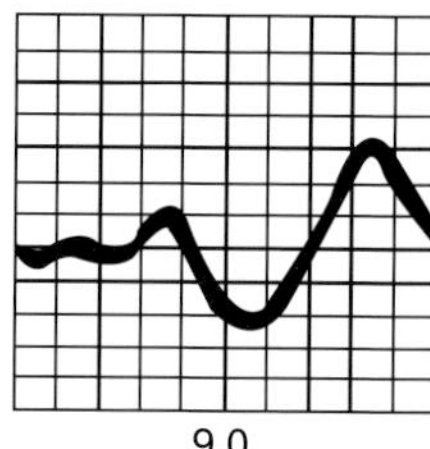

Fig. 19.4 Some ECG features of hyperkalaemia.

The ECG can begin to change when the serum potassium reaches 6.0 mEq/l, and it is always abnormal when the serum potassium reaches 8.0 mEq/l. As the hyperkalaemia progresses, the P wave amplitude decreases and the PR interval lengthens. The P waves eventually disappear and the QRS duration becomes prolonged. The final event is ventricular asystole.

Management of hyperkalaemia

Mild hyperkalaemia

Patients with plasma potassium <6 mmol/l and no ECG abnormalities may respond to diminished K intake or stopping potassium-elevating drugs. The addition of a loop diuretic enhances renal potassium excretion. Sodium polystyrene sulfonate can be given orally or rectally (15 g 3–4 times daily). It acts as a cation exchange resin and removes potassium through the GI mucosa. About 1 mEq of potassium is removed per gram of resin given.

Moderate to severe hyperkalaemia

Plasma K >6 mmol/l, especially with electrocardiographic changes, requires aggressive therapy to shift K into cells. The first two of the following measures are performed immediately:

(1) Administration of 10 to 20 ml 10% calcium gluconate IV over 5–10 min. Calcium antagonizes the effect of hyperkalaemia on cardiac muscle excitability. Calcium chloride can also be used but can be irritating and should be given through a central venous catheter. The effect occurs within minutes but lasts only 20 to 30 min. Calcium infusion is a temporizing measure while awaiting the effects of other treatments and may need to be repeated. When hyperkalaemia is accompanied by evidence of circulatory compromise, calcium chloride is preferred to calcium gluconate. One ampule (10 ml) of 10% calcium chloride contains three times more elemental calcium than one ampule of 10% calcium gluconate. Calcium must be given cautiously to patients on digitalis because hypercalcaemia can potentiate digitalis cardiotoxicity. If the hyperkalaemia is a manifestation of digitalis toxicity, calcium is contraindicated.

(2) Administration of regular insulin 5–10 units IV administered simultaneously with rapid infusion of 50 ml 50% glucose over 5–10 min. The effect on plasma potassium peaks in 1 hour and lasts for several hours. It will drop levels by 1 mmol/l for 1–2 hours.

(3) A high-dose β-agonist, such as salbutamol 10 to 20 mg inhaled over 10 min, can safely lower plasma potassium by 0.5–1.5 mmol/l and may be a helpful adjunct. The peak effect occurs in 90 min.

(4) Administration of IV $NaHCO_3$ is controversial. It may lower serum K over several hours. Reduction may result from alkalinization or the hypertonicity due to the concentrated Na in the preparation. The hypertonic sodium that it contains may be harmful for dialysis patients who also may have volume overload. $NaHCO_3$ is available in two concentrations: 1.26% and 8.4%, of which 1.26% is preferable as it is isotonic and causes less irritation.

(5) In addition to the above strategies for lowering K by shifting it into cells, manoeuvres to remove potassium from the body should also be performed early in the treatment of severe or symptomatic hyperkalaemia. Potassium can be removed via the GI tract by administration of Na polystyrene sulphonate or by haemodialysis. Haemodialysis should be instituted promptly after emergency measures in patients with renal failure or if emergency treatment is ineffective.

Magnesium

Main points

(1) Serum magnesium is not a sensitive marker of total body magnesium store because 99% of the magnesium in the body is inside cells.

(2) Magnesium depletion is very common in critically ill patients, particularly in patients with diarrhoea and patients receiving frusemide.

(3) Magnesium deficiency should be looked for daily in all critical care patients. Magnesium supplements are particularly important in patients receiving frusemide.

(4) Magnesium deficiency can cause resistant hypokalaemia, and magnesium replacement is necessary in these cases before the serum potassium will return to normal.

(6) The best indicator of magnesium replenishment is the urinary excretion of magnesium.

Magnesium plays an important role in the activity of electrically excitable tissues. Many enzymes are magnesium activated or dependent. Magnesium is required by all enzymatic processes involving ATP and by many of the enzymes involved in nucleic acid metabolism, so magnesium depletion could lead to defects in cellular metabolism. Magnesium is also related to calcium and potassium metabolism, the specifics of which are not fully understood. Magnesium also regulates the movement of calcium into smooth muscle cells and hence influences cardiac contractility and peripheral vascular tone.

Hypomagnesaemia

The maintenance of plasma Mg concentration is largely a function of dietary intake and effective renal and intestinal conservation. Plasma Mg concentration and either total body Mg or intracellular Mg content are not closely related. However, severe plasma hypomagnesaemia may reflect diminished body stores of Mg. Hypomagnesaemia is diagnosed by a serum Mg level <0.70 mmol/l. Severe hypomagnesaemia usually results in levels of <0.50 mmol/l.

Magnesium deficiency is common in hospitalized patients. It is probably the most underdiagnosed electrolyte disturbance. Hypomagnesaemia is seen very frequently in patients admitted to the intensive care unit and is present in about 65% of patients in this population. As serum Mg levels are still commonly used to reflect depleted stores of Mg this deficiency is still under diagnosed. Because serum Mg levels have a limited ability to detect Mg depletion, recognizing the conditions that predispose to Mg depletion may be the only clue to an underlying electrolyte imbalance. Magnesium depletion is often accompanied by depletion of other electrolytes, such as potassium, phosphate and calcium.

Common causes of magnesium deficiency

(1) Renal loss, due to (a) loop diuretics: frusemide; (b) nephrotoxins: aminoglycosides, amphotericin, cyclosporin, etc.; (c) diabetes mellitus: due to polyuria.

(2) Extrarenal loss, e.g. diarrhoea.

(3) Alcohol-related disease, e.g. malnutrition or diarrhoea.

Clinical features

The clinical manifestations of magnesium deficiency are not very specific. Magnesium has a membrane stabilizing effect and hence its deficiency is more likely to affect electrically active tissues, the heart and the central nervous system.

Magnesium deficiency makes the myocardium irritable and predisposes the heart to arrhythmias. One of the most serious arrhythmias associated with magnesium depletion is torsades de pointes (polymorphous ventricular tachycardia). It will potentiate digoxin toxicity and can cause ventricular arrhythmias. Intravenous magnesium can suppress digoxin toxicity induced arrhythmias, even when serum magnesium levels are normal.

The neurological manifestations of magnesium deficiency are not common and are non-specific; they include confusion, tremors, hyperreflexia and generalized seizures.

Diagnosis

Serum magnesium levels are not a sensitive indicator of magnesium stores. Diagnosing magnesium deficiency is difficult and will have to be assumed depending on the associated clinical features. In cases of magnesium depletion from a non-renal cause, the diagnosis of deficiency and replacement of magnesium can be guided by the urinary magnesium conservation for a given load of intravenous magnesium.

Urinary magnesium

When magnesium depletion is due to non-renal factors (e.g. diarrhoea), urinary magnesium excretion is a more sensitive test for magnesium depletion. However, because most cases of magnesium depletion are due to enhanced renal magnesium excretion, the diagnostic value of urinary magnesium excretion may be limited.

Under normal circumstances, only small quantities of magnesium are excreted in the urine. When magnesium intake is deficient, the kidneys conserve magnesium and urinary magnesium excretion falls to negligible levels. In the absence of renal magnesium wasting, the urinary excretion of magnesium in response to a magnesium load may be the most sensitive index of total body magnesium stores. Under normal conditions the rate of magnesium reabsorption is close to the maximum tubular reabsorption rate (T_{max}), so most of the infused magnesium will be excreted in the urine when magnesium stores are normal. However, when magnesium stores are deficient, the magnesium reabsorption rate is much lower than the T_{max}, so more of the infused magnesium will be reabsorbed and less will be excreted in the urine. When less than 50% of the infused magnesium is recovered in the urine, magnesium deficiency is likely, and when more than 80% of the infused magnesium is excreted in the urine, magnesium deficiency is unlikely. This test can be particularly valuable in determining the end-point of magnesium replacement therapy (i.e. magnesium replacement is continued until urinary magnesium excretion is at least 80% of the infused magnesium load). It is important to emphasize that this test will be unreliable in patients with impaired renal function or when there is ongoing renal magnesium wasting.

Magnesium replacement therapy

The magnesium preparations are available for oral and parenteral administration. The oral preparations can be used for daily maintenance therapy and for correcting mild, asymptomatic magnesium deficiency. However, because intestinal absorption of oral magnesium is erratic, parenteral magnesium is preferred for treating symptomatic or severe magnesium deficiency.

The standard intravenous preparation is magnesium sulphate. Each gram of magnesium sulphate has 4 mmol of elemental magnesium. Magnesium sulphate solution has an osmolarity of 4000 mOsm/l, so it must be diluted for intravenous use. Local protocols should be followed when replacing the deficiencies.

In severe, symptomatic hypomagnesaemia (e.g. generalized seizures, with Mg <0.5 mmol/l), 2–4 g of $MgSO_4$ IV is given over 5 to 10 min. If seizures persist, the dose may be repeated up to a total of 10 g over the next 6 hours. If seizures stop, 10 g can be infused over 24 hours, followed by up to 2.5 g every 12 hours to replace the deficit in total Mg stores and prevent further drops in plasma Mg. When plasma Mg is <0.5 mmol/l but symptoms are less severe, $MgSO_4$ may be given IV at a rate of 1 g/hour as slow infusion for up to 10 hours. In less severe cases of hypomagnesaemia, gradual repletion may be achieved by administration of smaller parenteral doses over 3–5 days until the plasma magnesium level is normal.

Hypermagnesaemia

Magnesium accumulation is very rare and may occur in patients with impaired renal function. Magnesium infusions are commonly used to treat eclampsia and pre-eclampsia on labour wards. The renal excretion of magnesium becomes impaired when the creatinine clearance falls below 30 ml/min. Toxicity is possible in these patients if they develop renal failure when they are receiving magnesium infusions. Other conditions that can predispose to mild hypermagnesaemia are diabetic ketoacidosis (transient), adrenal insufficiency, hyperparathyroidism and lithium intoxication.

Clinical features

Deep tendon reflexes disappear as the plasma Mg level approaches 5.0 mmol/l; hypotension, respiratory depression and narcosis develop with increasing hypermagnesaemia. Cardiac arrest may occur when blood Mg levels exceed 6.0–7.5 mmol/l. At plasma magnesium concentrations of 2.5–5 mmol/l, the ECG shows prolongation of the PR interval, widening of the QRS complex, and increased T wave amplitude. Most of the serious consequences of hypermagnesaemia are due to calcium antagonism in the cardiovascular system. Most of the cardiovascular depression is the result of cardiac conduction delays.

Management

Haemodialysis is the treatment of choice for severe hypermagnesaemia. Intravenous calcium gluconate (1 g IV over 2–3 min) can be used to antagonize the cardiovascular effects of hypermagnesaemia temporarily, until dialysis is started. if fluids are permissible and some renal function is preserved, aggressive volume infusion combined with frusemide may be effective in reducing the serum magnesium levels in less advanced cases of hypermagnesaemia.

Phosphorus

Main points

(1) Watch the plasma phosphate levels carefully when starting parenteral nutrition and while starting enteral nutrition in patients suffering prolonged malnutrition because of the risk of hypophosphataemia.

The average adult has 500–800 g of phosphorus. Most is contained in organic molecules such as phospholipids and phosphoproteins, and 85% is located in the bony skeleton. The remaining 15% in soft tissues is present as free, inorganic phosphorus. In soft tissues, PO_4 is mainly found in the intracellular compartment as an integral component of several organic compounds, including nucleic acids and cell membrane phospholipids.

Hypophosphataemia

Hypophosphataemia (serum PO_4 <0.8 mmol/l) occurs in 2% of hospitalized patients but is more prevalent in certain populations (e.g. it occurs in up to 10% of hospitalized patients with alcoholism). Hypophosphataemia has numerous causes, but clinically significant hypophosphataemia occurs in relatively few clinical settings, such as the recovery phase of diabetic ketoacidosis, acute alcoholism and severe burns. Hypophosphataemia may also occur in patients receiving TPN, during refeeding after prolonged malnutrition, and in severe chronic respiratory alkalosis. Hypophosphataemia is reported in 17% to 28% of critically ill patients and can be the result of an intracellular shift of phosphorus, an increase in the renal excretion of phosphorus, or a decrease in phosphorus absorption from the GI tract. Most cases of hypophosphataemia are due to movement of PO_4 into cells.

Causes

The movement of glucose into cells is accompanied by a similar movement of PO_4 into cells, and if the extracellular content of PO_4 is marginal, this intracellular PO_4 shift can result in hypophosphataemia. Glucose loading is the most common cause of hypophosphataemia in hospitalized patients, usually seen during refeeding in alcoholic, malnourished or debilitated patients. It can occur with oral feedings, enteral tube feedings or with TPN. In fact, hypophosphataemia may be responsible for the progressive weakness and inanition that characterizes the refeeding syndrome in malnourished patients.

Other causes of low phosphate levels include respiratory alkalosis, sepsis and use of β-receptor agonists for bronchodilatation.

Clinical manifestations

Hypophosphataemia is often clinically silent, even when the serum PO_4 falls to extremely low levels. In addition, serum PO_4 levels do not necessarily reflect the severity of tissue phosphorus deficit. In one study of patients with severe hypophosphataemia (i.e. serum PO_4 <1.0 mg/dl), none of the patients showed evidence of harmful effects. Despite the apparent lack of harm, phosphate depletion creates a risk of impaired energy production in all aerobic cells.

Muscle weakness

One of the possible consequences of impaired energy production from phosphate depletion is skeletal muscle weakness. Biochemical evidence of skeletal muscle disruption (e.g. elevated creatine kinase levels in blood) is common in patients with hypophosphataemia, but overt muscle weakness is usually absent. Some studies show that respiratory muscle weakness is common in hypophosphataemia but is not clinically significant in most patients. At present, the evidence linking phosphate depletion with clinically significant skeletal muscle weakness is scant.

Phosphate replacement

Oral PO_4 replacement is usually adequate in asymptomatic patients, even when the plasma concentration is very low. PO_4 can be given in doses ≤3 g/day PO in tablets containing Na or KPO_4. Oral Na or KPO_4 is usually poorly tolerated because of diarrhoea. Removal of the cause of hypophosphataemia, such as stopping PO_4-binding antacids or diuretics or correcting hypomagnesaemia, is preferable when possible.

Parenteral PO_4 should be administered when plasma PO_4 is <0.16 mmol/l; rhabdomyolysis, haemolysis or CNS symptoms are present; or oral replacement is not feasible due to underlying illness. IV administration of KPO_4 (as buffered mix of K_2HPO_4 and KH_2PO_4) is relatively safe if renal function is well preserved. The usual parenteral dose is 2 mg (8 mmol)/kg IV over 6 hours. Alcoholics may require ≥1 g/day during TPN.

Hyperphosphataemia

Most cases of hyperphosphataemia in the ICU are the result of impaired PO_4 excretion from renal insufficiency or PO_4 release from cells because of widespread cell necrosis (e.g. rhabdomyolysis or tumour lysis). Hyperphosphataemia can also be seen in diabetic ketoacidosis but, as described earlier, this disorder is almost always accompanied by phosphate depletion, which becomes evident after the onset of insulin therapy.

Clinical manifestations

Most patients with hyperphosphataemia are asymptomatic, although symptoms of hypocalcaemia, including tetany, can occur if concomitant hypocalcaemia is present. Soft-tissue calcifications are common in patients with chronic renal failure, especially if the plasma Ca × PO_4 product is chronically >70.

Management

There are two approaches to hyperphosphataemia. The first is to promote PO_4 binding in the upper GI tract, which can lower the serum PO_4 even in the absence of any oral intake of phosphate. Sucralfate or aluminium-containing antacids can be used for this purpose. The other approach to hyperphosphataemia is to enhance PO_4 clearance with haemodialysis. This is reserved for patients with renal failure, and is rarely necessary.

Calcium

Main points

(1) Because calcium infusions can be damaging, intravenous calcium should be reserved only for cases of symptomatic hypocalcaemia, or when ionized calcium levels fall below 0.65 mmol/l.

(2) Magnesium depletion, which is common in ICU patients, should always be considered as a possible cause of hypocalcaemia.

(3) For patients with hypoalbuminaemia, do not use any of the correction factors proposed for adjusting the plasma calcium concentration (because they are unreliable). You must measure the ionized calcium in these patients.

Calcium is required for the proper functioning of muscle contraction, nerve conduction, hormone release and blood coagulation. Maintenance of the body Ca stores depends on dietary Ca intake, absorption of Ca from the GI tract and renal Ca excretion. Cytosolic ionized Ca is maintained within the micromolar range (less than 1/1000 of the plasma concentration). Ionized Ca acts as an intracellular second messenger; it is involved in skeletal muscle contraction, excitation–contraction coupling in cardiac and smooth muscle, and activation of protein kinases and enzyme phosphorylation. Calcium is also involved in the action of other intracellular messengers, such as cyclic adenosine monophosphate (cAMP) and inositol 1,4,5-triphosphate, and thus mediates the cellular response to numerous hormones, including epinephrine, glucagon, ADH (vasopressin). Despite its important intracellular roles, roughly 99% of body Ca is in bone, mainly as hydroxyapatite crystals. Roughly 1% of bone Ca is freely exchangeable with the extracellular fluid and, therefore, is available for buffering changes in Ca balance.

Plasma calcium

Normal total plasma Ca levels range from 2.20 to 2.60 mmol/l. About 40% of the total blood Ca is bound to plasma proteins, primarily albumin. The remaining 60% includes ionized Ca plus Ca complexed with phosphate (PO_4) and citrate. The calcium assay used by most clinical laboratories measures all three fractions of calcium. Because albumin is responsible for 80% of the protein-bound calcium in plasma, a decrease in albumin decreases the amount of calcium in the protein-bound fraction. The total calcium in plasma decreases by the same amount, but the ionized calcium remains unchanged. Because the ionized calcium is the physiologically active fraction, the hypocalcaemia caused by hypoalbuminaemia is not physiologically significant. Acidosis decreases the binding of calcium to albumin and increases the ionized calcium, whereas alkalosis has the opposite effect.

The metabolism of Ca and of PO_4 are intimately related. The regulation of both Ca and PO_4 balance is greatly influenced by circulating levels of parathyroid hormone (PTH), vitamin D, and, to a lesser extent, calcitonin. Calcium and inorganic PO_4 concentrations are also linked by their ability to react chemically to form $CaPO_4$. The product of concentrations of Ca and PO_4 (in mEq/l) is estimated to be 60 normally; when the product exceeds 70, precipitation of $CaPO_4$ crystals in soft tissue is much more likely. Precipitation in vascular tissue accelerates arteriosclerotic vascular disease.

Hypocalcaemia

Ionized hypocalcaemia has been reported in 15% to 50% of admissions to the ICU.

Causes

Hypoparathyroidism is a leading cause of hypocalcaemia in outpatients, but is not a consideration in the ICU unless neck surgery has been performed recently. The common disorders associated with ionized hypocalcemia in ICU patients are listed below.

Renal failure

- Ionized hypocalcaemia can accompany renal failure as a result of phosphate retention and impaired conversion of vitamin D to its active form in the kidneys.
- The treatment is aimed at lowering the phosphate levels in blood with antacids that block phosphorus absorption in the small bowel.

Magnesium depletion

- Magnesium depletion promotes hypocalcaemia by inhibiting parathormone secretion and reducing end-organ responsiveness to parathormone. Hypocalcaemia from magnesium depletion is refractory to calcium replacement therapy, and magnesium repletion often corrects the hypocalcaemia without calcium replacement.

Sepsis

- Sepsis is a common cause of hypocalcaemia in the ICU. Septic shock can cause hypocalcaemia due to suppression of PTH release and decreased conversion of 25(OH)D to $1,25(OH)_2D$. But it may involve an increase in calcium binding to albumin caused by elevated levels of circulating free fatty acids.

Pancreatitis

- Severe pancreatitis can produce ionized hypocalcaemia through several mechanisms. The prognosis is adversely affected by the appearance of hypocalcaemia, although a causal relationship has not been proven.

Alkalosis

- As mentioned earlier, alkalosis promotes the binding of calcium to albumin and can reduce the fraction of ionized calcium in blood.
- Symptomatic hypocalcaemia is more common with respiratory alkalosis than with metabolic alkalosis.
- Infusions of sodium bicarbonate can also be accompanied by ionized hypocalcaemia because calcium directly binds to the infused bicarbonate.
- Other causes include drugs such as aminoglycosides, heparin, etc. Blood transfusions can reduce ionized calcium but the effects are transient and are more pronounced in patients with liver and kidney failure.

Clinical manifestations

The clinical manifestations of hypocalcaemia are related to enhanced cardiac and neuromuscular excitability and reduced contractile force in cardiac muscle and vascular smooth muscle.

Hypocalcaemia can be accompanied by tetany (of peripheral or laryngeal muscles), hyperreflexia, paraesthesias and seizures. The cardiovascular complications of hypocalcaemia include hypotension, decreased cardiac output and ventricular ectopic activity. These complications are rarely seen in mild cases of ionized hypocalcaemia (i.e. ionized calcium 0.8–1.0 mmol/l). However, advanced stages of ionized hypocalcaemia (i.e. ionized calcium <0.65 mmol/l) can be associated with heart block, ventricular tachycardia and refractory hypotension.

Chvostek's sign is an involuntary twitching of the facial muscles elicited by a light tapping of the facial nerve just anterior to the exterior auditory meatus. It is present in 10–25% of healthy people and in most people with acute hypocalcaemia but is often absent in chronic hypocalcaemia. Trousseau's sign is the precipitation of carpopedal spasm by reduction of the blood supply to the hand with a tourniquet or BP cuff inflated to 20 mmHg above systolic BP applied to the forearm for 3 min. Trousseau's sign also occurs in alkalosis, hypomagnesaemia, hypokalaemia and hyperkalaemia and in about 6% of people with no identifiable electrolyte disturbance. However,

Chvostek's sign is non-specific (it is present in 25% of normal adults), and Trousseau's sign is insensitive (it can be absent in 30% of patients with hypocalcaemia).

Calcium replacement therapy

The treatment of ionized hypocalcaemia should be directed at the underlying cause of the problem. However, symptomatic hypocalcaemia is considered a medical emergency, and the treatment of choice is intravenous calcium. The two most popular calcium solutions for intravenous use are 10% calcium chloride and 10% calcium gluconate. Both solutions have the same concentration of calcium salt (i.e. 100 mg/ml), but calcium chloride contains three times more elemental calcium than calcium gluconate. One 10-ml ampoule of 10% calcium chloride contains 272 mg of elemental calcium (2000 mOsmol/l), whereas one 10-ml ampoule of 10% calcium gluconate contains only 90 mg of elemental calcium (680 mOsmol/l).

Dosage recommendations

Intravenous calcium is indicated only for patients with symptomatic hypocalcaemia or an ionized calcium level below 0.65 mmol/l. The intravenous calcium solutions are hyperosmolar and should be given through a large central vein if possible. If a peripheral vein is used, calcium gluconate is the preferred solution because of its lower osmolarity. A bolus dose of 100 mg elemental calcium (diluted in 100 ml isotonic saline and given over 5–10 min) should raise the total serum calcium by 0.25 mmol/l , but levels will begin to fall after 30 min. Therefore, the bolus dose of calcium should be followed by a continuous infusion at a dose rate of 0.5–2 mg/kg/per hour (elemental calcium) for at least 6 hours. Individual responses will vary, so calcium dosing should be guided by the level of ionized calcium in blood.

Infusions of calcium are hazardous in patients receiving digoxin and should be given slowly and with continuous ECG monitoring. Aggressive calcium replacement can promote intracellular calcium overload, which can produce a lethal cell injury. Calcium infusions can promote vasoconstriction and ischaemia in any of the vital organs.

Hypercalcaemia

Hypercalcaemia is not a common problem in intensive care. In 90% of cases, the underlying cause is hyperparathyroidism or malignancy. Haematological cancers, most often myeloma, but also certain lymphomas and lymphosarcomas, cause hypercalcaemia. Other causes include granulomatous diseases like sarcoid. Less common causes include prolonged immobilization, thyrotoxicosis and drugs (lithium, thiazide diuretics).

Clinical manifestations

Clinical manifestations of hypercalcaemia include constipation, anorexia, nausea and vomiting, abdominal pain and ileus. Impairment of the renal concentrating mechanism leads to polyuria, nocturia and polydipsia. Elevation of plasma Ca >12 mg/dl (>3.00 mmol/l) causes emotional lability, confusion, delirium, psychosis, stupor and coma.

Management

Treatment is indicated when the hypercalcaemia is associated with adverse effects, or when the serum calcium is greater than 14 mg/dl (ionized calcium above 3.5 mmol/l). There are four main strategies for lowering plasma Ca: decrease intestinal Ca absorption, increase urinary Ca excretion, decrease bone resorption, and remove excess Ca through dialysis. The treatment used depends on both the degree and the cause of hypercalcaemia.

In mild hypercalcaemia (plasma Ca < 2.88 mmol/l), in which symptoms are mild, treatment is deferred pending definitive diagnosis. After diagnosis, the underlying cause is treated. If symptoms are significant, treatment aimed at lowering plasma Ca is necessary. Oral PO_4 can be used. Another treatment is increasing urinary Ca excretion by giving isotonic saline plus a loop diuretic. Initially, 1–2 l of saline is given over 2–4 hours because nearly all patients with significant hypercalcaemia are hypovolaemic. Frusemide 20 to 40 mg IV every 2–4 hours is given as needed to maintain a urine output of roughly 250 ml/hour (monitored hourly). Plasma Ca begins to decrease in 2–4 hours and falls to near-normal levels within 24 hours.

Moderate hypercalcaemia (plasma Ca >2.88 mmol/l and < 4.51 mmol/l) can be treated with isotonic saline and a loop diuretic as previously mentioned or, depending on its cause, agents that decrease bone resorption (usually calcitonin, bisphosphonates, or infrequently plicamycin or gallium nitrate), corticosteroids or chloroquine can be used.

Calcitonin

Calcitonin (thyrocalcitonin) is a rapidly acting peptide hormone normally secreted in response to hypercalcaemia by the C cells of the thyroid. Calcitonin appears to lower plasma Ca by inhibiting osteoclastic activity. A dose of 4–8 IU/kg SC every 12 hours of salmon calcitonin is safe. Its usefulness in the treatment of cancer-associated hypercalcaemia is limited by its short duration of action, the development of tachyphylaxis and the lack of response in ≥40% of patients. However, the combination of salmon calcitonin and prednisone may control plasma Ca for several months in some patients with cancer. If calcitonin stops working, it can be stopped for 2 days (while prednisone is continued) and then resumed.

In severe hypercalcaemia (plasma Ca >4.50 mmol/l or with severe symptoms), haemodialysis with low-Ca dialysate may be needed in addition to other treatments above. Although there is no completely satisfactory way to correct severe hypercalcaemia in patients with renal failure, haemodialysis is probably the safest and most reliable short-term treatment.

Intravenous PO_4 (disodium PO_4 or monopotassium PO_4) should be used only when hypercalcaemia is life-threatening and unresponsive to other methods and when short-term haemodialysis is not possible. No more than 1 g should be given IV in 24 hours; usually one or two doses over 2 days lower plasma Ca for 10 to 15 days. Soft-tissue calcification and acute renal failure may result.

Key points

- Crystalloids are solutions in water of inorganic ions and small organic molecules, used for intravenous therapy. They can be composed of either glucose or sodium chloride, and may be isotonic, hypotonic or hypertonic.
- Colloids contain large, poorly diffusible, solute molecules that create an osmotic pressure to keep water in the vascular space. They are more effective than crystalloid fluids for expanding the plasma volume.
- Disorders of sodium concentration are nearly always caused by excess free water (hyponatraemia) or free water loss (hypernatraemia). Severe or symptomatic acute hyponatraemia should be corrected at a steady rate (2 mEq/l per hour) because rapid correction risks ceretral swelling.
- When hypokalaemia is severe, potassium is replaced parenterally. Potassium solutions can irritate peripheral veins; the concentration should not exceed 40 mEq/l. The rate of correction of hypokalaemia is limited because of the lag in potassium movement into cells. Routine infusion rates should not exceed 10 mEq/hour.
- Moderate to severe hyperkalaemia with plasma K > 6 mmol/l, especially with electrocardiographic changes, requires aggressive therapy. 10% calcium gluconate IV should be given over 5–10 min. Calcium antagonizes the effect of hyperkalaemia on cardiac muscle excitability. Insulin 5–10 units IV is administered simultaneously with rapid infusion of 50 ml 50% glucose over 5–10 min. The effect on plasma potassium peaks in 1 hr and lasts for several hours.
- Magnesium depletion is very common in critically ill patients and should be looked for daily in all critical care patients.

Further reading

- Finfer S, Bellomo R, Boyce N *et al.* (2004) A comparison of albumin and saline for fluid resuscitation in the intensive care unit. *N. Engl. J. Med.* **350**: 2247–56.
- Fink MP, Edward Abraham E, Vincent J-L, Kochanek PM (2005) *Textbook of Critical Care*, 5th edn. Chapters 13–17. Philadelphia, PA: Elsevier.
- Marino, PL (2006) *The ICU Book*, 3rd edn. Chapter 32, Hypertonic and hypotonic conditions; Chapter 33, Potassium; Chapter 34, Magnesium; Chapter 35, Calcium and phosphorus; pp. 595–658. Baltimore, MD: Lippincott, Williams & Wilkins.

Chapter 20

Acid–base abnormalities

Prasad Bheemasenachar

Acid–base balance

With a normal caloric intake of a meat-based diet the average person will generate approximately 20 000 mmol of acid/day in the form of CO_2 as the end-product of carbohydrate and fat metabolism. This CO_2 will be excreted by the lungs. Protein catabolism produces about 1 mmol/kg (50–60 mmol/day) of inorganic acids (like sulphuric, phosphoric or hydrochloric acids) which must be excreted by the kidney. Normally these acids are eliminated very efficiently by the lungs and the kidneys which keep the hydrogen ion concentration within a very narrow range (Fig. 20.1). Concentration of H^+ is maintained within the nmol/l range (36–44 nmol/l). By contrast, most other ions are regulated in the mmol/l range. The physiological advantages of this tight control principally involve providing conditions for optimal intracellular function. A critically important aspect of the significance of pH involves proteins. The net protein charge is dependent on the pH and the function of proteins is dependent on this charge because it determines the 3-D shape of the molecule and its binding characteristics.

Disorders of acid–base equilibrium are common in critically ill and injured patients. The presence of these disorders often signals severe underlying pathophysiology and, particularly in the case of metabolic acidosis, is a significant marker of adverse outcome. Whether acid–base disturbances are independent contributors to morbidity and mortality in the ICU or rather are simply epiphenomena is still a topic of controversy. However, because accumulating evidence suggests that a significant proportion of these disturbances result from therapy, clinicians must understand why they occur and how to avoid them.

Hydrogen ion concentration and pH

Note that the hydrogen ion concentration in extracellular fluid is expressed in *nano*moles (nmol) per litre. A nanomole is *one-millionth* of a millimole, so there are millions more sodium, chloride and other ions measured in mmol than there are hydrogen ions. Because nanomoles represent such a small amount, the concentration of hydrogen ions is routinely expressed in pH units, which are derived by taking the negative logarithm (base 10) of the hydrogen ions in nmol/l.

The relationship between hydrogen ion concentration and the pH is as follows:

$$\text{pH } 7.4 \text{ equates to a hydrogen ion concentration } [H^+] \text{ of } 40 \text{ nmol/l}$$

For each additional point increase in the pH the corresponding $[H^+]$ is obtained by multiplying the H^+ concentration by a factor of 0.8:

$$H^+ \text{ at a pH of } 7.4 = 40$$
$$H^+ \text{ at a pH of } 7.5 = 40 \; ([H^+] \text{ at pH of } 7.4) \times 0.8$$
$$H^+ \text{ at a pH of } 7.6 = 32 \; ([H^+] \text{ at pH of } 7.5) \times 0.8$$
$$H^+ \text{ at a pH of } 7.7 = 26 \; ([H^+] \text{ at pH of } 7.6) \times 0.8$$

As can be seen, the $[H^+]$ concentration halves for a 3-point jump in pH value.

For each additional point decrease in the pH the corresponding H^+ is obtained by multiplying the H^+ concentration by a factor of 1.25:

$$[H^+] \text{ at a pH of } 7.4 = 40$$
$$[H^+] \text{ at a pH of } 7.3 = 40 \; ([H^+] \text{ at pH of } 7.4) \times 1.25$$
$$[H^+] \text{ at a pH of } 7.2 = 50 \; ([H^+] \text{ at pH of } 7.3) \times 1.25 = 63 \text{ nmol/l}$$
$$[H^+] \text{ at a pH of } 7.1 = 62 \; ([H^+] \text{ at pH of } 7.2) \times 1.25 = 79 \text{ nmol/l}$$
$$[H^+] \text{ at a pH of } 7.0 = 100$$

Core Topics in Critical Care Medicine, eds. Fang Gao Smith and Joyce Yeung. Published by Cambridge University Press.

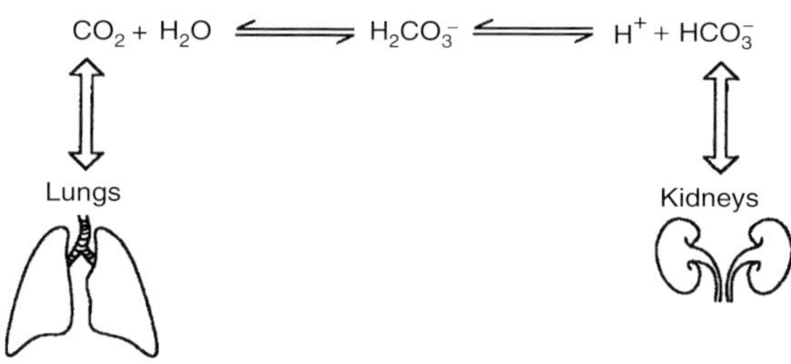

Fig. 20.1 Acid–base homeostasis maintained by lungs and kidneys.

As can be seen, the $[H^+]$ concentration doubles for a 3-point drop in pH value.

Changes in the $[H^+]$ by a factor of 2 cause a pH change of 0.3 – this provides us with a simple way to determine various pH–$[H^+]$ pairs of values if we know that pH 7.4 is 40 nmol/l. This useful relationship holds because log 2 is 0.3 so a doubling or a halving of $[H^+]$ means a change in pH by 0.3 either up or down.

There is a continuing discussion about the most appropriate symbol to represent the acidity of body fluids: pH or $[H^+]$.

The traditional versus the modern approach

There are two approaches, one traditional and the more recent physico-chemical (Stewart's) approach, which utilize different principles regarding the factors that influence the $[H^+]$ homeostasis.

The traditional theory makes us believe that the hydrogen ion concentration (pH) in blood is mainly influenced by balance between the carbon dioxide and the bicarbonate ions in the blood. The Henderson–Hasselbalch equation is central to this approach and demonstrates the relationship between key components of the blood that determine acid–base balance. The relationship among pH, $[HCO_3^-]$ and $PaCO_2$ is determined by the following equation:

$$pH = pKa + \log\left([HCO_3^-] \,/\, (PaCO_2 \times 0.03)\right)$$

An alternative approach derived from physico-chemical principles was proposed by a Canadian physiologist, Peter Stewart, in 1981. The two approaches are very similar in the way that acid–base disorders are classified and measured. The major difference between the approaches is conceptual; in other words, they differ in the way they explain the mechanism of the disturbance. In this approach the $[H^+]$ and the $[HCO_3^-]$ are dependent variables and their concentrations are determined by:

$PaCO_2$, partial pressure of carbon dioxide

SID (strong ion difference)

$= (Na^+ + K^+ + Ca^{2+} + Mg^{2+}) - (Cl^- + lactate^-)$

$=$ normally $40 - 42$

A_{TOT} = total weak acids 'buffers' concentration in blood (mainly consists of albumin and phosphates)

Neither $[H^+]$ nor $[HCO_3^-]$ can change unless one or more of these three variables changes. Hence, to understand how the body regulates pH, we need only ask how it regulates these three independent variables: SID, $PaCO_2$ and A_{TOT}.

The foundation of Stewart's theory is based on two fundamental laws of chemistry, the law of electro neutrality and the law of mass action. According to the law of electro neutrality all complex fluids achieve a status of electro neutrality and according to the law of mass action no new molecules (e.g. Na^+, K^+, Ca^{2+}, Mg^{2+}, Cl^-) can be formed or destroyed. Normally the SID_a (SID apparent: calculated by adding measured concentrations of strong ions $\{(Na^+ + K^+ + Ca^{2+} + Mg^{2+}) - (Cl^- + lactate^-)\}$) is matched by an equal and opposite negative charges contributed by the combined effects of weak ions, i.e. pCO_2 and the total weak acids (A_{TOT}). The combined charges of the weak ions is referred to as the effective strong ion difference: SID_e. When there are no unmeasured anions in blood the SID apparent is equal to SID effective; if there is a difference, this is referred to as the strong ion gap which predicts presence of unmeasured anions.

In health, blood achieves electro neutrality in its complex composition at an $[H^+]$ concentration of 40 nmol/l (pH of 7.4). When there is a change in one of the three independent variables the only way blood can maintain electro neutrality is to dissociate water to produce more H^+ ions or more OH^- ions which determines the new pH.

Both theories accept pCO_2 (respiratory component) as an independent variable that influences the $[H^+]$ homeostasis.

The role of plasma proteins, specifically albumin, in acid–base balance is neglected in the traditional approaches. This is addressed in Stewart's theory as the third independent variable, in the form of A_{TOT}.

Table 20.1 The major body buffer systems

Site	Buffer system	Comment
ECF	Bicarbonate	For metabolic acids
	Phosphate	Not important because concentration too low
	Protein	Not important because concentration too low
Blood	Bicarbonate	Important for metabolic acids
	Haemoglobin	Important for carbon dioxide
	Plasma protein	Minor buffer
	Phosphate	Concentration too low
ICF	Proteins	Important buffer
	Phosphates	Important buffer
Urine	Phosphate	Responsible for most of 'titratable acidity'
	Ammonia	Important – formation of NH_4^+
Bone	Calcium carbonate	In prolonged metabolic acidosis

This is important in the intensive care unit, as many patients suffer from hypoalbuminaemia. Reports have suggested that when using anion gap in the diagnosis of metabolic acidosis, unmeasured anions are missed in almost 50% of the critical care population as this is not taken into account. In this context using a corrected formula for measuring the anion gap which takes into account hypoalbuminaemia improves the accuracy of detecting unmeasured anions in the traditional approach.

The traditional approach attributes the reason for the metabolic disturbance to a change in the concentration of the bicarbonate ion, hence the measurement for this disturbance in the traditional approach is based on sodium bicarbonate measurements: the standard base excess, whilst in Stewart's approach the cause for a metabolic derangement is attributed to a change in the strong ion difference: the strong ion gap (the difference between the normal SID (40) and the measured SID ($Na^+ + K^+ + Ca^{2+} + Mg^{2+}$) – ($Cl^- +$ lactate$^-$)).

The standard base excess is mathematically equivalent to the change in the strong ion gap required to restore pH to 7.4 given a PCO_2 of 5.3 kPa. Thus, a standard base excess of −10 means that the strong ion difference is 10 mmol/l less than the strong ion difference that is associated with a pH of 7.4 when PCO_2 is 5.3 kPa. Hence whatever approach one uses neither the diagnosis nor the gravity of the derangement are different but what is different is the concept behind how these derangements happen.

Response to acid–base changes

Buffering

All acid or base challenges are buffered (see Table 20.1). In the ECF this is predominantly by the HCO_3^-/CO_2 buffer system, and inside cells the major buffers are proteins and PO_4. Buffering reactions are instantaneous and extremely effective: an acid load sufficient to reduce an unbuffered solution to a pH less than 2 only reduces the blood pH of an animal by 0.3 pH units.

The bicarbonate buffer system

The major buffer system in the ECF is the CO_2–bicarbonate buffer system. This is responsible for about 80% of extracellular buffering. It is the most important ECF buffer for metabolic acids but it cannot buffer respiratory acid–base disorders. The bicarbonate buffer system is an effective buffer system despite having a low pKa because the body also controls PCO_2.

The components are easily measured and are related to each other by the Henderson–Hasselbalch equation:

$$pH = pKa + \log10\ ([HCO_3]\ /\ 0.03 \times PCO_2)$$

On chemical grounds, a substance with a pKa of 6.1 should not be a good buffer at a pH of 7.4 if it were a simple buffer. The system is more complex as it is 'open at both ends' (meaning both $[HCO_3]$ and PCO_2 can be adjusted) and this greatly increases the buffering effectiveness of this system. The excretion of CO_2 via the lungs is particularly important because of the rapidity of the response. The adjustment of PCO_2 by change in alveolar ventilation has been referred to as physiological buffering.

The other buffer systems in the blood are the protein and phosphate buffer systems. These are the only blood buffer systems capable of buffering respiratory acid–base disturbances as the bicarbonate system is ineffective in buffering changes in H^+ produced by itself.

The phosphate buffer system

The phosphate buffer system is NOT an important blood buffer as its concentration is too low.

Phosphates are important buffers intracellularly and in urine where their concentration is higher.

Haemoglobin

Protein buffers in blood include haemoglobin (150 g/l) and plasma proteins (70 g/l). Haemoglobin is an important blood buffer particularly for buffering CO_2. Buffering is by the imidazole group of the histidine residue which has a pKa of about 6.8. This is suitable for effective buffering at physiological pH. Haemoglobin is quantitatively about 6 times more important than the plasma proteins as it is present in about twice the concentration and contains about three times the number of histidine residues per molecule.

Deoxyhaemoglobin is a more effective buffer than oxyhaemoglobin and this change in buffer capacity contributes about 30% of the Haldane effect. The major factor accounting for the Haldane effect in CO_2 transport is the much greater ability of deoxyhaemoglobin to form carbamino compounds.

Carbonate and phosphate salts

The carbonate and phosphate salts in bone act as a long-term supply of buffer especially during prolonged metabolic acidosis. Two processes are involved:

(1) Ionic exchange

(2) Dissolution of bone crystal.

Bone can take up H^+ in exchange for Ca^{2+}, Na^+ and K^+ (ionic exchange) or release of HCO_3^-, CO_3^- or HPO_4^{2-}. In acute metabolic acidosis uptake of H^+ by bone in exchange for Na^+ and K^+ is involved in buffering.

Compensation

Respiratory disorders evoke a compensatory renal response which will tend to correct the pH back towards normal. Metabolic disorders evoke a respiratory compensatory response.

Compensation is very important is maintaining a systemic pH compatible with life. Consider a severe metabolic acidosis which reduced HCO_3^- levels to 5 mEq/l. A normal respiratory response will be to increase ventilation, blow off CO_2, and reduce PCO_2 levels to approximately 2.5 kPa. The resulting pH is 7.07. If there had been no respiratory compensation the PCO_2 would remain at its normal value of 40, with a resulting pH of 6.70. The respiratory compensation therefore converts a life-threatening degree of acidaemia to much more tolerable level.

Across the Atlantic, a method commonly used to diagnose acid–base abnormalities is based on the measure of this compensation. This is called the Boston approach. There are six rules that this method follows to diagnose the acid–base derangements.

Rule 1: The 1-for-10 rule for acute respiratory acidosis

The $[HCO_3]$ will increase by 1 mmol/l for every 10 mmHg (1.3 kPa) elevation in PCO_2 above 40 mmHg:

$$\text{Expected } [HCO_3] = 24 + 4\ \{(\text{actual } PCO_2 - 40)\ /\ 10\}$$

Rule 2: The 4-for-10 rule for chronic respiratory acidosis

The $[HCO_3]$ will increase by 4 mmol /l for every 10 mmHg (1.3 kPa) elevation in PCO_2 above 40 mmHg:

$$\text{Expected } [HCO_3] = 24 + 4\ \{(\text{actual } PCO_2 - 40)/10\}$$

Rule 3: The 2-for-10 rule for acute respiratory alkalosis

The $[HCO_3]$ will decrease by 2 mmol/l for every 10 mmHg (1.3 kPa) decrease in PCO_2 below 40 mmHg:

$$\text{Expected } [HCO_3] = 24 - 2\ \{(40 - \text{actual } PCO_2)\ /\ 10\}$$

Rule 4: The 5-for-10 rule for chronic respiratory alkalosis

The $[HCO_3]$ will decrease by 5 mmol/l for every 10 mmHg (1.3 kPa) decrease in PCO_2 below 40 mmHg:

$$\text{Expected } [HCO_3] = 24 - 5\ \{(40 - \text{actual } PCO_2)\ /\ 10\}\ (\text{range} : +/-2)$$

Rule 5: The one and a half plus 8 rule for a metabolic acidosis

The expected PCO_2 (in mmHg) is calculated from the following formula:

$$\text{Expected } PCO_2 = 1.5 \times [HCO_3] + 8 \text{ (range : +/} - 2)$$

Rule 6: The 0.7 plus 20 rule for a metabolic alkalosis

The expected PCO_2 (in mmHg) is calculated from the following formula:

$$\text{Expected } PCO_2 = 0.7\,[HCO_3] + 20 \text{ (range : +/} - 5)$$

If the measured acid–base abnormality does not fit into one of these equations then a mixed disorder should be searched for.

Finally, every time we are dealing with an acid–base disorder, we have to check for appropriate compensations of the primary disturbance, so as to be able to distinguish simple from combined acid–base disorders, which are very frequent in ICU patients.

Acid–base disturbances

Disturbances of the acid–base equilibrium occur in a wide variety of critical illnesses and are among the most commonly encountered disorders in the ICU. In addition to reflecting the seriousness of the underlying disease, these disorders have their own morbidity and mortality.

A blood pH less than normal (normal range 7.35–7.45) is called acidaemia; the underlying process causing acidaemia is called acidosis. Similarly, alkalaemia and alkalosis refer to a raised pH and the underlying process, respectively. While an acidosis and an alkalosis may coexist, there can be only one resulting pH. Therefore, acidaemia and alkalaemia are mutually exclusive conditions.

The approach to acid–base derangements should emphasize a search for the cause, rather than an immediate attempt to normalize the pH. Many disorders are mild and do not require treatment. Treatment of the acid–base disorder per se may be more detrimental than the acid–base disorder itself. More important is a full consideration of the possible underlying pathological states, which may facilitate a directed intervention that will benefit the patient more than normalization of the pH would.

Physiological effects

Acidaemia can cause a decrease in cardiac contractility that is directly proportional to the degree of fall in pH. Both metabolic and respiratory acidaemia cause a similar degree of myocardial depression, but the effect of the latter occurs more promptly, presumably because of the rapid entry of CO_2 into the cardiac cell. Acidaemia also causes stimulation of the sympathetic–adrenal axis, and in severe acidaemia this effect is countered by a depressed responsiveness of adrenergic receptors to circulating catecholamines.

Acute respiratory acidaemia causes marked increases in cerebral blood flow. An acute elevation of PCO_2 to more than 8 kPa causes confusion and headache, and when it exceeds 9 kPa loss of consciousness and seizures can occur. However, chronic elevations in CO_2 are typically well tolerated, even when it is as high as 20 kPa.

The effects of acidaemia on electrolyte levels are quite complex.

Alkalaemia appears to increase myocardial contractility, at least to a pH of 7.7. Acute respiratory alkalaemia causes a decrease in cerebral blood flow, an effect that lasts only about 6 hours. It produces confusion, myoclonus, asterixis, loss of consciousness and seizures. Acute hypocapnoea causes a slight reduction in the serum levels of sodium, potassium and phosphorus. Alkalaemia also causes an increase in haemoglobin's affinity for oxygen. However, there is also an increase in the concentration of 2,3-DPG in red blood cells and a change in its morphology, which oppose this effect. The clinical effects of alkalaemia-induced changes in oxygen delivery are minimal, and only in patients with tissue hypoxia are the small, acute changes potentially relevant.

There are four primary disorders associated with acid–base abnormalities. They most commonly occur in isolation but multiple disorders can present at the same time.

- Metabolic acidosis – characterized by a decrease in plasma $[HCO^{3-}]$ through loss of HCO_3 or accumulation of $[H^+]$. Accompanied by compensatory fall in $[PCO_2]$ through hyperventilation.
- Respiratory acidosis – characterized by an increase in $[PCO_2]$ (hypoventilation), compensatory increase in $[HCO_3^-]$ via renal excretion of H^+; occurs slowly over days.
- Metabolic alkalosis – characterized by increase in plasma $[HCO_3^-]$ through $[H^{+]}]$ loss or $[HCO_3^-]$ gain accompanied by compensatory rise in $[PCO_2]$ through hypoventilation.

- Respiratory alkalosis – characterized by decrease in [PCO_2] (hyperventilation), compensatory decrease in [HCO_3^-] via renal excretion of NH_4.

See Figs. 20.2 and 20.3 for diagnostic approaches to these four disorders.

Metabolic acidosis

Metabolic acidosis is characterized by a primary decrease in bicarbonate [HCO_3^-] concentration and a compensatory decrease in the PCO_2 concentration. This decrease in bicarbonate levels shows up as base deficit. Traditionally metabolic acidosis is caused by either loss of bicarbonate or addition of hydrogen ion. Bicarbonate loss generally occurs through the kidneys or the bowel. Acidosis from decreased renal excretion is generally slow to develop. In contrast, acidosis from increased acid production, as in lactic acidosis or ketoacidosis, can exceed maximal renal excretion and cause a rapidly developing, severe acidosis.

In Stewart's approach the reason for developing acidosis is due to a drop in the SID. The SID drops when there is accumulation of organic anions (lactate, ketones) or due to loss of [Na^+] due to diarrhoea or from the kidneys (renal tubular acidosis). Similarly treating metabolic acidosis is achieved by efforts to increase the [Na^+] concentration compared to [Cl^-] to restore the SID and thereby restore the dissociation of water to yield a [H^+] concentration of 40 nmol/l.

The aetiologies of metabolic acidosis are divided into those that cause an increase in the anion gap, and those that cause an osmolar gap.

Anion gap

The *anion gap* (AG) is the difference between measured cations and measured anions. It is defined as:

$$[Na] - [Cl] - [HCO_3].$$

The AG is comprised largely of albumin and to a lesser extent, phosphate. Low albumin and phosphate will affect this value. To correct for this, the expected value can be calculated as AG = 2(albumin [g/dl]) × 1.5 (phosphate [mmol/dl]). The calculated AG using the traditional method [Na - (Cl + HCO_3)] is then compared to the expected AG. If the calculated AG is greater than the expected AG, the difference is attributed to unmeasured anions from non-volatile acids.

The normal value is 8–12 mEq/l. A normal anion gap acidosis occurs when chloride replaces the bicarbonate lost in buffering hydrogen ion. An increased anion gap acidosis occurs when the anion replacing the HCO_3 is not one that is routinely measured (albumin, phosphate, sulphates, lactate). Anions always equal cations, but if the anion is not chloride then the anion gap calculated from routine chemistries will increase. An increased anion gap does not always signify a metabolic acidosis. It increases in alkalaemia, because of an increase in the net anionic charge on plasma proteins. Dehydration will also increase it because of an increased protein concentration. However, if it is greater than 20 mEq/l, a metabolic acidosis should be pursued.

Normal anion gap acidosis occurs from loss of bicarbonate through the kidneys or the gut, or from the addition of an acid with chloride as the accompanying anion. The most common cause in the ICU is diarrhoea; in its absence, a renal tubular acidosis is likely. The other causes are usually obvious from the history and medication list. The aetiologies of normal anion gap metabolic acidosis are listed in Table 20.2. The aetiologies of increased anion gap acidosis are given in Table 20.3.

Osmolar gap

Determination of the presence of an *osmolar gap* may also be helpful in determining the aetiology of the metabolic acidosis:

$$\text{calculated serum osmolality} = 2[Na^+]$$
$$+\text{blood glucose in mmol}+\text{blood urea nitrogen in mmol.}$$

Osmolal gap = measured serum osmolality – calculated serum osmolality.

The presence of an elevated osmolal gap suggests the presence of an additional solute in the plasma.

Normal anion gap metabolic acidosis

Renal tubular acidosis

- The defect in all types of renal tubular acidosis (RTA) is the inability to excrete chloride in proportion to Na
- Type I (classic distal) RTA can present with profound hypobicarbonataemia and hypokalaemia and

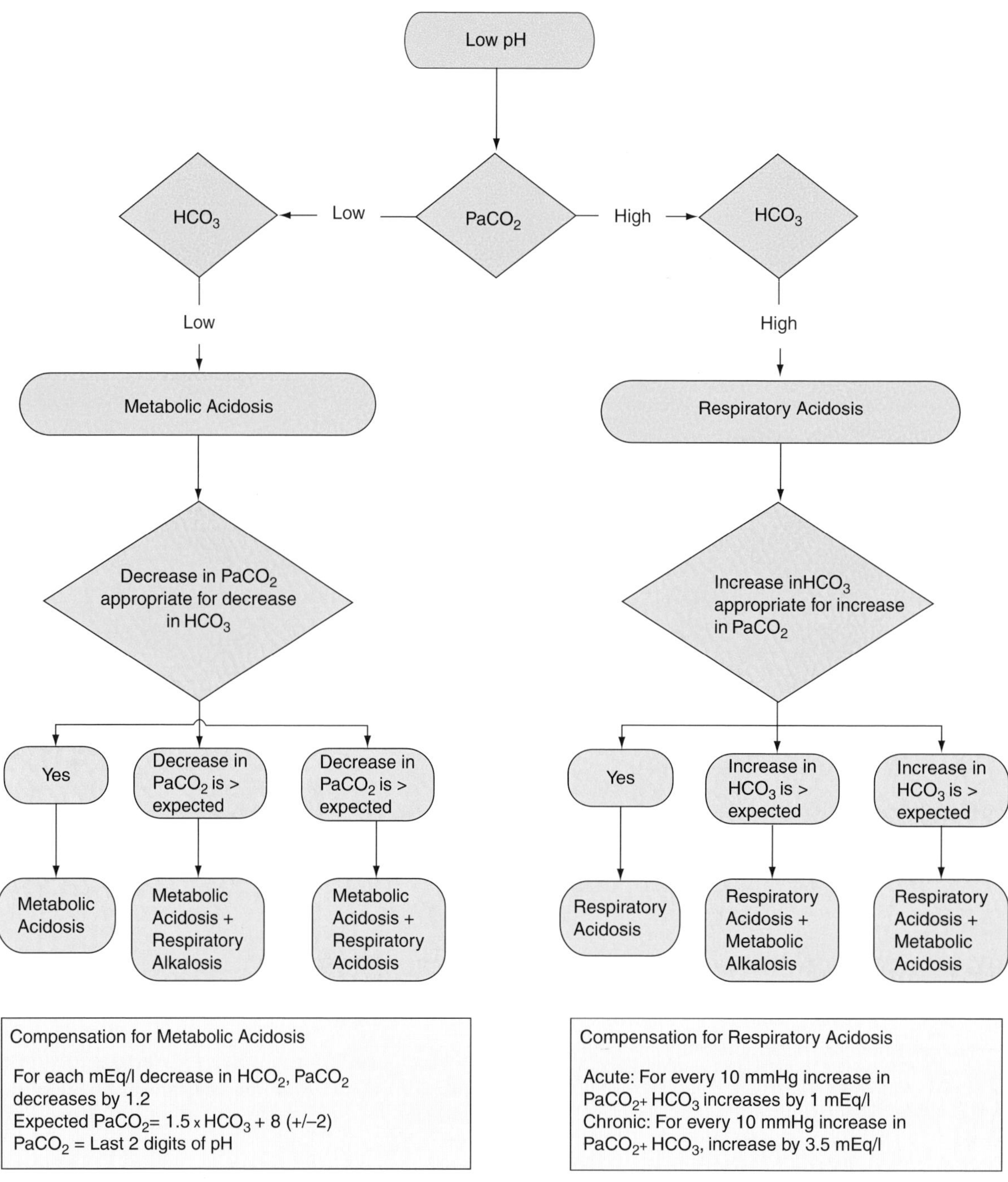

Fig. 20.2 Diagnostic approach to acidosis.

replacement with sodium bicarbonate and potassium infusion is usually required.

- Type IV RTA is associated with aldosterone deficiency or resistance. Clinical features include high serum potassium and low urine pH (<5.5). Treatment is directed at the underlying cause.

Diarrhoea

Loss of bicarbonate through the digestive tract is typically accompanied by losses of Na^+ that are out of proportion to the losses of chloride ions. This results in a non-AG hyperchloraemic metabolic acidosis.

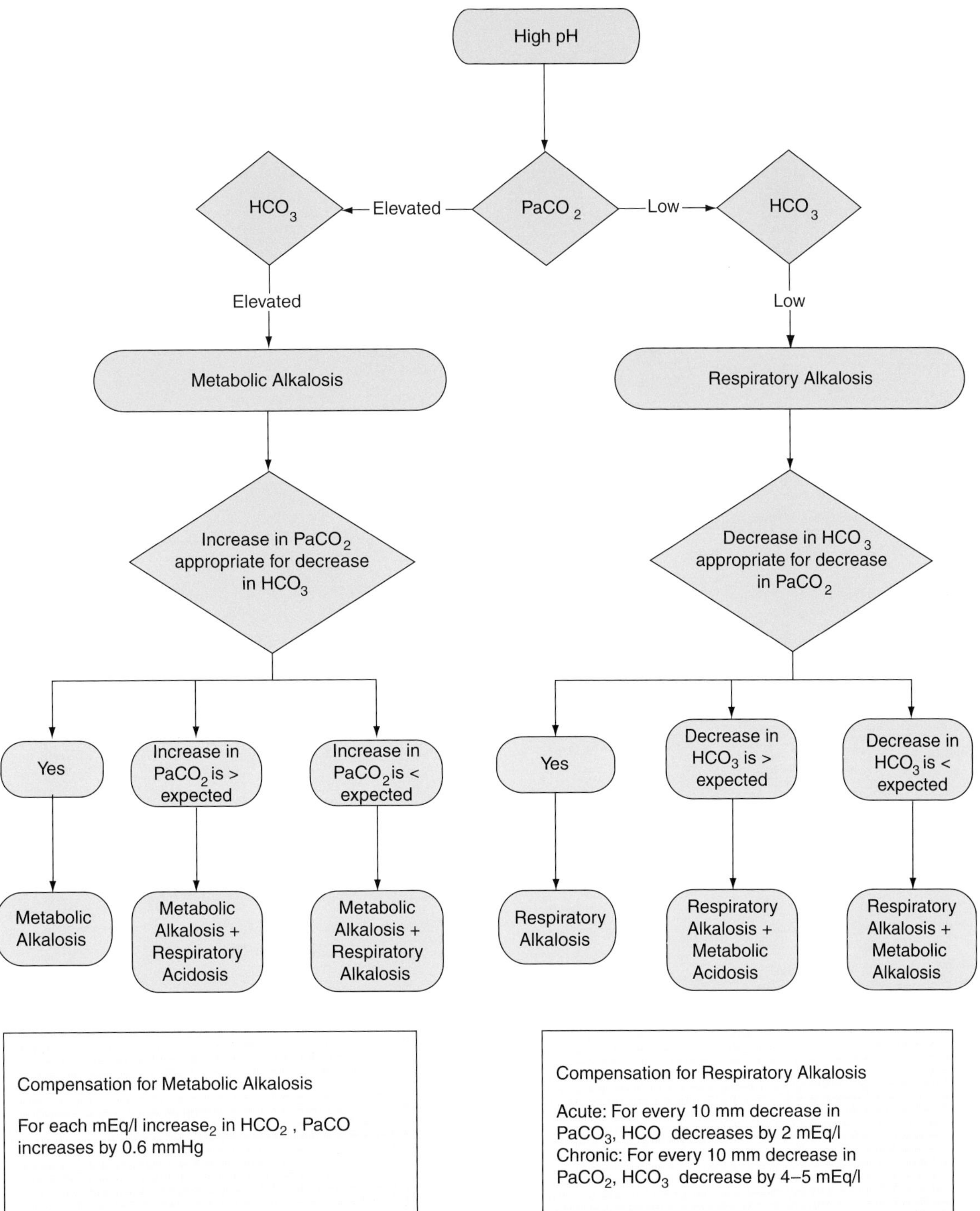

Fig. 20.3 Diagnostic approach to alkalosis.

Table 20.2 Aetiologies of normal anion gap metabolic acidosis

Gastrointestinal loss of bicarbonate
Diarrhoea
Urinary diversion
Small bowel, pancreatic or bile drainage (fistulas, surgical drains)
Renal loss of bicarbonate
Renal tubular acidosis
Recovery phase of ketoacidosis
Renal insufficiency
Iatrogenic
Large volume of saline infusion
Total parenteral nutrition

Table 20.3 Aetiologies of increased anion gap metabolic acidosis

Ketoacidosis
Diabetic
Alcoholic
Starvation
Metabolic errors
Lactic acidosis
Uraemia
Toxins
Ethylene glycol
Methanol
Salicylate
Rare causes
Dehydration
Decreased unmeasured cations
Hypomagnesaemia
Hypokalaemia
Hypocalcaemia

Increased anion gap metabolic acidosis

Lactic acidosis

Lactic acidosis is the most common and most important acidosis encountered in the ICU. The acidaemia has physiological significance and, perhaps most important, serves as a marker for a diverse group of serious underlying conditions. Its definition is somewhat arbitrary, but it is commonly defined as an arterial lactate level greater than 5 mmol/l, with an arterial pH less than 7.35. Increased lactate levels correlate well with increasing mortality in patients with cardiogenic shock and septic shock. Inadequate tissue oxygenation underlies the lactic acidosis in many patients. Therapy should focus on restoring circulation and tissue oxygenation while diagnosing and treating the underling aetiology (i.e. sepsis, haemorrhage or bowel infarction). Administration of sodium bicarbonate has not been shown to improve outcomes in patients with lactic acidosis.

Renal failure

Renal failure is often associated with a hyperchloraemic metabolic acidosis that is partially associated with an elevated AG. The AG reflects retained sulphates, phosphate and other organic ions. Haemodialysis will permit removal of these ions and will restore Na^+ and Cl^- balance.

Poisoning/ingestion

- Ethanol: alcoholic ketoacidosis is associated with both an elevated AG and an elevated osmolar gap.
- Methanol and ethylene glycol are both associated with elevated anion and osmolal gaps.
- Salicylate ingestion usually results in a mixed disturbance, a metabolic acidosis and a respiratory alkalosis. Respiratory alkalosis is caused by the direct stimulation of the respiratory centre by the salicylate and the metabolic acidosis is caused by lactate accumulation.

Metabolic alkalosis

Metabolic alkalosis is characterized by a primary increase in bicarbonate concentration and a compensatory increase in $PaCO_2$. Metabolic alkalosis occurs as either a loss of anions ($[Cl^-]$) from the stomach or an increase in cations, which is rare. It can be broadly divided into two categories.

Metabolic alkalosis according to Stewart's approach is brought about by excess loss of strong cations compared to anions (vomiting, nasogastric aspiration) due to an increase in the SID. Treatment approaches here would be to increase the strong anion $[Cl^-]$ by infusing saline or potassium chloride.

Chloride-responsive metabolic alkalosis

This is a consequence of temporary chloride loss. Urine chloride is typically below 20 mmol/l. Most common causes are vomiting, gastric drainage, volume contraction.

- Diuretic use is also chloride responsive but urine chloride may be >20 mmol/l.
- Treatment is replacement of chloride and volume loss. Saline with potassium supplementation is often given.

Chloride-resistant metabolic alkalosis

This is typically a consequence of a hormonal mechanism and is less easily corrected by the administration of chloride.

- Urine chloride is typically elevated (>20 mmol/l).
- Most common causes are processes involving excess mineralocorticoid activity. Examples include hypercortisolism, hyperaldosteronism, sodium bicarbonate therapy and severe renal artery stenosis.
- Treatment is directed at the underlying cause.

Other causes

Rarely, metabolic alkalosis is a consequence of cation administration rather than anion depletion.

Examples include the milk–alkali syndrome and massive blood transfusions or plasma exchange. The latter occurs because Na^+ is paired with citrate (a weak anion) instead of Cl^-.

Respiratory acidosis

Respiratory acidosis is characterized by a primary increase in $PaCO_2$ and a compensatory increase in bicarbonate. Respiratory acidosis represents ventilatory failure. Decreased alveolar ventilation arises from a decrease in minute ventilation or from an increase in dead space without a compensatory rise in minute ventilation. A rise in CO_2 production will produce hypercapnoea unless ventilation does not increase appropriately. The aetiologies can be classified according to which part of the respiratory system is affected (Table 20.4).

Table 20.4 Aetiologies for respiratory acidosis

Abnormalities of neural control
Drugs, e.g. opioids
CNS diseases
Neuromuscular diseases
Myasthenia gravis
Guillain–Barré syndrome
Electrolyte abnormalities
Hypophosphataemia
Hypokalaemia
Pulmonary disease
Chronic obstructive pulmonary disease
Obesity hypoventilation syndrome
Severe chest wall deformity

Treatment includes reversing causal disorders, increasing minute ventilation, decreasing dead space and decreasing CO_2 production. This often requires intubation and mechanical ventilation. In patients already on mechanical ventilation changes to ventilation should be instituted to increase alveolar ventilation.

Respiratory alkalosis

Respiratory alkalosis is characterized by a primary reduction in the arterial PCO_2, followed by a secondary two-phase reduction in bicarbonate, a small acute decrease due to tissue buffers and a larger chronic decrement due to a decrease in renal titratable acid excretion and an increase in renal bicarbonate excretion. It occurs when alveolar ventilation is increased relative to CO_2 production.

Treatment is that of the underlying cause. In sepsis, where a significant portion of cardiac output can go to respiratory muscles, intubation and muscle relaxation are often required to control hyperventilation and redirect blood flow.

The Stewart approach makes sense, and provides a better model of how acid–base balance works than does the conventional approach. For most acid–base disturbances, and for the foreseeable future, the traditional approach to acid–base balance seems certain to prevail. We need more evidence that using Stewart's approach will change clinical management. Under many, perhaps most circumstances, the old-fashioned approach works fine, but we should be aware of the exceptions (gross volume dilution with fluids which have a low SID; hypoalbuminaemia in association with metabolic acidosis) and invoke the physico-chemical approach in these circumstances. This new approach also helps us explain how our therapeutic interventions work. The new approach is discussed on many websites and has also appeared in standard textbooks of anaesthesia and intensive care.

Key points

- Acid–base homeostasis is important to maintain tissue and organ performance. Both acidosis and alkalosis can have harmful effects and when severe, can be life-threatening.
- pH or $[H^+]$ is tightly controlled in order to provide optimal conditions for the protein charge and structure which influence enzymatic reactions and thereby influence cellular metabolism.

- It is the nature of the condition responsible for the acid–base disturbance that largely determines the patient's prognosis.
- It is appropriate to focus on diagnosing and treating the underlying disorder, as most acid–base derangements do not benefit from specific correction of the abnormal pH.

Further reading

- Badr A, Nightingale P (2007) An alternative approach to acid–base abnormalities in critically ill patients. *Cotin. Educ. Anaesth. Crit. Care* 7(4): 107–11.
- Kellum JA (2005) Disturbances of acid–base balance. *Textbook of Critical Care*, 5th edn, eds. Fink MP, Abraham B, Vincent JL, Kochanek PM. Philadelphia, PA: Elservier.
- Neligan PJ, Deutschman, CS (2004) Acid–base balance. *Miller's Anasthesia*, 6th edn, ed. Miller RD. Philadelphia, PA: Elserver.
- Sirker A, Grounds RM, Bennet ED *et al.* (2002) Acid–base physiology: the traditional and the modern approaches. *Anaesthesia* **57**(4): 348–56.

Useful websites

1. www.acidbase.org
2. www.anaesthesiaMCQ.com

Post-operative critical care

Prasad Bheemasenachar

The main aim of post-operative care is prevention, early identification and treatment of post-operative complications. The immediate post-operative period is the crucial period when numerous physiological and pharmacodynamic changes occur due to surgical trauma and anaesthesia. There are a number of issues that must be addressed in the post-operative period to optimize recovery. Effective care in the peri-operative period should include attention to pain relief, maintenance of adequate tissue perfusion through careful fluid balance and optimized cardio-respiratory function (Fig. 21.1). This requirement can be effectively delivered in a critical care facility. Immediately after surgery the surgical team should write a detailed operation note, along with clear post-operative instructions. It is also essential that there are mechanisms in place for a clear and comprehensive handover of care from the anaesthetists and the operating team to the nurse in charge of the patient in the critical care unit to prevent ambiguity in the care provided.

The early post-operative period

Monitoring of vital parameters

The three factors hypotension, hypoxia and hypothermia which are interlinked to each other produce combined ill-effects leading to life-threatening complications. Monitoring the vital parameters like pulse, blood pressure, respiratory rate, ECG, oxygen saturation, temperature and the urine output are essential to diagnose any alterations in physiology and facilitate institution of appropriate measures to prevent post-operative complications. The invasiveness of the monitoring will depend on the extent of the surgery, patient's pre-operative physiological status and on anticipated complications.

Patients who are high risk and those who have undergone extensive surgical procedures require invasive measurements of their arterial and central venous pressure monitoring to optimize cardiovascular function. Some of these patients may require monitoring of cardiac output to optimize fluid management and to guide vasopressor/inotropic requirements. Whilst these invasive monitoring techniques provide information which guides therapy it is essential that clinicians are familiar with their limitations. Hence it is important that these patients are examined clinically, with special attention to cardio-respiratory and mental status, during each shift and their care is not based solely on monitored parameters. Arterial blood gases and laboratory investigations like electrolytes, liver and renal functions and chest X-rays should be targeted and not routinely performed.

Post-operative analgesia (see also Chapter 11)

Adequate management of pain is critical and decreases post-operative morbidity and reduces the hospital stay. Patient should be questioned frequently about their pain level. Pain medication should be given on a regular basis and whenever necessary (see also Chapter 11: Pain control).

There are various modalities available to provide effective pain relief after surgery. These therapies fall under two broad categories. One is to block the afferent nociceptive stimulus reaching the central nervous system by a peripheral nerve block or a neuraxial block (spinal or epidural) and the other is to use opioid and/or non-opioid painkillers. The method chosen depends on the region and the extent of surgery, the patient's pre-operative cardio-respiratory status, expertise of the anaesthetist and presence or absence of any contraindications for a regional block.

Core Topics in Critical Care Medicine, eds. Fang Gao Smith and Joyce Yeung. Published by Cambridge University Press.

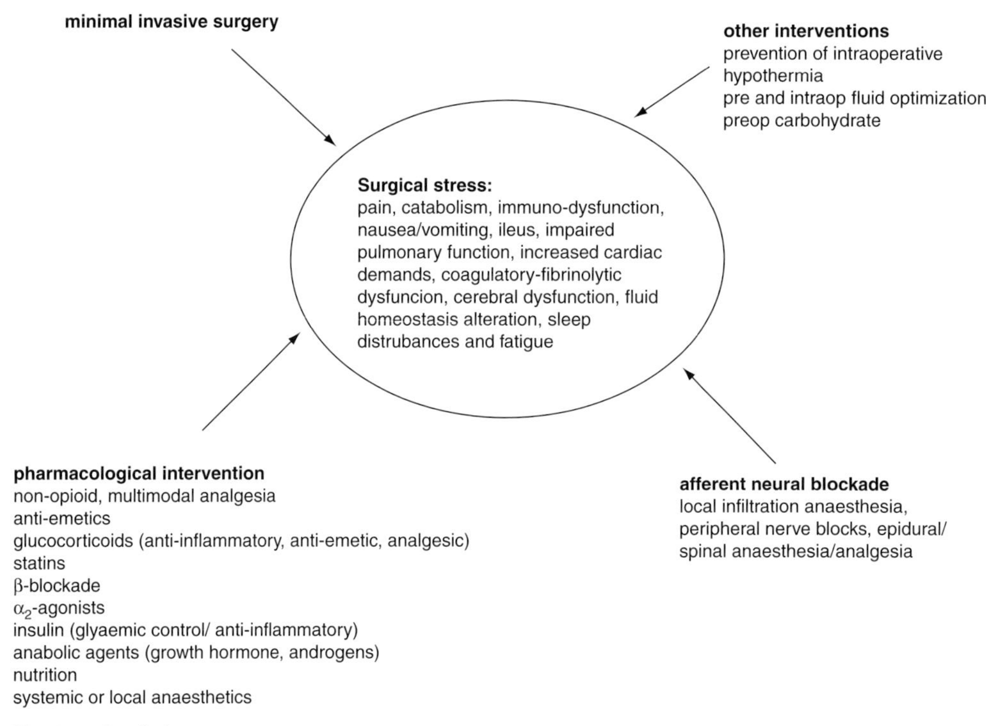

Fig. 21.1 Surgical stress.

Regional techniques

Epidural analgesia

Continuous epidural anaesthesia is valuable in patients having abdominal or thoracic surgery with poor respiratory function. This technique requires specialized equipment and trained staff to monitor and provide pain relief safely and effectively. Local anaesthetics and opioids in various combinations infused by dedicated pumps are used to provide continuous pain relief. When the epidural is ineffective early recognition and prompt request for expert help to optimize pain relief is important to prevent morbidity. There is still a debate as to where these patients should be cared for. Some hospitals provide care for this modality of pain relief on the wards with help from the acute pain service whilst others use an augmented care facility. The most common side effect of this technique is hypotension due to sympathetic blockade affecting both preload and afterload. The extent of hypotension is dictated by the expanse of the block; whilst most can be managed with judicious fluid replacement, some patients may require vasopressor support. Respiratory complications of epidurals are uncommon; high thoracic block can interfere with respiratory effort by paralysing intercostal muscles and if the block extends upwards beyond C3/C4, respiratory arrest will occur due to diaphragmatic paralysis.

Other complications include failure of adequate pain relief and very rarely neurological injury. Nerve injury can be caused during the performance of the technique or later due to haematomas or infections. Neurological injuries may be difficult to establish whilst the local anaesthetic infusion is in use. Any abnormal pattern in neurology should raise suspicion and prompt further investigations to diagnose and treat these complications spedily to prevent permanent damage.

Spinal analgesia

Many operations in the lower abdomen or the lower limbs can be performed with intrathecal blocks using local anaesthetics. It has been shown that addition of intrathecal opioids reduces the incidence of visceral pain intraoperatively and, when longer-acting drugs such as morphine and diamorphine are used, provides a few hours of post-operative analgesia.

Intrathecal preservative-free opioids like diamorphine and morphine are used as the main modality for providing pain relief in some centres. The pain relief is effective and the duration depends on the dose used. There is very little haemodynamic instability. These patients need close monitoring as they can suffer delayed respiratory depression. The peak incidence of respiratory depression is at around 4–5 hours post proceedure. It is important to bear this in mind whilst administering additional opioids for pain relief. Itch, nausea and vomiting are opioid-related side effects that can be distressing. Itch can be treated with small doses of naloxone, 20 μg IV. Nausea and vomiting can be treated with anti-emetics.

Nerve blocks

These include nerve blocks (sciatic, femoral) or plexus blocks (brachial plexus). They may be administered as the sole anaesthetic, to provide post-operative pain relief of varying duration depending on the drug used. They may also be used as part of a combined regional and general anaesthetic technique. These blocks require expertise to administer and are associated with complications, especially when performed with the patient anaesthetized.

Systemic pain relief

Opioids

Systemic opioids are the mainstay in proving pain relief after major surgery where regional techniques are not used. There are many ways of administering these drugs. Morphine is the most commonly used opioid. In the critical care setting it is administered mainly as a continuous infusion or as patient-controlled analgesia (PCA). PCA is preferred when patients are awake and compos mentis. PCA has the advantage of providing the patient with analgesia as and when they need it without having to wait for it to be administered. In addition, with PCA the patient determines the rate of intravenous administration of the drug thereby providing feedback control. It also provides safety in terms of how much can be self-administered due to lockout intervals between doses. PCA has been shown to provide greater patient satisfaction and to improve ventilation when compared with conventional routes. There should be clear guidelines regarding the actions to be taken in cases of inadequate analgesia and when side effects occur. Good risk management with PCA should emphasize the same drug, protocols and equipment throughout the hospital. PCA can cause nausea and vomiting in some patients which should be addressed with anti-emetics. Caution should be exercised in patients with renal failure who are on continuous infusion as the metabolites of morphine are not excreted and can cause respiratory depression.

Non-opioid drugs

Two main drugs that are used in this group are paracetamol and the non-steroidal anti-inflammatory drugs (NSAIDs). By themselves they are not adequate to provide good pain relief for patients undergoing major surgery. They can be administered by oral, intravenous or rectal route. Regular prescription of these drugs provides good background relief and they are effective in the multimodal approach to provide relief from pain. Caution should be exercised whilst administering NSAIDs in patients with renal failure, asthma, bleeding tendencies, etc.

Fluid balance

Meticulous fluid balance is important in the management of patients in the peri-operative period. Attention to this can be achieved only with a good working knowledge of the underlying physiology coupled with the information on the patient's maintenance needs and losses suffered during the peri-operative period.

In general, most maintenance requirements in the immediate post-operative period are met by administering salt-containing crystalloids based on body weight (1.5 ml/kg per hour). Whilst there is no advantage of one fluid over another, large volumes of normal saline infusion should be avoided to prevent hyperchloraemic acidosis.

Replacement of fluids lost should be like for like. It is important to note the volume and the site of loss, as fluids lost from different locations differ in their fluid and electrolyte composition. Most of the solutions lost from the body contain salt and should be replaced as such. Blood is administered to maintain haemoglobin around 8–10 g/dl.

Correction of hypovolaemia is important to maintain adequate cardiac output in order to meet the demands of the body. It is difficult to gain information on the adequacy of resuscitation of the interstitial and intracellular compartments. Clinical end-points like thirst, tissue turgor and core–peripheral temperature difference provide a rough guide to the needs of this compartment. An estimate of the fluid status of the intravascular compartment can be monitored by measuring heart rate, central venous pressure, stroke volume, blood pressure and central venous oxygen saturation which, when challenged dynamically, allow an assessment of the adequacy of resuscitation of the circulating volume. Serum lactate measurements may be used as a soft end-point for adequacy of resuscitation. When using this parameter as a surrogate for resuscitation, it is important that other pathologies that might increase serum lactate are ruled out. Patients on adrenaline infusion tend to have elevated lactate levels during the first 6–12 hours of infusion due to its effect on cellular metabolism in the skeletal muscle. Static pressure measurements are a poor guide to the adequacy of intravascular volume replacement. It is difficult to be absolutely sure about the adequacy of resuscitation as many measured parameters have fallacies. It is important to interpret values obtained from measured variables in conjunction with the findings on clinical examination to make an educated guess on the fluid status of the patient.

Urine output

Adequate hydration, good perfusion pressure and prevention of hypoxaemia are important to maintain good functioning kidneys. The medullar portion of the kidney is very sensitive to hypoxaemia as it normally works at very low levels of tissue oxygen tension. Urine output is an important indicator of the fluid status of patients. However in the first 24 hours after surgery, humoral response of the body to stress tends to conserve fluids and hence the patient may have low urine output during this period. Whilst it is logical to think about fluid resuscitation during times of poor urine output, it is also important that we look at the global picture. If patients are warm and well perfused, not acidotic and are haemodynamically stable further fluid challanges to improve urine output may not be necessary in the immediate post-operative period. The amount of urine output in the immediate peri-operative period is not a sensitive indicator of patients at risk of developing renal failure.

Pulmonary system

Post-operative pulmonary complications contribute significantly to overall peri-operative morbidity and mortality rates. Pulmonary complications occur much more often than cardiac complications in patients undergoing elective surgery to the thorax and upper abdomen. The frequency rate of these complications varies from 5% to 70%. Post-operative pulmonary complications prolong the hospital stay by an average of 1–2 weeks.

Atelectasis is common post-operatively. It causes pulmonary shunt and hypoxaemia, reduces lung compliance, increases the work of breathing and predisposes to pneumonia and respiratory failure. The diagnosis of atelectasis can be made clinically, but is more often made radiologically. It is common in obese patients, patients undergoing body cavity surgery, elderly patients especially if they suffer cognitive impairment, in patients who smoke and those with pre-existing respiratory disorder. Evidence suggests that cessation of smoking for more than 8 weeks and pre-operative physiotherapy with breathing exercises reduces the incidence of atelectasis.

Anaesthetic agents reduce respiratory muscle tone, causing a fall in functional residual capacity and collapse of small airways promoting atelectasis. There is good evidence to suggest that surgery lasting for more than 3–4 hours and surgery on the upper abdomen have a higher incidence of atelectasis. Manoeuvres used under anaesthesia to preserve lung volumes (PEEP), good tidal ventilation, avoiding high inspired concentrations of oxygen and providing good peri-operative pain relief go a long way in reducing the incidence of atelectasis.

Patients may need help to remove viscid tracheal secretions from tracheo-bronchial tree. When regular orotracheal or nasotracheal suction is poorly tolerated, use of a mini tracheostomy may assist sputum removal. If a blockage in a major bronchus is identified and physiotherapy is ineffective early bronchoscopy to remove secretions should be performed. In patients who develop hypoxaemia corrective measures to re-establish functional residual capacity (FRC) like attention to position and early recourse to continuous positive airway pressure (CPAP) should be considered. In patients who need CPAP to correct hypoxaemia chest physiotherapy and clearance of secretions can become difficult. In such circumstances, if the patient can tolerate it, a mini tracheostomy will help in clearing secretions. Antibiotics should be reserved for patients with established infection. In patients where there is a high index of suspicion of chest infection, broad-spectrum antibiotics after obtaining a sputum specimen for culture may be considered (in consultation with microbiologists). It is important to de-escalate antibiotic therapy once culture results are available.

Every effort should be made to prevent patients developing organ failure. Patients who develop single organ failures have a high risk of suffering multi-system failure leading to poor outcome. Patients who do develop respiratory failure should have early ventilatory support. This can be administered non-invasively or by traditional methods of ventilation.

Non-invasive ventilation

Non-invasive ventilation (NIV) refers to the delivery of mechanical ventilation using techniques that do not require an artificial airway (see also Chapter 31). The recent increase in NIV use in acute care settings has been encouraged by the desire to reduce the complications resulting from intubation and invasive ventilation. By avoiding these complications, NIV has the potential to reduce hospital morbidity, facilitate weaning from mechanical ventilation, and shorten the duration of hospitalization, thereby improving patient comfort.

The patient needs to be conscious and cooperative for NIV to be considered. Contraindications include risk of aspiration, severe hypoxaemia, trauma or surgery on face, upper gastrointestinal surgery and haemodynamic instability. NIV decreases the work of breathing and thereby improves alveolar ventilation while simultaneously resting the respiratory musculature. Patients in respiratory distress use as much as 30–40% of the cardiac output to support the oxygen cost of breathing. Early recourse to ventilator support not only relieves the respiratory load but also makes it possible for the cardiovascular system to divert cardiac output and use it to maintain blood flow to other vital organs. The recipe for success in using NIV is to use it early. Other important issues include the selection of the ventilation interface and the type of ventilator. Currently available interfaces include nasal, oronasal and facial masks, mouthpieces and helmets. Comparisons of the available interfaces have not shown one to be clearly superior. Both critical care ventilators and portable ventilators can be used for non-invasive positive-pressure ventilation; however, the choice of ventilator type depends on the patient's condition and therapeutic requirements and on the expertise of the nursing staff and the location of care.

There is good evidence from randomized trials to support the use of this modality in patients with acute exacerbation of chronic obstructive pulmonary disease (COPD) and in acute pulmonary oedema. Studies on the use of NIV in hypoxaemic respiratory failure in the absence of carbon dioxide retention have yielded conflicting results. Patients with a variety of diagnoses (e.g. pneumonia, congestive heart failure, acute respiratory distress syndrome) had been included in this category. A systematic review by Keenan and colleagues in 2004 analysed the efficacy of this technique in patients with hypoxaemic respiratory failure. Overall, NIV was associated with a significantly lower rate of intubation compared with standard management (absolute risk reduction 23%, 95% CI 10% to 35%). Also, NIV ventilation was associated with a reduction in mortality in intensive care units of 17% (95% CI 8% to 26%). This publication was followed by a study from Honrubia and colleagues who included 64 patients with acute respiratory failure from various causes. These patients were randomized to receive either non-invasive positive-pressure ventilation through a face mask with pressure support and positive end-expiratory pressure or to receive conventional invasive ventilation. Non-invasive ventilation reduced the need for intubation (relative risk reduction 43%). Mortality in intensive care units was 23% in the non-invasive group and 39% in the conventional therapy group ($p = 0.09$). The heterogeneity among studies suggests that the effectiveness of non-invasive positive-pressure ventilation varies among different populations and does not support its routine use in all patients with acute hypoxaemic respiratory failure.

Protocol for initiation of NIV in patients with acute respiratory failure (see also Chapter 30: Respiratory weaning)

(1) Position the head of the bed at a 45° angle.

(2) Choose the correct size of mask and initiate ventilator at CPAP (expiratory positive airway pressure; EPAP) of 0 cm H_2O with a pressure support (inspiratory positive airway pressure; IPAP) of 10 cm H_2O.

(3) Hold the mask gently on the patient's face until the patient is comfortable and in full synchrony with the ventilator.

(4) Apply wound care dressing on the patient's nasal bridge and other pressure points.

(5) Secure the mask with head straps, but avoid a tight fit.

(6) Slowly increase CPAP to more than 5 cmH_2O.

(7) Increase pressure support (IPAP, 10–20 cmH_2O) to achieve good exhaled tidal volume. Evaluate that ventilatory support is adequate, which is indicated by an improvement in dyspnoea, a decreased respiratory rate, achievement of desired tidal volume, and good comfort for the patient.

(8) Give oxygen supplementation to achieve an oxygen saturation of greater than 90%.

(9) A back-up rate may be provided in the event the patient becomes apnoeic.

Table 21.1 Clinical predictors of increased peri-operative cardiovascular risk

Major	Intermediate	Minor
Unstable coronary syndromes Acute or recent MI (>7 days, <30 days) with evidence of important ischaemic risk by clinical symptoms or non-invasive study Unstable or severe angina (Canadian class III or IV[a]) Decompensated heart failure Significant arrhythmias High-grade atrioventricular block Symptomatic ventricular arrhythmias in the presence of underlying heart disease Supraventricular arrhythmias with uncontrolled ventricular rate Severe valvular disease	Mild angina pectoris (Canadian class I or II[a]) Previous MI by history or pathological Q waves Compensated or prior heart failure Diabetes mellitus (esp. IDDM) Renal insufficiency	Advanced age (>75 years) Abnormal electrocardiography results (e.g. LVH, LBBB, ST-T abnormalities) Rhythm other than sinus (e.g. AF) Low functional capacity (e.g. inability to climb one flight of stairs with a bag of groceries) History of stroke Uncontrolled systemic hypertension

[a] Campeau L (1976) Grading of angina pectoris. *Circulation* **54**: 522–3.
Source: Adapted from Eagle KA, Berger PB, Calkins H, Chaitman BR, Ewy GA, Fleischmann KE *et al.* (2002) ACC/AHA guideline update for perioperative cardiovascular evaluation for noncardiac surgery: a report of the American College of Cardiology/American Heart Association Task Force on Practice Guidelines. *J. Am. Coll. Cardiol.* **39**: 546.

(10) In patients with hypoxaemia, increase CPAP in increments of 2–3 cmH_2O until FiO_2 is less than 0.6.

(11) Set the ventilator alarms and back-up apnoea parameters.

(12) Ask the patient to call for needs, and provide reassurance and encouragement.

(13) Monitor with oximetry, and adjust ventilator settings after obtaining arterial blood gas results.

NIV should be applied under close clinical and physiological monitoring for signs of treatment failure and, in such cases, endotracheal intubation should be promptly available. In patients who are not suitable for NIV and where NIV has failed prompt institution of invasive ventilation should be available for further support.

Cardiovascular system

The cardiovascular systems of patients who undergo general anaesthesia and surgical procedures are subject to multiple stresses and complications. A previously stable patient may decompensate post-operatively, leading to significant post-operative morbidity and mortality. A substantial number of all deaths among patients undergoing non-cardiac surgery are caused by cardiovascular complications. Approximately one-third of patients having non-cardiac surgery have cardiac disease or major cardiac risk factors. Current estimated rates of serious peri-operative cardiac morbidity vary from 1% to 10%. The incidence of peri-operative myocardial infarction (MI) is increased 10- to 50-fold in patients who have had previous coronary events.

Risk stratification

Cardiac risk stratification allows clinicians to group patients into various risk categories; thereby low-risk patients can be spared further testing, whereas intermediate- and high-risk patients should undergo pre-operative investigations and treatment to reduce overall cardiac peri-operative morbidity and mortality. A stepwise strategy that includes the assessment of clinical markers, prior cardiac evaluation and management, functional capacity in METs, and surgery-specific risks should be employed to stratify risk.

Clinical markers

The American College of Cardiology/American Heart Association guidelines recommend that an assessment begins with the patient's risk factors for perioperative morbidity and mortality which are classified into major, intermediate or minor clinical predictors (Table 21.1).

Functional capacity

- Poor functional class (<4 METS) – energy expended during activities, including dressing, eating, and walking around the house.
- Adequate functional class (>4 METS) – energy expended during activities, including walking up a flight of stairs, scrubbing floors and swimming.

Surgery-specific risk

The risk associated with the type of surgery can also be assessed and different surgery can be classified into high, intermediate and low risk (Table 21.2).

Table 21.2 Cardiac risk stratification for non-cardiac surgical procedures (combined incidence of cardiac death and non-fatal myocardial infarction)

High (cardiac risk often >5%)
Emergent major operations, particularly in patients older than 75 years
Aortic and other major vascular surgery
Peripheral vascular surgery
Anticipated prolonged surgical procedure associated with large fluid shifts and/or blood loss
Intermediate (cardiac risk generally 1% to 5%)
Carotid endarterectomy
Head and neck surgery
Intraperitoneal and intrathoracic surgery
Orthopaedic surgery
Prostate surgery
Low (cardiac risk generally <1%)
Endoscopic procedures
Superficial procedures
Cataract surgery
Breast surgery

Source: Adapted from Eagle KA, Berger PB, Calkins H, Chaitman BR, Ewy GA, Fleischmann KE *et al.* (2002) ACC/AHA guideline update for perioperative cardiovascular evaluation for noncardiac surgery: a report of the American College of Cardiology/American Heart Association Task Force on Practice Guidelines. *J. Am. Coll. Cardiol.* **39**: 547.

Stratification

Stratification allows the anaesthetist to employ techniques to minimize cardiovascular morbidity in the peri-operative period (Fig. 21.2). Peri-operative β blockade was advocated in high-risk patients as a means of reducing morbidity. However a recently concluded multi-centre trial has cast doubts on its routine use.

Hypotension

Haemodynamic instability in the post-operative period is common in patients who have multiple cardiac co-morbidities and in patients who have undergone extensive surgery. Hypotension in the post-operative period could be due to multiple aetiologies ranging from simple fluid depletion, to sepsis and cardiovascular failure. Invasive monitoring and clinical examination should help in searching for the cause and assist the clinician in instituting corrective measures.

Anaesthetic drugs cause myocardial depression and drop systemic vascular resistance. Central neuraxial blockade for pain relief may lead to profound vasodilatation. Major surgery can divert a lot of fluid to extracellular space. The metabolic response to surgical trauma leads to sodium and fluid retention. Managing fluid balance can sometimes be very challenging in these situations of complex interactions. Fluid administration should be used judiciously to optimize cardiac function. Fluid administration should be carefully monitored to avoid fluid overloading. Fluid overload is hazardous in patients with poor cardiac function and may lead to right heart failure. In patients with ischaemic heart disease haemoglobin concentration should be maintained above 10 g/dl.

In patients with persistent hypotension early institution of inotropic/vasopressor support is important. Fine tuning of fluid administration, the choice and dosage of vasoactive drugs should be guided by cardiac output measurements in high-risk patients with cardiovascular instability.

Routine cardiac medications should be started in the post-operative period as soon as possible. Patients who suffer ischaemic heart disease should be monitored closely. Post-operative ischaemia is well characterized, with its peak incidence within 48 hours of surgery. Post-operative ischaemia is clinically silent in more than 90% of cases and carries a grave prognosis. Haemodynamic instability in this group of patients should raise the suspicion of myocardial infarction. Appropriate measures to diagnose and institution of appropriate care early will result in favourable outcomes.

The management of patients with coronary artery stents during the peri-operative period is one of the most important patient safety issues clinicians confront. Peri-operative stent thrombosis is a life-threatening complication for patients with either bare-metal or drug-eluting stents. Non-cardiac surgery appears to increase the risk of stent thrombosis, myocardial infarction and death, particularly when patients undergo surgery early after stent implantation. The incidence of complications is further increased when dual antiplatelet therapy is discontinued pre-operatively. It is generally agreed that aspirin must be continued throughout the peri-operative period, except in circumstances when the risk of bleeding significantly outweighs the benefit of continued anticoagulation. Close liaison with the cardiology and surgical teams will help in managing these patients in the peri-operative period.

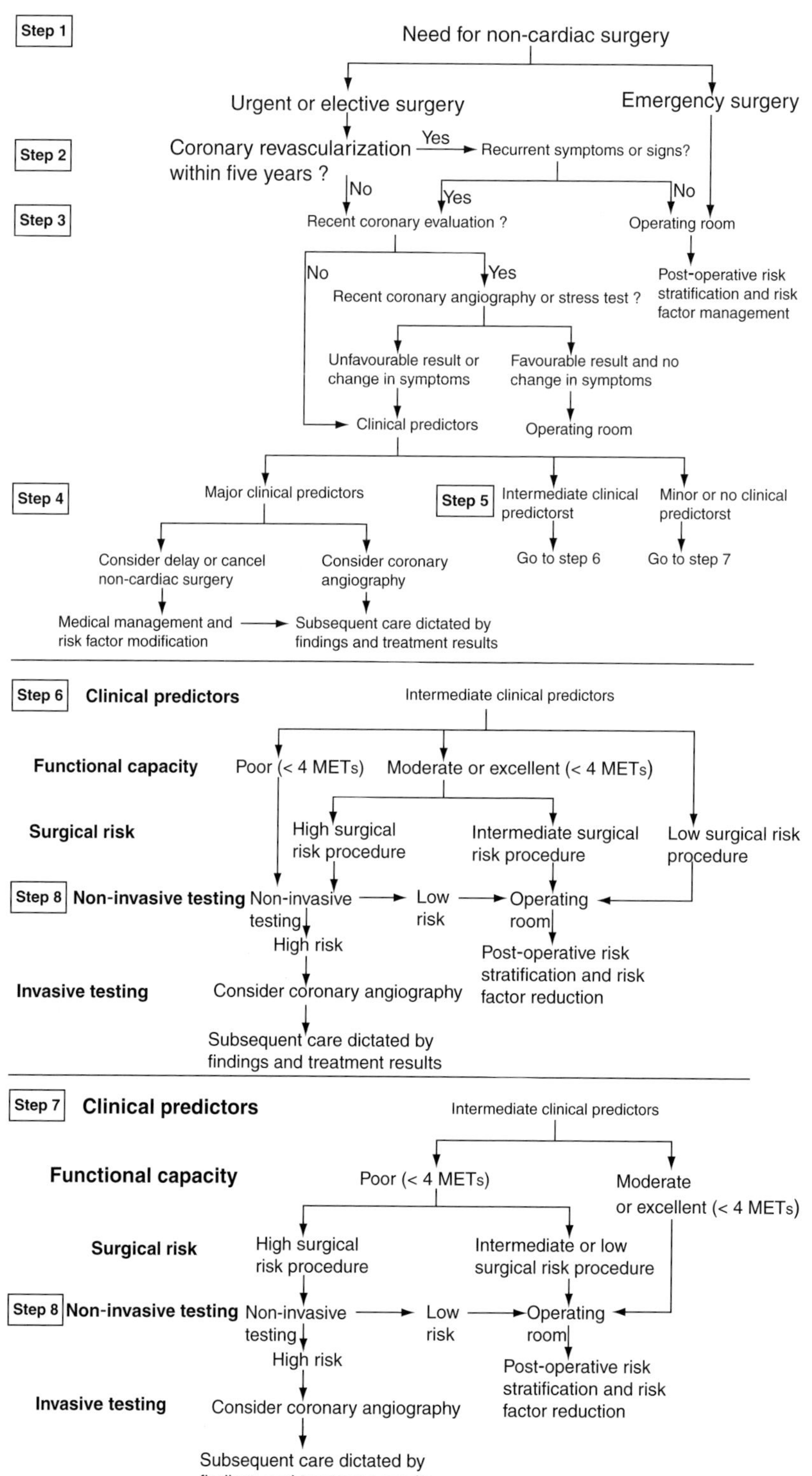

Major clinical predictors: unstable coronary syndromes, decompensated CHF, significant arrhythmias, severe valvular disease.
Intermediate clinical predictors: mild angina pectoris, prior myocardial infarction, compensated or prior CHF, diabetes mellitus, renal insufficiency.
Minor clinical predictors: advanced age, abnormal electrocardiography, rhythm other than sinus, low functional capacity, history of stroke, uncontrolled systemic hypertension.
Subsequent care may include cancellation or delay of surgery, coronary revascularization followed by non-cardiac surgery or intensified care.

Fig. 21.2 Pre-operative cardiac assessment.

Arrhythmias

Arrhythmias are common in the post-operative period and can compromise cardiovascular function. The incidence has been reported to vary from 16.3% to 61.7% with intermittent ECG monitoring and 89% with continuous Holter monitoring in patients undergoing non-cardiac surgery. Atrial fibrillation seems to be the most common form of arrhythmia seen in the peri-operative period. Common contributory factors include electrolyte abnormalities, mechanical irritation from central lines, hypoxaemia, hypercarbia, acidosis and ischaemia. Meticulous attention to electrolyte balance especially potassium and magnesium, removal of causative factors and measures to chemically cardiovert are successful in about 60% of patients. Drugs commonly advocated include β-blockers, calcium channel blockers and amiodarone. In haemodynamically unstable patients cardioversion is effective in most circumstances. In patients who are in atrial fibrillation beyond 48 hours systemic anticoagulation should be considered.

Nutrition

Nutritional support should be considered where return to normal feeding is expected to be delayed. This helps in preventing catabolism and also aids in the reparative process. Nutrition through the enteral route should be established at the earliest possible opportunity. In patients undergoing major upper gastrointestinal surgery placement of nasojejunal or jejunostomy tubes during surgery will help in establishing early enteral feeds. In situations where there is failure to establish enteral nutrition or when there are contraindications to enteral nutrition, parenteral nutrition should be considered early in the peri-operative period with recourse to enteral feeding at the earliest opportunity. Enterocytes obtain almost half of their nutritional requirements directly from the lumen. Hence, enteral feeding supports the integrity of the mucosal gut barrier and reduces bacterial translocation, thereby reducing the risk of suffering systemic infections leading to multi-organ failure.

Blood sugar

Controlling blood sugar levels in the peri-operative period reduces the risk of infections. Most patients who are diabetic would need sliding scale insulin for control of blood sugar levels following major surgery. Some patients who do not have a history of diabetes develop stress hyperglycaemia following major surgery and need insulin infusions.

Orientation

Immediately after surgery, many older patients are confused. Such confusion is more likely to last longer if they have been given long-acting sedative and amnesic drugs.

Confusion can be reduced by restoring spectacles and hearing aids, sitting patients up so that they can see the surroundings properly and returning them as soon as possible to their more familiar ward environment, and encouraging them to assume some sort of control over their life, e.g. allowing them to have drinks and food at the earliest safe opportunity and encouraging familiar visitors. A careful examination should always be made in delirious patients for underlying acute illness or the effects of drug excess or withdrawal.

Care of drains and wounds

After major surgery, drains are kept for draining the collected fluid, blood, etc. The amount of drainage should be carefully monitored and appropriate fluids/blood replaced. In case of large quantities of drainage in a short time, or severe blood loss, the wound should be re-explored. The wound should be dressed properly and kept clean and dry, and the change of dressing should be done aseptically if required. Drain sites are to be properly covered with adequate sterile pads.

Late post-operative period

Control of infection

It is very important to prevent spread of infection by adhering to strict infection control measures. Control of infection is done with appropriate antibiotics after culture and sensitivity if required.

If there is discharge from the wound, or respiratory or urinary infection is suspected, sputum and urine culture sensitivity tests should be done.

Deep vein thrombosis prophylaxis

Prophylaxis of deep vein thrombosis (DVT) is important following major surgeries and orthopaedic surgery. Low molecular weight heparin plays a vital role in prevention of deep vein thrombosis. Local protocols should be in place to prevent the development of this complication. Adherence to this protocol should be strictly implemented to prevent morbidity and mortality arising from this preventable complication. Early ambulation and maintenance of good hydration of the patient reduces incidence of deep vein thrombosis.

Early mobilization

Problems associated with immobility include atelectasis, pneumonia, deep vein thrombosis, constipation, decubitus ulceration, etc. Hence, the patient should be ambulated as early as possible. Good physiotherapy support in the post-operative period for lungs and mobilization helps prevent many complications associated with major surgery.

Prevention of pressure ulcers

Prevention of pressure ulcers is a critical part of post-operative management. The patient has to be turned frequently in the bed to prevent the pressure ulcers. Use of alpha beds and keeping the back dry as well as early mobilization prevents pressure ulcers. This is especially important where epidurals are used to provide pain relief as loss of sensory input prevents patients appreciating tissue injury.

Conclusion

With the current emphasis on promoting day case surgeries, surgeries requiring inpatient admission are becoming more complex. Advances in anaesthesia and surgical techniques have resulted in major surgeries being offered to patients with severe co-morbidities. In keeping with the trends towards longer life expectancy, we are seeing a more senior population with multiple co-morbidities having major surgical procedures. These patients need augmented care to provide ideal conditions for recovery from surgical trauma. Central to a good peri-operative outcome is a multi-disciplinary approach to promote effective and early therapy.

Key points

- The aim of post-operative care is prevention, early identification and treatment of post-operative complications.
- Post-operative pulmonary complications contribute significantly to overall peri-operative morbidity and mortality rates. Incidence of pulmonary complications varies from 5% to 70% and can lead to prolonged hospital stay.
- Attention should be paid to removing retained sputum, and the patient should be encouraged to breathe deeply to avoid atelectasis.
- Respiratory support may be needed in the form of CPAP or NIV.
- The cardiovascular system is placed under stress during the peri-operative period and cardiovascular complications contribute to a substantial number of all deaths among patients undergoing non-cardiac surgery. Incidence of serious peri-operative cardiac morbidity varies from 1% to 10%.
- Hypotension and arrhythmias should be diagnosed early and treated with fluid resuscitation, inotropes, replacement of electrolytes and anti-arrhythmic medications.
- Good post-operative care is attention to all organ systems and should include:
    - Monitoring of vital signs including urine output
    - Fluid balance
    - Effective analgesia
    - Control of blood sugar
    - DVT prophylaxis
    - Nutrition
    - Early mobilization.

Further reading

- Gandhi GY, Murad MH, Flynn DL *et al.* (2008) Effect of perioperative insulin infusion on surgical morbidity and mortality: systematic review and meta-analysis of randomized trials. *Mayo Clin. Proc.* **83**(4): 418–30.
- Honrubia T, García López FJ, Franco N *et al.* (2005) Noninvasive vs. conventional mechanical ventilation in acute respiratory failure: a multicenter, randomized controlled trial. *Chest* **128**: 3916–24.
- Keenan S, Sinuff T, Cook D *et al.* (2004) Does noninvasive positive-pressure ventilation improve outcome in acute hypoxemic respiratory failure? A systematic review. *Crit. Care Med.* **32**: 2516–23.
- Lawrence VA, Cornell JE, Smetana GW (2006) Strategies to reduce post-operative pulmonary complications after noncardiothoracic surgery: systematic review for the American College of Physicians. *Ann. Intern. Med.* **144** (8): 596–608.

- POISE Study Group (2008) Effects of extended-release metoprolol succinate in patients undergoing non-cardiac surgery (POISE trial): a randomised controlled trial. *Lancet* **371**: 1839–47.
- Spencer SL, Wu CL 2007 Effect of post-operative analgesia on major post-operative complications: a systematic update of the evidence. *Anesth. Analg.* **104**: 689–702.
- Squadrone V, Coha M, Cerutti E *et al.* (2005) Continuous positive airway pressure for treatment of post-operative hypoxcmia: a randomized controlled trial. *J. Am. Med. Ass.* **293**: 589–95.

Post-resuscitation care

Gavin Perkins

Incidence and outcome following cardiac arrest

Each year approximately 700 000 people in Europe sustain a cardiac arrest. In the UK there are approximately 50 000 treated sudden cardiac arrests annually of which about 20 000 occur in hospital. Overall survival from cardiac arrest is relatively poor. Data from European and American Cardiopulmonary Resuscitation (CPR) registries report initial survival rates of 10–20% for pre-hospital arrests and ≃40% from in-hospital arrests. Less than half of those that achieve an initial return of spontaneous circulation eventually leave hospital alive.

A significant proportion of patients will have a reduced consciousness level or other organ dysfunction after initial resuscitation from cardiac arrest. These patients will require assessment for potential admission to intensive care. The decision to admit a patient to intensive care following cardiac arrest, like many decisions in critical care, is challenging. There are no outcome prediction models with sufficient sensitivity or specificity upon which to base a treatment decision in an individual patient. Studies in this area are limited in number, usually observational in nature and often confounded by the effect of refusal to admit to intensive care being almost invariably associated with non-survival. Pre-arrest factors associated with poorer outcomes are increasing age, serious underlying illness, cardiac arrest location (out of hospital as opposed to in-hospital). Arrest related factors include down time prior to advanced life support; whether bystander CPR was performed; the cause of the cardiac arrest and initial rhythm (VF/VT have better outcomes) and the duration and quality of CPR performed.

The largest study to date to evaluate outcomes from cardiac arrest survivors specifically admitted to intensive care was conducted by Nolan *et al.* in 2007. This study performed a secondary analysis of the UK Intensive Care National Audit and Research Centre Case Mix Programme Database which included nearly 25 000 patients admitted to intensive care and requiring mechanical ventilation within 24 hours of a cardiac arrest from 1995 to 2005. This represented 5.8% of all ICU admissions. The study reported that 42.9% survived to leave the ICU, whilst 28.6% survived to hospital discharge. Most survivors (79.9%) were finally discharged to their normal residence implying a good neurological outcome in the majority of survivors. Long-term follow-up studies of cardiac arrest survivors demonstrate >80% are alive at 12 months.

Post-resuscitation syndrome

The concept of a post-resuscitation syndrome was first described by Negovsky, a Russian pathophysiolologist, in 1972. Current theories describe the development of a systemic inflammatory response/sepsis following resuscitation from cardiac arrest. The syndrome is characterized by multi-organ dysfunction due to direct ischaemic injury to organs and post-reperfusion activation of the systemic inflammatory response with upregulation of inflammatory cytokine cascades, endothelial activation, dysregulation of the coagulation/fibrinolysis pathways and adrenal dysfunction. Clinically, the post-resuscitation syndrome presents with neurological dysfunction, cardiovascular instability and multi-organ dysfunction.

Post-resuscitation care

The *Chain of Survival* describes a series of interrelated steps which can improve outcomes following cardiac arrest. In 2005, the Chain was updated to include the period of care after return of spontaneous circulation (known as post-resuscitation care) in response to the growing evidence that treatments in this phase have a significant influence on overall outcomes (Fig. 22.1).

Core Topics in Critical Care Medicine, eds. Fang Gao Smith and Joyce Yeung. Published by Cambridge University Press.

Patient assessment following cardiac arrest should use the ABCDE approach (Table 22.1). Critical care treatments during the post-resuscitation phase should focus on correcting hypoxia and hypercarbia, optimizing organ perfusion, identifying and treating the underlying cause of the cardiac arrest and optimizing neurological outcomes. In addition, specific therapeutic interventions listed below should be considered.

Table 22.1 Critical care for comatosed cardiac arrest survivor

Airway	Ensure clear airway Consider intubation in patients with obtunded consciousness level
Breathing	Examine chest and establish continuous pulse oximetry monitoring Place nasogastric tube to decompress the stomach/reduce diaphragmatic splinting Measure arterial blood gases (including lactate) and check electrolytes/glucose Obtain and review chest X-ray Aim for normal gas exchange (SpO_2 94–96% and normocarbia)
Circulation	Establish blood pressure and ECG monitoring Catheterize and monitor urine output (target >0.5 ml/kg) Optimize haemodynamic status with fluid/ inotropes (target MABP >65 mmHg) Record 12-lead ECG; consider reperfusion therapy
Disability	Assess initial neurological status including Glasgow Coma Score Treat seizure if present
Exposure	Measure and record temperature Consider therapeutic hypothermia Seek to identify and treat cause of cardiac arrest (if possible)

Therapeutic hypothermia

Hyperthermia is common following the return of a spontaneous circulation and is associated with adverse neurological outcomes. Several randomized controlled trials and a meta-analysis have shown that therapeutic hypothermia is associated with improved survival and neurological outcome in initially comatose survivors of cardiac arrest. The largest of these trials, the Hypothermia after Cardiac Arrest study conducted by Michael Holzer and colleagues, randomized comatose survivors of cardiac arrest (whose initial rhythm was ventricular fibrillation) to normal care or therapeutic hypothermia (core temperature of 32–34 °C). Cooling was commenced in the emergency department and continued for 24 hours. The study demonstrated improved neurological outcome and survival at 6 months in the group allocated to therapeutic hypothermia (see Fig. 22.2).

In 2003, the International Liaison Committee for Resuscitation introduced the recommendation that unconscious adult patients with spontaneous circulation after out of hospital cardiac arrest should be cooled to 32–34 °C for 12–24 hours when the initial cardiac arrest rhythm was ventricular fibrillation. This therapy may also be appropriate for other rhythms, or in-hospital cardiac arrests.

Complications of therapeutic hypothermia include increased risk of infection, cardiovascular instability, coagulopathy, reduced insulin sensitivity leading to hyperglycaemia, electrolyte abnormalities and prolonged reduced clearance of sedatives and muscle relaxants. Relative contraindications to thereuptic hypothermia include severe systemic infection, severe refractory

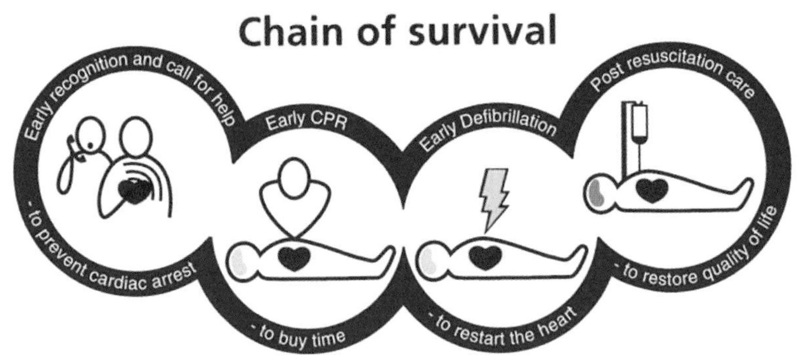

Fig. 22.1 The Chain of Survival describes evidence-based interventions that can improve survival from cardiac arrest. The concept of the Chain of Survival originated in the 1960s when it was used in an attempt to optimize outcome from pre-hospital cardiac arrest. In order to maximize the chances of a successful resuscitation attempt, each of the links of the chain must be in place and functioning. The Chain of Survival was revised in 2005 to include post-resuscitation care as the fourth link in light of the growing body of evidence demonstrating the impact good-quality post-resuscitation care can have on outcome. The brain of the victim is darker blue in the fourth link to emphasize the importance of therapeutic hypothermia after cardiac arrest.

Table 22.2 Methods for cooling patients after cardiac arrest

- **External cooling**
  - Ice packs; head cooling devices; surface cooling by circulation with cold air can all reduce core temperature. Responses to these methods are variable and precise temperature control can be difficult
- Cold intravenous fluids – 30 ml/kg ice-cold crystalloid can reduce core temperature by 1–2 °C and is associated with improved cardiovascular function
- Magnesium – intravenous magnesium increases rate of surface cooling, reduces shivering threshold, and may enhance the neuroprotective effects of hypothermia
- **Intravascular cooling**
  - A number of intravascular cooling devices have been developed. These devices allow rapid cooling and precise control of body temperature. They are particularly useful for controlling the rewarming and avoiding overshoot hyperthermia.

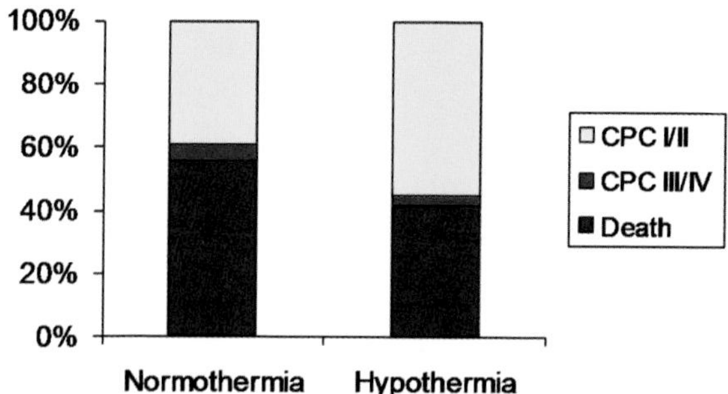

Fig. 22.2 The Hypothermia after Cardiac Arrest Study Group demonstrated improved neurological outcomes (55% vs. 39%, $P = 0.009$, number needed to treat (NNT) to prevent one adverse outcome = 6) and survival (59% vs. 45% $P = 0.02$, NNT = 7) at 6 months in patients randomized to receive therapeutic hypothermia compared to standard care. Neurological outcomes were assessed using the Pittsburgh Cerebral Performance Category (I, good recovery; II, moderate disability; III, severe disability; IV, vegetative state; V, death).

cardiogenic shock, established multiple organ failure and pre-existing medical coagulopathy.

There are a number of different strategies for reducing temperature after cardiac arrest (Table 22.2). The precise timing for initiating therapeutic hypothermia remains to be determined, but the general consensus is that it should be started as early as possible. If required, shivering should be treated with sedatives and muscle relaxants. Rewarming should be controlled, aiming to increase core temperature by 0.25–0.5 °C per hour. Care should be taken to avoid an overshoot hyperthermia which may be detrimental.

Glycaemic control

Observational studies in cardiac arrest survivors have shown that hyperglycaemia after return of spontaneous circulation is associated with an adverse outcome. A trial in patients following admission to a surgical intensive care reported improved survival in patients with tight glycaemic control (blood glucose 4.4–6.1 mmol/l). However, these results have not been reproduced in subsequent multi-centre trials. Indeed, the NICE–SUGAR trial found that a strategy of tight glycaemic control in general ITU patients was associated with increased mortality. A small trial in out of hospital cardiac arrest survivors ($n = 90$) failed to demonstrate improved outcomes with tight (<6 mmol/l) as opposed to moderate (6–8 mmol/l) glycaemic control. Current guidelines recommend avoiding hyperglycaemia by maintaining a blood sugar of <8 mmol/l. Therapeutic hypothermia causes insulin resistance, so control of glucose with an insulin sliding scale is often required in these patients.

Cardiac dysfunction

Myocardial dysfunction is common after cardiac arrest and usually starts to improve within 72 hours after return of spontaneous circulation. Supportive care with fluids and inotropes should be instituted when required to maintain adequate end-organ perfusion. Evidence of an acute coronary syndrome should be sought by recording a 12-lead ECG in all cardiac arrest survivors. Reperfusion therapy, ideally by percutaneous coronary intervention (PCI), should be considered when evidence of an ST elevation myocardial infarction is present. If PCI is not available, thrombolytic therapy is an appropriate alternative unless contraindicated for other reasons. An aggressive approach to optimizing end-organ perfusion and instituting reperfusion therapy as part of a post-resuscitation care bundle has been shown to be associated with improved outcomes. Dysrhythmias, if present, often improve after successful reperfusion treatment. Persistent dysrhythmias can be treated by restoring normal electrolyte concentrations (especially potassium and magnesium) and by using standard drug and electrical therapies. Assessment for an implantable cardioverter-defibrillator (ICD) or pacemaker should take place following discharge from ICU if the cardiac arrest occurred as a consequence of a dysrhythmia.

Acidosis

Most cardiac arrest survivors have an initially mixed respiratory and metabolic acidosis. The severity of the acidosis reflects the duration of the cardiac arrest and is related to the likelihood of subsequent survival. Early spontaneous clearance of the acidosis is a predictor of improved outcome. Treatment of the acidosis should be directed at the underlying cause. For a metabolic acidosis this will involve optimizing oxygen delivery to the tissues and for a respiratory acidosis increasing minute ventilation. Care should be taken to avoid hyperventilation and hypocarbia as this may have detrimental effects on coronary and cerebral perfusion. There is no role for the routine use of intravenous sodium bicarbonate. However, small amounts of bicarbonate may be given following cardiac arrest where there is profound acidaemia (pH <7.1, base deficit >10), if the excess hydrogen ions are thought to be contributing to depressed myocardial function. A failure to improve or worsening of the acid–base status after optimizing ventilation and oxygen delivery should direct the clinician to look for an underlying cause of the acidosis and treat accordingly.

Control of seizures

Seizures occur in 5–15% of those who achieve return of spontaneous circulation and in 40% of those remaining comatose. Seizures are associated with increased cerebral oxygen consumption and should be treated promptly. Benzodiazepines, phenytoin, barbiturates and propofol are the common choice of drugs in this scenario. There are no prospective randomized controlled trials demonstrating improved outcomes when anticonvulsants are administered prophylactically, so the routine use of prophylactic anticonvulsants is not recommended. The occurrence of seizures and myoclonic jerks alone is not associated with adverse outcomes. However, the development of status epilepticus, and in particular status myoclonus, is associated with poorer outcomes and can be particularly difficult to treat pharmacologically.

Prognostication

The ability to predict the likely neurological outcome of a patient following admission to critical care is important. Two-thirds of patients that die in intensive care following a pre-hospital cardiac arrest and a quarter of those following in-hospital arrest die as a consequence of poor neurological recovery. If reliable tests were available that could predict outcome shortly after admission to intensive care, they would help target aggressive treatment to patients likely to have a good outcome, whilst allowing early palliation and withdrawal of life-sustaining treatments in cases where continuing care is futile. Unfortunately, there are few prospective clinical studies in this area and at present no tests immediately after cardiac arrest have sufficient specificity at predicting outcome to be of use clinically. A major limitation of the studies that do exist is that most studies are confounded by knowledge of the test outcome affecting the decision making process around withdrawal, thus becoming a self-fulfilling prophecy.

To date a variety of clinical, electrophysiological and laboratory tests have been evaluated as predictors of outcome from 24 hours after cardiac arrest. Currently few centres have the facilities to perform routinely many of the electrophysiological or laboratory tests. The American Academy of Neurology conducted a systematic review of the evidence in 2006 and drew up practice recommendations for predicting neurological outcome after cardiac arrest. These are summarized in Fig. 22.3. The majority of studies evaluating prognostic markers after cardiac arrest took place prior to the widespread use of therapeutic hypothermia. Recent studies have shown that absence of a motor response to pain and brain enzymes within the first few days after cardiac arrest are unreliable after therapeutic hypothermia. The performance characteristics of these tests in patients that have received therapeutic hypothermia require further validation.

Organ donation

Clinical brainstem death occurs in up to 16% of comatose patients admitted to intensive care after cardiac arrest. With appropriate patient selection, studies have reported that transplant outcomes do not differ from those using organs obtained from other brain-dead donors.

Conclusion

Most patients achieving a return of spontaneous circulation after cardiac arrest will require assessment and potentially admission to critical care. The post-resuscitation syndrome is common in these patients and consists of haemodynamic, neurological and multi-organ dysfunction. Early and aggressive treatment during the post-resuscitation phase has the potential to significantly improve outcomes. There are no perfect clinical prediction models for predicting neurological outcome after cardiac arrest. Certain clinical and other tests can be used between 24 and 72 hours after cardiac arrest with a reasonable degree of certainty for detecting patients likely to have an adverse outcome.

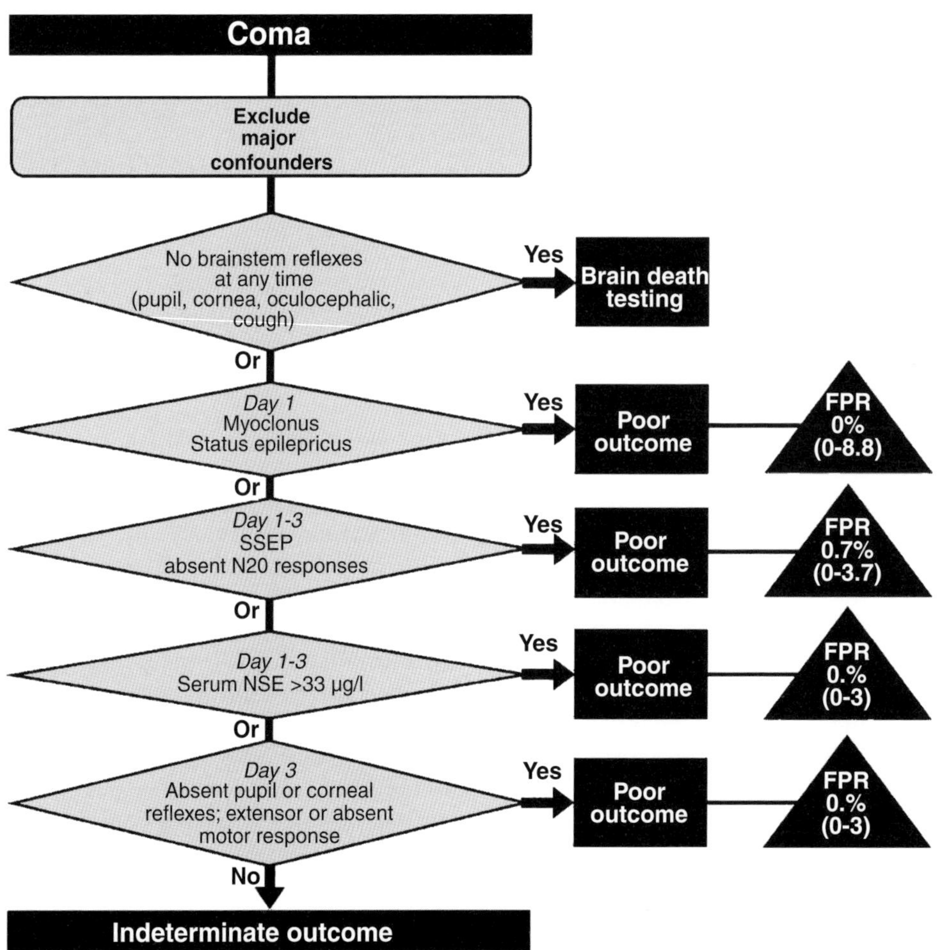

Fig. 22.3 Decision algorithm for use in prognostication of comatose survivors after cardiopulmonary resuscitation. The numbers in the triangles in parentheses are exact 95% CIs. Major confounders could include the use or prior use of sedatives or neuromuscular blocking agents, induced hypothermia therapy, presence of organ failure (e.g. acute renal or liver failure) or shock (e.g. cardiogenic shock requiring inotropes). Note that these tests have not been fully validated in patients that have received therapeutic hypothermia. Early studies are suggesting that motor response to pain and brain enzymes are less reliable early after cardiac arrest and therapeutic hypothermia has been used. (Adapted from Wijdicks, EFM *et al.* (2006) *Neurology* **67**: 203–10.)

Key points

- Survival from cardiac arrests is poor with estimates of 5–10% survival to hospital discharge from out of hospital arrests and 10–20% from in hospital arrests.
- Post-resuscitation syndrome presents the intensivists with the combined challenge of neurological dysfunction, cardiovascular instability and multi-organ dysfunction.
- Good quality post-resuscitation care is the fourth link in the Chain of Survival in resuscitation and can significantly improves outcome of patients. The strategies should include:
  - Therapeutic hypothermia of 32–34 °C for 12–24 hours has shown to improve outcome after in-hospital VF arrests and should be considered for other rhythms and out of hospital cardiac arrests
  - Supportive measures for cardiac dysfunction
  - Avoidance of hyperglycaemia
  - Correction of acidosis
  - Control of seizures.

Further reading

- Hypothermia after Cardiac Arrest Study Group (2002) Mild therapeutic hypothermia to improve the neurologic outcome after cardiac arrest. *N. Engl. J. Med.* **346**: 549–56.

- Nolan JP, Deakin CD, Soar J, Bottiger BW, Smith G (2005) European Resuscitation Council Guidelines for Resuscitation 2005 Section 4: Adult advanced life support. *Resuscitation* **67** (Suppl. 1): S39–S86.
- Nolan JP, Laver SR, Welch CA *et al.* (2007) Outcome following admission to UK intensive care units after cardiac arrest: a secondary analysis of the ICNARC Case Mix Programme Database. *Anaesthesia* **62**: 1207–16.
- Nolan JP *et al.* (2008) Post cardiac arrest syndrome: epidermiology, pathophysiology, treatment, and prognostication – a scientific statement from the International Liaison Committee on Resuscitation; the American Heart Association Emergency Cardiovascular Care Committee; the Council on Cardiovascular Surgery; Rand Anesthesia; the Council on Cardiopulmonary, Peri-Operative, and Critical Care; the Council on Clinical Cardiology; the Council on Stroke. *Resuscitation* **79**: 350–79.
- Wijdicks EF, Hijdra A, Young GB, Bassetti CL, Wiebe S (2006) Practice parameter: prediction of outcome in comatose survivors after cardiopulmonary resuscitation (an evidence-based review): report of the Quality Standards Subcommittee of the American Academy of Neurology. *Neurology* **67**: 203–10.

Section III Organ dysfunction and management

Chapter 23 Bleeding and clotting disorders

Nick Murphy

Normal haemostasis

Coagulation

Normal coagulation depends on the interaction of plasma proteins and circulating platelets with the vessel wall resulting in integrity of the circulation. It can fail leading to haemorrhage or be inappropriate resulting in disseminated intravascular coagulation or localized clotting.

Following injury, damaged vessels contract and the underlying matrix is exposed. Surface glycoproteins and other ligands, such as von Willebrand factor, bind to the exposed collagen. Simultaneously, the exposure of tissue factor (TF) on subendothelial cells initiates the production of thrombin which is amplified via a series of coagulation proteins. Circulating platelets also adhere to the exposed surface and are then activated. The activation of platelets initiates adhesion to each other and also to fibrin. The platelet aggregate forms a phospholipid surface for the contact activation clotting pathway thus linking the process of platelet activation and thrombin formation (see Fig. 23.1).

Classical coagulation cascade

The coagulation pathway functions as a result of the interaction between positive and negative feedback loops which control the activation process (Fig. 23.2).

The intrinsic pathway

The intrinsic pathway is initiated when blood comes into contact with subendothelial connective tissues exposed as a result of tissue damage. In the first step, factor XII binds to subendothelial surface and becomes activated. Activated factor XII, in turn, activates factor XI in a process that requires calcium. A complex of molecules containing activated factor IX, factor VIII, calcium and phospholipids then activates factor X.

The extrinsic pathway

The extrinsic pathway provides a quicker response to tissue injury, generating activated factor X almost instantaneously. The main function of the extrinsic pathway is to enhance the activity of the intrinsic pathway. The two components unique to the extrinsic pathway are TF and factor VII. Once activated, tissue factor binds to factor VII, which is then activated to form a complex in order to activate factor X.

Common pathway

The end result of the clotting pathway is the production of thrombin for the conversion of fibrinogen to fibrin. Cleaving of fibrinogen leads to formation of insoluble fibrin. The polymerized fibrin is then stabilized by the factor XIIIa. The fibrin and platelets aggregate to form a clot which blocks the damaged blood vessel and prevents further bleeding.

Cell-based model of coagulation

The elegant idea of the classical coagulation cascade has now been challenged. A cell-based model of coagulation better describes a series of overlapping stages in vivo (Fig. 23.3).

- The first phase, **initiation**, occurs on a cell surface expressing TF where small quantities of thrombin are produced. TF is a membrane-bound protein expressed on subendothelial cells such as fibroblasts and smooth muscle cells. Under normal circumstances endothelial cells do not express tissue factor but its production can be induced by inflammatory cytokines. TF binds with factor VII

Core Topics in Critical Care Medicine, eds. Fang Gao Smith and Joyce Yeung. Published by Cambridge University Press.

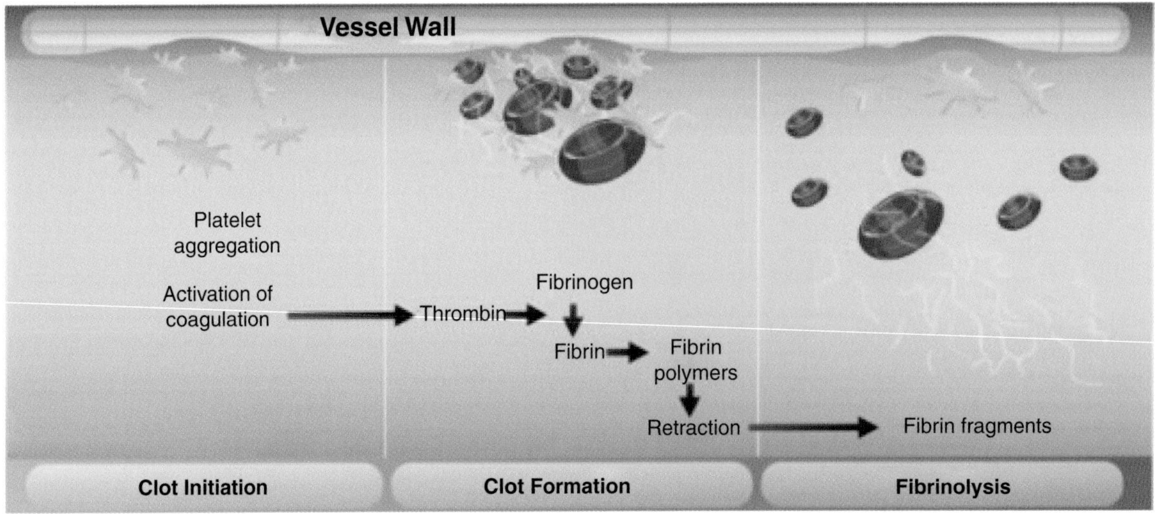

Fig. 23.1 An overview of normal haemostasis. (Courtesy of Novo Nordisk Inc., Princeton, USA.)

to activate it in the presence of calcium ions. Activated factor VII (VIIa) is a serine protease that induces the activation of circulating factor X into Xa. Xa coverts prothrombin into thrombin.

- **Amplification** of the production of thrombin-activated platelets and activated cofactors via a number of positive feedback loops to prepare for mass thrombin generation.
- **Propagation** occurs on the surface of platelets where large amounts of thrombin and a stable clot are formed. Thrombin is central to the coagulation haemostasis and has a number of actions. It cleaves circulating fibrinogen to fibrin which forms part of the stable clot. In addition, thrombin amplifies its own production by activating a number of circulating coagulation proteins. It also has a regulatory function by its interaction with thrombomodulin and protein C.

Regulation of coagulation

To prevent the obvious catastrophic consequence of uncontrolled coagulation throughout the vascular tree there are a number of mechanisms that regulate coagulation.

The antithrombin system

Antithrombin is a glycoprotein produced in the liver. It is a serine protease inhibitor that has activity against a number of factors that help amplify coagulation. These include the activated forms of factors X (Xa), IXa, VIIa, XIa, XIIa and thrombin (IIa). Antithrombin binds in an equimolar concentration to the complexes. Levels of antithrombin can be decreased due to increased consumption, decreased hepatic synthesis and degradation by neutrophil elastase. Heparin and heparan sulphate cause conformational change in the structure of antithrombin exposing the active site and increase its activity by up to 1000 times.

The protein C system

Thrombin combines with the endothelial cell surface protein thrombomodulin. The resulting complex activates the circulating zymogen, protein C. Protein C is a vitamin K dependent protein synthesized in the liver. Activated protein C (APC), with its cofactor protein S, proteolytically inactivates factor Va and factor VIIIa, rapidly inactivating the coagulation process as a result. Levels of protein C and protein S are reduced in septic patients due to increased consumption and downregulation of thrombomodulin on the endothelial surface.

Tissue factor pathway inhibitor

Tissue factor pathway inhibitor (TFPI) is a protein which circulates in the blood bound to lipoprotein (LDL, HDL). It has three inhibitory domains which inhibit factor Xa and the factor VIIa–T Factor complex. A small percentage is carried in combination with platelets. Its function is enhanced by heparin but not to the same extent as antithrombin.

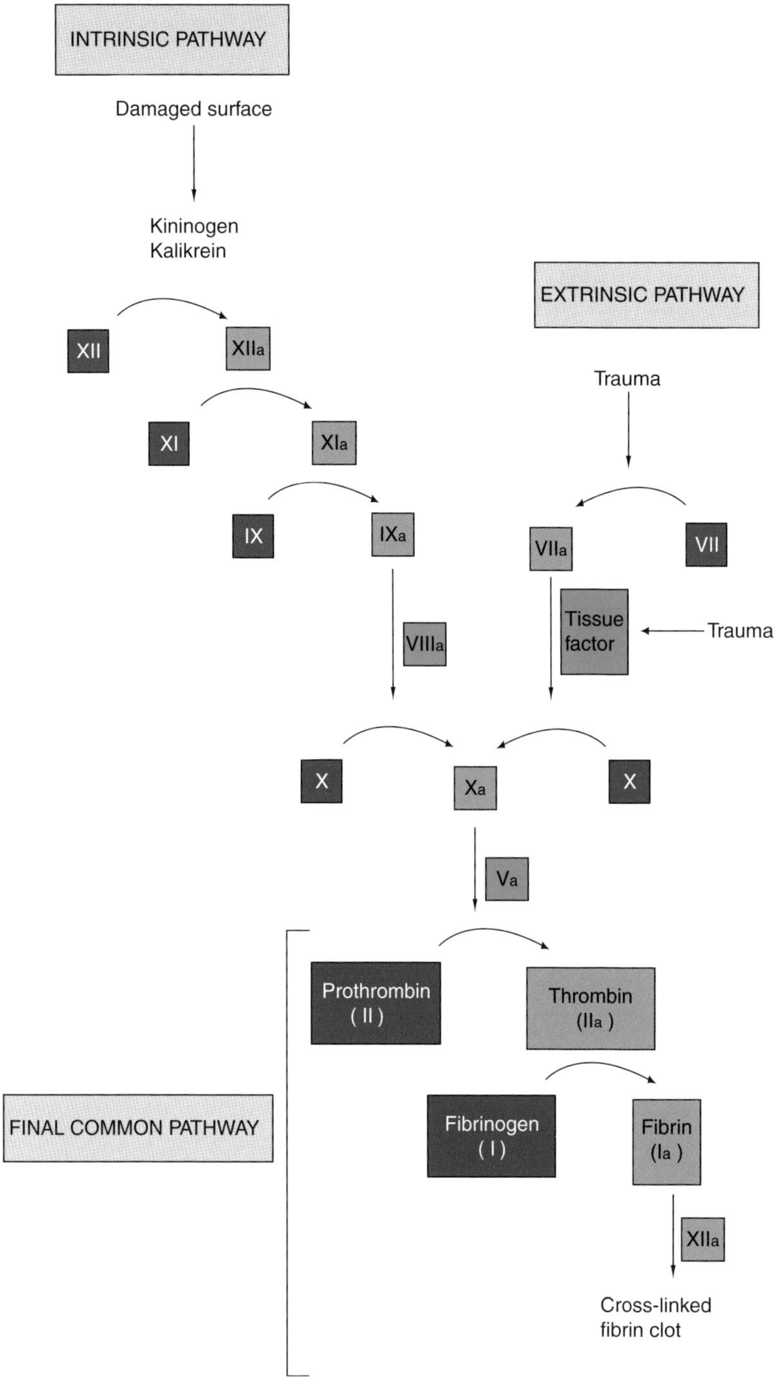

Fig. 23.2 Classical coagulation pathway.

Bleeding disorders

Congenital disorders

Patients with congenital coagulation defects can present to the intensive care unit. The most common of these will relate to isolated factor deficiencies such as haemophilia A (factor VIII deficiency), haemophilia B (factor IX deficiency) and von Willebrand disease (von Willebrand factor deficiency). The mainstay of treatment is to stop the bleeding in

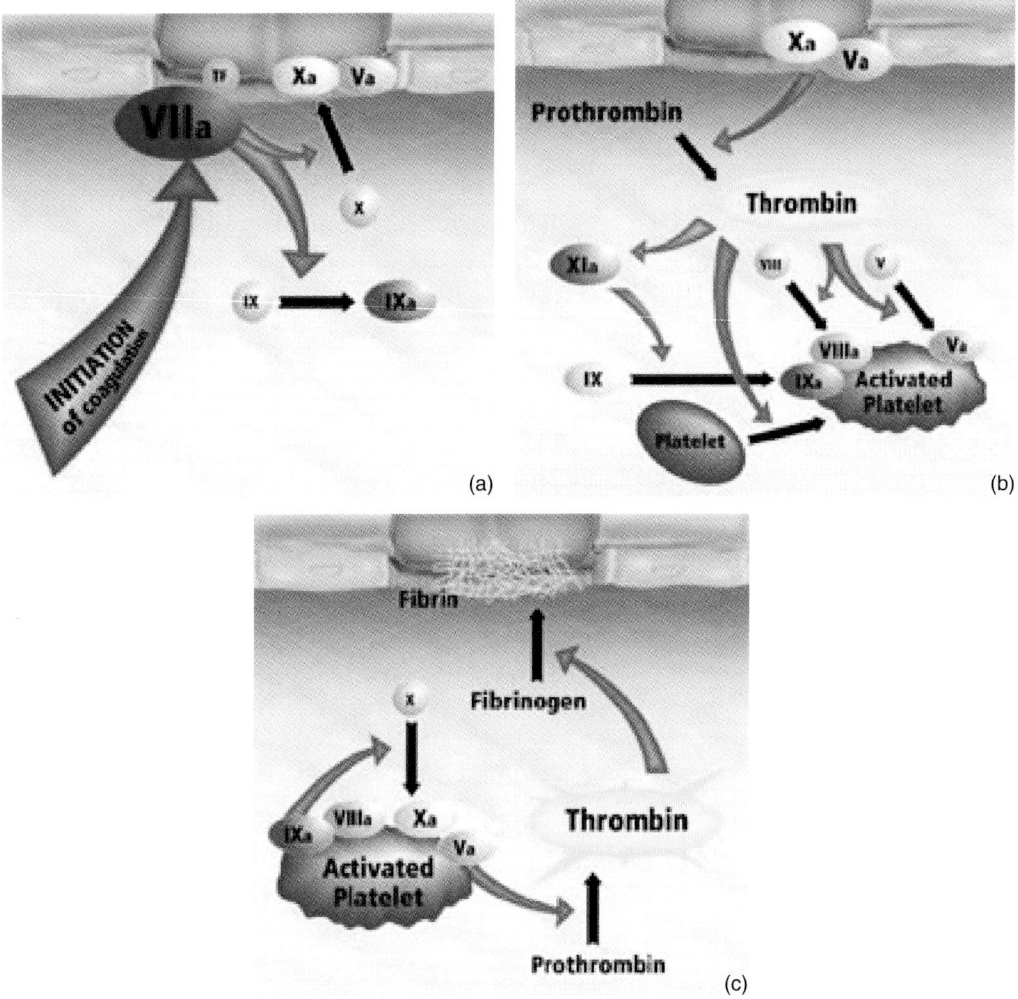

Fig. 23.3 Cell-based model of initiation: (a) initiation; (b) amplification; (c) propagation.

these patients, which may include transfusion of clotting products and need close consultation with the haematology department.

Acquired disorders

Thrombocytopenia

Thrombocytopenia is common in patients in the intensive care unit. This may occur because of:

- impaired production
- sequestration
- increased consumption
- enhanced degradation.

Depending on the definition used, the incidence of thrombocytopenia (platelet count $<150 \times 10^9$/l) in critically ill patients has been reported to be up to 50% of patients. Low platelet count is associated with an increased risk of bleeding and mortality. Severely reduced count ($<50 \times 10^9$/l) increases the risk of spontaneous bleeding by about 4–5 times compared to patients with higher counts.

Spontaneous intracerebral bleeding is rare in critically ill patients but it is almost always associated with severe thrombocytopenia. In a retrospective review, Oppenheim-Eden *et al.* found nine patients out of a total of 2198 patients in a tertiary university hospital had spontaneous intracerebral bleeding. Seven of the nine had a primary haematological malignancy or recent

Table 23.1 Causes of thrombocytopenia in critical care

Sepsis
Disseminated intravascular coagulation
Massive blood loss
Heparin-induced thrombocytopenia
Immune thrombocytopenia
Drug-induced thrombocytopenia

bone marrow transplant. The median platelet count was 10×10^9/l. All had bled from other sites prior to the intracerebral bleed. The study concluded that the severity and length of sustained thrombocytopenia are both associated with an increase in mortality (Table. 23.1).

Sepsis is the most common cause for thrombocytopenia in the critically ill and occurs in about 30% of patients. The cause of thrombocytopenia in sepsis is not completely clear but is probably caused by a combination of all the possible mechanisms.

Disseminated intravascular coagulation

Disseminated intravascular coagulation (DIC) is not a disease in itself and is always the result of some underlying disorder. The syndrome can range from mild to severe and is characterized by widespread activation of the coagulation system. This results in reduced blood flow and localized ischaemia in organs and the peripheries of the circulation. Excessive consumption of coagulation factors and platelets often results in an increased tendency to bleed. Actual bleeding is, however, much less common than the associated organ dysfunction.

Activation of inflammatory cytokines is the main initiating factor in DIC. Inflammatory cytokines induce the expression of TF which, together with activated factor VII, initiate the coagulation cascade within blood vessels. Despite this, widespread coagulation will not occur without the concomitant reduction in the innate anticoagulant pathways. Impairment of these pathways is invariable during DIC in sepsis. All the major pathways including antithrombin III, protein C and TF inhibitor pathway are decreased during sepsis. In addition it appears that the fibrinolytic pathways are impaired just as the coagulation system is activated and homeostatic regulation is disrupted. About 5–10% of patients with severe DIC associated with sepsis have clinically significant bleeding. It is the severity of thrombocytopenia that dictates this rather than any of the other coagulation parameters.

Management of DIC is essentially supportive while therapy is directed at the underlying cause. Transfusion of blood products should be based on clinical indicators rather than laboratory findings. The transfusion of platelets remains a controversial issue. Bleeding should be aggressively managed to maintain a platelet count between 50 and 100×10^9/l. If the patient is not showing signs of bleeding then a lower transfusion trigger is usually tolerated, somewhere between 10 and 20×10^9/l. The use of other coagulation factors is also controversial as their use could exacerbate the intravascular coagulation, thereby worsening the situation. A pragmatic stance is usually taken in which fresh frozen plasma or factor concentrates are used if the patient is bleeding actively. Even if the patient is not bleeding, there is still a theoretical advantage and there is some evidence to suggest that enhancing the regulatory anticoagulant activity can improve outcome.

Antithrombin (AT) is the main natural inhibitor of thrombin and is well known to be reduced in DIC. Many studies have investigated increasing the levels of AT during DIC and sepsis. In Kypercept, a large multicentre trial of the use of AT in sepsis, AT was not shown to improve survival at 30 or 90 days. Post-hoc analysis of the patients with DIC and sepsis did show improvement in survival in those patients that received AT but not heparin. It has been suggested that heparin may impair the anti-inflammatory properties of AT by competing with the naturally produced heparin sulphate residues on endothelial cells. In the natural course of events AT is bound to the endothelium via the heparin sulphate bridges. Bound AT increases endothelial epoprostenol production and has other anti-inflammatory effects. Exogenous unfractionated heparin prevents this process from occurring.

Activated protein C has been shown to reduce mortality in sepsis in the recent PROWESS trial, a large randomized controlled trial looking at the efficacy and safety of recombinant human activated protein C for severe sepsis. This effect was more pronounced in patients with DIC and in those with multi-organ failure. Prothrombotic agents are not recommended as, theoretically, they exacerbate the reduction in thrombolysis seen in DIC. That being said, in situations of uncontrolled bleeding, they are sometimes tried. Activated factor VII (VIIa) has been used in this setting without any obvious exacerbation of thrombotic events or severity of bleeding in most patients.

Microangiopathic haemolytic anaemia

Thrombotic thrombocytopenia purpura (TTP) and haemolytic uraemic syndrome (HUS) are similar syndromes which fall at either end of a spectrum and it is important to recognize that TTP and HUS are not diseases in themselves but descriptions of pathological processes with many different causes. The main problem with these syndromes is not bleeding per se but micro and macro thrombosis leading to ischaemia and organ failure.

HUS typically affects children and is associated with a diarrhoeal illness, often induced by Shiga toxin producing bacteria such as *E. coli*. It classically consists of microangiopathic haemolytic anaemia, thrombocytopenia and acute renal failure. These children are described as having D+HUS or typical HUS. HUS can occur in adults when renal failure is prominent, although it cannot be clinically differentiated from TTP.

TTP was recognized earlier than HUS and has a different spectrum of signs and symptoms. Early descriptions of TTP emphasized the addition of fever and neurological symptoms and signs for the diagnosis. The need for early initiation of therapy and the absence of these factors in many patients led to the present definition of microangiopathic haemolytic anaemia and thrombocytopenia. The differentiation between the two conditions remains pertinent as it distinguishes which patients should benefit from plasma exchange. TTP should be treated with plasma exchange whereas typical or childhood HUS often only requires supportive care.

The most prominent finding in all patients is haemolytic anaemia with red cell fragmentation caused by turbulent flow. This is due to widespread microthrombi within the circulation causing organ damage associated with the illness. The pathogenesis is variable but has been described in some patients. Acquired TTP has been shown to be the failure of von Willibrand factor cleavage resulting in large multimers that readily activate platelets. The underlying pathology appears to be a neutralizing antibody to the cleavage enzyme, a disintegrin and metalloproteinase with a thrombospondin type 1 metif, member 13 (ADAMTS 13). This observation provides the rationale for plasma exchange which, at the same time, removes the neutralizing autoantibody and provides exogenous ADAMTS 13. Rarely, congenital reduction in ADAMTS 13 can lead to the syndrome. In these patients infusion of plasma has a similar effect. Other causes include drug reactions, pregnancy and autoimmune disorders such as systemic lupus erythematosus.

TTP has a poor prognosis without therapy. In early reports approximately 90% of patients died. Patients can present with a fulminating course but often the diagnosis is difficult to make. Mild to severe neurological signs are present in about two-thirds of presentations and evidence of early renal dysfunction in about half of presentations. It is more common in females and has a much higher incidence in Afro-Caribbean people. The diagnosis is usually made on a combination of full blood count and blood film. Lactase dehydrogenase levels are often markedly elevated suggesting both haemolysis and ischaemia.

Major haemorrhage and massive transfusion

During the resuscitation of patients who have suffered a major haemorrhage, a number of factors can contribute to associated coagulopathy.

- Hypothermia is common as a result of the injury or trauma, exposure during operation or resuscitation of with cold intravenous fluids. Hypothermia exacerbates coagulopathy by affecting both the performance of platelets and coagulation enzymes. The effects of hypothermia on platelet function are much more severe than on other coagulation factors. The activity of the platelet glycoprotein Ib/IX is highly temperature dependent resulting in inadequate interaction with von Willebrand factor. By about 30 °C, 75% of platelet activity is lost. In contrast, the coagulation enzymes remain fairly resistant with a reduction of about 10% for every degree centigrade reduction.
- Metabolic acidosis is common due to increased lactate production and also hyperchloraemia if a copious amount of normal saline has been used in fluid resuscitation. Metabolic acidosis is the most consistent predictor of coagulopathy following major trauma. Hydrogen ion concentration itself appears to affect actions of a number of the coagulation factors and platelet function resulting in a severe coagulopathy as the pH approaches 7.
- Consumption of clotting products if injuries sustained are severe and the dilution of the patients' plasma and platelets due to crystalloid and colloid resuscitation. Major transfusion will

inevitably result in dilutional coagulopathy when one considers that normal transfusion ratios (1: 1: 1, blood, platelets and plasma) result in a platelet and factor count below normal.

Management of massive transfusion and the resulting coagulopathy requires laboratory assessment of the nature of the clotting abnormality. Under these circumstances functional assessments such thromboelastography (TEG) are very useful in directing the focus of replacement. Treating hypothermia is important as is warming of fluids and products given to the patient. Localized surgical factors are important. There is no point filling the bucket up if the holes are not patched! In addition to traditional methods, fibrin glue and other topical haemostatics are often used in certain circumstances. Antifibrinolytics such as aprotonin and tranexamic acid are often used, especially if there are signs of enhanced thrombolysis in a TEG graph. Finally factor VIIa has been shown to reduce bleeding in severe trauma and following major surgery and often has a dramatic effect when used.

Drug-induced thrombocytopenia

Heparin

Heparin-induced thrombocytopenia (HIT) usually occurs 5–10 days following exposure to heparin. It is a pro-thrombotic disorder and can lead to significant venous and arterial thrombosis. Presentation can vary in severity ranging from a mild reduction in platelet count without any overt thrombotic events to a severe form in which thrombosis and organ failure are prevalent. The pathophysiological mechanism involves the formation of antibodies to platelet factor 4 (PF4) proteins and heparin complex. Heparin binds to PF4 and induces a conformational change that renders the complex immunogenic. Many patients exposed to heparin will express antibodies to the PF4/heparin complex but only a small number will develop thrombocytopenia and an even smaller number of thrombotic problems. The longer the exposure is, the greater the prevalence of antibody production. For example cardiac surgical patients following bypass will have a high incidence of antibody production although the incidence of thrombocytopenia is much lower, in the order of 2%.

The correct diagnosis of HIT is difficult as thrombocytopenia can be seen in up to 50% of critically ill patients. Of the tests currently available the most specific is a platelet activation assay such as serotonin release assay. These tests are more specific than the measurement of antibody to the protein complex as these can be present without clinical disease. HIT usually resolves following the discontinuation of heparin over a few days. Management includes the prompt removal of all heparin containing medication and the substitution of a direct thrombin inhibitor to control clotting.

Other drugs

There are many drugs which can cause thrombocytopenia. Some examples are:

- Antimicrobials
  - cephalosporins
  - ciprofloxacin
  - clarithromycin
  - fluconazole
  - gentamicin
  - penicillins
  - rifampin
  - vancomycin
- NSAIDs
- Cardiac medications and diuretics
  - digoxin
  - amiodarone
  - captopril
  - frusemide
  - spirolactone
- Benzodiazepines
  - diazepam
- Anti-epileptic drugs
- H_2-antagonists
- Iodinated contrast agents
- Antihistamines
- Lidocaine
- Morphine.

Key points

- The incidence of thrombocytopenia in critically ill patients is high and it is associated with an increased risk of bleeding and mortality.

- DIC is characterized by widespread activation of the coagulation system and results in reduced blood flow and ischaemia in organs. Consumption of coagulation factors and platelets results in an increased tendency to bleed.
- Activated protein C has been shown to reduce mortality in sepsis especially in patients with DIC and multi-organ failure.
- Massive transfusion can lead to hypothermia, metabolic acidosis and dilutional coagulopathy. Blood bank should be alerted and clotting products should be available.
- HIT is a prothrombotic disorder that occurs following exposure to heparin. It can lead to significant venous and arterial thrombosis. All heparin-containing medication should be stopped and substituted with a direct thrombin inhibitor to control clotting.

Further reading

- Bernard GR, Vincent J-L, Laterre P-F *et al.* (2001) Recombinant Human Protein C Worldwide Evaluation in Severe Sepsis (PROWESS) Study Group: Efficacy and safety of recombinant human activated protein C for severe sepsis. *N. Engl. J. Med.* **344** (10): 699–709.
- Bombeli T, Spahn DR (2004) Updates in perioperative coagulation: physiology and management of thromboembolism and haemorrhage. *Br. J. Anaesth.* **93**(2): 275–87.
- Hoffman M (2003) A cell-based model of coagulation and the role of factor VIIa. *Blood Rev.* **17** (Suppl. 1): S1–5.
- Hoffman M, Monroe DM III (2001) A cell-based model of haemostasis. *Thromb. Haemost.* **85**(6): 958–65.
- Oppenheim-Eden A, Glantz L, Eidelman LA, Sprung CL (1999) Spontaneous intracerebral hemorrhage in critically ill patients: incidence over six years and associated factors. *Intens. Care Med.* **25** (1): 63–7.
- Warren BL, Eid A, Singer P *et al.* (2001) High-dose antithrombin III in severe sepsis: a randomized controlled trial. *J. Am. Med. Ass.* **286**: 1869–78

Acute coronary syndromes

Harjot Singh and Tony Whitehouse

Definition

The consensus document of European Society of Cardiology (ESC), American College of Cardiology (ACC), American Heart Association (AHA) and World Heart Federation's (WHF) task force defines myocardial infarction (MI) as evidence of myocardial necrosis in a clinical setting which is consistent with myocardial ischaemia.

Under this definition any one of the following criteria will meet the diagnosis of acute coronary syndrome:

- Detection of the rise and/or fall of cardiac biomarkers (preferably troponin) with at least one value above the 99th percentile of the upper reference limit (URL) with evidence of myocardial ischaemia with at least one of the following:
  - Symptoms of ischaemia (see below)
  - ECG changes indicative of new ischaemia (new ST changes) or new left bundle branch block (LBBB)
  - Development of pathological Q waves in the ECG
  - Imaging evidence of new loss of viable myocardium or new regional wall motion abnormality.

The consensus document also defines other clinical situations in which patients may suffer MI such as following cardiac surgery and percutaneous coronary intervention (PCI). A rise in cardiac biomarkers greater than three times above the 99th percentile of URL following surgery and five times above the 99th percentile for PCI is indicative of peri-procedure MI. This is also the basis of a clinical classification of the types of MI as shown in Table 24.1.

Clinically, patients with acute coronary syndrome (ACS) are classified into two groups based on the ST segment changes (ST segment elevation or non-ST segment elevation MI). This gives not only the initial working diagnosis but helps decide the treatment arm and provides prognostic information.

Pathophysiology

The commonest cause of MI is disruption of arterial supply to the myocardium through thrombus formation on an atherosclerotic plaque. The three mechanisms that cause this are plaque rupture, plaque erosion and thrombus on the calcified nodule. Uncommon causes of regional myocardial ischaemia are coronary artery spasm, emboli, arteritis, dissection and allograft vasculopathy.

Diagnosis

History and examination

Presentation can be variable; patients may present with central or retrosternal, crushing or tight, chest pain or discomfort which may radiate to left shoulder, left arm, the jaw or between the shoulder blades. It may be associated with dyspnoea, diaphoresis, nausea, vomiting, palpitation or syncope. In diabetic patients and the elderly, the presentation may not be classic and can be subtle. The spectrum of signs may vary widely from no significant clinical findings to haemodynamic compromise with signs of right and left ventricular failure or even cardiac arrest. Severe bradycardia occurs in up to 25% of patients with inferior MI and cardiogenic shock in up to 4% of patients with ST elevation MI. The clinical picture can evolve with time following presentation and, as a result, risk stratification should be a continuous process after hospitalization. The clinician should also consider other causes of chest pain that are non-ischaemic and non-cardiac.

Core Topics in Critical Care Medicine, eds. Fang Gao Smith and Joyce Yeung. Published by Cambridge University Press.

ECG

An ECG should be obtained on admission and the ST segments monitored. If the initial ECG is normal or mildly abnormal and there is high suspicion of myocardial ischaemia, serial ECGs should be obtained. In absence of LBBB and left ventricular hypertrophy (LVH), the criteria are as follows:

ST elevation	New ST elevation at the J point in two contiguous leads with the cut-off points: ≥0.2 mV in men or ≥0.15 mV in women in leads V2–V3 and/or ≥0.1 mV in other leads
ST depression and T wave changes	New horizontal or down-sloping ST depression ≥0.05 mV in two contiguous leads; and/or T inversion ≥0.1 mV in two contiguous leads with prominent R wave or R/S ratio >1 (see Figs. 24.1 and 24.2)

A patient with new LBBB or presumed new LBBB with history consistent with myocardial ischaemia should be treated as ST elevation ACS. In the presence of LBBB, the diagnosis of ACS is difficult even when marked ST–T abnormalities or ST elevation are present as the LBBB morphology distorts the ST segments. A previous ECG may be helpful and the following ECG criteria are of diagnostic value (see Figs. 24.3 and 24.4):

Table 24.1 Clinical classification of different types of myocardial infarction

Type 1	Spontaneous myocardial infarction related to ischaemia due to a primary coronary event such as plaque erosion and/or rupture, fissuring or dissection
Type 2	Myocardial infarction secondary to ischaemia due to either increased oxygen demand or decreased supply, e.g. coronary artery spasm, embolism, anaemia, arrhythmias, hypertension or hypotension
Type 3	Sudden unexpected cardiac death with symptoms suggestive of myocardial ischaemia and death occurring before blood samples could be obtained
Type 4a	Myocardial infarction associated with PCI
Type 4b	Myocardial infarction associated with stent thrombosis as documented by angiography or at autopsy
Type 5	Myocardial infarction associated with coronary artery bypass grafting

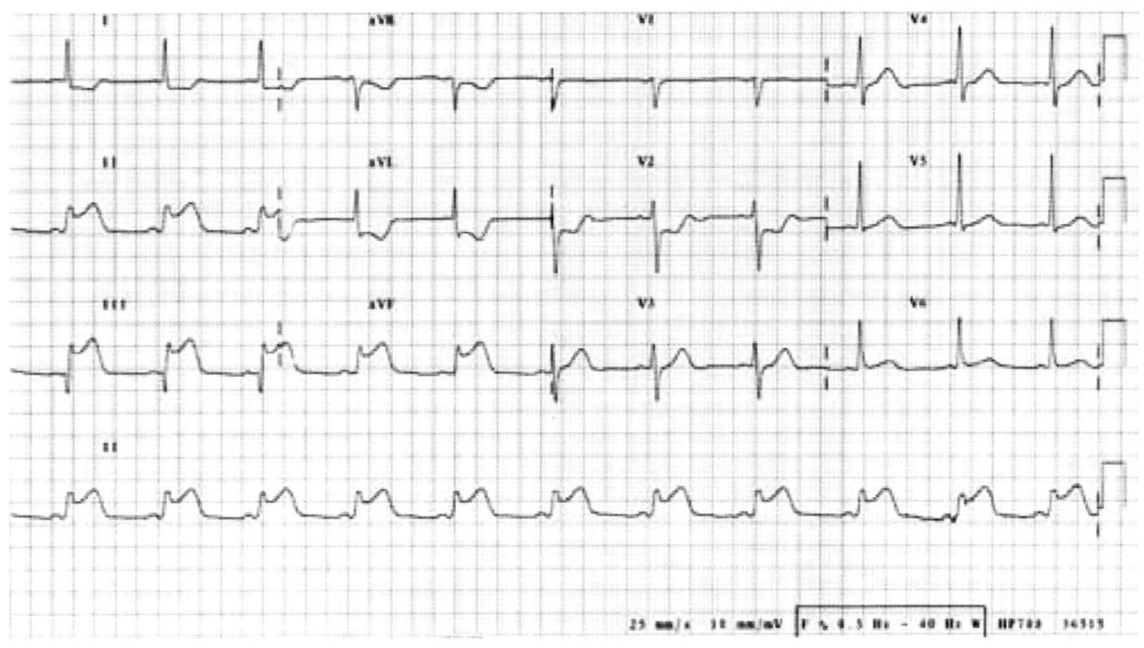

Fig. 24.1 ECG showing ST elevation in II, III, aVF and reciprocal changes in I, aVL and V2, indicating ST-elevated MI (inferior).

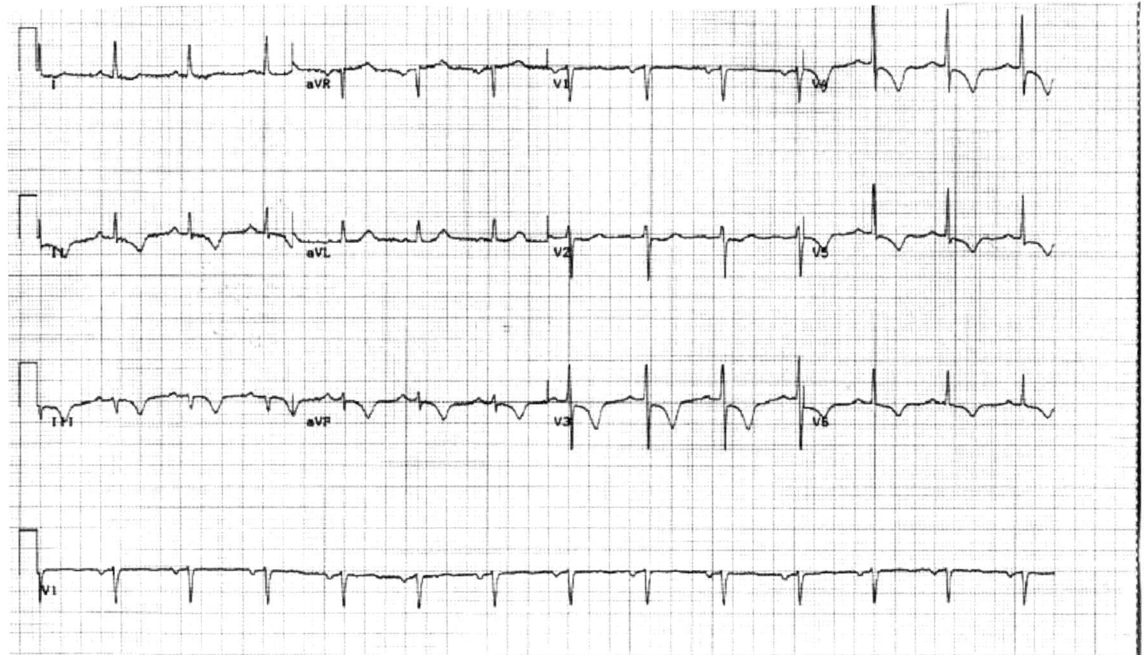

Fig. 24.2 ECG showing ST depression and T wave inversion in V3–6, II, III and aVF indicating myocardial ischaemia.

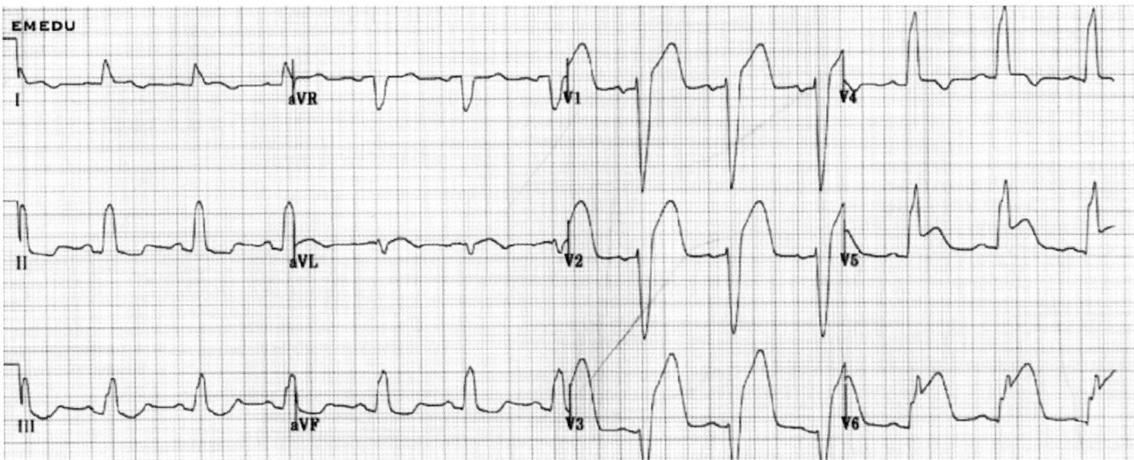

Fig. 24.3 ECG showing LBBB with ST elevation.

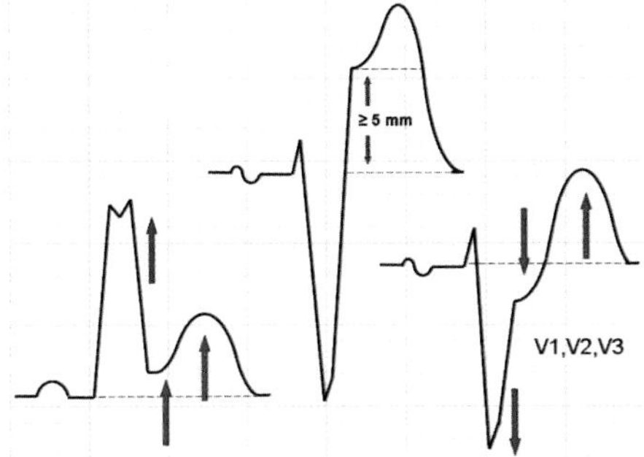

Fig. 24.4 Diagnostic criteria for ACS in LBBB.

ST elevation ≥ 0.1 mV with a positive QRS complex
ST depression ≥ 0.1 mV in leads V1–V3
ST elevation ≥ 0.5 mV in leads with a negative QRS complex

In patients with right bundle branch block (RBBB), ST–T abnormalities in leads V1–V3 are common. However, when ST elevation or Q waves are present, ACS should be considered (see Figs. 24.5 and 24.6):

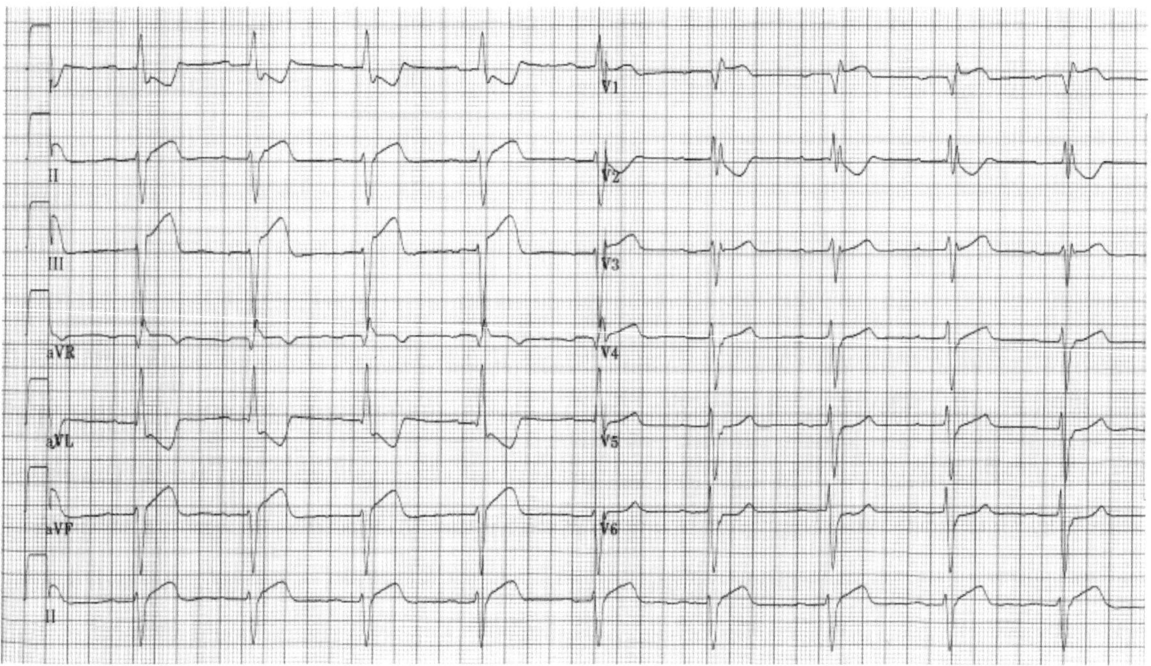

Fig. 24.5 ECG showing acute myocardial infarction in presence of RBBB. Note ST depression I, aVR and ST elevation II, III, aVL, aVR.

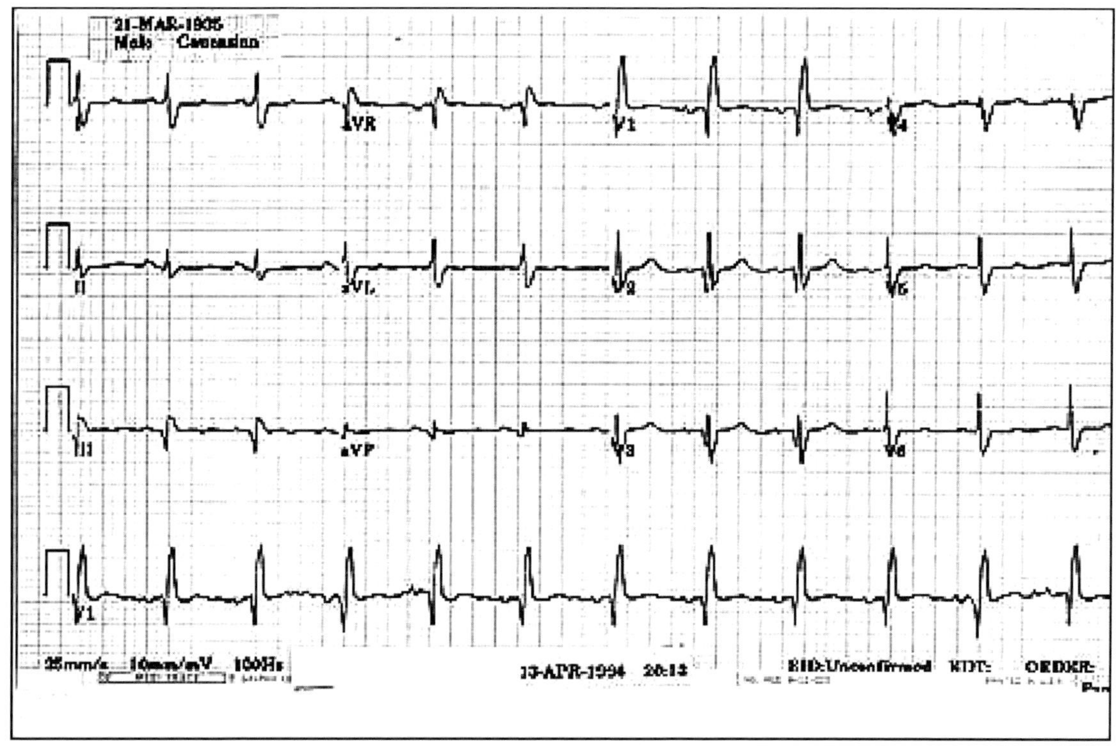

Fig. 24.6 ECG showing pathological Q waves seen in leads II, III, aVF (inferior MI) and in leads V1–V3 (anteroseptal MI). RBBB is characterized by the wide QRS (>0.12 s) and the anterior/rightwards orientation of terminal QRS forces.

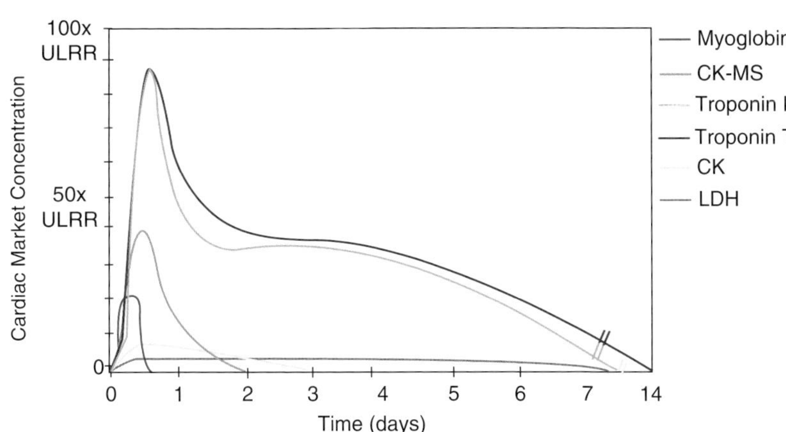

Fig. 24.7 Graph showing the serum levels of cardiac biomarkers post MI.

Development of any Q waves in leads V2−V3 ≥0.02 s
Development of a Q wave ≥0.03 s and ≥0.1 mV deep in leads I, II, aVL, aVF and V4−V6
in any two leads of a contiguous lead grouping

The ECG by itself is insufficient to diagnose ACS since ST deviation may be observed in other conditions such as pericarditis, paced rhythm, LVH, LBBB, Brugada syndrome (sudden unexpected cardiac death in apparently healthy individuals caused by severe rhythm disturbances) and some non-cardiac aetiologies such as subarachnoid haemorrhage. It is important to remember that the ECG may be normal in non-ST elevation ACS.

Patients with ST segment depression have a poorer prognosis when compared with patients with T wave abnormalities. The magnitude of ST depression and number of leads in which it occurs is also a prognostic marker.

Biomarkers

Troponin

An elevation in biomarkers indicates myocardial necrosis (Fig. 24.7). The preferred biomarker is cardiac **troponin** (I or T) which has a sensitivity of 100% 6 hours after the onset of MI. The specificity of troponin T is high except in acute skeletal muscle disease and chronic renal failure, where troponin I is more helpful as it is not influenced by these conditions. An increased value is defined as value exceeding the 99th percentile of URL. Troponins are raised for 7 to 10 days in the case of troponin I and up to 10 to 14 days in the case of troponin T, after the index event, making interpretation difficult in cases of re-infarction within this time frame.

Creatine kinase

Creatine kinase (CK) is found in all striated muscle and has three isoforms: CK-MM (found in skeletal muscle), CK-BB (found in brain) and CK-MB (found in myocardium). CK-MB is the best alternative when troponin is either unsuitable or not available. A blood sample should be taken at the time of first assessment and 6–9 hours later to demonstrate rise and/or fall. CK-MB remains elevated for only 3 to 4 days.

Re-elevations in CK-MB by more than 50%, can be used to diagnose re-infarctions as early as 18 hours after the index event. The role of troponin is controversial but a greater than 20% increase of the value over the immediate pre-infarct value may indicate re-infarction.

Other markers

Other markers of inflammation such as C-reactive protein, interleukin-6 and CD40 ligand provide prognostic information but are not routinely employed in assessment of patients with ACS. B type natriuretic peptide (BNP) is also an independent prognostic marker, and a low level of BNP and negative troponin may identify patients at low risk of having suffered MI.

Table 24.2 Risk stratification of patients with ST-elevation acute coronary syndrome

		Risk score	Odds of death at 30 days (95% CI)
History			
Age 65–74	2 points	0	0.1 (0.1–0.2)
Age >75	3 points	1	0.3 (0.2–0.3)
Examination			
SBP 100 mmHg	3 points	2	0.4 (0.3–0.5)
HR >100	2 points	3	0.7 (0.6–0.9)
Killip II–IV heart failure	2 points	4	1.2 (1.0–1.5)
Weight 67 kg		5	2.2 (1.9–2.6)
Presentation			
Anterior ST elevation	1 point	6	3.0 (2.5–3.6)
or LBBB	1 point	7	4.8 (3.8–6.1)
Time to treatment		8	5.8 (4.2–7.8)
>4 hours		8	8.8 (6.3–12)

CI, confidence interval; SBP, systolic blood pressure; HR, heart rate; LBBB, left bundle branch block.

Other laboratory tests

For optimal management, other laboratory tests (glucose, urea and electrolytes, lipid profile and coagulation) are requested.

Imaging

Chest radiography should form part of the initial routine diagnostic investigation. More sophisticated imaging techniques such as echocardiography, radionuclide imaging, magnetic resonance imaging and computed tomography may be applied depending upon the clinical situation. Echocardiography is the imaging technique of choice for detecting the complications of MI (see below). A normal echocardiogram or resting ECG gated scintigram (imaging by radionuclide) has 95–98% predictive value for excluding MI in a patient with a probable history but non-diagnostic ECG findings.

Risk stratification

Patients can be risk stratified in ST-elevation ACS to predict 30-day mortality according to Table 24.2. In non-ST-elevation ACS prognosis may guided according to risk strata shown in Table 24.3.

Management

ST-elevation ACS

PCI or fibrinolysis

Urgent reperfusion is the therapeutic goal to minimize myocardial loss. The choice is between fibrinolysis and primary PCI. In a recent meta-analysis of 23 trials comparing PCI with fibrinolysis, PCI was found to be superior in reducing short-term mortality and rates of re-infarction and stroke. However, there is some evidence to suggest that very early administration (within 3 hours of symptom onset) of fibrinolysis offers similar survival rate. In late presentation ST-elevation ACS the choice is less clear, although where available, PCI is probably advantageous (Fig. 24.8).

Among the various fibrinolytic agents, fibrin-specific agents such as Tenecteplase or Alteplase are the agents of choice especially in situations where (1) the patient has an anterior ST elevation ACS who presents within 12 hours of onset of symptoms, (2) where saphenous vein graft is considered to be the conduit of blood supply to the infarcted area and (3) in patients who previously had streptokinase. In all other situations, streptokinase can be used although full regional myocardial reperfusion at 90 min is achieved in fewer patients.

Heparin therapy

Patients treated with thrombolytic therapy after acute MI are at risk of early recurrence of ischaemia. Administration of heparin and aspirin is indicated following thrombolysis. Low-molecular-weight heparin (LMWH) for 48 hours is preferred although if unfractionated heparin is used, activated partial thromboplastin time is monitored and heparin infusion is titrated. LMWH dose interval is increased to 24 hours in presence of renal dysfunction.

Antiplatelet therapy

Aspirin (loading and maintenance) is used in all patients if not contraindicated. Clopidogrel should be considered in all ST-elevation ACS. Patients should receive a loading dose if less than 75 years old. For patients undergoing PCI, clopidogrel (loading dose) can be given at presentation or after defining the coronary anatomy and maintained for up to 12 months, depending upon the type of stent used.

Table 24.3 Risk stratification of patients with non-ST-elevation acute coronary syndrome

Feature	High risk – at least 1 of the following	Intermediate risk – No high risk features but 1 of the following	Low risk – no high or intermediate risk features but may have any of the following
History	Accelerating tempo of ischaemic symptoms in preceding 48 hours	Prior MI, peripheral or cerebrovascular disease, or CABG, prior aspirin use	
Character of pain	Ongoing prolonged (>20 min) rest pain	Prolonged rest pain, now resolved, or ongoing, short duration rest pain, which resolves spontaneously or with NTG, with moderate or high likelihood of CAD	New-onset or progressive CCS Class III/IV angina in the past 2 weeks without prolonged pain but with moderate or high likelihood of CAD
Clinical findings	Pulmonary oedema likely be due to ischaemia; new or worsening mitral regurgitation murmur, S3 or new/worsening crackles, hypotension, bradycardia, tachycardia, diabetes, PCI within 6 months and age >75 years	Age >70 years	
ECG	Angina at rest with transient ST changes >0.05 mV, new or presumed new bundle branch block, sustained ventricular tachycardia	T wave inversions >0.2 mV, pathological Q waves	Normal or unchanged ECG during an episode of chest discomfort
Cardiac markers	Elevated	Normal	Normal

CABG, coronary artery bypass grafting; CAD, coronary artery disease; CCS, Canadian Cardiological Society classification of angina; MI, myocardial infarction; NTG, nitroglycerine; PCI, percutaneous coronary intervention.

Rescue PCI

Ongoing ischaemia (pain or lack of resolution of ST changes by 50%) or haemodynamic instability after fibrinolytic therapy is indication for rescue PCI.

Surgical revascularization

The patients who are unsuitable for pharmacological or PCI reperfusion, failed primary or rescue PCI and patients who fulfil the criteria of the SHOCK (Should We Emergently Revascularize Occluded Coronaries for Cardiogenic Shock) trial should be put forward for urgent CABG. The surgery is also indicated in case of complications like severe mitral regurgitation, septum or free wall rupture. All other cases, CABG is delayed for several days until myocardial stunning is resolved.

Non-ST-elevation ACS

The treatment strategy depends upon the risk group.

Low-risk patients

Patients are monitored and if stable with no elevation in markers, they are investigated for inducible ischaemia.

Intermediate and high-risk patients

Aggressive antithrombotic therapy followed by early angiography and revascularization may be indicated. In high-risk patients, a glycoprotein IIb/IIIa inhibitor (such as abciximab (ReoPro®)) should be included. Clopidogrel should be avoided in patients with high likelihood of urgent CABG surgery.

Adjunctive therapy

Oxygen and pain relief are given to all the patients along with an antiemetic agent.

- Nitroglycerin – Sublingual nitroglycerin for pain relief and intravenous for control of hypertension and management of pulmonary oedema may be used.
- Beta-blockers – In ST elevation ACS, beta-blockers have been shown to reduce the rate of re-infarction and arrhythmias. However, utmost care with titration is required and these are avoided if there is high risk (compromised haemodynamics or Killip class III or IV failure). The role of beta-blockers in non-ST elevation ACS is less clear, but is usually

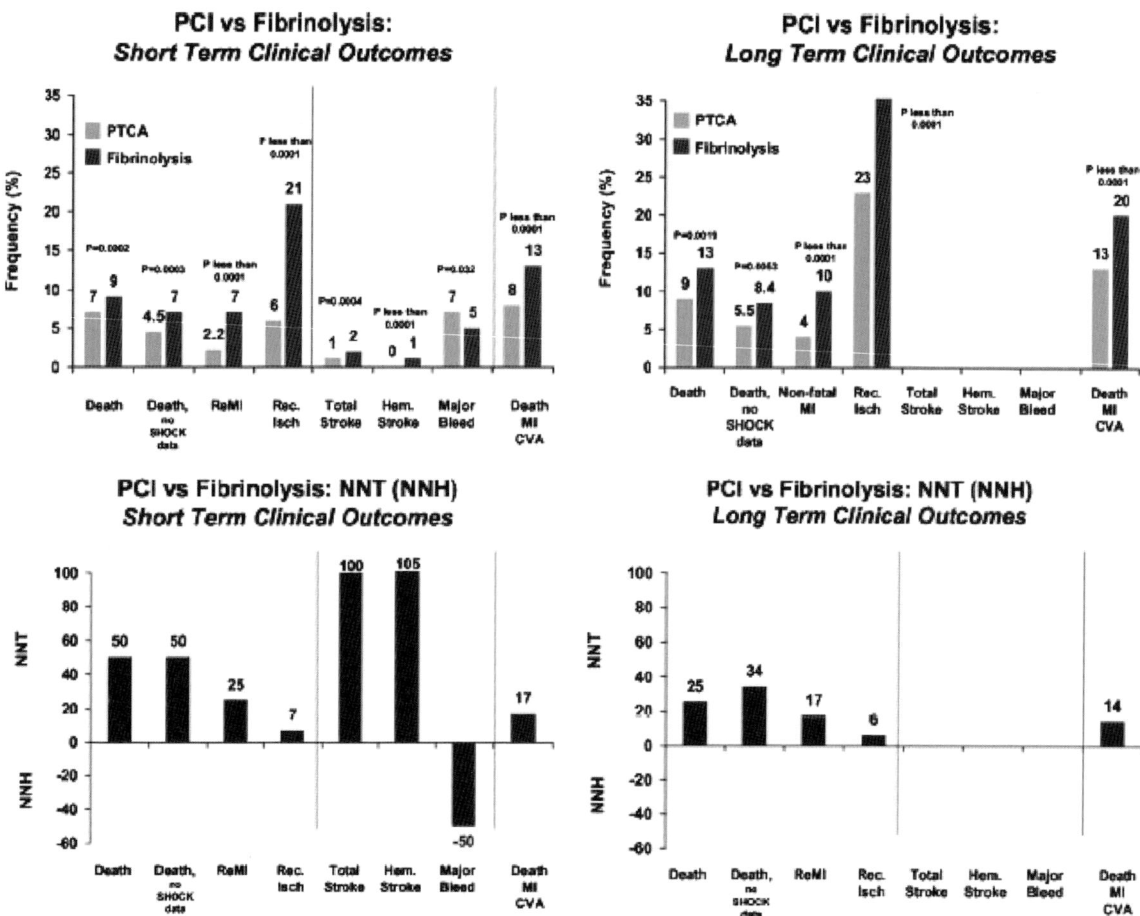

Fig. 24.8 Keeley *et al.* carried out a quantitative review of 23 randomized controlled trials in 2003 and found that primary PTCA was better than thrombolytic therapy at reducing overall short-term death (7% ($n = 270$) vs. 9% ($n = 360$); P = 0.0002), non-fatal re-infarction (3% ($n = 80$) vs. 7% ($n = 222$); $P > 0.0001$), stroke (1% ($n = 30$) vs. 2% ($n = 64$); $P = 0.0004$). The results seen with primary PTCA remained better than those seen with thrombolytic therapy during long-term follow-up, and were independent of both the type of thrombolytic agent used, and whether or not the patient was transferred for primary PTCA. They concluded that primary PTCA is more effective than thrombolytic therapy for the treatment of ST-elevated MI. From *Lancet* (2003) **361**: 13–20; (reproduced with permission).

recommended. In the post-infarct period, beta-blockers reduce mortality.

- Angiotensin-converting enzyme inhibitors (ACEIs) are administered for their indirect anti-ischaemic benefit by reducing ventricular workload. They may be used in high risk patients, diabetics, patients with anterior infarct, tachycardia or overt LV failure. As with beta-blockers, there is a risk of producing hypotension.
- Statin therapy – Intense statin therapy should be commenced as soon as practical and titrated towards optimal lipid levels.
- Glucose control – Optimal short- and long-term glucose control reduces infarct size.
- Respiratory support – in addition to supplemental oxygen, non-invasive respiratory support such as continuous positive airway pressure (CPAP) is of benefit in patients with pulmonary oedema where it improves oxygenation and reduces left ventricular afterload.
- Patients should be advised about cessation of smoking during their rehabilitation.

Complications

Acute common complications of ACS are acute heart failure, arrhythmias including heart block and cardiac arrest. Mechanical complications such as mitral regurgitation, ventricular septal defect and free wall rupture may also occur. Long-term complications are chronic heart failure due to ischaemic cardiomyopathy and ventricular remodelling, formation of left ventricular aneurysm and pseudo-aneurysms.

Key points

- The diagnosis of ACS requires that there is elevated cardiac biomarker with either symptoms of ischaemia, ECG showing new ischaemic changes or imaging demonstrating loss of myocardium.
- The commonest cause of MI is disruption of arterial supply to the myocardium through thrombus formation on an atherosclerotic plaque caused by plaque rupture, plaque erosion and thrombus on the calcified nodule.
- In ST-elevated ACS, there is evidence to suggest that PCI was superior in reducing short-term mortality and rates of re-infarction and stroke than fibrinolysis.

Further reading

- Anderson JL, Adams CD, Antman EM *et al.* (2007) ACC/AHA 2007 guidelines for the management of patients with unstable angina/non ST-elevation myocardial infarction. *J. Am. Coll. Cardiol.* **50**: 1–157.
- Antman EM, Anbe DT, Armstrong PW *et al.* (2004) ACC/AHA guidelines for the management of patients with ST-elevation myocardial infarction. *J. Am. Coll. Cardiol.* **44**(3): E1–E211.
- Keeley EC, Boura JA, Grines CL (2003) Primary angioplasty versus intravenous thrombolytic therapy for acute myocardial infarction: a quantitative review of 23 randomised trials. *Lancet* **361**: 13–20.
- Morrow DA, Antman EM, Charlesworth A *et al.* (2000) TIMI risk score for ST-elevation myocardial infarction: a convenient, bedside, clinical score for risk assessment at presentation: an intravenous nPA for treatment of infarcting myocardium early II trail substudy. *Circulation* **102**: 2031–7.
- Raffel CO, White H (2007) Acute coronary syndromes. In *Cardiothoracic Critical Care*, eds. Sidebotham D, McKee A, Gillham M, Levy J H. Philadelphia, PA: Elsevier, pp. 257–77.
- Thygesan K, Alpert JS, White HD (2007) Joint ESC/ ACCF/AHA/WHF Task Force for Redefinition of Myocardial Infarction: Universal definition of myocardial infarction. *Eur. Heart J.* **28**: 2525–38.

Cardiac arrhythmias

Khai Ping Ng and George Pulikal

Introduction

Cardiac arrhythmia encompasses an array of cardiac electrical rhythm derangements. It is frequently encountered by the healthcare professionals in the intensive care setting, among which the two most common arrhythmias are atrial fibrillation and ventricular tachyarrhythmia. Cardiac arrhythmias raise concerns not only owing to their possible detrimental effect on patients' already vulnerable haemodynamic systems, but also it is suggested to be associated with longer ITU stay and higher mortality.

Arrhythmogenic mechanisms

Normal sinus rhythm initiates as the sinus node (SN) generates an electrical impulse, which relays along internodal pathway before arriving at the atrioventricular node (AV node). The electrical impulse is delayed at the AV node before transmission is continued along the atrioventricular bundle, left and right bundle branch, the Purkinje fibres and eventually concludes in contraction of the myocytes in the ventricles (Fig. 25.1).

Reduction or failure of the automaticity of the SN (i.e. sick sinus syndrome) or interruption of the propagation of electrical impulses along the conduction pathway (i.e. bundle branch block) gives rise to bradyarrhythmia. On the other hand, enhanced automaticity, re-entry and triggered activity are the three main mechanisms which lead to tachyarrhythmia. Often, more than one mechanism results in the occurrence and ongoing event of the cardiac arrhythmias.

Automaticity

Automaticity is the ability to generate spontaneous electrical activity. All conduction tissues exhibit various degree of automaticity, notably the SN which possesses the greatest automaticity. The automaticity may be suppressed or enhanced by numerous cardiac or non-cardiac influences, i.e. hypoxia, metabolic disturbance, sympathetic and parasympathetic nervous system, drugs as well as myocardial infarction and cardiomyopathies.

Re-entry

Re-entry is responsible for many types of tachyarrhythmia and it occurs when two or more conduction pathways link up to allow indefinite propagation of electrical impulses within in a closed loop of circuit. Presence of fibrous scar tissue due to previous myocardial infarction or post-surgical intervention increases likelihood of re-entry as it usually occurs around the conduction barrier. It may also occur around the orifice of venous drainage into the atrium, atrial septum and valvular regions. Other risk factors include dilated cardiomyopathy which encourages the formation of a macro-re-entrant circuit.

Atrial flutter and atrial fibrillation are the results of intra-atrial macro-re-entrant and micro-re-entrant circuits respectively. Similarly, AV nodal re-entrant tachycardia and AV re-entrant tachycardia are the consequence of additional conduction pathways connecting between the right atrium and AV node or connecting between the atrium and ventricle respectively.

Triggered activity

Membrane potential displays minute degrees of fluctuation of electrical amplitude following depolarization. In abnormal circumstances, especially under the influence of anti-arrhythmic drugs, this fluctuation may gather significant amplitude beyond threshold potential to trigger an action potential.

Core Topics in Critical Care Medicine, eds. Fang Gao Smith and Joyce Yeung. Published by Cambridge University Press.

Table 25.1 List of arrhythmogenic factors

Oxygenation	Hypoxia
Temperature	Hypothermia
Electrolyte imbalances	Hyper/hypokalaemia, hypomagnesaemia, hypocalcaemia, acidosis
Drugs	Anti-arrhythmic agents, antihistamines, tricyclic antidepressants, gastrointestinal motility agents, antimalarials, antibiotics such as erythromycin
Endocrine disturbances	Hypo/hyperthyroidism, phaeochromocytoma
Autonomic disturbances	Sympathetic or parasympathetic overdrive
Genetic disorders	Long QT syndrome (e.g. Romana Ward syndrome, Jervell and Lange Nielsen syndrome), Brugada syndrome, short QT syndrome, catecholaminergic polymorphic VT
Cardiac abnormalities	Ischaemic heart disease, cardiomyopathies, valvular heart disease

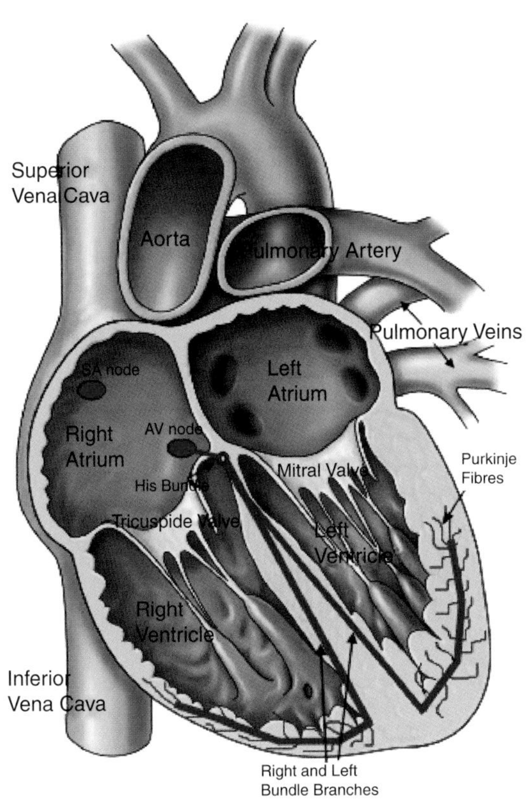

Fig. 25.1 Electrical conduction in normal sinus rhythm.

Triggered activity leads to ectopic beats, which may cause perpetual arrhythmia if sustained by further re-entry circuit. Adrenergic state and medication such as digitalis are common causes of triggered activity.

Arrhythmogenic factors

Overall, electrolytes and acid imbalances, hypoxia, numerous medications, pre-existing cardiac structural abnormalities or genetic disorders which interfere with automaticity, create re-entry circuit, alter the duration of QT interval or increase the likelihood of triggered activity may all contribute to cardiac arrhythmia (Table 25.1).

Classification of arrhythmias and anti-arrhythmia drugs

Classification of arrhythmias

Cardiac arrhythmias can be broadly classified based on the heart rate as bradyarrhythmia (<60 bpm) and tachyarrhythmia (>100 bpm). Physiological bradycardia can often be found in athletes whilst pathological bradycardia signifies sinus node or conduction pathway abnormalities, which may or may not be associated with drugs, autonomic or endocrine dysfunction (Fig. 25.2).

Bradyarrhythmias

ECG appearance of different bradyarrhythmias:

- Sick sinus syndrome – HR<60 bpm, PR interval 0.12–0.2 s
- 1st degree AV block – P wave precedes each QRS complex, PR interval >0.2 s (Fig. 25.3)
- Mobitz type I AV block – cycles of increasing PR interval with each subsequent QRS complex;

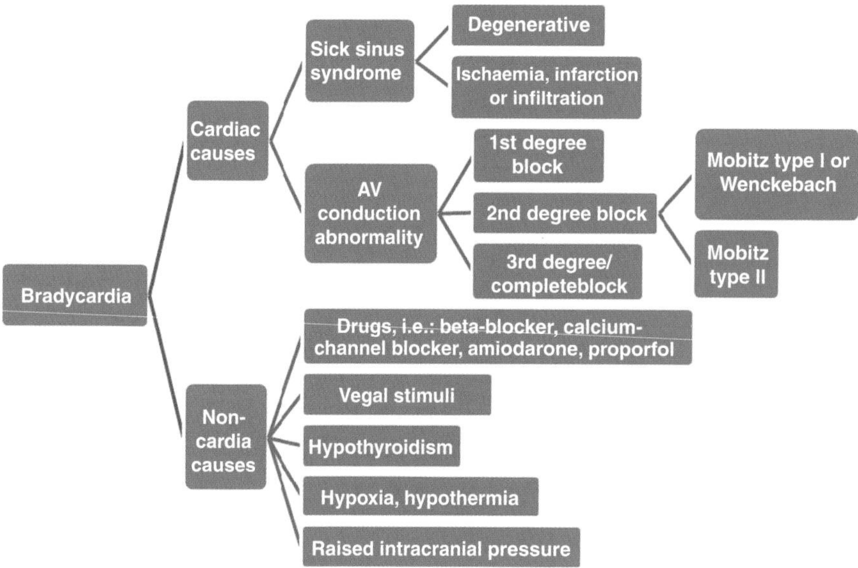

Fig. 25.2 Causes of bradyarrhythmias.

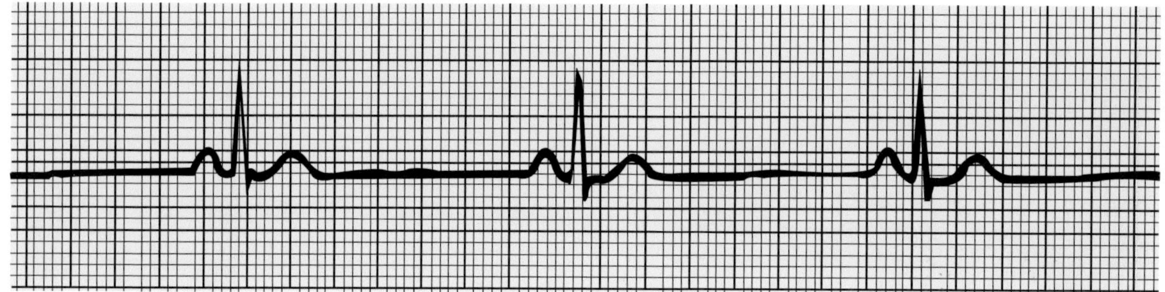

Fig. 25.3 Sinus bradycardia.

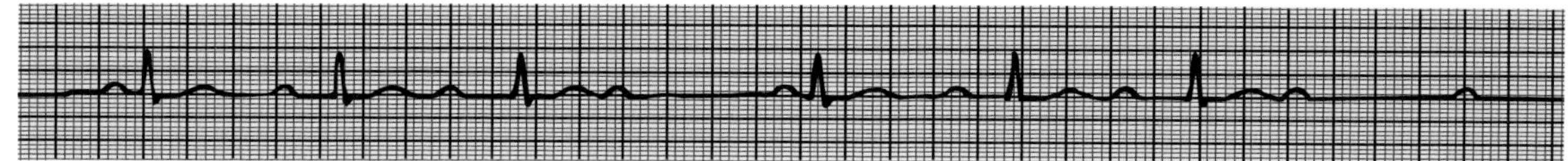

Fig. 25.4 Mobitz type I AV block.

P wave eventually will fail to be followed by a QRS complex ('dropped beats') before a normal PR interval begins the whole cycle again (Fig. 25.4)

- Mobitz type II AV block – QRS complexes preceded by 2 or 3 P waves (2 : 1 or 3 : 1 block) (Fig. 25.5)
- 3rd degree AV block – complete dissociation of P wave and QRS complexes (Fig. 25.6)

Tachyarrhythmias

Anatomically, tachyarrhythmia can broadly be divided into supraventricular (includes atrial or junctional tachyarrhythmia) or ventricular tachycardia. Other methods of classification include narrow complex arrhythmia (QRS ≤0.12 s) (Fig. 25.7) and broad complex arrhythmia (QRS >0.12 s) (Fig. 25.8) based on ECG morphology. All supraventricular tachycardias

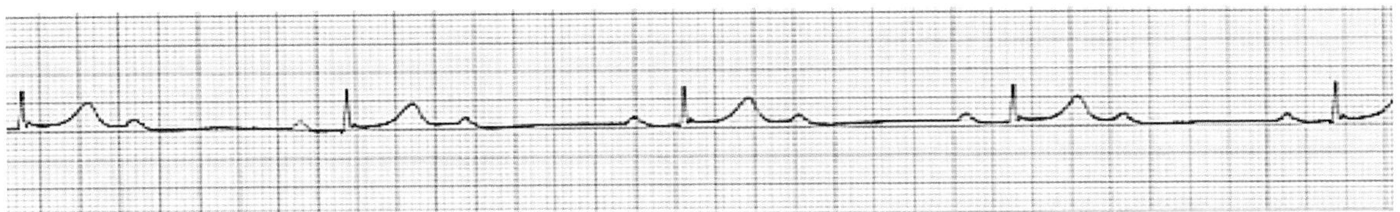

Fig. 25.5 Mobitz type II AV block.

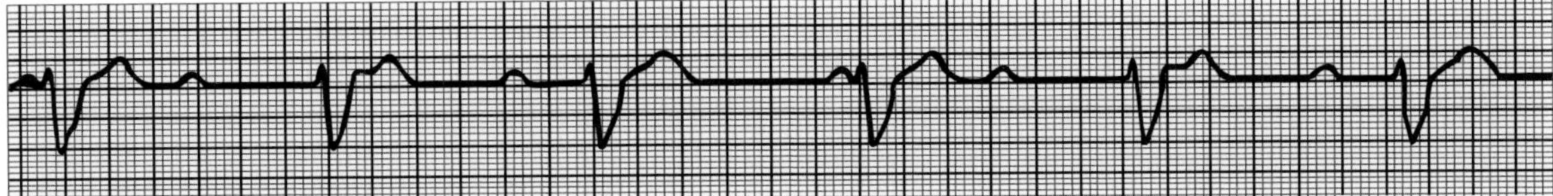

Fig. 25.6 3rd degree AV block.

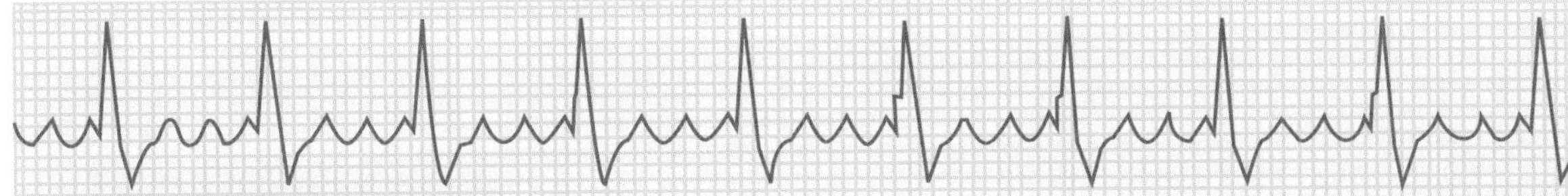

Fig. 25.7 Narrow-complex arrhythmia (atrial flutter).

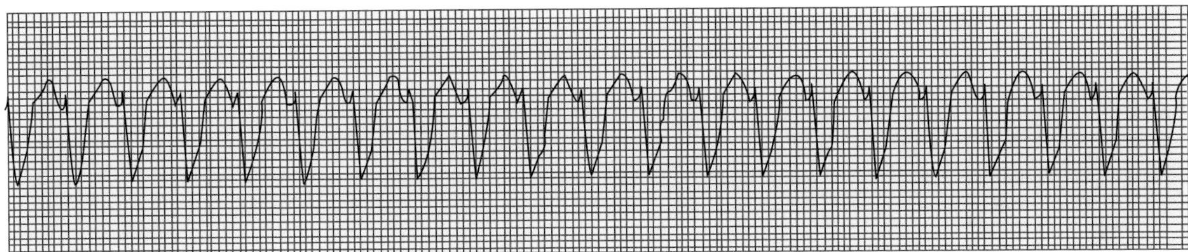

Fig. 25.8 Broad-complex arrhythmia (ventricular tachycardia).

(SVT) are narrow complex tachycardias except for SVT which occurs concurrently with aberrant pathway or AV block, which will be of the appearance of broad complex tachycardia.

SVT encompasses atrial tachycardia, atrial flutter, atrial fibrillation, AV nodal re-entrant tachycardia (AVNRT) and AV re-entrant tachycardia (AVRT). Atrial tachycardia is associated with enhanced automaticity and is often related to digoxin toxicity. Atrial flutter has a sawtooth baseline appearance on ECG with the regular QRS rate of 300 bpm (1 : 1 conduction), 150 bpm (2 : 1 block) or even 100 bpm (3 : 1 block, especially after vagal manoeuvre or adenosine). Atrial fibrillation is associated with micro-re-entry which produces chaotic, ineffective atrial depolarization (atrial fibrillation wave) at the rate of 300–500 bpm and results in irregularly irregular heart rate. Both AVNRT and AVRT are due to accessory conduction pathways connecting either between atrium and AV node in AVNRT or between atrium and ventricles in AVRT. They are usually paroxysmal in nature with a narrow complex tachycardia appearance on ECG in most cases and P waves may not be visible. A classic example of AVNRT is Wolff–Parkinson–White syndrome (WPW) where there is a presence of the bundle of Kent between atrium and ventricle. This results in slurred upstroke of the R wave (delta wave) on the ECG. This accessory pathway may give rise to orthodromic SVT (narrow complex) if impulses are conducted antegradely through the AV node and retrogradely via the accessory pathway or antidromic SVT (broad complex) if conduction occurs in the opposite direction (Fig. 25.9).

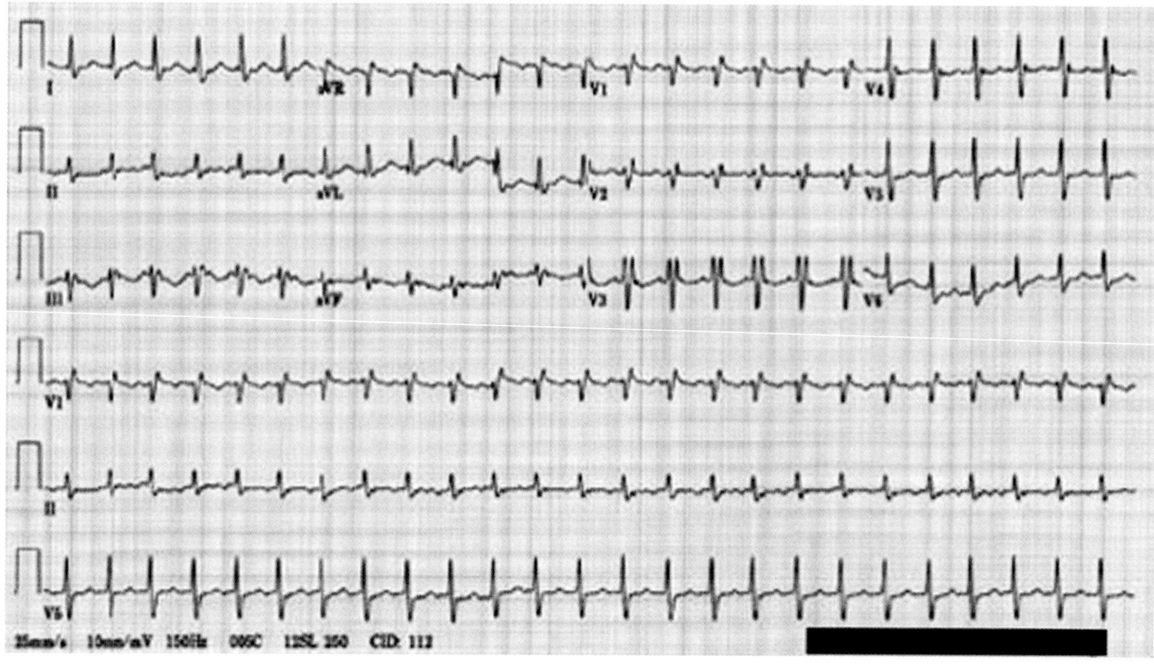

Fig. 25.9 AV nodal re-entrant tachycardia (AVNRT).

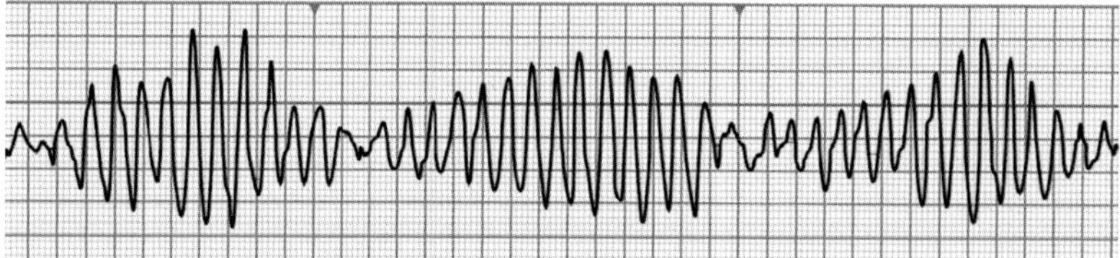

Fig. 25.10 Torsade de pointes.

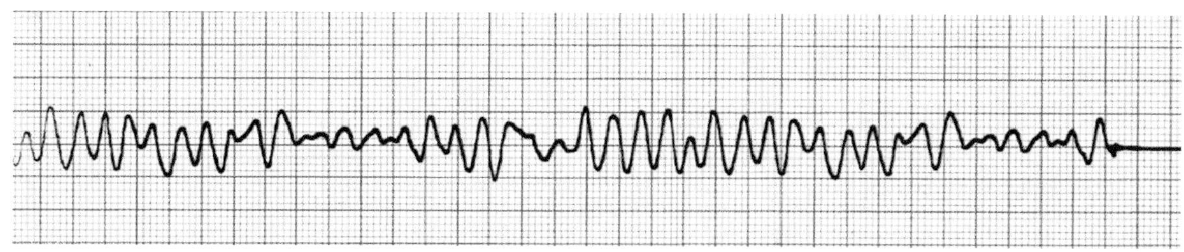

Fig. 25.11 Ventricular fibrillation.

Broad complex tachycardia includes SVT with aberrant pathway or bundle branch block (BBB), ventricular tachycardia (VT), torsade de pointes and ventricular fibrillation (VF). VT can appear rather similar to SVT with aberrant pathway or BBB on the ECG. AV dissociation, concordance of QRS complexes on chest leads (all QRS deflections are either positive or negative on all chest leads), extreme axis deviation, presence of fusion or capture beat and wider QRS complexes of >0.14 s and failure to response to vagal manoeuvre or adenosine support the diagnosis of VT. Torsade de pointes is a variant of VT which is related to prolonged QT. It is characterized by the varying of the amplitude of QRS complexes around the isoelectric baseline (Fig. 25.10). VT ECG shows a chaotic irregular fibrillatory baseline and absence of QRS complex. All VFs result in cardiac arrest as no effective cardiac output can be maintained (Fig. 25.11).

Table 25.2 Anti-arrhythmic agents – classification, mechanism of action, clinical use and examples

Class	Mechanism of action	Clinical use	Examples
I	Membrane stabilizer		
Ia	Block voltage-sensitive Na^+ channels (moderate dissociation)	SV and V Relatively obsolete due to its side effect	Quinidine Procainamide Disopyramide
Ib	Block voltage-sensitive Na^+ channels (fast dissociation)	SV and V	Lidocaine
Ic	Block voltage-sensitive Na^+ channels (slow dissociation)	SV and V, i.e. paroxysmal atrial fibrillation (AF); flecainide should be avoided in LV dysfunction and coronary artery disease	Flecainide
II	Block beta-adrenoceptor	SV and V, i.e. paroxysmal AF, post-myocardial infarction	Propanolol Esmolol Metoprolol
III	Affect K^+ efflux	SV and V, i.e. Amiodarone is a common treatment for various SVT and VT. It may also be used in Wolff–Parkinson–White syndrome (WPW). However, its potential effect on thyroid and liver function, formation of corneal deposits, pulmonary fibrosis and neuropathy need to be considered and monitored especially in long-term use.	Amiodarone Sotalol
IV	Block Ca^{2+} channel	SV, i.e. effective for SVT and also used to prevent recurrent of paroxysmal SVT; concomitant use of Class II and Class IV may results in severe AV block/bradycardia and should be avoided	Verapamil Diltiazem
V	Unclear or other action	SV; adenosine (intravenously given) has very short half-life of <10 s – it is widely used in acute setting to terminate SVT which failed to responds to vagal manoeuvre. It can provoke severe bronchospasm in patient with asthma Digoxin is commonly used in AF in non-acute setting; it is contraindicated in WPW as it can results in VT/VF and its therapeutic range is narrow especially in hypokalaemia	Adenosine Digoxin

SV, supraventricular arrhythmia; V, ventricular arrhythmia.

Anti-arrhythmia drugs

Based on their primary electrophysiological mechanism on the action potential, Vaughan-Williams' four classifications of anti-arrhythmia agents have been widely used for the past four decades. Nonetheless, some of the agents have multiple electrophysiological effects on the action potential, such as Class IA agents. In addition, Class V was later added in to take into account other commonly used anti-arrhythmic agents, whose mechanisms of action are either unclear or do not belong to the four original classes (Table 25.2).

Essentially, all anti-arrhythmic agents are found to have various degrees of pro-arrhythmic effect. For instance, Class 1A and III agents, which prolong the action potential, increase the risk of torsades de pointes (Fig. 25.12).

Management of common arrhythmias in ICU

Assessment

Acute management of arrhythmias depends on the haemodynamic status of the patient and the type of arrhythmia. Patients who exhibit adverse features will require urgent treatment to resolve the arrhythmia. These features include (Fig. 25.13):

- hypotensive (systolic blood pressure of <90 mmHg)
- extreme heart rate (<40 or >150 bpm)
- ventricular arrhythmias
- heart failure
- chest pain
- reduced consciousness

In addition to supporting the patient's airway, breathing and circulation, it is also paramount to rectify any associated arrhythmogenic factors, such as electrolyte imbalances, hypovolaemia, hypoxia, sepsis, myocardial infarction, as most arrhythmias are triggered and sustained by their underlying causes.

Bradyarrhythmia

Patients who show any of the above adverse signs or are at risk of asystole (i.e. recent asystole, Mobitz type II block, complete heart block with broad QRS complex or ventricular pause >3 s) require active treatment with atropine IV 500 µg to be given up to 3 mg. If bradycardia persists, adrenaline 2–10 µg/min or transcutaneous pacing can be employed whilst awaiting transvenous pacing to be arranged. A permanent pacemaker may be required if bradycardia persists in the long term.

Tachyarrhythmias with adverse signs

All patients with pulseless VF and VT should be managed according to cardiac arrest guidelines.

However, for patients with other tachyarrhythmias with heart rate of above 150 bpm and exhibiting any adverse sign, synchronized DC cardioversion should be given up to three attempts under sedation. This should then be followed by amiodarone infusion (300 mg over 20 min) and rectification of any electrolyte imbalances to reduce the recurrence of the tachyarrhythmia. The initial success rate for electrical cardioversion in patients with AF is approximately 75–93%. This depends strongly on the duration of AF, left atrial size and coexisting structural heart disease. Repeat synchronized cardioversion may be required followed by further amiodarone infusion (900 mg over 24 hours) if tachyarrhythmia persists.

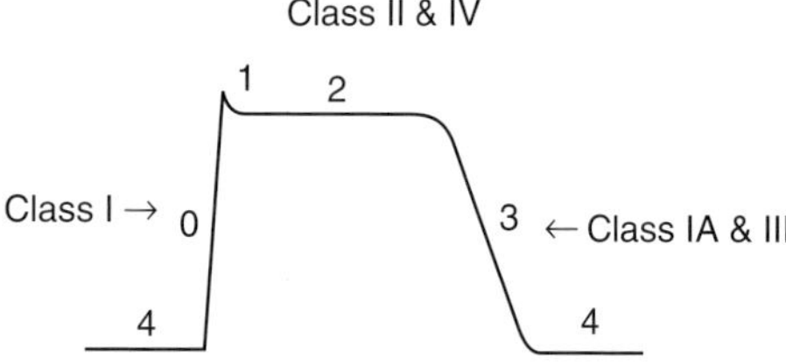

Fig. 25.12 Phase 4: resting membrane potential. Phase 0: rapid depolarization (rapid influx of Na^+). Phase 1: inactivation of fast sodium ion channel. Phase 2: plateau (influx of Ca^{2+} and efflux of K^+). Phase 3: repolarization (closure of Ca^{2+} channel).

Tachyarrhythmias without adverse signs

Narrow complex and broad complex tachyarrhythmias without adverse signs are managed differently in the acute setting.

Most sinus tachycardias are related to underlying causes and will resolve once the cause is rectified. Other narrow complex tachycardias include irregular rhythm of AF and regular rhythm of atrial flutter or junctional tachycardias (AVNRT and AVRT). They can be difficult to differentiate on the ECG especially with excessive tachycardias. Vagal manoeuvres (i.e. Valsava manoeuvre or carotid sinus massage after excluding any carotid bruits) or intravenous adenosine (6 mg, 12 mg, 12 mg) which increase the AV nodal block often terminate junctional arrhythmias and slow down the heart rate of atrial flutter to reveal its flutter wave. Rate control agents such as beta-blockers are used in the further management of atrial flutter. Atrial fibrillation (AF) does not respond to AV nodal block manoeuvre. In acute onset stable AF, IV amiodarone or beta-blockers are used. One randomized study supported the use of magnesium sulphate infusion but further evidence to support its routine use will be required. Persistent rate-controlled atrial fibrillation will require anticoagulation to prevent thromboembolic events in the long term.

Broad complex tachycardias are due to a number of underlying rhythms. In haemodynamically stable patients, ventricular tachycardia and pre-excited AF can be treated with IV amiodarone. Magnesium infusion (2 g over 10 min) is used in torsade de pointes. However, if the patient has a previously established

Systolic blood pressure < 90 mmHg	Reduced consciousness
Heart rate < 40 bpm or >150 bpm	Recent asystole
Ventricular arrhythmia	Mobitz type II block
Heart failure	Complete heart block
Chest pain	Ventricular pause > 3 s

Fig. 25.13 Adverse features.

bundle branch block, a new onset AF or junctional tachyarrhythmia may present as broad complex tachyarrhythmia. If adverse signs are absent, they can be treated as per the narrow complex tachyarrhythmia algorithm. In the long term, implantable cardiovertor-defibrillator (ICD) insertion is beneficial for patients who have structurally abnormal hearts with ventricular arrhythmias as it has been shown to be associated with lower mortality rates compared to amiodarone in randomized studies.

Key points

- Atrial fibrillation and ventricular tachyarrhythmia are the two most common arrhythmias in the intensive care setting.
- Reduction or failure of the automaticity of the SN or interruption of the propagation of electrical impulses along the conduction pathway gives rise to bradyarrhythmias.
- Bradyarrhythmias are classified into sick sinus syndrome, 1st degree AV block, Mobitz type I/II AV block and 3rd degree AV block.
- Enhanced automaticity, re-entry and triggered activity are the three main mechanisms leading to tachyarrhythmias.
- Tachyarrhythmias are classified into supraventricular and ventricular tachyarrhythmias.
- All anti-arrhythmic agents have pro-arrhythmic side effects.
- Management of arrhythmias depends on the type of arrhythmia and the presence or absence of adverse features.
- Associated arrhythmogenic factors should be identified and rectified.

Further reading

- Antzelevitch C (2007) Mechanism of cardiac arrhythmias and conduction disturbance. In *The Heart*, 12th edn, eds. Fuster V, O'Rourke RA, Walsh RA, Richard A, Poole-Wilson P. New York: McGraw-Hill, pp. 913–45.
- Bardy GH, Lee KL, Mark DB *et al.* (2005) Amiodarone or an implantable cardioverter-defibrillator for congestive heart failure. *N. Engl. J. Med.* **352**: 225–37.
- Davey MJ, Teubner D (2005) A randomised controlled trial of magnesium sulphate, in addition to usual care, for rate control in atrial fibrillation. *Ann. Emerg. Med.* **45**: 347–53.
- Guyton AC, Hall JE (2000) Chapter 13, Cardiac arrhythmias and their electrocardiographic interpretation. In *Textbook of Medical Physiology*, 10th edn. London: W. B. Saunders, pp. 134–42.
- Nathan AW, Sullivan ID, Timmis AD (1997) Chapter 11, Cardiac arrhythmia. In *Essential Cardiology*, 3rd edn, Oxford: Blackwell Science, pp. 228–54.
- Reinelt P, Delle Karth G, Geppert A, Heinz G (2001) Incidence and type of cardiac arrhythmias in critically ill patients: a single centre experience in a medical-cardiological ICU. *Intens. Care Med.* **27**: 1466–73.
- Resuscitation Council (2005) *Advanced Life Support*, 5th edn. London: Resuscitation Council.
- Vaughan-Williams EM (1970) Classification of anti-arrhythmia drugs. In *Symposium on Cardiac Arrhythmias*, eds. Sandfte E, Flensted-Jensen E, Olesen KH. Stockholm: AB ASTRA, Sodertalje, pp. 449–72.

Acute heart failure

Harjot Singh and Tony Whitehouse

Definition and aetiology

Heart failure can be defined as failure of the heart to maintain a cardiac output sufficient to meet the metabolic demands of the body. Decline in cardiac function may be de novo or acute decompensation due to chronic cardiac failure. Acute heart failure (AHF) may arise from systolic or diastolic dysfunction, rhythm disorder or preload and afterload mismatch from various aetiologies (Table 26.1).

Clinical syndromes and classifications

The European Society of Cardiology describes the following AHF syndromes:

- Mild acute decompensated heart failure, where there is fluid overload but no cardiogenic shock, pulmonary oedema or hypertension.
- Hypertensive AHF, where there is hypertension with relatively preserved left ventricular function and pulmonary oedema.
- AHF with pulmonary oedema.
- Cardiogenic shock.
- High-output failure, usually with tachycardia, warm peripheries, pulmonary congestion and sometimes low blood pressure.
- Right heart failure, characterized by low cardiac output, jugular venous distension, hepatomegaly and hypotension.

There may be overlap between these clinical presentations.

Various classifications of AHF syndrome are used:

- The Killip classification is based on clinical signs and chest X-ray findings; it was designed to provide a clinical estimate of the severity of myocardial derangement (Table 26.2).
- The Forrester classification is based on invasive haemodynamic assessment, employing cardiac index (CI) and pulmonary capillary wedge pressure for categorization of patients with myocardial infarction (MI) (Fig. 26.1). The original mortality figures may not be directly relevant in modern medicine, but these classifications still serve as an important prognostic tool.

Clinicians should bear in mind that pulmonary oedema can have non-cardiogenic aetiologies such as neurogenic pulmonary oedema, transfusion-related acute lung injury and acute respiratory distress syndrome (ARDS). Cardiogenic pulmonary oedema is defined by a pulmonary artery wedge pressure value greater than 18 mmHg, and when it occurs after MI is often associated with left ventricle systolic dysfunction. AHF may also present with flash pulmonary oedema due to diastolic dysfunction where there is associated acute hypertension and relatively preserved systolic function.

Cardiogenic shock is a state of tissue hypoperfusion due to heart failure despite the correction of preload. Although there are no set haemodynamic parameters for its definition, generally agreed parameters include hypotension (systolic blood pressure (SBP) below 90 mmHg for more than 90 min or above 90 mmHg with ionotropic/vasopressor support) in association with tissue hypoperfusion; or cardiac index of less than 2.2 l/min/m^2 in clinical context.

Presentation

Signs and symptoms can vary in AHF depending upon the underlying cause and include dyspnoea, tachycardia, tachypnoea, central cyanosis, third heart sound (S3)/gallop rhythm, rhonchi and rales on auscultation. There may be raised jugular venous pressure (JVP) due to right-sided heart failure. Classic 'frothy pink' sputum is found in frank pulmonary oedema. Respiratory alkalosis

Core Topics in Critical Care Medicine, eds. Fang Gao Smith and Joyce Yeung. Published by Cambridge University Press.

Table 26.1 Causes and precipitating factors in acute heart failure

(1) Decompensation of pre-existing chronic heart failure (e.g. cardiomyopathy)

(2) Acute coronary syndromes
- (a) Myocardial infarction/unstable angina with large extent of ischaemia and ischaemic dysfunction
- (b) Mechanical complication of acute myocardial infarction
- (c) Right ventricular infarction

(3) Hypertensive crisis

(4) Acute arrhythmias

(5) Valvular regurgitation (endocarditis, ruptured papillary muscle or worsening of pre-existing valvular regurgitation)

(6) Severe aortic valve stenosis

(7) Acute severe myocarditis

(8) Pericardial effusion or cardiac tamponade

(9) Aortic dissection

(10) Post-partum cardiomyopathy

(11) Non-cardiovascular precipitating factors
- (a) Lack of compliance with medical treatment
- (b) Volume overload
- (c) Infections, particularly pneumonia or septicaemia
- (d) Severe brain insult
- (e) After major surgery
- (f) Reduction in renal function
- (g) Asthma
- (h) Drug abuse
- (i) Alcohol abuse
- (j) Phaeochromocytoma

(12) High-output syndromes
- (a) Septicaemia
- (b) Thyrotoxicosis crisis
- (c) Anaemia
- (d) Shunt syndromes

is common with hypercarbia and respiratory acidosis as late signs indicating imminent cardio-respiratory arrest. Signs of tissue hypoperfusion include cool peripheries, altered consciousness and oliguria. Biochemistry may reveal a lactic acidosis from tissue hypoperfusion, increased urea and creatinine from impaired renal function and increased transaminase levels from portal hypertension.

After a myocardial infarction, about 25% of patients with inferior MI may have right ventricular infarction and a proportion of these patients develop right-sided heart failure. Most patients who develop cardiogenic shock do so early after the event (within 24 to 36 hours). Late development should raise the possibility of mechanical complications of MI (see Chapter 24: Acute coronary syndromes).

Table 26.2 Killip classification and mortality rates from Global Utilization of Streptokinase and Tissue Plasminogen Activator for Occluded Coronary Arteries (GUSTO-I) trial

Stage	Signs	Mortality rate (odds ratio)
I	No heart failure. No clinical signs of cardiac decompensation	5.1
II	Heart failure. Diagnostic criteria include rales, S3 gallop and pulmonary venous hypertension. Pulmonary congestion with wet rales in lower half of the lung fields	13.6 (2.95)
III	Severe heart failure. Frank pulmonary oedema with rales throughout the lung fields	32.2 (8.91)
IV	Cardiogenic shock. Signs include hypotension (SBP ≤90 mmHg), and evidence of peripheral vasoconstriction such as oliguria, cyanosis and diaphoresis	57.8 (25.68)

Source: Data adapted from Kerry L *et al.* (GUSTO-I Investigators) (1995) Predictors of 30-day mortality in the era of reperfusion for acute myocardial infarction: results from an international trial of 41 021 patients. *Circulation* **91**: 1659–68.

Pathophysiology

Impaired left ventricular (LV) function leads to increased left ventricular end diastolic pressure (LVEDP) and reduced stroke volume. The increased LVEDP causes back pressure on lung capillaries and causes interstitial and alveolar oedema. Low cardiac output causes activation of sympathetic nervous system, renin–angiotensin system and endothelin secretion as a result of which there is tachycardia, vasoconstriction, sodium and water retention. The release atrial (A type) and brain (B type) natriuretic peptide (ANP/BNP), which are secreted by atria and ventricles, partly offset this response and can be used as a prognostic marker.

Hypoperfusion of kidneys leads to renal dysfunction and systemic hypoperfusion leads to metabolic acidosis and lactic acid accumulation. Impaired hepatic perfusion combined with venous congestion exacerbates lactic acidosis and is a grave sign. There may be systemic inflammatory response with profound

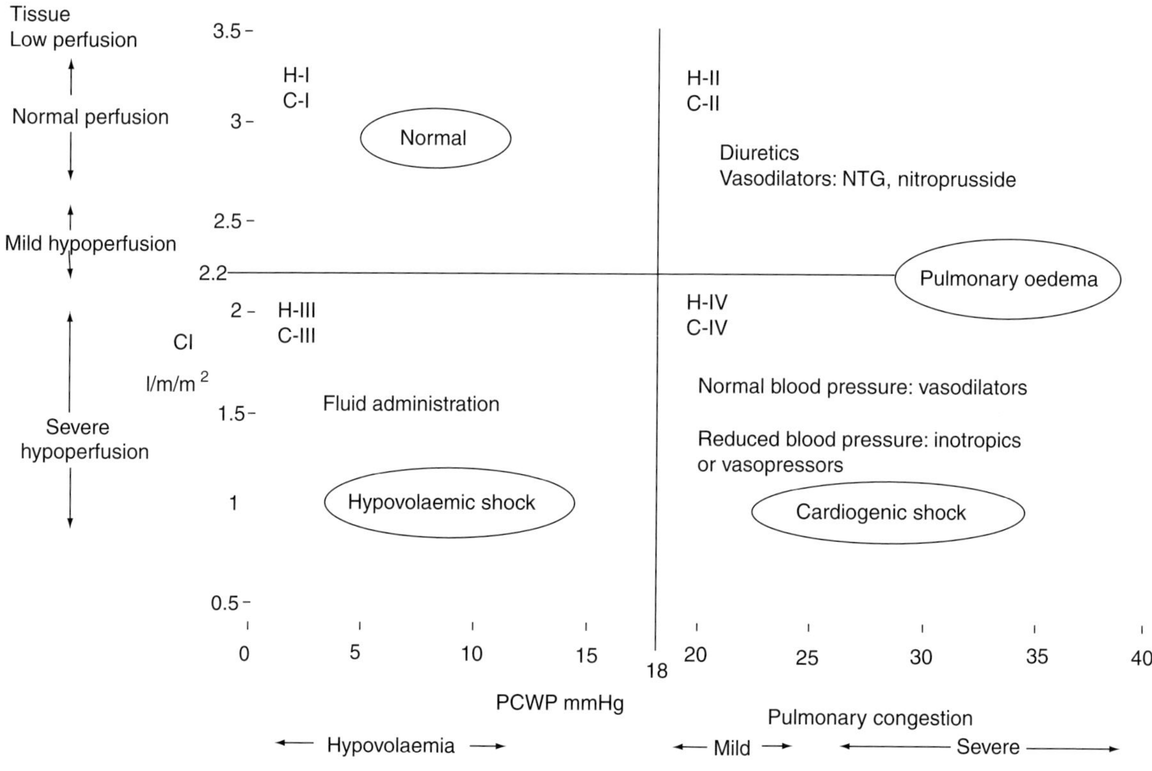

Fig. 26.1 The Forrester classification.

haemodynamic compromise and vasodilatation which resembles septic shock. Mortality is high in these patients as underlying myocardial dysfunction inhibits the increase in cardiac output seen in non-cardiomyopathic patients. A vicious cycle of further myocardial depression due to acidosis and various inflammatory mediators may then occur (Fig. 26.2).

Diagnosis

Clinical evaluation

The strongest sign is presence of a S3 (gallop rhythm) on auscultation. Interpretation of JVP must be done with caution as high values might represent decreased venous compliance and reduced right ventricular (RV) compliance despite low RV filling pressure (Fig. 26.3). The assessment of LV filling pressure clinically by auscultation for rales changes rapidly with quickly evolving clinical condition or coughing and is present in other non-cardiogenic pulmonary oedemas. Other clinical signs depend on the aetiology of AHF and its correlation with the history helps guide further investigation and treatment.

Electrocardiogram

A normal ECG is uncommon in AHF and it may indicate aetiology of AHF, e.g. pre-existing cardiac abnormalities, rhythm disorders, loading conditions of the heart, perimyocarditis, etc. (Fig. 26.4). The presence of Q wave indicates previous myocardial damage. Small QRS complexes may be a sign of a loss of functioning myocardium but also pericardial effusion.

Imaging techniques

Chest X-ray

Chest X-ray is performed early to confirm diagnosis, monitor the progress of the treatment of AHF and to look for pulmonary causes of respiratory distress (Fig. 26.5). A widened mediastinum should prompt further investigation (such as CT scan or transoesophageal echocardiography) to exclude aortic dissection.

Computed tomography

CT pulmonary angiography is a gold standard for diagnosing pulmonary embolism but transoesophageal echocardiogram is commonly used.

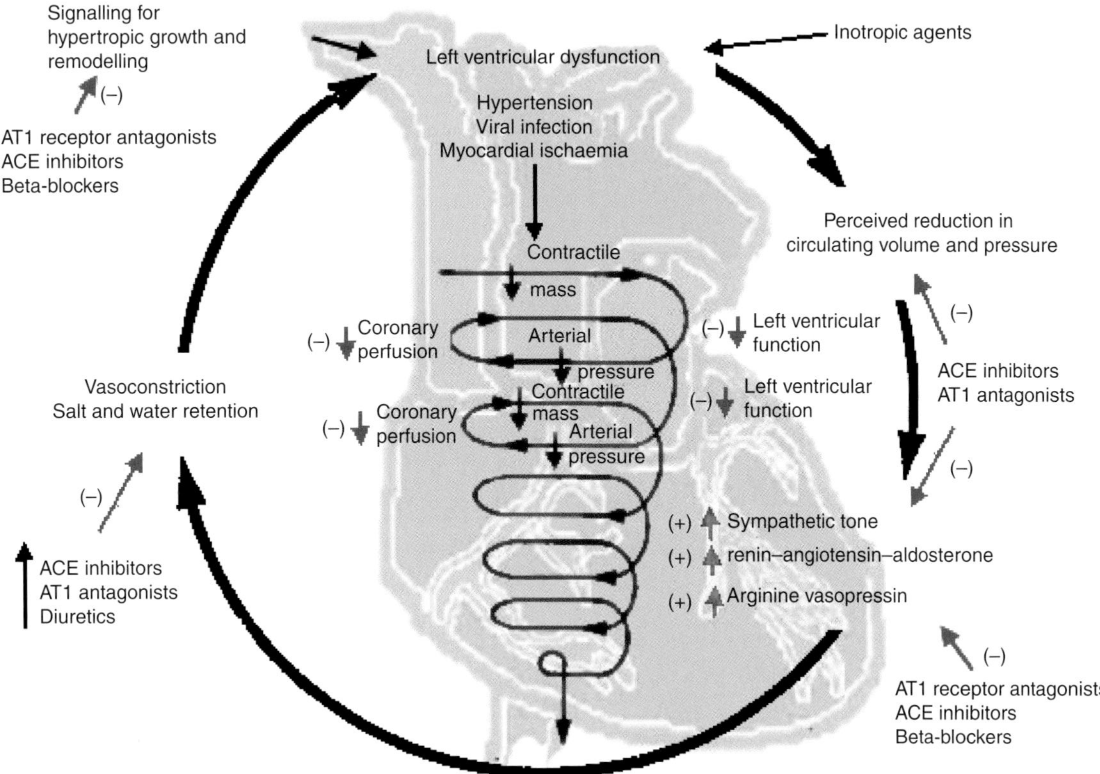

Fig. 26.2 Pathophysiology of heart failure.

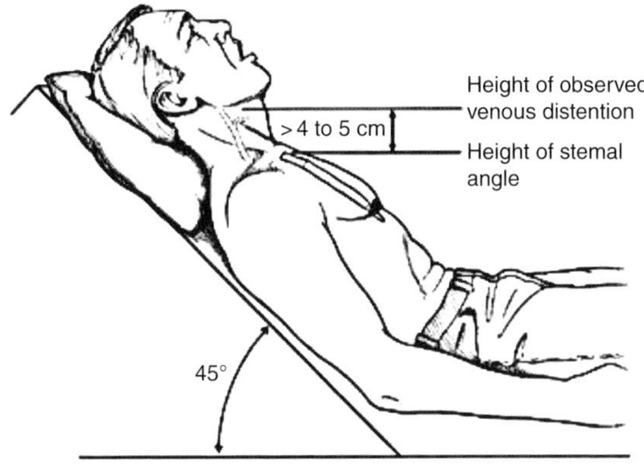

Fig. 26.3 Correct assessment of the JVP.

Echocardiography

Echocardiography has received class 1 recommendation as an essential tool for evaluation of the structural and functional changes underlying or associated with AHF. It can evaluate right and left ventricular systolic (global and regional) and diastolic function, valvular structure and function, pericardial pathology, thrombus or lesions, complications of MI and aortic dissection, preload and pulmonary artery pressure assessment (Fig. 26.6).

Laboratory investigations

For optimal management, full blood count, clotting, urea and electrolytes, blood glucose, cardiac enzymes, inflammatory markers and arterial blood gas analysis are recommended.

Both ANP and BNP levels correlate inversely with ejection fraction, and positively with pulmonary artery pressure. Although BNP is secreted by both atrial and ventricular tissue, in heart failure there is upregulation of ventricular production which is more important for BNP than ANP, and circulating BNP levels are consistently elevated in untreated heart failure compared to normals. Studies have demonstrated that BNP and the N-terminus of pro-BNP (N-BNP) is useful in determining the cause of acute dyspnoea (cardiac vs. non-cardiac). Cut-off values of 300 pg/ml for N-BNP and 100 pg/ml for BNP have been proposed. The diagnostic accuracy of BNP at this level is 83.4% and the negative predictive value of BNP at the value less than 50 pg/ml is 96%. The interpretation of BNP values requires caution and they may be elevated in a variety of conditions such as aortic stenosis, pulmonary embolus, renal failure, ARDS and septic shock. In addition, BNP may be normal in early phase of flash

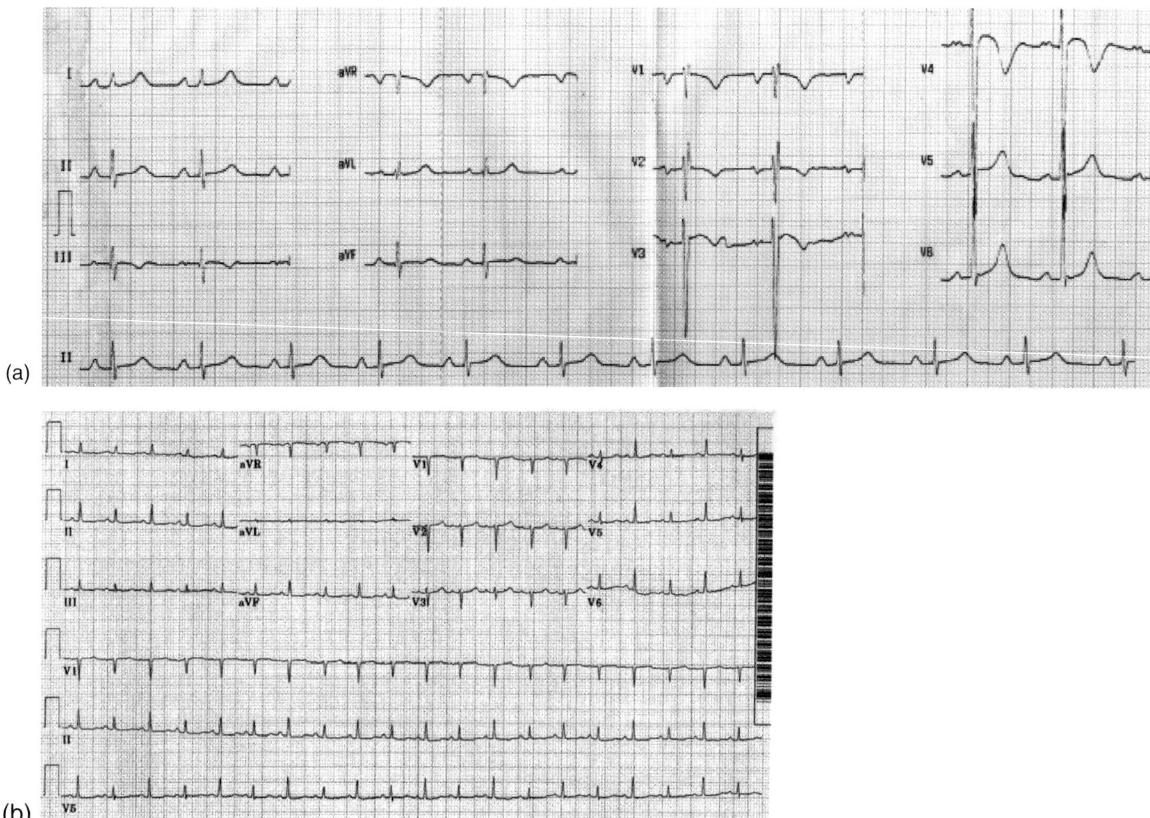

Fig. 26.4 Examples of ECG in heart failure. (a) Volume overload. Prominent negative component of P waves in lead V1 indicates left atrial overload. There is an rSr′ pattern in leads V1 and V2. This pattern can be seen in incomplete right bundle branch block and right ventricular volume overload situations like atrial septal defect. T waves are inverted in anterior leads. (b) Pericardial effusion. This ECG shows low voltage and electrical alternans seen in pericardial effusion.

pulmonary oedema. If AHF is confirmed, its level serves as important prognostic marker.

Other investigations

- Coronary angiography may be indicated if coronary artery disease is suspected or in prolonged AHF unexplained by other investigations.
- Endomyocardial biopsy may be required to diagnose acute cardiomyopathy in case of normal angiogram and severe biventricular dysfunction.
- CT angiogram can be used to assess the renal arteries. An uncommon cause of flash pulmonary oedema is bilateral renal artery stenosis.

Invasive monitoring

- Arterial line is used for close monitoring of blood pressure.
- Central venous lines are frequently used but central venous pressure (CVP) should be interpreted with caution as it may not represent a true reflection of left-sided filling pressure. CVP is also affected by tricuspid regurgitation and positive pressure ventilation.
- Pulmonary artery flotation catheter (PAFC) has been used extensively in the past. Mixed venous saturation (SvO_2) can be obtained through PAFC and maintaining SvO_2 above 65% suggests adequate global oxygen delivery. However, the ESCAPE trial did not show improvement in outcome in patients with acute decompensation of heart failure in whom PAFC was used.
- Echocardiography (both transthoracic and transoesophageal) may also be used to monitor myocardium and valvular integrity and has low complication rates.

(a)

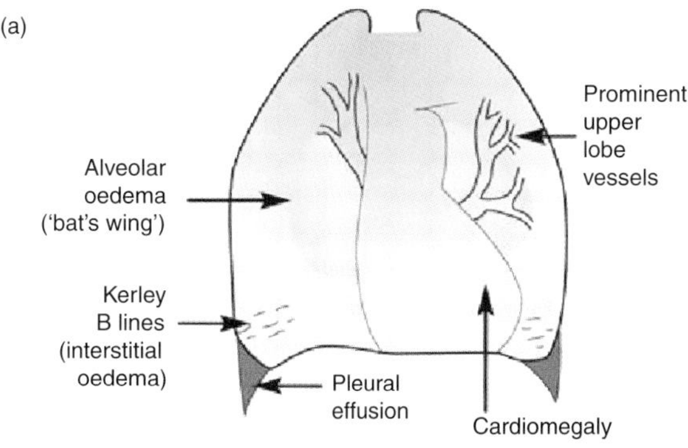

(b)

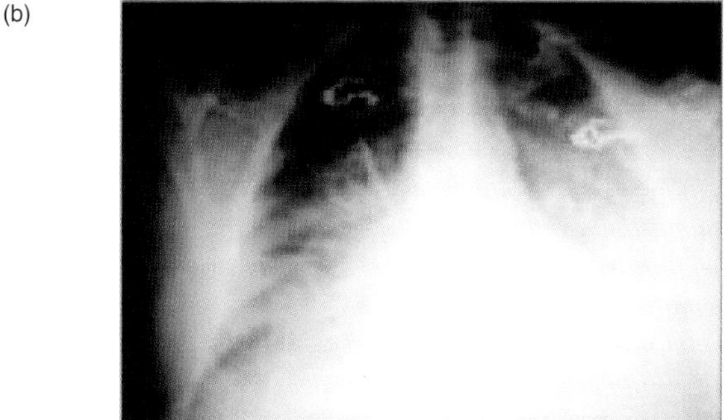

Fig. 26.5 Chest X-ray changes seen in heart failure. (a) Underlying pathology; (b) appearance in X-ray.

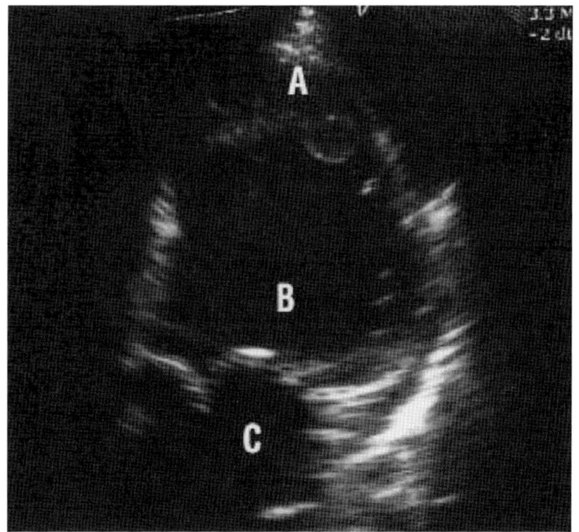

Fig. 26.6 Echocardiogram showing thrombus at left ventricular apex in patient with dilated cardiomyopathy. A, thrombus; B, left ventricle; C, left atrium.

Treatment

Immediate resuscitation

Acute heart failure is a medical emergency and diagnosis and resuscitation must be simultaneous. This should involve giving high-flow oxygen, establishing intravenous access, obtaining blood for laboratory investigation, urinary catheterization, ECG, chest X-ray and echocardiography at the earliest possible opportunity. In case of MI, thrombolysis or coronary angiography with or without coronary artery dilatation may be indicated and only life-saving interventions (such as intubation) should take precedence. Respiratory support (non-invasive or invasive) might be required for respiratory distress and haemodynamic shock. Evidence in patients admitted to ICU suggests that the use of continuous positive airway pressure (CPAP) and inodilator support may be superior to conventional treatment with glyceryl trinitrate (GTN) and frusemide in the acute phase. Monitoring should be escalated depending upon the response to the initial treatment.

Respiratory support

Supplemental oxygen is required in patients with hypoxia to maintain SaO_2 and maximize oxygen delivery. In a recent meta-analysis, non-invasive CPAP was found to reduce the need for mechanical ventilation and was associated with a lower mortality. In acute decompensated heart failure, non-invasive ventilation works by reducing the preload to the heart. In MI with respiratory distress, invasive ventilation may be more appropriate in anticipation of transfer for cardiac catheterization. Invasive ventilation is also required if non-invasive strategy fails or results in respiratory fatigue.

Analgesia

Morphine should be administered intravenously in aliquots for pain relief. It also induces venodilatation and mild arteriolar dilatation, and has a beneficial effect on heart rate. This is partly a direct effect but may also act through an anxiolytic effect and reduce sympathetic drive.

Haemodynamic support

Inodilators such as dobutamine, milrinone (phosphodiesterase enzyme inhibitors (PDEIs)) or levosimendan (calcium sensitizer and potassium channel opener – not currently licensed in the UK) are appropriate choices for starting treatment in mild cardiogenic shock. The loading doses of milrinone and levosimendan are either reduced or omitted in patients who are hypotensive. These medications may also need low-dose norepinephrine to offset the vasodilatation which is titrated to achieve a desired mean

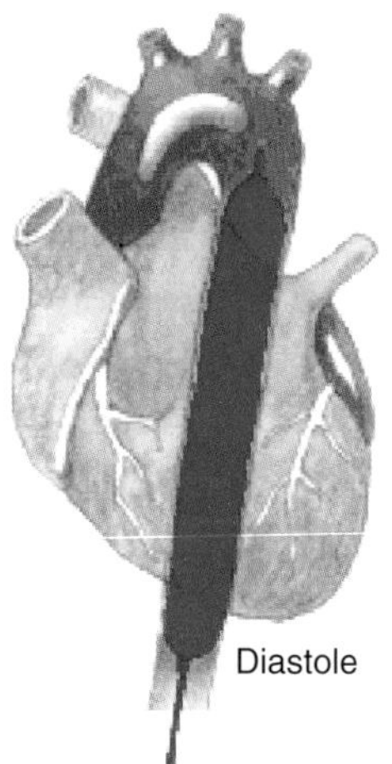

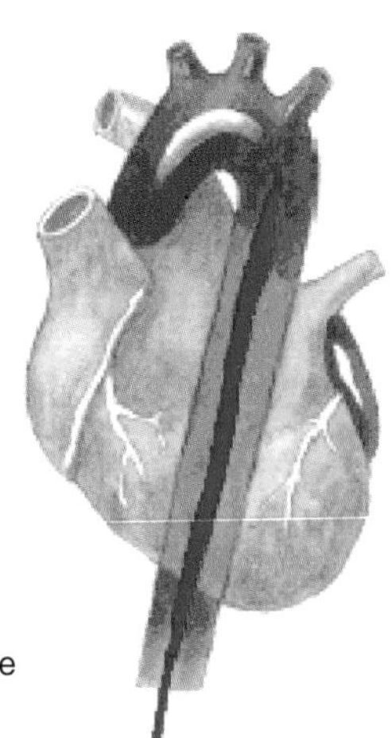

The IABP rapidy shuttles helium gas in and out of the balloon, which is located in the descending aorta. The balloon is inflated at the onset of cardiac diastole and deflated at the onset of systole.
Systole

Fig. 26.7 Diagram illustrating the mechanics of how the intra-aortic balloon pump works.

arterial pressure. The effect of PDEI and dobutamine is additive and these drugs may be used simultaneously. When norepinephrine is used, cardiac output should be measured as its use can adversely affect cardiac output by increasing afterload. Signs of end-organ hypoperfusion should be monitored and avoided. If there is failure of response, the doses of inodilator should be cautiously titrated upwards, and monitoring made more intense; additional inotropic support (such as epinephrine) may be required. It should be borne in mind that these patients have a finite and reduced cardiac output and that overuse of inodilators may simply induce over-vasodilatation and hypotension without concomitant increases in cardiac output.

Acute use of digoxin is not well defined but is best continued if the patient is on long-term therapy. Clinicians should remember that digoxin is renally cleared and that acute reduction in renal function may cause digoxin toxicity. Digoxin in AHF may be indicated if there is a tachycardia such as fast atrial fibrillation (AF). In addition to renal dysfunction, other factors which predispose to digoxin toxicity are coronary artery disease, cor pulmonale and metabolic disorders such as hypokalaemia, hypomagnesaemia and uncorrected hypothyroidism. Digoxin clearance is reduced by quinidine, spironolactone and verapamil.

Mechanical assist devices

Circulatory assist devices are indicated when there is failure to respond to conventional therapy and there is potential recovery of myocardium or as a bridge to cardiac transplantation.

Intra-aortic balloon counterpulsation

Mechanism

The intra-aortic balloon pump (IABP) is a mechanical device that is used to decrease myocardial oxygen demand while at the same time increasing cardiac output by counterpulsation. The device consists of a cylindrical balloon that sits in the aorta which deflates in systole increasing forward blood flow by reducing afterload and inflates in diastole increasing blood flow to the coronary arteries (Fig. 26.7). By increasing cardiac output it increases coronary blood flow and myocardial oxygen delivery (Fig. 26.8). Helium is used because of its low viscosity and has a lower risk of causing an embolism if the balloon were to rupture.

Indications

- Patient does not respond to optimization of preload, ionotropic support or vasodilatation.
- When there is significant mitral regurgitation or rupture of interventricular septum to achieve haemodynamic stabilization for a definitive treatment.
- In context of myocardial ischaemia, in preparation for angiography and revascularization.

Contraindications

- There is severe aortic regurgitation.
- Aortic dissection.

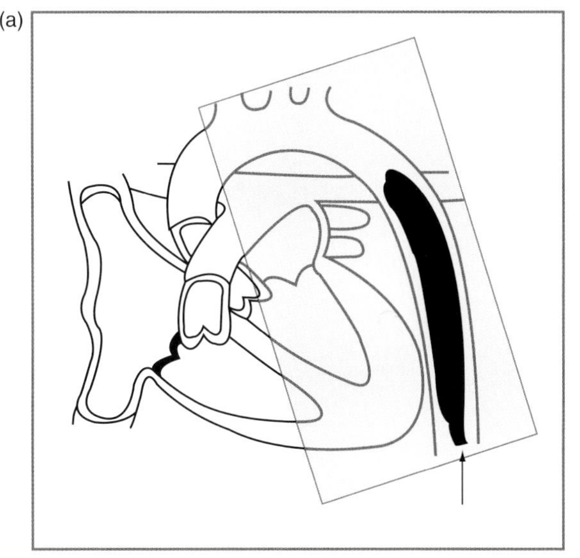

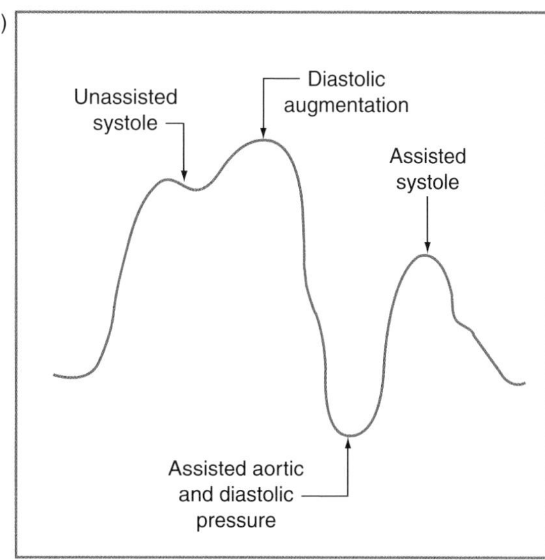

Fig. 26.8 Diagram illustrating the effect of (a) intra-aortic balloon pump on (b) aortic blood pressure.

- Severe (mobile) atheroma in descending thoracic aorta.
- Severe occlusive vascular disease involving distal aorta, iliac or femoral arteries

Ventricular assist devices

Ventricular assist devices (VADs) are mechanical pumps that partially replace the mechanical work of the ventricle either in anticipation of recovery from the acute insult or as a bridge to transplant (Fig. 26.9). Such use may need complex surgery and the patient needs to be anticoagulated whilst the device is in the use. Thromboembolism, bleeding, infection, haemolysis and device malfunction are some of the problems associated with these.

Diuretics

Volume overload is central to pathophysiology of most episodes of AHF. There is a lack of any large prospective randomized trail on use of diuretics in AHF. Diuretics are clearly indicated in volume overloaded patients and, in combination with vasodilators, probably facilitate weaning from ventilatory support. Careful monitoring is recommended to avoid overdiuresis resulting in hypotension and renal dysfunction. There is growing interest in use of ultrafiltration in control of volume overload. The Ultrafiltration versus Intravenous Diuretics for Patients Hospitalized for Acute Decompensated Heart Failure (UNLOAD) trial showed greater weight loss at 48 hours, decreased need for vasoactive drugs and reduced readmission rates at 90 days.

Vasodilators

Nitrate therapy is used for reduction in preload and results in reducing congestion and improvement in dyspnoea. A reduction in afterload may be achieved by nitroprusside although its use, even in low doses, can cause hypotension. Invasive blood pressure monitoring is mandatory for its safe use. It is particularly helpful when pulmonary oedema is associated with hypertensive crisis. Transition to angiotensin converting enzyme inhibitor or angiotensin II receptor blocker is recommended as soon as renal function and blood pressure allow. The combined use of hydralazine and isosorbide dinitrate is an alternative in patients who have significant renal dysfunction.

Natriuretic peptides

Nesiritide, a recombinant B-type natriuretic peptide, is a mixed vein and arteriolar vasodilator with mild diuretic effect. After an initial promising report in Vasodilation in Management of Acute Congestive Heart Failure (VMAC) trial, its use is being re-examined in patients with acutely decompensated heart failure for its possible benefits on renal function and mortality.

Treatment of underlying disease and co-morbidities

The underlying acute morbidity leading to de novo or acute decompensation of heart failure will also need to be addressed. A few examples are acute coronary syndromes (ACS) (revascularization may need to be

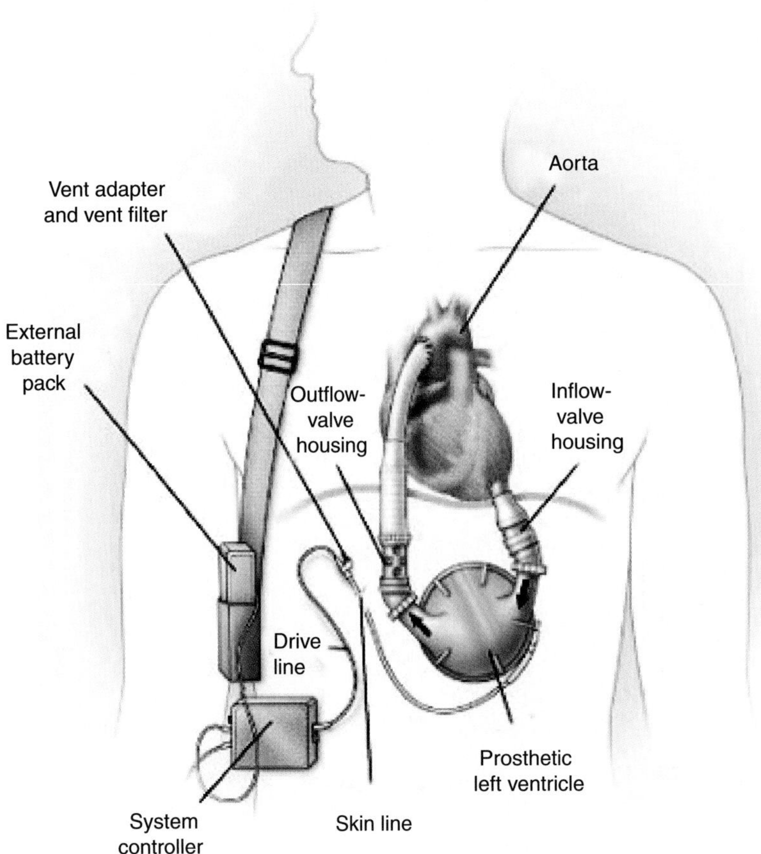

Fig. 26.9 Ventricular assist device (VAD). There are three parts: an electrically driven mechanical pump, an electronic controller and a power supply. The VAD is placed in the abdominal cavity and acts by taking blood from the left ventricle and pumping it into the aorta. The VAD normally pumps at a rate of 60–80 bpm, but can increase to 120 bpm with exercise. Power to the pump is supplied by two external batteries which can be carried in a backpack by the patient.

considered), complications of ACS (such as acute papillary rupture or septal rupture), aortic dissection, treatment of hypertensive crisis (such as phaeochromocytoma) and arrhythmia control (such as fast AF, bradycardic or other decompensating rhythms). Anticoagulation is well established as adjunctive therapy in ACS and AF. Prophylactic doses of anticoagulants to prevent deep vein thrombosis should also be used.

Renal dysfunction is independently associated with poor prognosis and measures should be taken to preserve renal function and treat optimally when the dysfunction is severe. Studies suggest that so-called 'renal dose dopamine' may have an effect by improving cardiac output but does not preserve renal function. Utmost care should be taken to prevent and treat infection. Hyperglycaemia should be controlled with short acting insulin. Calorie and nitrogen balance should be maintained.

Heart transplantation

This is considered where AHF is known to have poor prognosis, e.g. in severe acute myocarditis, postpuerperal cardiomyopathy or patients with large MI with poor initial outcome after revascularization. The patient should be stabilized initially with the aid of vasoactive drugs and assist devices until a suitable donor is available.

Future agents

Vasopressin receptor antagonists (tolvaptan and conivaptan), adenosine A1 receptor antagonists, endothelin receptor antagonists (tezosentan and bosentan) are potential agents that may be added to the armamentarium of the treatment of AHF.

Prognosis

Acute, severe AHF may be partially reversed when the myocardium is ischaemic, stunned or hibernating. However, mortality is high in AHF associated with acute MI (30% mortality in 12 months). Acute pulmonary oedema has 12% in-hospital mortality with 40% mortality at 1 year. Patients who are successfully treated have a significant 12 month readmission rate.

Key points

- Acute heart failure may arise from systolic or diastolic dysfunction, rhythm disorder or preload and afterload mismatch from various aetiologies.
- Pulmonary oedema can have non-cardiogenic aetiologies such as neurogenic pulmonary oedema, transfusion-related acute lung injury and ARDS.
- Management aims to support the perfusion to major organs and can include ventilatory support, the use of inotropes and renal replacement therapy.

Further reading

- Allen LA, O'Connor CM (2007) Management of acute decompensated heart failure. *Can. Med. Ass. J.* **176**(6): 797–805.
- Binanay C, Califf RM, Hasselblad V *et al.* (2005) Evaluation study of congestive heart failure and pulmonary artery catheterization effectiveness: the ESCAPE trail. *J. Am. Med. Ass.* **294**: 1625–33.
- Maisel AS, Krishnaswamy P, Nowak RM *et al.* (2002) Rapid measurement of B-type natriuretic peptide in the emergency diagnosis of heart failure. *N. Engl. J. Med.* **347**(3): 161–7.
- McMurray JJV, Pfeffer MA (2005) Heart failure. *Lancet* **365**: 1877–89.
- Mieiniczuk LM, Haddad H, Davies RA (2009) Ultrafiltration in the management of acute decompensated heart failure. *Curr. Opin. Cardiol.* Dee. 5 (Epub ahead of print).
- Nieminen MS, Bohm M, Cowie MR *et al.* (2005) The Task Force on Acute Heart Failure of the European Society of Cardiology: Executive summary of the guidelines on the diagnosis and treatment of acute heart failure. *Eur. Heart J.* **26**: 384–416.
- Peter JV, Moran JL, Phillips-Hughes J, Graham P, Bersten AD (2006) Effect of non-invasive positive pressure ventilation (NIPPV) on mortality in patients with acute cardiogenic pulmonary oedema: a meta-analysis. *Lancet* **367**(9517): 1155–63.

Chapter 27

Mechanical ventilation

Bill Tunnicliffe

This chapter deals with the practice of invasive positive pressure ventilation in adults within the critical care setting. Advanced airway skills, weaning from mechanical support and non-invasive ventilation are dealt with separately in Chapters 2, 30 and 31 respectively and will not be dealt with further.

Introduction

Mechanical ventilation (MV) is used to replace or supplement the work carried out by the respiratory muscles, usually with the aim of achieving or maintaining adequate gas exchange.

Mechanical ventilation is a supportive intervention rather than a therapeutic one; it is hazardous and potentially injurious to the ventilated lung especially in the presence of intrinsic lung disease or lung injury. Initiating mechanical ventilation should therefore only be undertaken when the balance of risk of not intervening is considered greater than the risk of proceeding; once initiated, mechanical ventilation should in general be applied for as short a duration as is possible and as 'gently' as possible. It is now recognized that ventilatory strategies should be chosen on the basis of clinically important outcomes rather than on the basis of their ability to alter gas exchange in the short term.

History and development of mechanical ventilation

Despite the recognition by Galen in the second century AD that the lungs served both to supply some property of air to the body and to discharge a waste product from the blood, it is only relatively recently, chiefly consequent to the development of technology, that the role for mechanical ventilatory support has become established. Bjorn Ibsen successfully applied positive pressure ventilation to a population of patients with polio-induced respiratory paralysis during the 1952 Copenhagen outbreak, reducing their overall mortality from around 85% in July 1952 to 15% in March the following year. This intervention is now seen as the birth of modern mechanical ventilation as a method to manage acute respiratory failure, and also heralded the development of the modern intensive care unit.

The provision of respiratory support by positive pressure ventilation is now a core function of the intensive care unit; internationally around a third of patients admitted to intensive care units currently receive mechanical ventilation for more than 12 hours. Recent international epidemiological studies have revealed that the median age of patients receiving mechanical ventilatory support is 63 years (interquartile range 48 to 73 years), and almost 40% of patients are female. The majority of ventilated patients (>65%) receive less than 24 hours ventilatory support as a component of their routine anaesthetic and post-operative management following major surgery such as cardiac, aortic or neurosurgery. The other major patient groups include the critically ill with severe primary respiratory disease (<13%), patients with head or chest trauma (<10%) and those with poisoning/deliberate self-harm (<8%), in which the duration of mechanical ventilation is more variable.

Indications for initiating mechanical ventilation

Respiratory homeostasis can be thought about in terms of the equilibrium between respiratory load, respiratory capacity and respiratory drive. Respiratory failure develops when one or more of these elements is out of balance, and is defined as the inability of the body's breathing apparatus to maintain adequate gas exchange for its metabolic needs; this usually equates to the presence of a PaO_2 below 8 kPa and/or a $PaCO_2$ above 6.7 kPa when breathing room air.

Core Topics in Critical Care Medicine, eds. Fang Gao Smith and Joyce Yeung. Published by Cambridge University Press.

Table 27.1 Indications for mechanical ventilation

Criteria for starting mechanical ventilation are difficult to define and the decision is often a clinical one. Indicators include:

- Respiratory rate >35 or <5 breaths/minute
- Exhaustion, with laboured pattern of breathing
- Hypoxia – central cyanosis, SaO_2 <90% on oxygen or PaO_2 <8 kPa
- Hypercarbia – $PaCO_2$ >8kPa
- Decreasing consciousness level
- Significant chest trauma
- Tidal volume <5 ml/kg or vital capacity <15 ml/kg

Other indications for ventilation:

- Control of intracranial pressure in head injury
- Airway protection following drug overdose
- Following cardiac arrest
- For recovery after prolonged major surgery or trauma

Mechanical ventilation is in general indicated where established or impending respiratory failure exists. While respiratory failure can be precisely defined in terms of blood gas tensions as above, impending respiratory failure has no clear definition. Here clinical judgement is required and frequently a decision to commence mechanical ventilation will need to be made in the absence of arterial blood gas results. There are a multitude of clinical presentations that prompt the consideration of mechanical ventilation; they range from patients presenting with severe respiratory distress or apnoea to patients with relatively minor clinical signs of increased work of breathing though with clearly limited reserve. Increased work of breathing causes signs of respiratory distress: nasal flaring, accessory muscle recruitment, tracheal tug, intercostal recession, tachypnoea, tachycardia, hyper- or hypotension and changes in mental status. In patients with acute respiratory failure their increased work of breathing may account for up to 20% of their total oxygen consumption, whereas at rest this fraction is between 1% and 3% (see Table 27.1).

Respiratory failure

Respiratory failure occurs when pulmonary gas exchange is sufficiently impaired to cause hypoxaemia with or without hypercarbia. The causes of respiratory failure are diverse and the problem may occur due to disease at the alveolar/endothelial interface (e.g. pulmonary oedema) or in the respiratory pump mechanism resulting in inadequate minute ventilation (e.g. flail segment accompanying fractured ribs). It can be classified into two broad categories, Type 1 (or hypoxaemic) and Type 2 (or hypercarbic) respiratory failure.

Type 1 or hypoxaemic respiratory failure

The pathophysiological mechanisms responsible for hypoxaemia can be grouped into two categories, defined by the presence or absence of an increased alveolar–arterial O_2 gradient (A–aDO_2) (Fig. 27.1). An increased A–aDO_2 results from either ventilation–perfusion abnormalities or excessive right-to-left shunt. Patients with hypoxaemic respiratory failure and a normal A–aDO_2 typically have alveolar hypoventilation or inadequate inspiratory partial pressure of O_2. The most common causes of hypoxaemic respiratory failure are pulmonary conditions such as severe pneumonia, pulmonary oedema and acute respiratory distress syndrome (ARDS), causing ventilation–perfusion mismatch and shunt. The goal of mechanical ventilation in hypoxaemic respiratory failure is to provide adequate arterial oxygen saturations through a combination of supplemental oxygen and specific patterns of ventilatory support that enhance oxygenation.

Type 2 or hypercarbic respiratory failure

Type 2 respiratory failure results from disease states causing either a decrease in minute ventilation or an increase in physiological dead space such that, despite adequate minute ventilation, alveolar ventilation is inadequate to meet metabolic demands. Common causes include neuromuscular diseases such as myasthenia gravis, Guillain–Barré syndrome and myopathies, as well as diseases that cause respiratory muscle fatigue due to increased workload such as asthma, acute exacerbations of chronic obstructive pulmonary disease and restrictive lung disease. Acute hypercarbic respiratory failure is characterized by an arterial CO_2 tension >6.7 kPa and an arterial pH <7.35, whereas chronic hypercarbic respiratory failure is characterized by elevated arterial CO_2 tensions but with a relatively normal arterial pH consequent on metabolic compensation. Mechanical ventilation should generally be instituted in acute hypercarbic respiratory failure. In contrast, the decision to institute mechanical ventilation when components of both acute and chronic respiratory failure are present is less clear and will depend on both blood gas parameters and clinical evaluation. In general, the goal of ventilatory support in hypercarbic respiratory failure should be to

A–a gradient = $PAO_2 - PaO_2$
PaO_2 (partial pressure of O2 in the artery) from ABG
PAO_2 (partial pressure of O_2 in the alveoli from the alveolar gas equation

Alveolar gas equation:
$PAO_2 = P_iO_2 - (PaCO_2 / R)$
$P_iO_2 = F_iO2\ (P_B - P_{H2O})$
or using common values:
$PA0_2 = (FiO2 * (760 - 47)) - (PaCO_2 / 0.8)$
*P_iO_2 = partial pressure of O_2 in the central airways
*F_iO_2 (fraction of inspired oxygen) F_iO_2 on room air = 0.21
*$PaCO_2$ (value from ABG)
*P_B = barometric pressure (760 mmHg at sea level)
$P_B = P_{N_2} + P_{O_2} + P_{CO_2} + P_{H_2O}$
*P_{H_2O} = Water vapour pressure (47 mm Hg at 37°C)
*R = Respiratory quotient = $V_{CO_2} / V_{O_2} = 0.8$
(ratio of carbon dioxide production to oxygen consumption.)

Estimating A–a gradient:
Normal A–a gradient = (Age + 10) / 4
A–a increases 5 to 7 mmHg for every 10% increase in F_iO_2

Fig. 27.1 Calculation of alveolar–arterial oxygen gradient. Normal A–a gradient 20–65 mmHg, severe distress >400 mmHg.

normalize arterial pH through changes in CO_2 tensions, rather than to normalize CO_2 tensions per se.

Mechanical ventilators, airway pressure, flow and delivered volumes

Although modern mechanical ventilators are highly complex pieces of equipment, most are conceptually very simple in design. Sources of high-pressure air and oxygen are connected via appropriate regulators to a gas blender, and the flow from the blender is via a valve under microprocessor control. The operator defines the characteristics of the inspiratory and expiratory phase of the ventilator, which then delivers the breath through the valve to the patient, and checks measured parameters such as flow and pressure.

Airway pressure is dependent chiefly on two factors: how stiff the lungs are and resistance to airflow. As gas enters the lung, the pressure in the airway has to overcome flow resistance within the branching airways whilst also trying to overcome the elastic recoil of the lung. In doing so, net inflow of gas occurs and the lungs inflate. The elastic recoil or stiffness of the lungs and chest wall is called its compliance pressure being proportional to volume × 1/total compliance. Airway pressure related to the flow of gas through the branching airways is proportional to flow × resistance:

$$\text{airway pressure} = (\text{volume} \times 1/\text{total compliance}) + (\text{inspiratory flow} \times \text{resistance})$$

or

$$P_{aw} = (V \times 1/C_{rs}) + (\mathrm{F} \times \mathrm{R})$$

The relationship between airway pressure, flow and compliance is known as the equation of motion and is expressed as three simultaneous graphs of pressure, flow and volume running simultaneously versus time. Most modern ventilators display these graphs at the bedside, giving the operator potentially important information to support decision making. During mechanical ventilation, most modes control only one of the variables of the equation of motion, with the remaining variables being dependent.

Modes of ventilation

The classification and nomenclature describing modes of ventilation are confusing. A working group is currently being established with the aim of unifying the terms used internationally.

As ventilation is under microprocessor control, there are numerous potential patterns of breath delivery, with more than 20 modes in clinical use. Although the range is wide, very few clinical trials have been performed exploring whether the mode of ventilation is related to clinically relevant outcomes, making rational choice quite difficult.

Table 27.2 Descriptive classification of the modes of ventilation

- How does the ventilator control the breath?
  - Pressure control
  - Volume control
  - Timed
- Are mandatory breaths being delivered to the patient?
  - All breaths are mandatory
  - Some breaths are mandatory
  - No breaths are mandatory
- What type of inspiratory trigger is used?
  - Pressure triggering
  - Flow triggering
  - Other
  - No triggered breaths
- Are the spontaneous breaths supported?
  - Is pressure support in use
- Is expiration assisted or augmented?
  - Continuous positive airway pressure (CPAP)/positive and expiratory pressure (PEEP)

Source: Adapted from: Goldstone JC (2002) Mechanical ventilation: the basics. In *Respiratory Critical Care*, eds. Davidson C and Treacher D. London: Arnold, pp. 21–31.

An example of a classification system that helps make sense of what the ventilator is doing is outlined in Table 27.2. Its use helps unravel the components of ventilator control available to the operator and can form a logical basis for decision making around ventilator adjustments.

Volume control ventilation

In volume control ventilation (VCV) the operator determines the tidal volume to be delivered over a set duration, and the other factors in the equation of motion (i.e. flow and pressure) will vary dependent on the mechanics of the system. The ventilator will effectively deliver a predetermined minute volume, which is an advantage when the patient is unable to make an inspiratory effort and the underlying lung mechanics are normal. Pressure in the airway will be dependent on resistance to airflow and the compliance of the respiratory system; if the airway resistance is high or the lungs and/or chest wall are stiff, excessive airway pressure may result with potentially damaging effects. To avoid this, pressure limits can be set to provide pressure-limited volume control ventilation (Fig. 27.2).

Traditional guidelines for determining the tidal volume to be delivered to a particular patient were based on a value of 10–15 ml/kg lean body weight. While this may be reasonable in the otherwise normal lung, there is now compelling evidence that delivering such volumes in the injured lung is deleterious and a value of 6–8 ml/kg lean body weight is preferable.

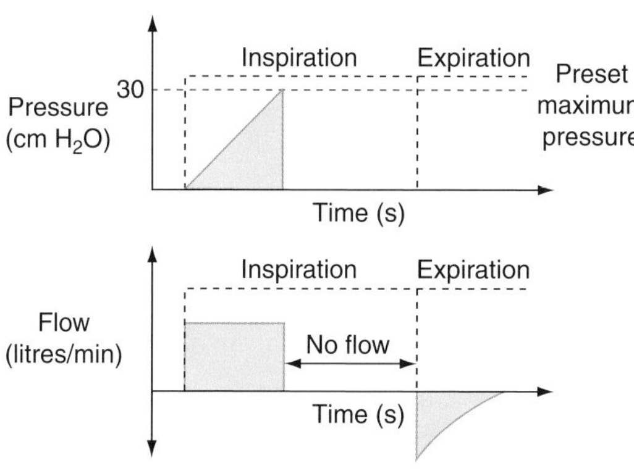

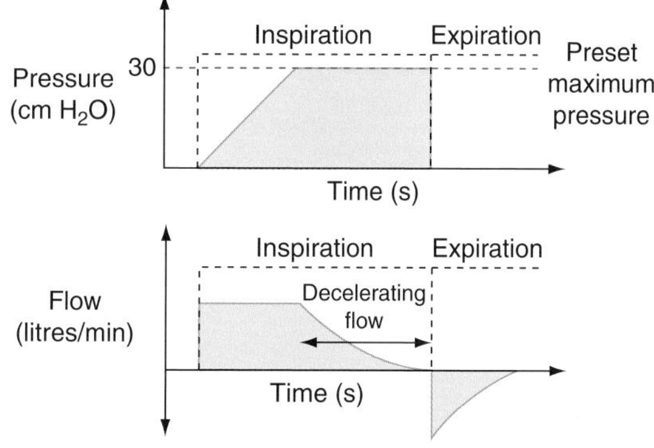

Fig. 27.2 Pressure-limited volume control ventilation.

In volume control ventilation, the operator can select the shape of the inspiratory flow waveform, usually either a square wave (i.e. constant flow) or a decelerating waveform. The selection of one over the other may influence airway pressures, and also may affect the homogeneity of ventilation throughout the lungs; a decelerating waveform showing improved homogeneity, versus a constant flow profile delivering the same tidal volume over the same time duration.

Pressure control ventilation

During pressure control ventilation (PCV), the operator defines the inspiratory pressure to be delivered over a set duration, and the other factors in the equation of motion (i.e. flow and volume) will vary, again dependent on the mechanics of the system. As a consequence, the delivered tidal volumes will vary with alterations in the airway resistance or compliance (Fig. 27.3). As pressure is pre-set, potentially injurious high airway pressures will be avoided; however, the target minute ventilation may not necessarily be achieved. This means that the relationship between clinician-set variables and ventilation targets may not be quite as intuitive or straightforward as with VCV.

In the critically ill, lung compliance due to lung injury is often dyshomogeneous. Achieving ventilation in the stiffer lung segments may require prolonged inspiratory times and delivering this is generally conceptually more easily achieved with PCV than with VCV (Table 27.3).

Table 27.3 Comparison of volume control ventilation and pressure control ventilation

	Volume control ventilation	Pressure control ventilation
Advantages	Maintains constant tidal volume	Reduced peak airway pressure and risk of barotraumas
	Control of $PaCO_2$	Improved gas exchange with decelerating flow More homogeneous ventilation in distribution disorders
Disadvantages	Potential high airway pressure and lung injury	Hypoventilation secondary to changes in lung compliance and resistance
	Cannot compensate for leaks	

Mandatory breaths and spontaneous breaths

During continuous mandatory ventilation (CMV), the operator selects a breath frequency that the ventilator then delivers. CMV is typically employed during elective general anaesthesia, particularly when muscle relaxants are used. It requires no interaction between the ventilator and the patient, in fact during CMV the ventilator will continue to deliver what the operator has set, regardless of whether the patient is making any respiratory effort or not. However when caring for the critically ill, it is desirable for patients to initiate some or all of their breaths. Spontaneous breathing on the whole delivers better regional distribution of ventilation while requiring less sedation.

At each extreme, that is either of complete mandatory breath delivery and that of no mandatory breath delivery (spontaneous breathing), there is no need for the ventilator to take into account the patient's own inspiratory effort in timing its own delivered breaths. In between those extremes there is a need for the ventilator to be responsive to the patient's efforts when determining when to deliver a breath. If the ventilator attempts to deliver a mandated breath while the patient is beginning to exhale, very high airway pressures may result; similarly problems might arise if the ventilator attempts to deliver a mandated breath just when the patient had completed an inspiration. To avoid these problems the ventilator needs to be able to detect when a patient is breathing in or out and time the mandatory breath delivery appropriately. The ventilator can detect what the patient is doing by measuring either changes in flow or pressure within the breathing circuit. This ventilation mode is called synchronized intermittent mandatory ventilation (SIMV).

During SIMV, the ventilator is inhibited from delivering a mandatory breath during the initial phase of exhalation. The amount of inhibition is related to expiratory time; progressively the ventilator becomes more sensitive to inspiratory effort as the expiratory time lengthens, resulting in the next mandatory breath being delivered in synchrony with a

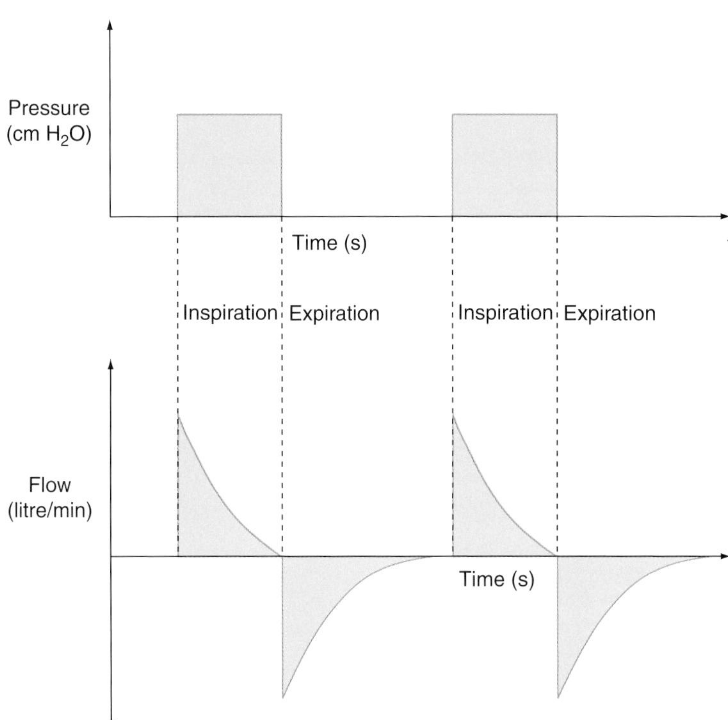

Fig. 27.3 Pressure control ventilation.

spontaneous breath. Of note, during SIMV, the ventilator is only responsive to whether the patient is breathing when it is *not* delivering a breath, that is, once a mandatory breath is triggered and being delivered, what the patient is doing becomes immaterial to the ventilator.

An alternative mode used to deliver a proportion of mandatory breaths is bi-level ventilation. This mode is similar to pressure control SIMV, except that the ventilator remains sensitive to the patient's own respiratory efforts throughout its respiratory cycle, in principle allowing for greater synchrony between the patient and the ventilator.

Triggers

How a ventilator senses an inspiratory effort is termed its trigger. The sensitivity of the trigger and its response time can impact on the work of breathing of a patient breathing on a ventilator. All systems have a degree of delay from the beginning of inspiration to the point when the ventilator responds to that signal; any significant delay means that at the beginning of inspiration, the patient will be trying to breathe in against a closed valve.

Historically, there have been two broad types of triggers, pressure and flow. More recently, an experimental technique termed neurally adjusted ventilatory assistance (NAVA) has been developed where the diaphragm's electrical activity, detected by an oesophageal probe, is used to signal inspiratory effort.

Pressure triggers remain most commonly used, chiefly because of their simplicity. A pressure transducer measuring airway pressure continuously is programmed to detect a fall in pressure consequent on inspiratory effort, signalling this to the ventilator. The trigger sensitivity can usually be adjusted, so that it reacts to smaller falls in pressure, potentially enabling the ventilator to trigger closer to the beginning of the breath.

Flow triggering can be achieved either by measuring absolute changes in flow within the breathing circuit, or by detecting differences in an applied bias flow. The latter technique offers potentially improved sensitivities and response times, which may be important in patients with lung disease such as chronic obstructive pulmonary disease.

Auto cycling can occur with both flow and pressure triggers. This phenomenon usually reflects oversensitive trigger settings, allowing other physiological events (such as cardiac contractions) to trigger the ventilator.

Supporting spontaneous breaths and pressure support ventilation

When the ventilator is in an assist-control mode, the patient has the opportunity of initiating additional machine supported breaths when the ventilator rate set by the operator is insufficient to meet the patient's own rate demand. The support is triggered by the patient making an inspiratory effort; the ventilator then provides positive inspiratory pressure to augment the patient's effort. The operator can determine the level of support offered thereby influencing the contribution spontaneous breaths make to the patient's overall minute ventilation.

In pressure support ventilation (PSV), the only operator-set variable is the target inspiratory pressure. The patient determines their respiratory rate and inspiratory time; when inspiration is sensed, the target pressure is delivered and as inspiration continues the constant pressure is maintained. The signal that marks the nearing of the end of inspiration is a fall in the inspiratory flow (usually to a value of 25% of the maximum inspiratory flow achieved during that breath), and this cycles the ventilator to end the delivery of the target inspiratory pressure. During PSV, the delivery of a specific tidal volume is not assured. It is possible that PSV may deliver more assistance than is needed or that the support is insufficient as it is inherently difficult to judge the correct amount of pressure support needed by an individual patient at any particular time

PSV is a popular weaning mode for adults. Weaning from mechanical ventilation should be a gradual process. The work of breathing through an endotracheal tube may be unreasonably high and could lead to respiratory muscle failure in susceptible patients. There is no evidence however to support this view, in fact several large clinical trials have demonstrated equivalence between PSV and T-piece weaning.

Support during expiration

During normal spontaneous breathing, at the end of expiration the tendency of the lungs to collapse is balanced by the outward elastic recoil of the chest wall. The resting end-expiratory lung volume is termed the functional residual capacity (FRC). FRC is reduced in the supine position, during sedation and anaesthesia, and in critical illness. The effect of a reduced FRC depends on the state of the small dependent airways and alveoli; at some point airways will close and hypoxaemia may follow. Applying a positive pressure throughout the respiratory cycle can mitigate these effects: a positive pressure when a patient is breathing spontaneously is termed continuous positive airway pressure (CPAP), and positive end expiratory pressure (PEEP) when the patient is receiving positive pressure mechanical ventilation.

The application of PEEP is used widely in the prevention and management of hypoxaemia during mechanical ventilation, and is an important component in the 'open lung' ventilation strategy. PEEP can achieve recruitment of collapsed alveoli, but is probably best conceived as a means of preventing de-recruitment.

The application of PEEP does not only have pulmonary effects, but by raising the mean intrathoracic pressure, it may also influence cardiac function. Originally PEEP was thought to act chiefly through reductions in venous return, potentially reducing ventricular filling and cardiac output. It is now recognized that the relationships between the heart and lungs during mechanical ventilation are considerably more complex than this. Nevertheless it is important to consider that although the application of PEEP may improve the oxygen content of arterial blood, it may also have the potential to reduce oxygen delivery to the tissues by its effects on cardiac output.

Alternative ventilation modes

Inverse ratio ventilation

Inverse ratio ventilation (IRV) is the use of extended inspiratory times during mechanical ventilation so that the inspiratory period extends beyond 50% of the total cycle time. IRV can be applied in either volume (VC) or pressure control (PC) ventilatory modes; though more commonly now as PC-IRV. The rationale for the use of IRV centres on achieving and maintaining an open lung in acute lung injury (ALI)/ARDS. The concept is that in the injured lung the spectrum of alveolar time constants (slower and faster alveolar compartments) is increased. Intrinsic PEEP is generated by deliberately shortening expiratory times thereby preventing collapse of the slower alveolar compartments, and improving oxygenation. This implies using regional gas trapping to prevent alveolar collapse, with an increased risk of barotrauma. The delivery of IRV requires profound sedation and frequently the use of neuromuscular blockers. In addition the technique inevitably raises mean intrathoracic pressures with potentially adverse consequences to cardiac output; any perceived benefits to oxygenation may well be offset by consequent reductions in oxygen delivery. Overall, clinical studies have failed to demonstrate any benefit in outcomes associated with IRV.

Proportional assist ventilation

Proportional assist ventilation (PAV) is in essence an extension of PSV, but the key difference is that the operator defines the proportion of the work of breathing that the ventilator should deliver. The ventilator in real time measures compliance and resistance and then determines the amount of support to offer, proportional to the patient's effort, for a particular breath, in practice trying to solve the equation of motion rather than just control one of its variables. Measures of patient comfort and breathing pattern variability favour PAV over PSV, but in clinical trials, mainly during non-invasive ventilation, these effects did not produce any outcome benefits.

Airway pressure release ventilation

Airway pressure release ventilation (APRV) is a form of bi-level ventilation utilizing CPAP with periodic pressure releases, either to a lower CPAP pressure or to atmospheric pressure. These periodic releases provide for a tidal volume and respiratory rate enabling CO_2 clearance, while the periods of sustained CPAP produce a high mean airway pressure resulting in lung recruitment and effective oxygenation. Unrestricted spontaneous breathing throughout the ventilator cycling also enables CO_2 clearance. Advantages claimed over conventional ventilation include superior lung recruitment, higher mean airway pressure but lower peak airway pressure, superior haemodynamic and renal/splanchnic perfusion, and the patient's ability to breathe spontaneously from the time of intubation to the point of extubation. Protagonists suggest a theoretically lower risk of biotrauma and accelerated weaning, but these claims remain unproven. Currently in the UK, APRV is typically used as a rescue technique for those failing to achieve adequate oxygenation with conventional ventilation. Its safe application requires considerable knowledge and skill as ventilator adjustments may seem counter-intuitive.

There is currently insufficient evidence supporting the use of any particular mode of ventilation over another in the critically ill. To date there is no conclusive evidence to suggest any mode of ventilation will improve patient centred outcomes such as mortality or physiological outcomes such as gas exchange or work of breathing.

Practical aspects of mechanical ventilation

Intubation

The provision of invasive positive pressure mechanical ventilation requires a sealed connection between the ventilator and the patient's airway, usually via an endotracheal tube or a tracheostomy tube. Complications of intubation can occur not only at the time of intubation, but also while the patient remains intubated and following extubation.

Tracheal intubation is a hazardous procedure even when undertaken electively, but is particularly so for the critically ill (see Chapter 2). Anaesthetic drugs in general depress cardiovascular function and their administration often results in hypotension; neuromuscular paralysis removes laryngeal reflexes that would normally protect against aspiration. Even when pre-oxygenation has been meticulously provided rapid desaturation is often encountered, all in the presence of an already unstable patient.

Tracheal intubation in the critically ill may not be technically straightforward and often needs to be undertaken in a suboptimal setting, where skilled support and specialized equipment might not be available. Rapid sequence induction is typically used to minimize some of these risks, but it is important to remember that the risks of precipitating life-threatening hyperkalaemia when using suxamethonium are considerably increased in the critically ill.

Endotracheal tubes

The internal diameter of an endotracheal tube is an important determinant of resistance to airflow and in general, larger diameter tubes are preferable to smaller ones. Good nursing care is needed to ensure endotracheal tubes remain clear of secretions not only to prevent sudden occlusion but also to keep tube-associated resistance to airflow at a minimum. The position of the endotracheal tube within the airway requires considerable vigilance; the effect of body heat is often to soften the tubes allowing them to kink and occlude. Tube displacement is also possible, either with the cuff migrating above the vocal cords with its associated risks of loss of the airway and aspiration, or the tip slipping beyond the carina resulting in endobronchial intubation.

Tracheostomy

About 10% of critically ill patients receiving mechanical ventilation undergo a tracheostomy. Most of these patients are either anticipated to require or have received ventilation for a long time. Tracheostomies are performed to avoid laryngeal and tracheal problems associated with prolonged translaryngeal intubation. Other benefits include ease of tube reinsertion, improved secretion removal, patient comfort and tolerance. Disadvantages include perioperative complications, long-term airway injury and higher cost. Controversy remains as to what is the optimal time to perform the procedure, whether to employ a surgical or percutaneous technique, and whether it does in fact facilitate weaning.

Humidification

Maintaining adequate humidification of the bronchial tree is very important, not only for mucosal integrity, but also for adequate mucus transport. In health, the upper airway conditions the inspired gas very effectively. During invasive mechanical ventilation the upper airway is bypassed and the gas sources used by mechanical ventilators can be very dry. To overcome this two different approaches are commonly used: active humidification of the ventilator delivered gases, and the use of a heat and moisture exchange unit (HME) within the ventilator circuit. HMEs are simpler and are now widely used; they avoid the potential risks of infection associated with humidifier use and have been shown to have similar efficacy.

Sedation

Patients undergoing mechanical ventilation usually require some form of sedation and analgesia to maintain an acceptable level of comfort and safety. The level of sedation required varies with the patient's clinical state and the type of ventilatory support they require. Regular review of the goals of sedation and the levels achieved are very important so that the minimal amount of sedation required is used. Over-sedation will delay weaning and prolong ventilation days and ICU length of stay. Typical sedation regimens consist of a benzodiazepine and opiate administered intravenously when ventilation is likely to continue for more than a few hours, or continuous infusions of shorter-acting anaesthetic agents (such as propofol) or the use of volatile anaesthetic agents where more rapid awakening is desirable.

Thromboprophylaxis

Relatively immobile patients receiving mechanical ventilation in ICUs are at increased risk of thromboembolic events, and thromboprophylaxis should be carefully considered for each individual. Low-molecular-weight heparin is used for its effectiveness and a lower incidence of heparin-induced thrombocytopenia compared to unfractionated heparin. Mechanical methods of deep vein thromboprophylaxis such as thromboembolic stockings and calf compression devices should also be considered.

Gastric protection

Historically, diffuse gastrointestinal mucosal injury and bleeding used to frequently occur in mechanically ventilated patients. The practice of establishing early enteral feeding has dramatically reduced the incidence of this problem. Where feeding can be established early, ongoing gastric prophylaxis is not indicated unless there are other risk factors such as a history of active peptic ulceration or oesophagitis, spinal cord injury, and for those receiving non-steroidal anti-inflammatory drugs (NSAIDs). For those for whom enteral feeding cannot be established and other at-risk groups, gastric protection should probably continue for at least the duration of mechanical ventilation. There is still considerable debate regarding which is the optimal prophylactic regime for critically ill patients. Acid-suppressive treatment with either proton pump inhibitors or H_2 antagonists is commonly used but their use is associated with an increased risk of ventilator-associated pneumonia.

Complications of mechanical ventilation

Haemodynamic effects

Positive pressure ventilation can decrease venous return and right ventricular ejection through its effects on the pulmonary vascular tree, resulting in a decreased cardiac output. Mean airway pressure rather than peak airway pressure, or the level of PEEP, is likely to be the most important determinant of this effect. The intermittent decrease in venous filling associated with the positive pressures during breath delivery produces a variation in system arterial pressures, typically producing pulse pressure variation. The magnitude of this effect will depend not only on the respiratory mechanics, but also on the haemodynamic state of the patient. If signs of decreased peripheral perfusion occur with mechanical ventilation, intravenous fluids should be given until the pressure variations are minimized or intracardiac filling is shown to be adequate.

Ventilator-induced lung injury

The potential for mechanical ventilation to affect the lung adversely has long been recognized. The injuries that result from mechanical ventilation can be divided into those that are radiologically visible and those that are not. Injury is thought to result from high transpulmonary pressures, overdistension of lung units and shear forces being applied to alveoli. Air leaks, manifested by the presence of extra-alveolar air (pneumothorax, surgical emphysema pneumomediastinum, pneumopericardium, intra-abdominal air) are the most common radiologically detectable lung injuries; they were initially considered to be caused by high airway pressure and were collectively termed barotrauma. With greater understanding of likely mechanisms, the term volutrauma has now been coined, reflecting the fact that air leaks usually result from the effects of regional overdistension of relatively compliant lung units embedded in a dyshomogeneously non-compliant lung. The term atelectrauma has also been proposed to describe lung injury thought to follow repeated cyclical episodes of regional atelectasis.

Microscopic ventilator-induced lung injuries are probably very common. Considerable interest has recently focussed on them as it is thought that they might contribute to the systemic inflammatory response, potentially leading to multiple organ dysfunction and a higher mortality. It has been suggested that the process of mechanically ventilating the lung can result in the release of proinflammatory mediators which can trigger or contribute to the inflammatory cascade. The mechanisms proposed include pressure, volume and shear stresses acting through changes in epithelial and microvascular permeability plus cytokine release.

The recognition of the potential importance of ventilator-induced lung injury (VILI) in the pathogenesis of ALI/ARDS and the systemic inflammatory response syndrome has been very important in the development of the concept of lung protective ventilation.

Ventilator-associated pneumonia

There is no universal definition of ventilator-associated pneumonia (VAP), but it is often defined as pneumonia that develops 48 hours or more after intubation with an endotracheal or tracheostomy tube, and that was not present before intubation. The quoted incidence of VAP ranges from around 9% to 50% of mechanically ventilated patients, with duration of ventilation, presence of a tracheostomy and case mix being important determinants of risk. It is now thought that VAP accounts for around 80% of all nosocomial pneumonias and that an artificial airway is associated with a 21-fold increased risk of developing pneumonia. Patients who develop VAP are at risk of serious complications and have a significantly longer duration of mechanical ventilation and ICU stay. Data from the USA indicate that the mortality rate of patients who have developed VAP is between 38% and 50%, although the true attributable risk of VAP is not clear.

It is thought that VAP is initiated by colonization of the upper respiratory tract with potentially pathogenic bacteria and that secretions contaminated by these bacteria are aspirated into the lungs around the cuff of the endotracheal tube (Fig. 27.4). If the lung's antibacterial defences are unsuccessful, pneumonia may develop.

A care bundle approach has been recommended to try to reduce the magnitude of this problem. Elements of the care bundle include elevation of the head of the bed to 30–45°, sedation holding/review, avoidance of gastric acid suppression therapy where possible, appropriate ventilator tubing management, suctioning of respiratory secretions and routine oral hygiene. Other interventions including the use of selective digestive tract decontamination (SDD) and subglottic drainage of secretions have been proposed but remain controversial. A multidisciplinary approach involving microbiologists and physiotherapists should be employed in patient management (Fig. 27.5).

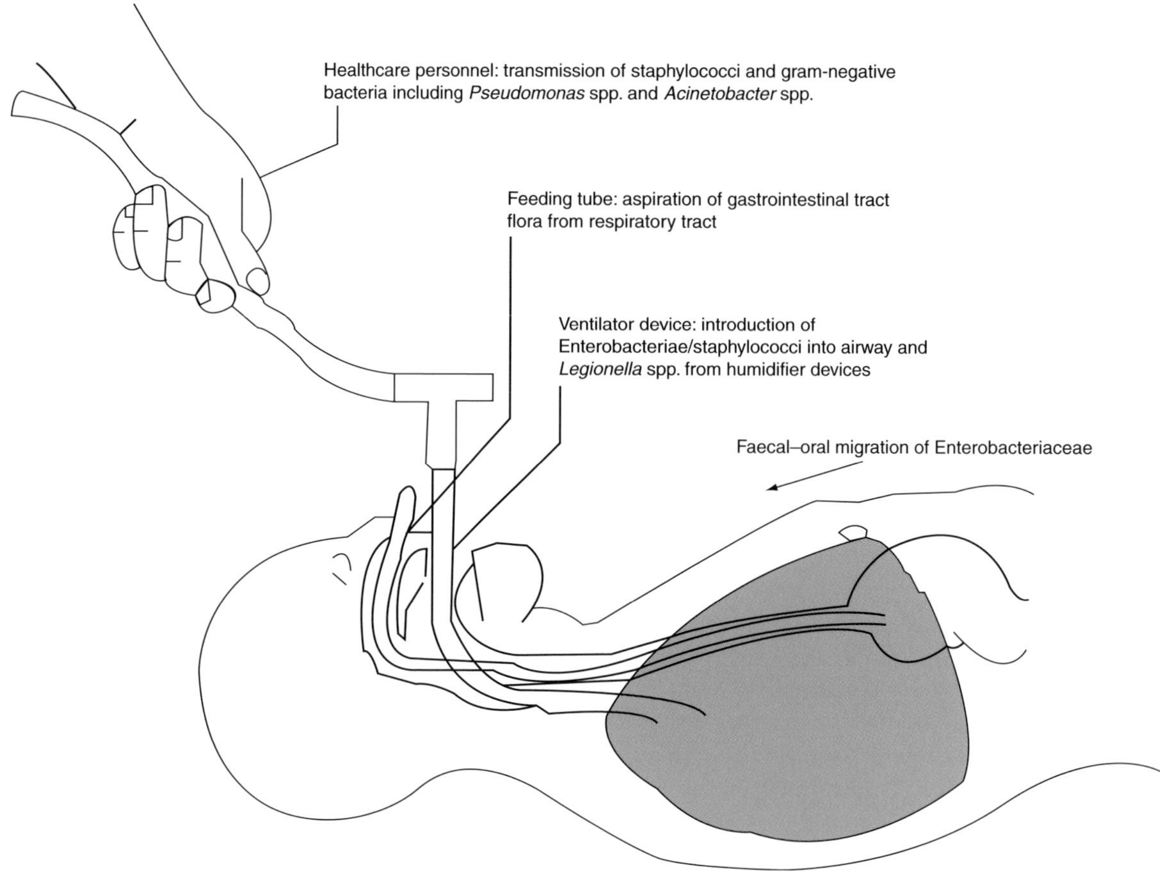

Fig. 27.4 Possible routes of infection for ventilator-associated pneumonia.

Ventilatory strategies for specific conditions

Appropriate goal setting is vitally important in determining a ventilatory strategy for each individual patient. While ventilation can be life-saving, it is at best a supportive intervention, and it carries significant risks. If mechanical ventilation is initiated, it should be continued for as short a period as possible in a way that is least likely to cause harm. While short-term improvements in arterial blood gas parameters can often be achieved by making adjustments to the ventilator, these short-term gains are often at the expense of lung injury.

Acute lung injury/acute respiratory distress syndrome

In ALI and early ARDS, pulmonary membrane permeability is critically increased as a result of an acute systemic inflammatory response, resulting in non-cardiogenic pulmonary oedema. Under the influence of gravity, dependent lung regions become compressed and the surface area for gas exchange is reduced, typically resulting in severe impairment of oxygenation. Gas exchange is still maintained in the non-dependent areas of the lung although these may become damaged through the effects of overdistension through mechanical ventilation, due to the dyshomogeneity of the condition.

The key principles are:

- The 'open lung approach'. PEEP should be applied with the aim of reducing repeated recruitment–de-recruitment in partially consolidated areas avoiding their exposure to shear stress and minimizing biotrauma. In addition, the use of PEEP may enable lower inspired oxygen concentrations, hopefully reducing the likelihood of oxygen toxicity. How best to select the optimal

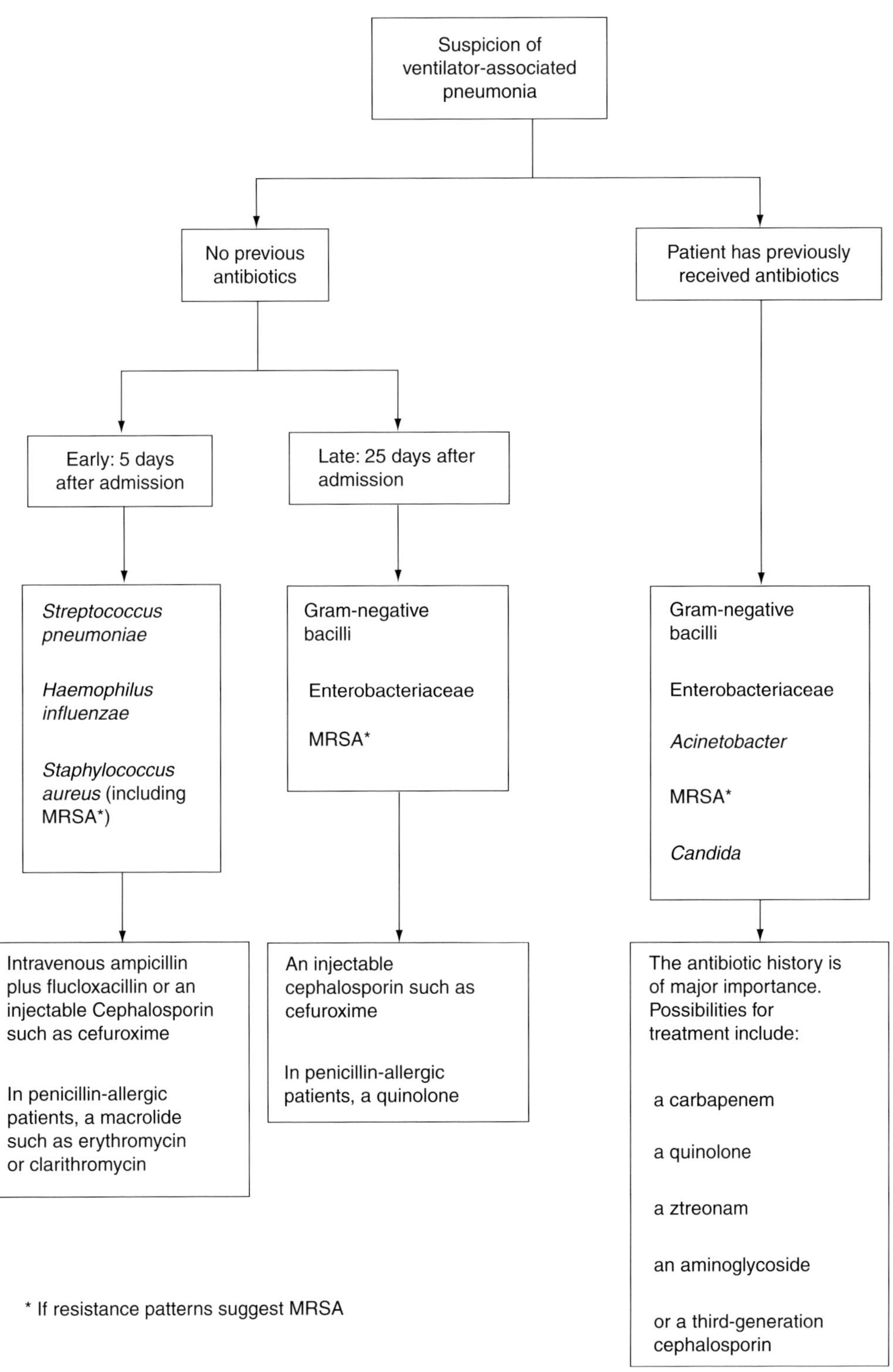

Fig. 27.5 A sample treatment algorithm for ventilator-associated pneumonia.

level of PEEP is hotly debated, the pragmatic fixed table approach adopted in the ARDSnet study is attractive because of its simplicity, but may be suboptimal.

- Limit airway pressure and tidal volume. Transpulmonary pressures should be kept as low as is feasible; this corresponds to a maximum plateau airway pressure target of <35 cm H_2O. In ARDS the consequence is a need to reduce tidal volumes to avoid high inflation pressures and minimize regional alveolar overdistension. Tidal volumes of 6–8 ml/kg lean body weight are now recommended. The consequence might well be hypercapnia, and this can be managed in part by increasing breath frequency up to a maximum of 25 breaths/min.
- Permissive hypercapnia. Accepting high $PaCO_2$ values allows overall minute ventilation targets to be considerably reduced. This technique has been shown to be very well tolerated. The magnitude of the resultant respiratory acidosis should guide interventions, with target pH values of between 7.2 and 7.3.
- Encourage spontaneous breathing as early as possible.

Chronic obstructive pulmonary disease

In COPD, decompensation is usually accompanied by dynamic hyperinflation and respiratory muscle fatigue, resulting in impairment of pulmonary gas exchange. The insult producing decompensation may be relatively slight, but in the presence of very little respiratory reserve can have life-threatening consequences.

The key principles are:

- Non-invasive ventilation should be considered as first line management in all patients with acute respiratory decompensation consequent on an exacerbation of COPD unless there is a compelling reason to intubate.
- The decision to offer invasive ventilatory support in the presence of chronic respiratory disability requires very careful judgement.
- Minimize dynamic hyperinflation. Aggressive medical management, using controlled mechanical ventilation initially accepting low minute ventilation targets with resultant hypercapnia and avoiding PEEP, and increasing expiratory times will reduce dynamic hyperinflation.
- Early return to spontaneous breathing where possible. Here patient–ventilator interactions become important, low trigger sensitivities and the application of modest external PEEP is likely to be of value. Inspiratory flows must be able to meet the patient's flow demands.
- Consider elective extubation on to non-invasive ventilation as an aid to weaning. If not, early percutaneous tracheostomy may be of benefit to weaning.

Acute asthma

As with COPD, decompensation in acute severe asthma is characterized by dynamic hyperinflation, respiratory muscle fatigue and impaired gas exchange. In general, the patient's respiratory reserve is often greater than that of a patient with COPD, so the insult producing decompensation is often disproportionately larger.

The key principles are:

- Mechanical ventilation in acute severe asthma is exceptionally hazardous and hypercapnia per se is not an indication for intubation. Absolute indications include coma, apnoea, cardiac arrest and severe hypoxaemia despite high FiO_2.
- Minimize dynamic hyperinflation. Aggressive medical management, using controlled mechanical ventilation initially accepting low minute ventilation targets with resultant hypercapnia and avoiding PEEP, and increasing expiratory times will reduce dynamic hyperinflation.
- In the context of cardiac arrest, permissive hypercapnia is relatively contraindicated unless intracranial pressure measurements are available. Extracorporeal CO_2 clearance and/or extracorporeal membrane oxygenation (ECMO) (see Chapter 32: Unconventional strategies for respiratory support) should be considered under these circumstances.
- Early return to spontaneous breathing where possible. Here patient–ventilator interactions become important, and low trigger sensitivities and the application of modest external PEEP is likely to be of value. Inspiratory flows must be able to meet the patient's flow demands.

- Volatile anaesthetic agents should be considered if bronchospasm is poorly responsive to standard treatments.

Brain injury

Mechanical ventilation in brain injury poses significant challenges. Hypoxia is the second most important cause of mortality and morbidity following traumatic brain injury. In addition, secondary brain injury in patients with raised intracranial pressure may occur consequent on episodes of hypoxia, hypercapnia or hypotension.

The key principles are:

- In the emergency situation, clearing the airway, providing oxygenation and adequate ventilation must be achieved without delay.
- Intubation can be hazardous. Head injuries are often accompanied by cervical spine injuries. In suspected or proven cervical spine-injured patients, manual in-line axial stabilization with the cervical collar removed is regarded as the safest approach.
- Ensure that targets of normocarbia and normoxia are achieved. The application of PEEP is considered potentially problematic in patients with raised intracranial pressure. When patients require PEEP to achieve adequate arterial oxygenation, monitoring of intracranial pressure and cerebral perfusion pressure is recommended.

Key points

- Mechanical ventilation can be a life-saving intervention; however, it carries many risks.
- Ventilatory goals should be set for each patient to reduce the potential for harm while maximizing the benefits of ventilation.
- A care bundle approach for the care of the ventilated patient should include thromboprophylaxis, gastric protection and evaluation of sedation status.

Further reading

- Davidson C, Treacher D (eds.) (2002) *Respiratory Critical Care*. London: Arnold.
- Esteban A, Anzueto A, Cook D (2005) *Evidence-Based Management of Patients with Respiratory Failure: Updates in Intensive Care Medicine*. Berlin: Springer-Verlag.
- Hedenstierna G (1998) *Respiratory Measurement*. London: BMJ Books.
- Mackenzie I (ed.) (2008) *Core Topics in Mechanical Ventilation*. Cambridge: Cambridge University Press.
- Mancebo JM, Net A, Brochard L (2003) *Mechanical Ventilation and Weaning: Updates in Intensive Care Medicine*. Berlin: Springer-Verlag.
- Tobin MJ (ed.)(2006) *Principles and Practice of Mechanical Ventilation*. New York: McGraw-Hill.

Failure of ventilation

Darshan Pandit and Joyce Yeung

Introduction

Ventilation concerns the process of taking in oxygen from inhaled air and releasing carbon dioxide by exhalation. This chapter will begin with an overview of lung volumes, and the control of ventilation, and then discuss common disorders of ventilation.

Lung volumes and capacities

Static lung volumes are measured by spirometer. The sum of two or more lung volume subdivisions constitutes a lung capacity (Fig. 28.1).

Tidal volume (VT) is the volume of air that is inhaled or exhaled with each cycle in normal respiration. It is normally 350–500 ml or 5–7 ml/kg but can vary with the conditions, for example at rest, during exercise or change in posture. When a person takes a maximal inspiration followed by maximal expiration, the exhaled volume is called vital capacity (VC). But not all gas can be exhaled and the remaining gas is termed residual volume (RV). The volume of gas in the lung after a normal expiration is called functional residual capacity (FRC). It is equal to the sum of VT and ERV. The functional residual capacity is the combination of expiratory reserve volume and residual volumes.

Inspiratory reserve volume (IRV) is the maximal volume of air that can be inhaled. Expiratory reserve volume (ERV) is the maximal volume of air that can be exhaled after a normal tidal exhalation.

Total lung capacity (TLC) is the volume of air in the lung at the end of a maximal inspiration. It is usually calculated by the sum of RV and VC. It cannot be measured directly but by gas dilution or body plethysmography. Total lung capacity when expanded by voluntary effort is 5–6 litres in the average adult.

Principles of control of respiration

There are three parts of the respiratory control system: (1) sensors, (2) central control and (3) respiratory muscles.

Sensors

Sensors gather information and feed it to the brainstem and cortex. There are two types of sensors:

(1) Central receptors are present on the ventral surface of the medulla surrounded by brain extracellular fluid and respond to changes in H^+ ion concentration (increase in H ions stimulates ventilation and decrease inhibits it). These receptors are involved in the minute-by-minute control of ventilation.

(2) Peripheral chemoreceptors are located in the carotid bodies in the bifurcation of the common carotid arteries and the aortic bodies above and below the aortic arch. These receptors respond to fall in arterial pH and are mainly responsible for respiratory compensation in patients with metabolic acid. They also respond to increases or decreases in arterial PO_2.

Central control

Neurons in the pons and medulla are divided into three respiratory centres:

(1) The medullary respiratory centre located in the reticular formation of the medulla beneath the floor of the fourth ventricle, divided further into the dorsal (controls inspiration) and ventral (controls expiration) respiratory centres.

(2) The apneustic centre in the lower pons – role unclear.

Core Topics in Critical Care Medicine, eds. Fang Gao Smith and Joyce Yeung. Published by Cambridge University Press.

(3) The pneumotaxic centre in the upper pons regulates volume and rate of inspiration by its ability to switch off inspiration.

Respiratory muscles

In inspiration, the main respiratory muscle is the diaphragm and it is controlled by the phrenic nerves originating in the cervical segments 3, 4 and 5. When the diaphragm contracts, the abdominal contents are forced downwards and chest cavity expands. External intercostal muscles pull ribs upward and outwards and increase the diameter of the chest cavity during inspiration.

Expiration, on the other hand, is mainly passive and relies on elastic recoil of the lungs and chest wall, and relaxation of the diaphragm (Fig. 28.2).

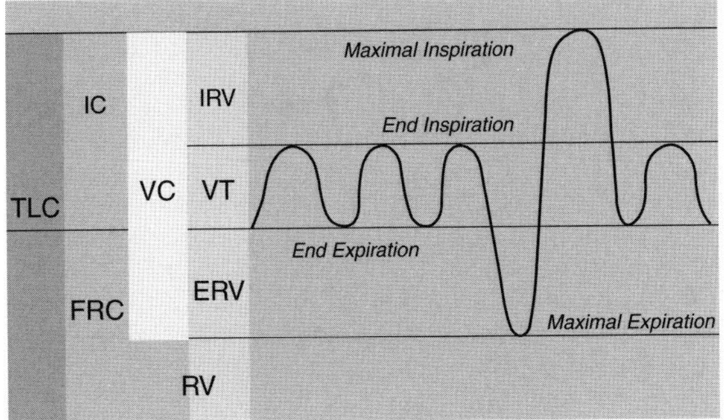

Fig. 28.1 Diagram illustrating lung volume and capacities. TLC, total lung capacity; IC, inspiratory capacity; FRC, functional residual capacity; IRV, inspiratory reserve volume; VC, vital capacity; VT, tidal volume; ERV, expiratory reserve volume; RV, residual volume.

Monitoring pulmonary function

Spirometry

Spirometry assesses the mechanical properties of the respiratory system by measuring expiratory volumes and flow rates. This test requires the patient to make a maximal inspiratory and expiratory effort and needs to be repeated to ensure reproducibility of results and it has no place in the critical care setting.

Flow volume loop

Many modern ventilators can display the flow volume loop which can provide a graphical real-time illustration of a patient's spirometric efforts. Flow is plotted

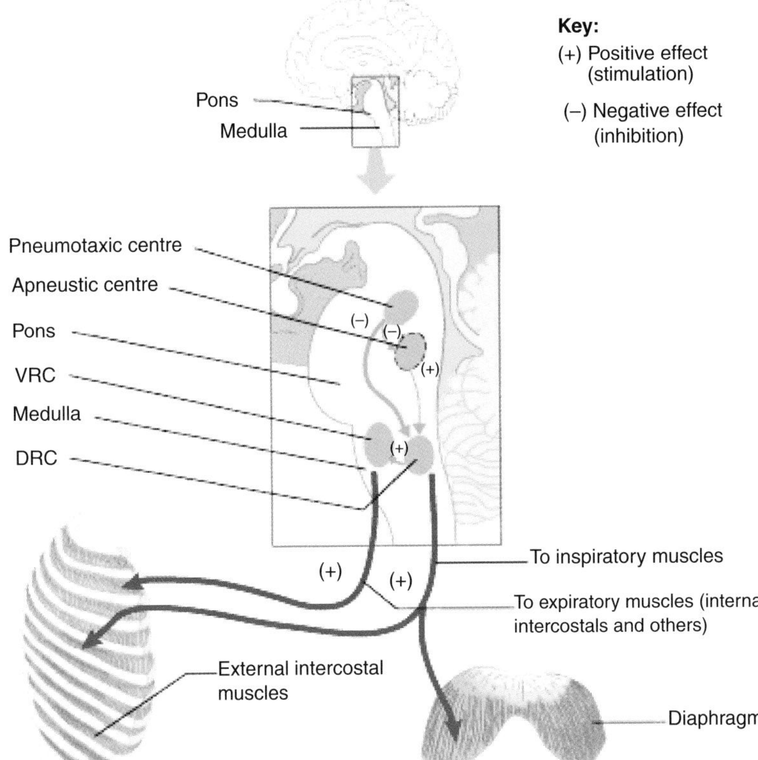

Fig. 28.2 Schematic diagram illustrating the control of respiration. VRC, ventral respiratory centre; DRC, dorsal respiratory centre.

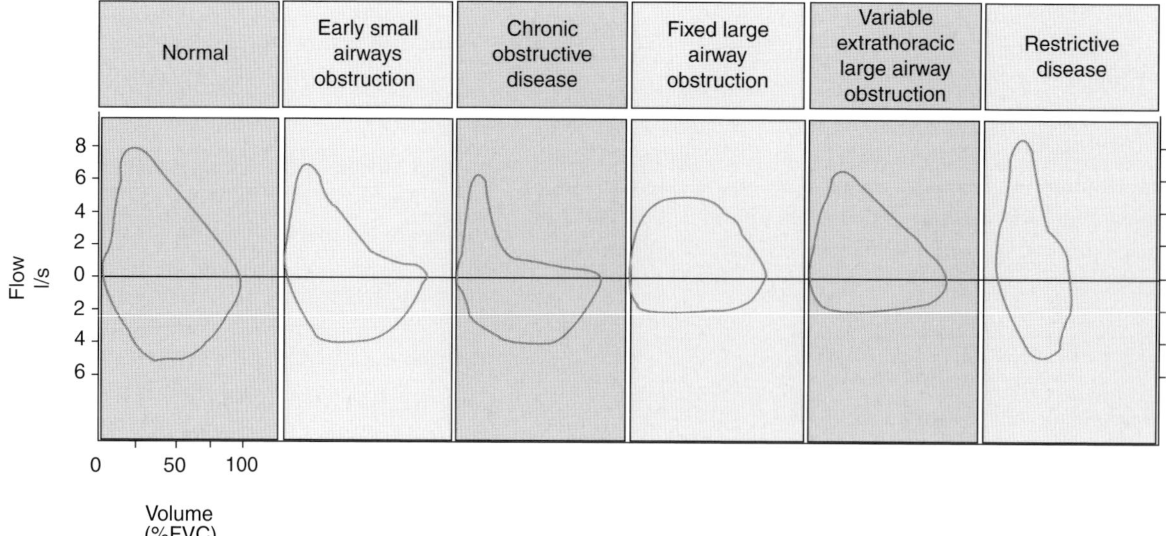

Fig. 28.3 Examples of flow volume loop.

against volume to display a dynamic loop from inspiration to expiration. The overall shape of the flow volume loop is important in interpreting results. In restrictive lung diseases, the maximum flow rate and the total volume are both reduced. The flow is abnormally high in the latter part of expiration because of increased recoil leading to a tall and narrow loop. In obstructive airway diseases, the flow rate is low in relation to lung volume, resulting in a scooped-out appearance of the loop (Fig. 28.3).

Other assessments of lung mechanics and neuromuscular function are discussed in detail in Chapter 30: Respiratory weaning.

Alveolar ventilation

At rest alveolar ventilation is adjusted to maintain PCO_2 close to 5.3 kPa. Arterial PCO_2 depends mainly on the minute ventilation whereas arterial PO_2 depends on the efficiency of ventilation/perfusion matching.

Alveolar ventilation is the volume of air passing in and out of the alveoli each minute and dead space is the volume of inspired air that does not reach the alveoli where the gas exchange is taking place (see Chapter 29).

$$\begin{aligned}\text{Alveolar ventilation} &= \text{frequency of breathing} \\ &\quad \times \text{alveolar volume} \\ &= \text{frequency of breathing} \\ &\quad \times (\text{tidal volume} - \text{dead space})\end{aligned}$$

Alveolar concentration of CO_2 and hence the arterial PCO_2 is proportional to the rate of production of CO_2 and is inversely proportional to alveolar ventilation. In reality a raised PCO_2 is caused by underventilation and only occasionally does increased production of PCO_2 contribute.

Disorders of ventilation

Hypoventilation

Hypoventilation syndromes are divided into (1) acute hypoventilation, which is a life-threatening emergency, and (2) chronic hypoventilation which involves a defect in either in the metabolic respiratory control, the respiratory neuromuscular system or the ventilatory apparatus (Table 28.1).

Pathophysiology

The key component of all hypoventilation syndromes is an increase in alveolar PCO_2 and a rise in arterial PCO_2 causing respiratory acidosis. This then leads to a compensatory rise in plasma bicarbonate and a decrease in chloride concentration. In turn this will result in a decrease in PaO_2 causing hypoxaemia which if severe can manifest as cyanosis. If this hypoxia becomes chronic, it can cause pulmonary hypertension and congestive cardiac failure.

Table 28.1 Causes of hypoventilation

Mechanism	Disorder
Central causes/ impaired respiratory drive	Prolonged hypoxia Carotid body dysfunction Brainstem causes (encephalitis, demyelination, infarction, drugs, primary hypoventilation syndrome)
Defective neuromuscular system	Spinal cord and peripheral nerves (high cervical lesion, motor neuron disease) Respiratory muscles (myasthenia gravis, muscular dystrophies)
Impaired ventilatory apparatus	Chest wall (kyphoscoliosis, ankylosing spondylitis, obesity hypoventilation) Airway and lungs (upper airway obstruction, tracheal stenosis, obstructive sleep apnoea, chronic obstructive airways disease, cystic fibrosis, asthma)

Clinical features

The clinical features of chronic hypercapnia result from cerebral vasodilatation causing morning headaches, poor sleep quality, morning fatigue, daytime sleepiness and intellectual impairment.

Diagnosis

Central causes

- Sleep studies would show evidence of central apnoeas.
- As the neuromuscular system and ventilatory apparatus are normal, patients will hyperventilate normally and generate normal inspiratory and expiratory pressures against an occluded airway and have normal lung volumes on spirometry.
- Response to chemical stimuli is impaired.
- Alveolar–arterial gradient (A–a gradient) is normal.

Defects in neuromuscular system

- Patients are unable to hyperventilate voluntarily.
- Patients are unable to generate normal static respiratory muscle pressures, lung volumes or flow rates.
- Impaired responses to chemical stimuli may be present.
- In early stages, compliance and resistance of the respiratory system and A–a gradient will be normal.

Impaired ventilator apparatus

- Abnormal resistance and compliance.
- Wide A–a gradient.
- Abnormal spirometry (restrictive defect).

Hypoventilation syndromes

There are three main types of hypoventilation syndromes: (1) obesity hypoventilation syndrome, (2) respiratory neuromuscular disorders and (3) primary alveolar hypoventilation.

Obesity hypoventilation syndrome

In obese patients, there is increased mechanical load to the rib cage by the abdomen, reducing the compliance of the chest wall and functional residual capacity. Breathing at lower lung volumes leads to collapse and underventilation of the lung bases and tidal volumes may encroach on closing volumes, widening the A–a gradient.

Most obese patients have sufficient respiratory drive to maintain a normal $PaCO_2$. Only a small proportion of obese patients develop hypoxaemia, chronic hypercapnia, pulmonary hypertension and right-sided heart failure. Most patients present to sleep clinics and are started on nocturnal non-invasive ventilation (NIV) but they could present with acute Type 2 respiratory failure requiring short-term NIV. Treatment should focus on weight reduction, smoking cessation and NIV during sleep to improve daytime sleepiness. Supplemental oxygen may be needed to achieve appropriate oxygenation.

Respiratory neuromuscular disorders

These disorders are related to spinal cord, peripheral respiratory nerves and respiratory muscles. These conditions could present insidiously over months or years or acutely if a sudden extra stress such as airway obstruction occurs. It could also present as late feature in conditions like motor neuron disease, myasthenia gravis or muscular dystrophies.

Clinical features become apparent when diaphragmatic weakness develops and paradoxical movement of the diaphragm and orthopnoea ensue. Treatment should include treating or optimizing the underlying condition and assessment for long-term mechanical ventilation via a tracheostomy.

Primary alveolar hypoventilation

Primary alveolar hypoventilation is a defect characterized by hypoxaemia, chronic hypercapnia and respiratory acidosis. Blood gas analysis will reveal a raised bicarbonate as carbon dioxide can be normal during daytime or if the patient voluntarily hyperventilates. Diagnosis is confirmed once neuromuscular dysfunction or disorders of ventilatory apparatus have been excluded. The defect is then postulated to be in the metabolic respiratory control system.

The condition occurs at all ages but mainly has been reported in men aged between 20 and 50 years old. It is often brought to attention when there is severe respiratory depression after administration of standard doses of sedatives or general anaesthetic agents.

Hyperventilation syndromes

Alveolar hyperventilation exists when $PaCO_2$ decreases below 4.5 kPa. It is not the same as hyperpnoea which is increased minute ventilation with a normal $PaCO_2$.

Pathophysiology

The underlying mechanism is an increase in the respiratory drive which can be due to disorder in the metabolic or behavioural respiratory control systems. Possible causes are:

- Hypoxaemia drives ventilation by stimulating the peripheral chemoreceptors (Fig. 28.4).
- Metabolic acidosis increases the sensitivity of peripheral chemoreceptors to coexistent hypoxaemia (Fig. 28.5).
- Low cardiac output and hypotension stimulate the peripheral chemoreceptors and inhibit baroreceptors resulting in an increase in ventilation.
- Hepatic failure produces hyperventilation by metabolic stimuli acting on peripheral and central chemoreceptors.
- Progesterone in pregnancy causes hyperventilation by acting on the respiratory neurons.
- Neurological and psychological disorders can drive ventilation through the behavioural respiratory control system such as anxiety, severe cerebrovascular insufficiency.

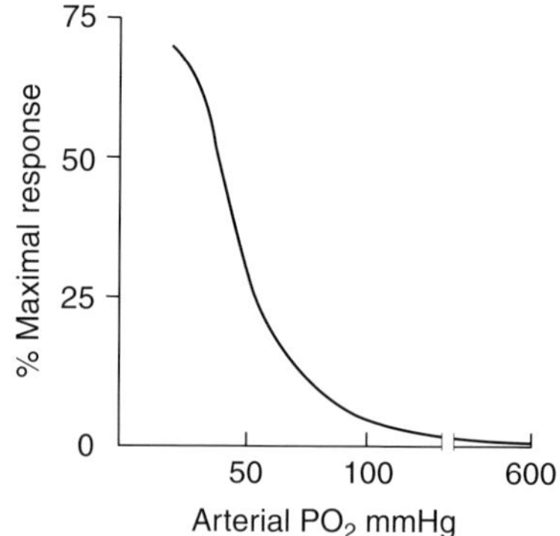

Fig. 28.4 Chemoreceptor responses to arterial PO_2.

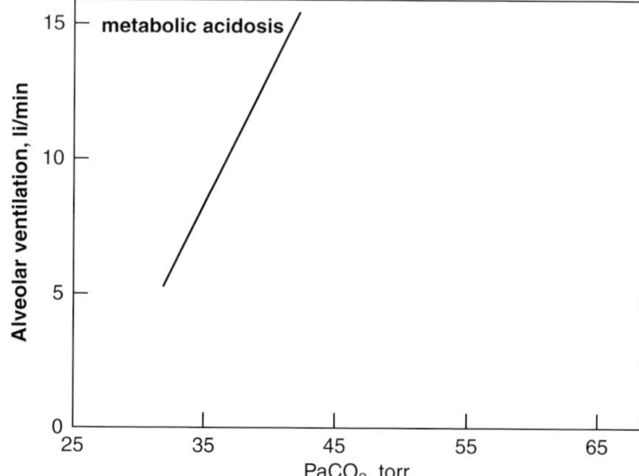

Fig. 28.5 Effects of metabolic acidosis on alveolar ventilation.

- Drugs such as salicylates, β-agonists or aminophylline can cause hyperventilation by stimulating the central and peripheral chemoreceptors or by direct action on the respiratory neurons.

Diagnosis

Detailed history and clinical examination along with knowledge of coexistent disorders can provide clues to the cause of hyperventilation.

Investigations should begin with a blood gas analysis:

- $PaCO_2$ is decreased in alveolar hyperventilation.
- An elevated pH is suggestive of a primary respiratory alkalosis; a low pH will show a metabolic acidosis.
- Widened A–a gradient suggests presence of a primary pulmonary disorder.
- Low bicarbonate suggests a chronic nature of the disorder and implies an organic cause.

- Transcutaneous PCO_2 or arterial PCO_2 during sleep studies can help to exclude psychogenic hyperventilation, as hyperventilation cannot be maintained during sleep.

Treatment

Treatment of the underlying cause is essential.

Key points

- Static lung volumes are unhelpful in the critical care setting. Dynamic measurements such as flow volume loop are more useful in identifying abnormal pulmonary physiology.
- Chemoreceptors act as sensors to gather information regarding ventilation and send signals to respiratory control centre in the medulla. Changes in oxygenation and acid–base balance will result in changes in respiration.
- Arterial PCO_2 quantifies ventilation.
- There are three main causes of hypoventilation: defect in the metabolic respiratory control, the respiratory neuromuscular system or the ventilatory apparatus.
- Alveolar hyperventilation exists when $PaCO_2$ decreases below 4.5 kPa. The main cause is an increase in the respiratory drive.

Further reading

- Dakin J, Kourteli E, Winter J (2003) *Making Sense of Lung Function Tests*. Oxford: Oxford University Press.
- Philipson EA (2005) Disorders of ventilation. In *Harrison's Principles of Internal Medicine*, 17th edn, eds. Fauci A, Braunwald E, Kaspar DL *et al.* New York: McGraw-Hill, pp. 1569–75.
- West JB (2001) *Pulmonary Physiology and Pathophysiology: The Essentials*. Baltimore, MD: Lippincott Williams & Wilkins.

Failure of oxygenation

Darshan Pandit and Joyce Yeung

Introduction

Oxygen is vital to life and its role in the metabolic process should be remembered when considering its importance in monitoring critically ill patients. Most cellular activities require energy in the form of oxygen primarily obtained from the degradation of adenosine triphosphate (ATP) and other high-energy compounds. Oxygen has to be present to maintain adequate concentrations of ATP by the electron transport system. If oxygen availability is reduced cellular oxygen consumption will fall leading initially to cellular dysfunction followed by cell death and organ failure.

Oxygen cascade

Oxygen cascade describes the transfer of oxygen from inspired air, to respiratory tract, to alveolar gas, the arterial blood, capillaries and finally to the mitochondria in the cell.

Atmosphere

Air is made up of 21% oxygen, 78% nitrogen and small quantities of CO_2 and noble gases. At atmospheric pressure, the total pressure is 760 mmHg and PO_2 of dry air is $21/100 \times 760 = 159$ mmHg.

Trachea

By the time air reaches the trachea, it has been warmed and humidified by the upper respiratory tract. Water vapour exerts a pressure of 47 mmHg at 37 °C. PO_2 in trachea is $(760 - 47) \times 21/100 = 150$ mmHg.

Alveoli (PAO_2)

PO_2 is about 100 mmHg as PO_2 in alveoli (PAO_2) is a balance between the removal of oxygen by pulmonary capillaries and its own supply by alveolar ventilation.

Blood from pulmonary arteries (PaO_2)

Blood returning to heart has a low PaO_2 of about 40 mmHg. Oxygen diffuses down the gradient from the high concentration in alveoli (100 mmHg) to the lower concentration in pulmonary arterial blood (40 mmHg). Oxygenated blood will now be returned to the heart via the pulmonary veins to be circulated to the systematic system. In the perfect lung, PO_2 in pulmonary veins (PvO_2) would equal PaO_2; however, three factors can lead to a lower PvO_2: ventilation/perfusion mismatch, shunt and slow diffusion.

Mitochondria

By the time oxygen is delivered to the cellular level, PO_2 has dropped significantly due to a lengthened diffusion path. PO_2 in mitochondria is only 4–20 mmHg. This delivery of oxygen to the mitochondria of metabolically active cells also depends on an adequate circulation. Therefore adequate fluid resuscitation is important in management of critically ill patients, as opposed to fluid overload which may impair the diffusion of oxygen across the alveolar pulmonary membrane and the metabolically active cells they supply (Fig. 29.1).

Monitoring gas exchange

Pulse oximetry

The principle of pulse oximetry is based on the red and infrared light absorption characteristics of oxygenated and deoxygenated haemoglobin. Oxygenated haemoglobin absorbs more infrared light and allows more red light to pass through. Conversely, deoxygenated haemoglobin absorbs more red light and allows more infrared light to pass through. Red light is in the 600–750 nm wavelength band. Infrared light is in the 850–1000 nm wavelength band. A light emitter with red and

Core Topics in Critical Care Medicine, eds. Fang Gao Smith and Joyce Yeung. Published by Cambridge University Press.

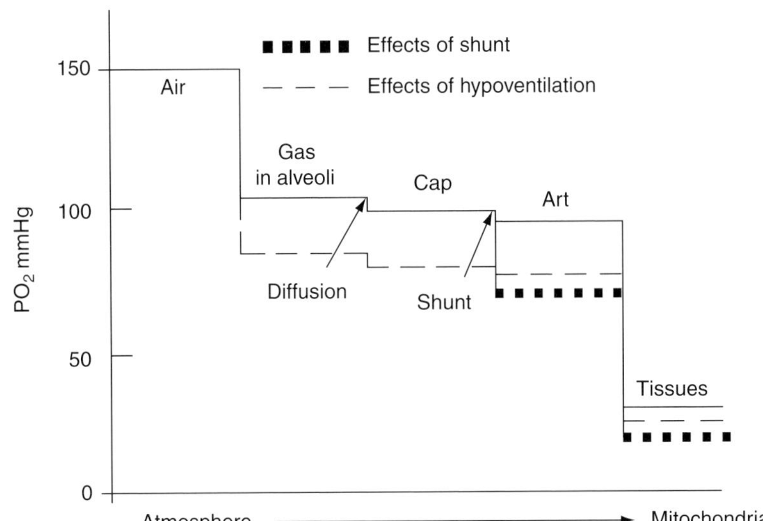

Fig. 29.1 The oxygen cascade. (With permission of *World Anaesthesia Online*, (1999) Issue 10, Article 3, The physiology of oxygen delivery.)

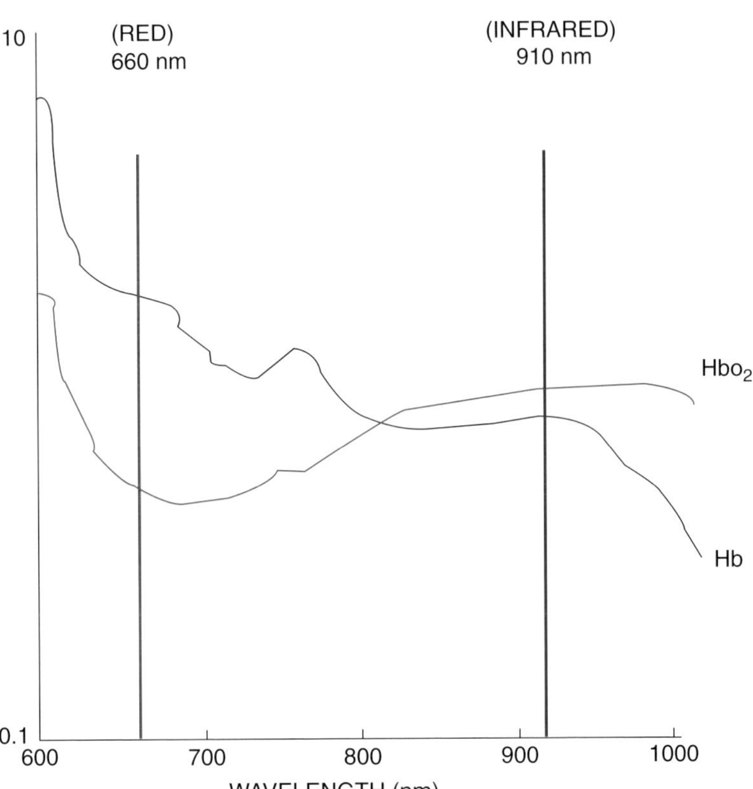

Fig. 29.2 Diagram illustrating the absorption of red and infrared light by oxygenated and deoxygenated haemoglobin.

infrared light-emitting diode (LEDs) shines through either a finger or earlobe with pulsatile blood flow. A photodetector is on the opposite side and receives the light that passes through the measuring site (Fig. 29.2).

After the transmitted red (R) and infrared (IR) signals pass through the measuring site and are received at the photodetector, the R/IR ratio is calculated. The R/IR is then compared to a table that converts the ratio to an SpO_2 value. SpO_2 is displayed as a percentage. It is averaged over 3–6 s and is updated every 0.5–1 s. The accuracy of SaO_2 can have bias of <1% in the 90–97% saturation range but suffers from

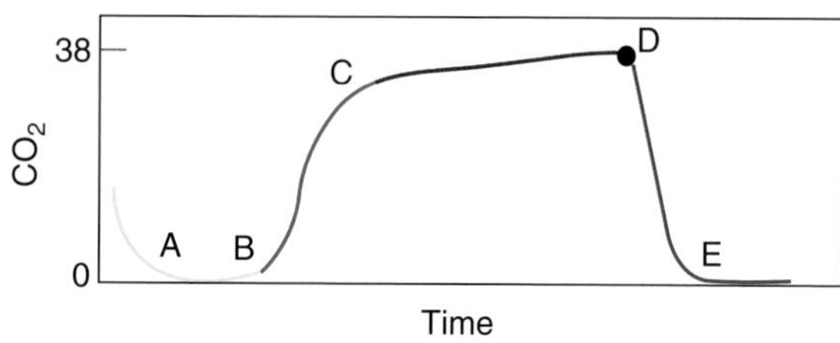

Fig. 29.3 A normal capnograph trace. Phase 1, A to B; Phase 2, B to C; Phase 3, C to D; Phase 4, D to E.

significant imprecision and tendency to a negative bias when it is less than 80%.

Causes of errors in SpO_2 readings:

- The presence of carboxyhaemoglobin and methaemoglobin may give an erroneously high reading.
- Low pulsatile signal caused by shock, arrhythmias, vasoconstriction and limb ischaemia.
- Significant venous pulsation from tricuspid regurgitation or venous congestion can give false readings.
- Dark nail polish can cause a falsely low SpO_2.
- Tremor and movement can cause interference.
- Sunlight, ambient lighting or flickering light can cause interference.

Capnography

Respiratory gases are sampled continuously and CO_2 is measured by the amount of infrared absorption in the gas sample. The capnogram is a display of CO_2 concentration (Fig. 29.3). Expired CO_2 has four phases:

Phase 1 Early part of exhaled breath which consists of mainly anatomical dead space that does not take part in gas exchange. There is negligible CO_2 normally and if there is a significant amount of CO_2 in this phase then there is rebreathing of exhaled gas.

Phase 2 Alveolar gas containing CO_2 causes a rapid increase in slope.

Phase 3 Alveolar plateau represents CO_2 concentration in mixed expired alveolar gas. There is normally a slight increase as gas exchange continues to take place. A steep slope may represent ventilation/perfusion mismatch when poorly ventilated but well-perfused alveoli empty late in the respiratory cycle. It is also seen in patients with auto positive end expiratory pressure (PEEP) and airway obstruction.

Phase 4 Inspiration begins with a rapid fall in CO_2.

Table 29.1 Normal values obtained by blood gas analysis

pH	7.35–7.45
pCO_2	4.6–6 kPa
pO_2	10–13.3 kPa (on air)
HCO_3	22–26 mmol/l
Base excess	−2 to +2
SaO_2	95–98%
SvO_2	70–75%
Lactate	<1

It is important to remember that PCO_2 only approximates $PaCO_2$ in healthy lungs due to mixing of dead space gas. In critically ill patients, end tidal CO_2 will be a poor representation of the true $PaCO_2$.

Blood gas analysis

A sample of heparinized blood is analysed by blood gas machine with three separate electrodes, measuring pH, PO_2 and PCO_2 (Table 29.1). It is useful in identifying hypoxaemia, hypercapnia and hypocapnia and allowing the ventilator setting to be adjusted accordingly. Measurements of pH and base deficit allow for monitoring of the patient's acid–base status with lactate being an indication of tissue perfusion. Mixed venous saturation can also be measured to calculate oxygen delivery and consumption. A co-oximeter where blood is haemolysed can give an accurate measurement of total haemoglobin and different fractions of COHb, deoxyHb and fetal Hb.

Blood gas analysis which measures arterial PaO_2 is accurate but errors in measurement could arise due to:

- Air bubbles in sample.
- Flush fluid contamination from arterial line.
- High white cell count could cause pseudohypoxaemia by excessive in vitro oxygen consumption.
- Inter-analyser variability could be significant with 8% measurement variation on the same sample.
- Electrode temperature maintenance is within narrow limits as PO_2 changes by 7% for every °C temperature change.

Pathophysiology of hypoxia

Hypoventilation

Hypoventilation is a reduction in the volume of gas delivered to the alveoli causing hypoxia. Alveolar hypoventilation also causes a rise in $PaCO_2$ as $PaCO_2$ is inversely proportional to alveolar ventilation:

$$PaCO_2 = (VCO_2/VA) \times K$$

where VCO_2 is CO_2 production, VA is alveolar ventilation and K is a constant.

The hypoxia of hypoventilation can be reversed by the administration of a higher inspired oxygen concentration as demonstrated by the alveolar gas equation:

$$PAO_2 = PIO_2 - (PACO_2/R)$$

where PIO_2 is the partial pressure of inspired oxygen.

Ventilation/perfusion mismatch

Ventilation/perfusion mismatch is responsible for the hypoxaemia seen in pulmonary oedema, chronic obstructive pulmonary disease, pulmonary embolism and interstitial lung disease.

Relative ventilation and perfusion are unequal in different areas of the lung, resulting in inefficient gas transfer. The distribution of blood flow through the lung is uneven due to the low pressures in the pulmonary circulation and gravity affects the distribution. In the erect patient there is greater ventilation towards the apex of the lungs than to the bases but pulmonary blood flow is greater at the bases than the apices. In the supine position, the lower dependent alveoli are preferentially ventilated and perfused. Although both perfusion and ventilation increase from the apices to the bases the increase in ventilation is less than that of perfusion. At rest, ventilation is at approximately 4 l/min and pulmonary blood flow at 5 l/min, giving an overall ratio of 0.8 throughout the whole lung.

Hypoxic pulmonary vasoconstriction (HPV) is a potent regulator of the distribution of blood flow to match areas of ventilation. HPV normally acts to improve gas exchange by reducing the blood flow to lung regions with low V/Q ratios. In sepsis and trauma, the released inflammatory mediators mean that HPV is less effective in redistribution of blood flow and results in hypoxia. Hypoxic pulmonary vasoconstriction can also be abolished in the presence of raised pulmonary artery pressures leading to V/Q mismatch and hypoxia.

Shunt

A shunt represents blood that does not come into contact with ventilated alveoli therefore remaining deoxygenated. Hypoxia is therefore not corrected by increasing oxygen as there is a lack of contact between blood and oxygen. The common causes of shunt are consolidation, pulmonary contusion, atelectasis, pulmonary oedema or extrapulmonary shunts such as congenital heart disease.

The degree of shunting may be calculated by referring to the shunt equation:

$$Q_s/Q_t = C_c - C_a/C_c - C_v$$

where Q_s and Q_t are the shunt and total blood flows, and C_c, C_a and C_v represent the oxygen concentrations of end-capillary, arterial and mixed venous blood.

Dead space

Dead space refers to the proportion of the tidal volume that does not take part in gas exchange. Dead space is divided into:

- Anatomical dead space – the volume of the conducting air passages that does not reach alveoli. It is increased by bronchodilator use.
- Alveolar dead space – the gas that reaches alveoli but does not take part in gas exchange. It is increased by ventilation/perfusion mismatch, pulmonary embolism and reduced cardiac output.

Diffusion impairment

Equilibration between alveolar gas and pulmonary capillary blood is normally fast with blood PO_2 almost reaching that in the alveolus after about one-third of the contact time of 0.75 s in the capillary. There is a large physiological window for gas exchange to take place and it only becomes a problem in disease states causing thickening of the alveolar membrane and in high cardiac output states where the contact time between the red cell and alveolar interface is reduced. Impaired diffusion between alveoli and pulmonary capillaries can be caused by inflammation and fibrosis of the alveolar membrane. The thickening of blood–gas barrier means that PO_2 in pulmonary capillary blood cannot equilibrate with alveolar gas. Common causes are cardiac failure, interstitial lung fibrosis, connective tissue diseases and emphysema. In general, this diffusion impairment can be corrected by

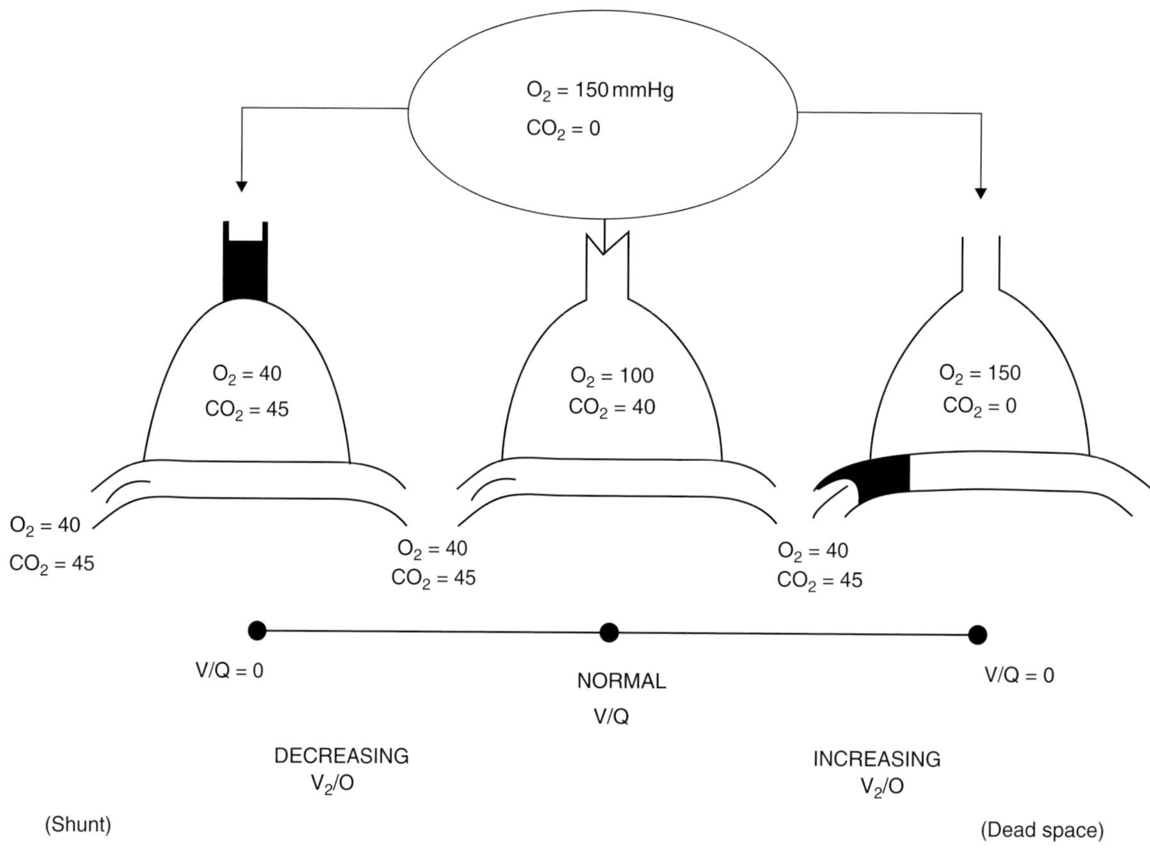

Fig. 29.4 Diagram illustrating the concept of shunt and dead space. (With permission from *World Anaesthesia Online* (1999) Issue 10, Article 3 The physiology of oxygen delivery.)

increasing FiO_2. Diffusion impairment does not affect carbon dioxide elimination. Carbon dioxide is more soluble in blood than oxygen and it is also carried in carbamino compounds and as bicarbonate ions.

Acute respiratory distress syndrome

Acute lung injury (ALI) and acute respiratory distress syndrome (ARDS) describe a spectrum of a critical illness syndrome involving severe inflammatory disease of the lung. It is characterized by the sudden onset of pulmonary oedema and respiratory failure, usually in the setting of other acute medical conditions resulting from local or distant injury. Severe sepsis is the leading cause, followed by pneumonia, aspiration, massive blood transfusion and trauma. ALI and ARDS develop within 12–72 hours after the precipitating event and often within 6 hours.

The incidence of ALI and ARDS is 86.2 and 58.7 per 100 000 person-years respectively, and they are associated with an in-hospital mortality rate estimated 38.5% for ALI and 41.1% for ARDS (Table 29.2).

Table 29.2 The causes of ARDS

Direct/local	Indirect/distant
Pneumonia	Sepsis
Aspiration	Trauma
Pulmonary contusion	Massive transfusion
Inhalational injury	Acute pancreatitis
Fat emboli	Drug overdose
Near drowning	Pregnancy-related ARDS
Reperfusion pulmonary oedema	

Source: Adapted from Ware and Matthay (2000).

Pathophysiology

ALI and ARDS develop when inflammatory cytokines cause damage to the endothelium and epithelium of the lung. These inflammatory insults can occur locally in the lung or be part of a systemic inflammatory syndrome. Irrespective of the precipitating cause, the pathophysiological mechanisms driving the process are the same and progress through phases.

Initial phase

- Severe oxygenation defect.
- Reduced lung compliance.
- Bilateral pulmonary infiltrates.
- Endothelial and epithelial cell injury.
- Leak of protein-rich fluid in interstitium.
- Abnormal surfactant/inactivation of surfactant.
- Neutrophil sequestration in lung.

Sub-acute phase

- Oxygenation defect.
- Reduced lung compliance.
- Increased alveolar dead space.
- Interstitial fibrosis with proliferation of type II alveolar cells.
- Widespread disruption of the pulmonary microcirculation.

Chronic phase

- Reduced lung compliance.
- Increase in dead space ventilation.
- Pulmonary fibrosis.
- Destruction of normal alveolar architecture.
- Emphysema and bullae.

Diagnosis

In 1994, the American–European Consensus Conference Committee proposed definitions for ALI and ARDS:

- Acute onset.
- Bilateral infiltrates on chest radiographs.
- Pulmonary artery occlusion pressure (PAOP) <18 mmHg and absence of clinical signs of left atrial hypertension.
- ARDS = PaO_2 / FiO_2 <200 mmHg (<26.7 kPa).
- ALI = PaO_2/ FiO_2 <300 mmHg (<40 kPa).

Management

Fluid Management

The goal is to use intravenous fluids and inotropes to maintain the intravascular volume at the lowest level that is consistent with adequate organ perfusion. Oxygen delivery is dependent on cardiac output:

$$\text{oxygen delivery } (DO_2) = \text{cardiac output (CO)} \times \text{Hb} \times SaO_2$$

Lung protection ventilation strategies

These strategies use smaller tidal volumes both to protect the lung from overdistension and to prevent any further release of inflammatory mediators. A higher PCO_2 and respiratory acidosis is tolerated as permissive hypercapnia. The ARDSnet conducted a randomized controlled trial to compare the use of traditional ventilation (VT of 12 ml/kg, plateau pressure $<50\,cmH_2O$) with low tidal volumes (VT 6 ml/kg, plateau pressure $<30\,cmH_2O$) in ARDS. Results showed that the lower tidal volume group has a significantly lower 28-day mortality rate, more ventilator-free days and a lower incidence of non-pulmonary organ failure. Alternative ventilation strategy with high-frequency oscillation ventilation (HFOV), liquid ventilation and extracorporeal membrane oxygenation (ECMO) have been used in patients with severe ARDS but have so far failed to demonstrate any superiority over current recommendations (see Chapter 32: Unconventional strategies for respiratory support).

PEEP is used to improve oxygenation and prevent lung shear-stress injury associated with the opening and closing of collapsed alveoli. However, PEEP can also cause cardiovascular compromise and increased airway pressures and overdistension. Current recommendation is to use PEEP of 5–20 cmH_2O with lower tidal volumes when ventilating patients with severe ARDS to maintain oxygenation.

Positioning the patient

ARDS classically affects the lung in a non-homogeneous manner and CT scans taken during the initial phases can show striking asymmetry of lung involvement. Dependent posterior regions are preferentially infiltrated, consolidated or collapsed. Anterior areas are often normally or even excessively aerated during mechanical ventilation. Proning has been used to improve oxygenation in patients with ARDS; however, it has failed to demonstrate any improved clinical outcome. There are also the added risks of displaced endotracheal tubes, invasive monitoring lines and chest drains.

Surfactant

There are reduced production and biochemical alterations of endogenous surfactant in ARDS. The lack of surfactant contributes to atelectasis, shunts, poor gas exchange and increased risks of ventilator associated pneumonia. Despite benefits seen in neonates with idiopathic respiratory distress syndrome, the use of artificial surfactant in adults with ARDS has failed to improve outcome, and its use is not justified.

Vasodilatation

Both nitric oxide and prostacyclin can selectively vasodilate the pulmonary vasculature and potentially reduce pulmonary hypertension, decrease shunting and improve gas exchange in ARDS. However, the improvement of oxygenation does not improve clinical outcome and their use is not recommended.

Prognosis

As ARDS progresses, the cardiovascular system and renal system are commonly affected and multi-organ failure follows. Patients with only lung involvement have 15–30% mortality but this increases to greater than 80% if three or more organs are involved. If multi-organ failure persists beyond 4 days, mortality is 100%.

Pulmonary embolism

The incidence of pulmonary embolism (PE) is estimated at 60–70 cases per 100 000 in the general population in the UK. Half of these patients develop PE while they are in hospital or in long-term care.

Pulmonary embolism can be classified by its clinical effects:

- Small pulmonary emboli are defined as emboli that do not cause pulmonary hypertension and do not affect right ventricular function.
- Submassive PE is characterized by right ventricular dysfunction in a patient who remains normotensive.
- Massive PE, on the other hand, results in acute right ventricular dysfunction, systemic hypotension, collapse or even cardiac arrest.

Immediate consequences of large PEs are from occlusion of pulmonary arteries, release of vasoactive mediators (e.g. 5HT and thromboxane A2) and neurogenic reflexes. These cause vasoconstriction of pulmonary and coronary arteries and vasodilation of peripheries. The result is V/Q mismatch leading to hypoxia.

Haemodynamic effects

- Increased right ventricular afterload.
- Increased pulmonary arterial pressure leading to right ventricular dilatation.
- Reduced pulmonary blood blow and Bernheim effect (displacement of interventricular septum into left ventricle, causing a fall in stroke volume) lead to a reduction in CO and hence a fall in blood pressure.

Clinical features

- Chest pain, shortness of breath, collapse.
- There may not be any abnormal breath sounds.
- Jugular venous pressure engorgement.
- Hypotension and gallop rhythm.

Diagnosis

Diagnosis is often made on clinical grounds.

- Arterial blood gases can be unhelpful, as hyperventilation causes hypocapnoea with hypoxaemia.
- Chest X-ray can also be normal, or there may be vascular shadows and enlarged hilum.
- ECG often shows sinus tachycardia. Signs of right ventricular strain can also be indicated by the classic S wave in lead I, Q wave in III, and inverted T in III (S1, Q3, T3).
- D-dimers are a degradation product produced by plasmin-mediated proteolysis of cross-linked fibrin. They have a low sensitivity for diagnosing PE as they can be raised by many different causes.
- V/Q scan of the lung is the mainstay of hospital diagnostics in PE. It compares the ventilation (V) to perfusion (Q) of the lungs. The inherent

inaccuracy of V/Q scans is demonstrated by the imprecision of the reports:

- Normal scan rules out significant PE.
- High-probability scan establishes the diagnosis.
- Low-probability scan without symptoms would mean the diagnosis is unlikely.
- Medium-probability scan, or a low-probability scan with PE symptoms, is unhelpful, and the patient should then have pulmonary angiography.

- Pulmonary angiography is the gold standard of diagnosis of PE but is not widely available.
- CT scan may be useful when pulmonary angiography is not available as it provides more accurate information than chest X-ray.

Treatment

- ABC. Give high flow oxygen. Treat hypotension with intravenous fluids and give analgesia for pain.
- In small PE, the treatment is anticoagulation with heparin; aim for activated partial thromboplastin time (APTT) 2–3 times normal. This is continued until adequate anticoagulation with warfarin is achieved.
- In massive PE, thrombolysis with streptokinase or recombinant tissue plasminogen activator may be used. To date, there has been only one randomized controlled trial of thrombolysis versus heparin in massive PE. The trial was stopped prematurely after just eight patients when all four patients who had received thrombolysis survived and the other four who had been given heparin died. In patients with both right heart intraventricular or intra-atrial thrombus and PE, mortality with thrombolysis was found to be one-third of that with heparin alone. There is no evidence to support the use of thrombolysis in submassive PE. The current British Thoracic Society guideline recommends that 'thrombolysis should be reserved for patients with clinically massive PE'.
- Percutaneous thrombectomy can be carried out by placing a percutaneous catheter in the pulmonary arterial tree to remove any thrombi by suction or by dissolving with locally administered thrombolytic agents. The result can be assessed immediately by pulmonary angiography using the same catheter. Several small case series suggest both a high efficacy in restoring pulmonary perfusion and a low rate of complications. Complications can include cardiac arrhythmias, pulmonary reperfusion injury and pulmonary haemorrhage.
- Open surgical embolectomy can only be offered in specialist centres, and is usually reserved as a last resort when other methods have failed. Some case reports have reported that when surgical embolectomy has been used early in patients with massive PE, results have generally been encouraging.
- An inferior vena cava (IVC) filter is indicated when anticoagulation cannot be undertaken because of active bleeding, recent surgery or recurrent or persistent PE despite adequate anticoagulation.
- In animal studies, both intravenous magnesium sulphate and inhaled nitric oxide have been shown to be efficacious in decreasing pulmonary artery pressure and increasing cardiac output in acute PE. However, there is no evidence of any clinical benefits of these interventions in humans.

Key points

- Hypoxaemia caused by hypoventilation is easily treated with higher concentrations of oxygen. Hypoxia caused by ventilation/perfusion mismatch, shunts, dead space and impairments of diffusion does respond to simple oxygen therapy.
- In ARDS, mechanical ventilation with smaller tidal volumes (6 ml/kg body weight) is associated with improved survival. Prone positioning and low-dose inhaled nitric oxide both improve oxygenation but are not associated with improved survival. Oxygenation is improved by application of positive end expiration pressure, optimization of cardiac output, keeping haemoglobin level adequate.
- In small, uncomplicated PE anticoagulation remains the treatment of choice.
- In suspected massive PE with associated hypotensive shock, thrombolysis should be given unless there is a significant risk of major bleeding complications.
- Surgical and catheter-based thrombectomy are alternative strategies in the management of massive PE and must be considered when thrombolysis is either contraindicated or has failed.

Further reading

- Acute Respiratory Distress Syndrome Network (2000) Ventilation with lower tidal volumes as compared with traditional tidal volumes for acute lung injury and the acute respiratory distress syndrome. *N. Engl. J. Med.* **342**: 1301–8.
- Bernard GR, Artigas A, Brigham KL *et al.* (1994) The American–European Consensus Conference on ARDS: definitions, mechanisms, relevant outcomes, and clinical trial coordination. *Am. J. Resp. Crit. Care Med.* **149**: 818–24.
- British Thoracic Society Standards of Care Committee Pulmonary Embolism Guideline Development Group (2003) British Thoracic Society guidelines for the management of suspected acute pulmonary embolism. *Thorax* **58**: 470–84.
- Eichacker PQ, Gerstenberger EP, Banks SM, Cui X, Natanson C (2002) Meta-analysis of acute lung injury and acute respiratory distress syndrome trials testing low tidal volumes. *Am. J. Resp. Crit. Care Med.* **166**: 1510–14.
- Jerjes-Sanchez C, Ramirez-Rivera A, Garcia MM *et al.* (1995) Streptokinase and heparin versus heparin alone in massive pulmonary embolism: a randomised controlled trial. *J. Thromb. Thrombolysis* **2**: 227–9.
- Moloney ED, Griffiths MJD (2004) Protective ventilation of patients with acute respiratory distress syndrome. *Br. J. Anaesth.* **92**: 261–70.
- Pinsky M, Brochard L, Mancebo J *et al.* (2006) *Applied Physiology in Intensive Care Medicine,* 2nd edn. New York: Springer-Verlag.
- Simonneau G, Sors H, Charbonnier B *et al.* (1997) A comparison of low molecular-weight-heparin with unfractionated heparin for acute pulmonary embolism: The THESEE Study Group. *N. Engl. J. Med.* **337**: 663–9.
- Vincent JL (2006) DO_2 /VO_2 relationships In *Functional Hemodynamic Monitoring*, eds. Pinsky MR, Payen D. Basel, Switzerland: Birkhaüser, pp. 251–257.
- Ware LB, Matthay MA (2000) The acute respiratory distress syndrome. *N. Engl. J. Med.* **342**: 1334–48.

Respiratory weaning

Darshan Pandit

Introduction

Weaning is the process of liberating the patient from mechanical support and from the endotracheal tube. It is important to remember the goals of mechanical ventilation, which are to provide adequate arterial oxygenation, achieve carbon dioxide clearance and relieve the work of breathing. At the same time, it is important to try to avoid barotrauma, multiple organ dysfunction, atelectasis, haemodynamic depression, nosocomial infection and muscular dystrophy associated with mechanical ventilation, and these factors will all have to be taken into consideration while attempting to wean from ventilator support (Table 30.1).

Time spent in the weaning process can make up 40–50% of total duration of mechanical ventilation. As many as 20% mechanically ventilated patients will fail at their first attempt of weaning; hence choosing the right time to discontinue mechanical ventilation is a challenge as failed extubation followed by reintubation is associated with increased morbidity and mortality.

It is important to recognize that there are stages from the initiation of mechanical ventilation to liberation from the ventilator and these include:

Stage 1 – Treating the cause of acute respiratory failure
Stage 2 – Suggestion that weaning may be possible
Stage 3 – Assessment of readiness to wean
Stage 4 – Spontaneous breathing trials (SBT)
Stage 5 – Extubation
Stage 6 – Reintubation

It is important to ensure progress is made from one stage to the other as delay in weaning will expose the patient to discomfort and complications, and will inevitably increase the cost of care.

Definitions

Simple weaning – Those patients who proceed from initiation of weaning to successful extubation on the first attempt without difficulty

Difficult weaning – Those patients who fail initial weaning and require up to three SBT or as long as 7 days from their first SBT to achieve successful weaning

Prolonged weaning – Those patients who fail at least three weaning attempts or require up to 7 days of weaning after first SBT.

Assessment of readiness to wean

It is important to consider weaning as early as possible using both clinical and objective assessments.

A patient should meet four criteria in order to be considered ready for weaning:

(1) Clear evidence of reversal or stability of cause of acute respiratory failure.
(2) Adequate gas exchange as indicated by PaO_2/FiO_2 between 150 and 200 at a positive end expiratory pressure (PEEP) level between 5 and 8 cmH_2O and pH above 7.25.
(3) Cardiovascular stability (no active myocardial ischaemia or clinically significant hypotension requiring inotropes).
(4) Ability to make an adequate inspiratory effort.

Core Topics in Critical Care Medicine, eds. Fang Gao Smith and Joyce Yeung. Published by Cambridge University Press.

Table 30.1 Clinical and objective assessments used in considering patients for respiratory wean

Clinical assessments

- Adequate cough and minimal tracheobronchial secretions
- Resolution of the acute phase of disease
- Optimize posture

Objective assessments

- Stable cardiovascular and metabolic status
- Adequate oxygenation (SaO_2 >90% or FiO_2 <40%)
- Maximum inspiratory pressure <20–25 cmH_2O
- Airway occlusion pressure <4 cmH_2O
- Tidal volume >5 ml/kg
- Vital capacity >10 ml/kg
- Respiratory frequency(f)/tidal volume(VT) <105/min (RSBI – rapid shallow breathing index)
- No significant respiratory acidosis
- No sedation and the patient is compos mentis

Vital capacity and tidal volume

Vital capacity (VC) is the greatest volume of gas that a patient is able to exhale in taking a maximal inspiration from residual volume. Tidal volume (VT) is the volume of gas moved during a normal respiratory cycle. A vital capacity of 10–15 ml/kg and tidal volume of 5–8 ml/kg is considered as a positive factor predictive of weaning.

Minute ventilation and maximal voluntary ventilation

Normal minute ventilation (MV) for an adult is 6 l/min and as long as $PaCO_2$ is adequate a value below 10 l/min with minimal ventilatory support (pressure support of 5 cmH_2O) is desirable in weaning.

Maximal voluntary ventilation (MVV) (normal values 50–200 l/min) is a measure of respiratory reserve. A measurement of MVV that is twice the value of the resting MV is desirable.

Frequency/tidal volume ratio (f/VT) or rapid shallow breathing index

The rapid shallow breathing index (RSBI) is measured over 1 min during a T-piece trial (e.g. pressure support of 5 cmH_2O or continuous positive pressure of 5 cmH_2O) that has been in place for 30–60 min. Values of frequency/VT ratio (f/VT) above 105 breaths/l per minute suggest a high likelihood of failure to wean. The advantages are that this ratio is easy to measure and not dependent on patient cooperation or effort.

Measuring muscle strength – maximum inspiratory pressure

This assesses the total strength of respiratory muscle but does not take into account the demands placed on respiratory muscles, so a good maximum inspiratory pressure (MIP) in the presence of increased work of breathing due to poor lung compliance may still lead to failure to wean.

An MIP of less than −30 cmH_2O is associated with successful extubation but an MIP greater than −20 cmH_2O is associated with an inability to maintain spontaneous breathing. These values have a better negative predictive value than positive predictive value.

Respiratory centre function – airway occlusion pressure

The negative pressure generated by inspiratory muscle contraction against an occluded airway is directly related to neural input and is proportional to the diaphragmatic electromyographic signal. Values of greater than 4–6 cmH_2O mean that the patient is not ready to be weaned from the ventilator.

Other parameters such as transdiaphramatic pressure are unhelpful as they show considerable variability in normal subjects.

Spontaneous breathing trial

It is important to understand the concept of a spontaneous breathing trial (SBT) as it is the next step towards discontinuation of mechanical support after an RSBI test. Before the start of SBT, a cuff leak test to indicate the absence of laryngeal oedema should be considered in all patients. The initial SBT should last for at least 30 min and should be with one of the modes below with PEEP of 5 cmH_2O.

There are three choices of ventilator setting during an SBT:

- T-piece circuit that provides a constant flow of oxygen past the endotracheal tube with an extension downstream to prevent entrainment of room air.
- Low levels of pressure support of 5–6 cmH_2O.
- Continuous positive airway pressure (CPAP).

The use of automated tube compensation (ATC) which adjusts for the assumed resistance of the endotracheal tube may be used in SBT to compensate for a narrow endotracheal tube. The criteria for passing an

SBT include good respiratory pattern, adequate gas exchange, haemodynamic stability and subject comfort. Failure during an SBT is likely to occur within the first 20 min and the patient should be put back on to full ventilatory support. A comprehensive review of potential contributing factors to the failure should then be made.

Successful completion of an SBT does not necessarily guarantee that the patient is ready for extubation as reintubation rates are still as high as 13–19% using this protocol, with a higher rate for those intubated for >48 hours. The risk factors include old age, increased severity of underlying illness and cardiac failure.

Methods of weaning

When the patient successfully completes the SBT, weaning can then be started using one of the three ways:

(1) Move from assist control to higher levels of pressure support ventilation which can be decreased as tolerated.
(2) Use synchronized intermittent mandatory ventilation with an initial higher rate which can be decreased over time.
(3) Continue full ventilatory support with intermittent trials of low levels of pressure support or CPAP.

Once a pressure support level of less than 10 cmH_2O is reached, the patient could be considered as extubatable from a ventilatory point of view. Success or failure of weaning will then depend on respiratory muscle function, central nervous system drive and work of breathing required.

The role of tracheostomy in weaning

A trachoestomy tube decreases airway resistance due to its shorter length compensating for the turbulent flow and resistance generated by the smaller radius of curvature of the tube. There is a reduction of 10–20 ml of dead space and tracheostomy tubes are also less prone to progressive occlusion due to more effective suctioning.

Other advantages of tracheostomy include:

- Easier airway management.
- Improved patient comfort and communication.
- Reduction of sedation required.
- Improved respiratory mechanics.
- Earlier transition to oral feeding.
- Prevention of ventilator-associated pneumonia.

Why patients fail

If patients fail attempts at weaning the goals should be:

(1) Choose appropriate modes of ventilation to provide a balance between respiratory load and capacity.
(2) Prevent diaphragm muscle atrophy.
(3) Reassess reversible factors preventing weaning (Table 30.2).

Role of non-invasive ventilation in weaning

Non-invasive ventilation (NIV) could be used in three different scenarios for weaning (see also Chapter 31: Non-invasive ventilation).

- As treatment for patients who have been extubated but have developed acute respiratory failure within 48 hours.
- As a prophylactic measure after extubation for those who are at high risk for reintubation.
- To wean those patients who are intolerant of an initial weaning trial.

Newer modalities for weaning

Proportional assist ventilation

Proportional assist ventilation (PAV) is a form of synchronized partial ventilatory support in which the ventilator generates support in proportion to the patient's instantaneous effort. This proportionality also applies from breath to breath as well as continuously throughout each inspiration. The objective of PAV is to allow the patient to use the breathing pattern that the patient finds most comfortable. To achieve these objectives the machine provides pressure assistance in proportion to ongoing inspiratory flow (flow assist, FA) and volume (volume assist, VA).

Adaptive support ventilation

Adaptive support ventilation (ASV) is based on a computer-driven closed loop regulation system of

Table 30.2 Factors that can prevent successful weaning

System	Causes
Respiratory	Increased resistive load during SBT – endotracheal tube and post-extubation glottic oedema, increased airway secretions, sputum retention, airway bronchoconstriction Reduced compliance due to pneumonia, cardiogenic or non-cardiogenic pulmonary oedema, diffuse pulmonary infiltrates Increased work of breathing, inappropriate ventilator settings, ventilator induced diaphragm dysfunction
Cardiac	Increased cardiac workload due to structural heart disease, systolic or diastolic dysfunction which may be only apparent when exposed to workload of breathing
Metabolic	Electrolyte disturbances (hypophosphataemia, hypomagnesaemia, hypokalaemia) Corticosteriod use and hyperglycaemia
Gastrointestinal	Obesity Malnutrition
Neurological	Depressed central drive – encephalitis, brainstem haemorrhage, neurosurgical complications Abnormalities of upper airway control Peripheral dysfunction – Guillain–Barré syndrome, myasthenia gravis, motor neuron disease Critical illness polyneuropathy Anxiety, depression
Haematological	Anaemia
Endocrine	Hypothyroidism, hypoadrenalism

ventilator settings which are responsive to changes in both the respiratory system mechanics and spontaneous breathing efforts.

At the onset of mechanical ventilation the clinician enters the patient's body weight and sets the desired percentage of minute ventilation (100% equals 100 ml/kg body weight) as well as the FiO_2, the level of PEEP and the MIP. The algorithms generated are based on real-time determination of expiratory time constant. Adjustment of inspiratory pressure and minute ventilation can improve patient–ventilator interaction. Spontaneous breathing efforts can trigger either a pressure-controlled breath or a spontaneous breath with inspiratory pressure support at the level suitable for the target respiratory rate and tidal volume.

Trials have compared the use of ASV with synchronized intermittent mandatory ventilation (SIMV) as a weaning mode in post cardiac surgery patients but have failed to conclude which is the better weaning mode, so further studies are needed to compare ASV with other weaning modes.

Knowledge-based expert system

This system is incorporated into a standard ICU ventilator (Evita XL Smartcare) and follows two main goals. The first goal is a real-time adaptation of the level of pressure support to maintain the patient within a comfort zone (respiratory rate between 15 and 30 breaths/min). The second goal is to keep the tidal volume above the minimum threshold of 250 ml if body weight <55 kg and 300 ml if >55 kg.

The pressure support level is periodically adapted by the system in steps of 2–4 cmH_2O. There is also provision to automatically perform a spontaneous breathing trial as the pressure support decreases.

Specialized weaning units have the personnel (consisting of specialized teams of respiratory therapist, nurses, nutritionist) and the organizational structure to care for patients with prolonged weaning problems. About 35–60% of patients in such units can be weaned successfully.

Key points

- Consider weaning as soon as various pathophysiologies that may impact on weaning have been corrected.
- There are both clinical and objective criteria in assessing readiness of patients to wean and these should be evaluated daily.

- Daily interruptions of sedation, muscle paralysis and spontaneous breathing trials are important.
- Weaning protocols are important and along with lessons learnt from specialized weaning units could have a major impact on the success of weaning.

Further reading

- Boles JM, Bion J, Connors A *et al.* (2007) Weaning from mechanical ventilation: statement of the Sixth International Consensus Conference on Intensive Care Medicine. *Eur. Respir. J.* **29**: 1033–56.
- Eskandar N, Apostolakos M (2007) Weaning from mechanical ventilation. *Crit. Care Clinic* **23**: 263–74.

Non-invasive ventilation

David Thickett

Introduction

Over the last 10–15 years there has been a dramatic increase in the number of patients treated with non-invasive ventilation (NIV) both in the setting of critical care and as a ward-based/home therapy. This has occurred as a result of the relative ease of its application, improvement in mask and ventilator technology, and clearly established efficacy in terms of relevant clinical outcomes such as mortality in chronic obstructive pulmonary disease (COPD) as well as improving cost effectiveness. In this chapter we will outline the principals of NIV, the indications and discuss the practicalities of managing cases – with particular emphasis upon proper patient selection.

Definition

Non-invasive ventilation represents the provision of ventilatory assistance without an artificial airway. The vast majority of patients receiving NIV now use positive pressure ventilation, but the term also encompasses other forms of ventilatory assistance such as negative pressure ventilation which avoids direct airway intubation.

Mechanism of action

Non-invasive ventilation has been shown to improve the work of breathing by assisting the patient's respiratory effort and reducing the negative pressure needed to generate a breath. It improves oxygenation by reducing trans-diaphragmatic pressure and increasing functional respiratory capacity. The result of this is a rise in tidal volume, reduced respiratory rate and consequent improved minute ventilation.

Indications

Many applications of NIV have been tried in the acute clinical setting. Only four are supported by multiple controlled trials or meta-analysis, and some of these remain controversial.

(1) Acute exacerbation of COPD

The clinical data for exacerbations of COPD strongly support the use of NIV in hypercapnic respiratory failure, especially for those with systemic acidosis. Non-invasive ventilation has been shown to improve vital signs and gas exchanges as well as reducing the need for formal intubation, decreasing both mortality and length of hospital stay. Based upon these data, NIV should be considered the first line treatment for acute hypercapnic respiratory failure caused by exacerbations of COPD. It can successfully be used in critical care or high dependency unit (HDU) as well as general ward areas.

(2) Cardiogenic pulmonary oedema

Continuous positive airway pressure ventilation (CPAP) and non-invasive positive pressure ventilation (NPPV) are accepted treatments in acute cardiogenic pulmonary oedema (ACPE). However, it remains unclear whether NPPV is better than CPAP in reducing the need for endotracheal intubation (NETI) rates, mortality and other adverse events.

A recent pooled analysis of 10 studies of CPAP compared to standard medical therapy (SMT) showed a significant 22% absolute risk reduction (ARR) in NETI and 13% in mortality. Six studies of NPPV compared to SMT showed an 18% ARR in NETI and 7% in mortality (95% CI, −14% to 0%). Seven studies of NPPV compared to CPAP showed a non-significant 3% ARR in NETI (95% CI, −4% to 9%) and 2% in mortality (95% CI, −6% to 10%). None of these methods increased AMI risk.

In light of these findings, 3CPO, a large-scale, open, randomized, controlled multi-centre trial, was designed

Core Topics in Critical Care Medicine, eds. Fang Gao Smith and Joyce Yeung. Published by Cambridge University Press.

Table 31.1 Physiology data at 1 hour and mortality data at 7 and 30 days in the 3CPO study

	Baseline	Standard therapy	Non-invasive ventilation	*P* value
Heart rate (bpm)	113	102	96	<0.001
Respiratory rate (per min)	32	26	25	0.023
pH	7.22	7.30	7.32	<0.001
Oxygen saturation (%)	90	94	93	0.044
Mortality at 7 days		9.8%	9.5%	NS
Mortality at 30 days		16.7%	15.4%	NS

NS, not significant.
Reproduced with permission of the *European Journal of Heart Failure.*

to evaluate the effect of NIV on mortality compared with SMT, and also to compare the effectiveness of CPAP vs. NPPV. Although currently reported only as abstracts and conference proceedings this large randomized controlled trial has failed to confirm the meta-analysis results with mortality at 30 days being 16.7% in the standard treatment arm and 15.4% in the non-invasive ventilation group (see Table 31.1). Clearly analysis of the effects of NIV in cardiogenic pulmonary oedema requires further clarification.

(3) The immunocompromised patient

Immunocompromised patients such as those with haematological malignancies or following solid organ transplant are at high risk of infectious complications of endotracheal intubation. Hilbert *et al.* performed a randomized controlled trial of intermittent NIV, as compared with SMT with supplemental oxygen and no ventilatory support, in 52 immunosuppressed patients with pulmonary infiltrates, fever and an early stage of hypoxaemic acute respiratory failure. Early initiation of NIV was associated with significant reductions in the rates of endotracheal intubation and serious complications and an improved likelihood of survival to hospital discharge.

(4) Failure to wean from ventilation

Switching to NIV as a way of facilitating extubation has been successfully used as a strategy for COPD patients who are 'persistent' weaning failures (failure of three consecutive T-piece trials). The use of NIV compared to conventional methods resulted in shorter duration of intubation, ICU and hospital stay and nosocomial pneumonia, and improved ITU and 90-day survival.

When to use NIV?

It is essential before NIV is initiated that arterial blood gas measurements be available. The patient should be established upon appropriate oxygen therapy and interpretation must be made in the context of the FiO_2. Pulse oximetry should not be used alone to assess the need for NIV as it can provide false reassurance in those patients in whom oxygenation is maintained but who have deteriorating hypercapnia.

Arterial blood gas tensions improve rapidly in many patients with acute hypercapnic respiratory failure when they receive maximum medical treatment and appropriate supplementary oxygen. A repeat sample should usually be taken after a short interval to see if NIV is still indicated.

Patient selection for NIV

Correct patient selection is essential for the success of NIV: it is a complementary not alternative therapy to IPPV. Nevertheless NIV has several potential advantages over IPPV (see Table 31.2).

Contraindications

- Respiratory arrest.
- Inability to use mask because of trauma or surgery in the face or upper airway.
- Excessive secretions.
- Haemodynamic instability or life-threatening arrhythmia.
- High risk of aspiration or inability to protect airway.
- Impaired mental status.

Table 31.2 Advantages (+) and disadvantages (–) of NIV and IPPV

	IPPV	NIV
Ventilator related infection	–	+
Tracheal injury	–	+
Sedation	–	+
Intermittent application	–	+
Protection of airway	+	–
Access to airway	+	–
Eating	–	+
Facial pressure effects	+	–
Leaks	+	–

- Uncooperative or agitated patient.
- Life-threatening refractory hypoxaemia (alveolar–arterial difference in PaO_2 <60 mmHg with FiO_2 of 1).

Instituting NIV

Important questions to consider prior to instituting NIV

- Is the patient receiving optimal medical therapy?
- Is there a reversible cause, and what is it?
- Is benefit from the intervention likely?
- Does the patient want active treatment?

If proceeding, consider:

- In what setting should NIV take place – ward, HDU, ITU?
- How should the patient be monitored?
- What are we going to do if NIV fails?
- Define what constitutes failure.

Practical tips for successful NIV

The successful instigation of NIV is very dependent upon establishing a good rapport with the patient and inspiring confidence in what will feel like a very unusual treatment. It is useful for all physicians initiating NIV to have experienced the feeling themselves in order to understand this. The procedure should be established in an appropriate environment where the staff is familiar with the technique and the equipment.

Table 31.3 Factors associated with success or failure in NIV

Success
Younger age
Moderate hypercapnia ($PaCO_2$ >45mm Hg but <92 mmHg) with low A–a oxygen gradient
Moderate acidaemia/pH 7.25–7.35 (H^+ 56–45 nmol/l)
Improvement in pH, $PaCO_2$ and respiratory rate after 1 hour of NIV
Good level of consciousness
Failure
Pneumonia
Copious respiratory secretions
Edentulous
Poor nutritional status
Confusion or impaired consciousness

- Set up equipment before taking it to the bedside. The following settings are appropriate:
  - *IPAP* 12 cmH_2O
  - *EPAP* 5 cmH_2O
  - *RR* 12–15 breaths/min
  - *Triggers* maximum sensitivity
  - *Back-up rate* 15 breaths/min
  - *Back-up I : E ratio* 1 : 3
- Position patient sitting at 45°.
- Take time selecting interface and explaining procedure.
- Titrate O_2 to achieve saturations of 88% to 92%.
- Introduce mask gradually – allow the patient or a nurse to hold the mask in place before securing straps.
- Regularly review the fit of straps and mask in order to improve comfort and compliance with NIV.
- Expect changes in physiology to be relatively slow.
- Initial pressures should be increased as tolerated up to 20 cmH_2O. IPAP can be gradually increased (up to 30 to 35 cmH_2O) to control hypercapnia.
- Increase FiO_2 and EPAP (8 to 12 cmH_2O) to control hypoxia.

Factors associated with success or failure in NIV are outlined in Table 31.3.

Table 31.4 Guidelines for NIV. (Adapted from the British Thoracic Society's *NIV Guidelines*, with permission.)

Is the treatment of the underlying condition optimal?

- Check medical treatment prescribed and that it has been given
- Consider physiotherapy for sputum retention

Have any complications developed?

- Consider a pneumothorax, aspiration pneumonia, etc.

$PaCO_2$ remains elevated

Is the patient on too much oxygen?

- Adjust FiO_2 to maintain SpO_2 between 85% and 90%
- Is there excessive leakage?
- Check mask fit
- If using nasal mask, consider chin strap or full-face mask

Is the circuit set up correctly?

- Check connections have been made correctly
- Check circuit for leaks
- Is rebreathing occurring?
- Check patency of expiratory valve (if fitted)
- Consider increasing EPAP (if bi-level pressure support).

Is the patient synchronizing with the ventilator?

- Observe patient.
- Adjust rate and/or I:E ratio (with assist/control).
- Check inspiratory trigger (if adjustable).
- Check expiratory trigger (if adjustable).
- Consider increasing EPAP (with bi-level pressure support in COPD).

Is ventilation inadequate?

- Observe chest expansion.
- Increase target pressure (or IPAP) or volume.
- Consider increasing inspiratory time.
- Consider increasing respiratory rate (to increase minute ventilation).
- Consider a different mode of ventilation/ventilator, if available.

$PaCO_2$ improves but PaO_2 remains low

- Increase FiO_2
- Consider increasing EPAP (with bi-level pressure support).

Complications of NIV

Complications may include:

- Mild gastric distension.
- Pressure effects of the mask and straps causing facial tissue damage.
- Eye irritation, sinus pain or nasal congestion.
- Significant haemodynamic effects resulting from NIV are unusual although hypotension may occur.

Troubleshooting

When a patient is establish successfully upon NIV and the treatment appears to be failing, a number of possible causes should be considered (outlined in Box below). Sometimes the treatment of the underlying condition has not been optimized in part because of focus upon the ventilation aspects. Check that medication has been given if a patient is on a full face mask and consider complications such as pneumothorax or aspiration pneumonia.

If the $PaCO_2$ remains elevated, check that the circuit for the ventilator has been set up correctly and check the circuit for leaks. Ensure that if there is an expiratory valve upon the mask that it is patent. Consider increasing EPAP. In COPD patients, consider if the FiO_2 is too high – aim to maintain saturations between 88% and 90%. Clinically assess the adequacy of ventilation and if inadequate increase the IPAP and or inspiratory time. If the PaO_2 remains low despite ventilation consider increasing the FiO_2 or EPAP. Close monitoring is essential, and respiratory rate, comfort and synchrony with ventilation as well as oxygen saturation should be recorded (Table 31.4).

Key points

- NIV is safe and highly effective therapy provided it is used in the correct patients and an appropriate environment.
- The success of NIV is dependent upon the establishment of clear goals of therapy.
- A definite management plan for what to do if it fails should always be in place prior to initiation of the therapy.

Acknowledgement

David Thickett is supported by the Wellcome Trust.

Further reading

- 3CPO Study http://clintrialresults.org/Slides/Newby_3CPO.ppt
- British Thoracic Society Standards of Care Committee (2002) BTS Guideline: Non-invasive ventilation in acute respiratory failure. *Thorax* **57**: 192–211.
- Cleland JG, Freemantle N, Coletta AP. *et al.* (2007) Clinical trials update from the European Society of Cardiology Congress 2007: 3CPO, ALOFT, PROSPECT and statins for heart failure. *Eur. J. Heart Fail.* **9**(10): 1070–3.
- Hilbert G, Gruson D, Vargas F *et al.* (2001) Noninvasive ventilation in immunosuppressed patients with pulmonary infiltrates, fever, and acute respiratory failure. *N. Engl. J. Med.* **344**(7): 481–7.
- Nava S, Hill N (2009) Non-invasive ventilation in acute respiratory failure. *Cancer* **374**: 250–9.
- Winck JC, Azevedo LF, Costa Percira A *et al.* (2006) Efficacy and safety of non-invasive ventilation in the treatment of acute cardiogenic pulmonary edema: a systematic review and meta-analysis. *Crit. Care* **10**(2): R69.

Unconventional strategies for respiratory support

Bill Tunnicliffe

Introduction

Conventional mechanical ventilation is a critical element of the management of patients with respiratory failure. It must be remembered that it is a supportive rather than therapeutic intervention, and that its application has limitations. It is also potentially injurious to the ventilated lung, particularly in the presence of intrinsic lung diseases or acute lung injury (see Chapter 27: Mechanical ventilation). A range of interventions has been devised to try to extend the potential range for conventional ventilation, as well as alternative strategies to support patients with respiratory failure beyond the current limits of conventional ventilation. Clinical evidence supporting the use of these interventions is generally limited.

Prone positioning during mechanical ventilation

In patients with severe respiratory failure associated with acute respiratory distress syndrome (ARDS), failure of oxygenation despite optimal conventional ventilatory strategies can occur and often leads to death. Given that in the majority of patients ARDS is reversible, interventions that can improve oxygenation failure in this setting, hence allowing further time for lung healing to occur, have attracted considerable interest. One of these interventions is placing the patient in the prone position during conventional ventilation. An attraction of this intervention is that it is relatively simple to undertake and does not require any specific equipment.

Improvements in oxygenation are observed in around two-thirds of patients with ARDS and refractory hypoxaemia when they are placed in the face-down position. It is thought to work principally by reordering VQ relationships in previously dependent lung units. While these improvements have been impressive, clinical trials have to date failed to demonstrate any survival benefit from this technique when it is used routinely, rather it is now principally used for short-term rescue or as 'a last resort' particularly when other interventions such as high-frequency oscillatory ventilation (HFOV) are not available.

Placing a patient in the prone position is not without difficulties; complications include amongst others inadvertent extubation, loss of central venous access and chest drains, delayed cardiopulmonary resuscitation and blindness. It also places a considerable extra physical burden on nursing staff as well as potentially having adverse psychosocial effects on carers and visitors.

Using the prone position is not limited to conventional ventilation, it can also be applied during HFOV when adequate oxygenation at an FiO_2 of <0.6 cannot be achieved or maintained, or when bronchorrhoea makes supine HFOV challenging. Experience with this combination is limited, but unexpected survival of a number of patients has been observed.

Use of inhaled nitric oxide

Nitric oxide (NO) is a selective pulmonary vasodilator that improves blood flow to ventilated lung units and improves oxygenation in around two-thirds of adult patients when it is added to the inspired gases of patients with refractory hypoxaemia undergoing conventional ventilation, or HFOV, for ARDS. Unfortunately, despite considerable early enthusiasm for its routine use, clinical trials have failed to demonstrate any survival benefit from NO in this setting; on the contrary, three trials have shown a trend towards increased mortality with its use.

Administration of NO requires specific equipment for its safe use and it is costly; it is also contraindicated

Core Topics in Critical Care Medicine, eds. Fang Gao Smith and Joyce Yeung. Published by Cambridge University Press.

in methaemoglobin reductase deficiency (congenital or acquired).

In the adult setting, while NO may still have an important role in the management of pulmonary hypertension, it cannot currently be recommended for the management of refractory hypoxaemia in ARDS.

Recruitment manoeuvres (RMs)

Recruitment manoeuvres (RMs) are used to improve the volume of aerated lung, and consequently hypoxaemia, principally in patients receiving conventional ventilation for ARDS. They generally involve the application of a static pressure to the lung that would be considered hazardous during tidal ventilation. Both the magnitude of the pressure applied and its duration seem to be important in determining their effects.

Protagonists see RMs as complementary to the process of 'optimal PEEP' selection; they argue that applied PEEP will be unable to 'keep open' lung units that were not open at an earlier point in the respiratory cycle. They suggest that these refractory units of the acutely injured lung may require pressures considerably higher than 25 cmH_2O to open. Once opened, however, these lung units are believed to close at lower pressures, allowing ventilation to be achieved with the same tidal volume and PEEP though in the context of a more open lung.

Various techniques have been described; one of the simplest is the static application of 40 cmH_2O pressure to the airway for 40 s, if tolerated, followed by the re-instatement of PEEP 2 to 5 cmH_2O higher than the initial value.

When sustained pressure is applied to the airway, through its effects principally on right ventricular afterload (and to a lesser degree its preload) it may produce significant falls in cardiac output and result in hypotension. There is also a significant risk of barotrauma. Clinicians performing an RM should remain vigilant to these effects and be prepared to both rapidly reinstate typical mechanical ventilation and perform resuscitation, and manage a pneumothorax.

Currently there are no data demonstrating clinical benefit from RMs, or to support the use of one manoeuvre over another, and their use remains controversial. Given this it would seem reasonable to suggest that RMs should in general be limited to those patients with ARDS who require an FiO_2 >0.6 despite an apparently adequate level of applied PEEP. In terms of timing, again it is probably reasonable to attempt recruitment earlier rather than later in the course of ARDS, and that the ability of the patient to tolerate attempts at recruitment should be carefully monitored. If benefits accrued through recruitment are maintained, further attempts at recruitment should probably not be attempted. If initial benefits are lost (despite an increase in PEEP) then it is probably reasonable to have further attempts at recruitment, with further increases in PEEP if successful. Failure to re-recruit or repeated de-recruitment, and the requirement for an FiO_2 >0.6 to achieve adequate oxygenation should prompt consideration of alternative forms of ventilatory support.

High-frequency oscillatory ventilation

High-frequency oscillation (HFOV) is an unconventional mode of ventilation that can be thought of as an extension of the 'open lung' approach to mechanical ventilation. By eliminating the need for the bulk gas flow of tidal ventilation, it tends to avoid problems of cyclical overinflation and collapse in differing lung zones that may accompany conventional ventilation.

In adult practice in the UK, HFOV is generally used as a rescue for ARDS patients with refractory hypoxaemia on conventional ventilation. Clinical trial data are accumulating suggesting that it is at least as safe and effective as conventional ventilation in this setting. Whether HFOV applied as the primary ventilatory strategy in ARDS might improve outcomes is currently being investigated in the OSCAR trial, a multi-centre randomized controlled trial in the UK.

A specific ventilator is required for HFOV; in the UK currently only two models are available for adult use, the SensorMedics 3100B and the Novalung Vision Alpha.

The principles of the HFOV are relatively simple; oxygenation and carbon dioxide clearance are in essence disconnected from one another and are controlled through generally independent mechanisms. Oxygenation is determined by the delivered FiO_2 and the degree of alveolar recruitment that is achieved and maintained by the mean airway pressure (MAP). This acts like 'super CPAP', with pressures of up to 55 cmH_2O being used, and is controlled by the fresh gas flow into the circuit, and a variable (operator-controlled) resistance to outflow from the circuit. Carbon dioxide clearance is managed principally through an oscillating diaphragm that has both active inspiratory and expiratory travel; it causes symmetrical oscillations of intrapulmonary pressure around the mean airway pressure at a frequency of 3 to 15 Hz (range dependent on machine type used), which equates to 180 to 900 cycles per minute. The amplitude of the pressure excursions is proportional to the cycle volume (and the inspiratory time), but *inversely* proportional to the frequency. This process, when applied at the airway opening, induces rapid gas mixing within the lungs with net gas transport occurring along the partial pressure gradients for oxygen and carbon dioxide.

At initiation, an FiO_2 of 1 is selected and the starting mean airway pressure determined by adding 5 cmH_2O pressure to the plateau pressures being generated with conventional ventilation. Sequential increases in the mean airway pressure, in 5 cmH_2O increments up to a maximum of 55 cmH_2O, are then applied to achieve alveolar recruitment. Successful recruitment is demonstrated by improved oxygenation; overdistension is usually signalled by a fall in indices of oxygenation. When alveolar recruitment is achieved, the FiO_2 is sequentially reduced to achieve the target PaO_2, with the goal of achieving adequate oxygenation with an FiO_2 below 0.6. The time course of recruitment varies between patients, but tends to occur more rapidly when HFOV is initiated early in the course of ARDS. Sequential reductions in the mean airway pressure, in 2 cmH_2O decrements, are then attempted to exploit the hysteresis of the lungs, with the aim of maintaining alveolar recruitment but at a lower distending pressure. De-recruitment will occur if pressures are reduced by too much, and is generally indicated by a fall in PaO_2. If this happens, the MAP can be increased transiently by 8 to 10 cmH_2O to achieve re-recruitment, and then lowered again to an intermediate value.

Arbitrary starting settings for the oscillating piston are usually selected at the initiation of HFOV. These values are machine type specific, reflecting the differing dimensions and characteristics of the diaphragms used on the HFOV ventilators currently available. Unless hypercarbia and the resultant respiratory acidosis are extreme, adjustments are delayed until adequate recruitment is achieved; in general if adequate recruitment is achieved, managing carbon dioxide clearance is relatively straightforward. To increase carbon dioxide clearance power/cycle volume tends to be increased initially in steps that produce an increase in amplitude (ΔP) of 5 cmH_2O. Power/cycle volume increments are generally halted when amplitude exceeds 100 to 120 cmH_2O or the adjustment reaches its maximum value. If this fails to produce adequate carbon dioxide clearance then sequential reductions in frequency can be made, to a minimum of 3 Hz. For optimal lung protection, the lowest cycle volume (power) and highest frequency that achieve adequate $PaCO_2$ should be used. Carbon dioxide elimination can also be increased by deliberately causing a leak around the endotracheal tube cuff, exploiting the resultant bulk gas flow out of the lungs. This is generally safe and can reduce the cycle volume needed to achieve relative normocapnia by up to half. Creating a deliberate cuff leak should probably be thought about at the time HFOV is initiated, and certainly should be considered before reductions in frequency below 6 Hz are undertaken.

High-frequency oscillatory ventilation is a sensitive detector of hypovolaemia; volume resuscitation and increased vasopressor support are often required at the time of initiation. Concerns about an increased risk of air leaks with HFOV have in general been discounted; in experienced hands the incidence of pneumothorax is no higher than with conventional ventilation.

A major limitation to the use of HFOV is the need to develop and maintain HFOV skills in medical and nursing staff; they tend to only encounter HFOV rarely and then when it is being used as a late intervention or as a measure of last resort.

Extracorporeal membrane oxygenation

Extracorporeal membrane oxygenation (ECMO), or extracorporeal life-support, is the use of a cardiopulmonary bypass device in a critically ill patient who has inadequate pulmonary and/or cardiac function, with the intention of 'buying time' to allow their underlying problem to improve. In adults in the UK, it is still seen as an experimental treatment for patients with severe respiratory failure, although its application in neonatal and paediatric practice is more established. The following discussion limits itself to the use of ECMO in adults with severe respiratory failure in the UK.

Extracorporeal membrane oxygenation involves the continuous drainage of venous blood to a pump and membrane oxygenator and its reinfusion to a major vein or artery. High blood flows through the extracorporeal circuits are required for ECMO to achieve adequate oxygenation. *Venoarterial* bypass used to be used most commonly, but now tends to be reserved for patients who require haemodynamic support. Typically the inferior vena cava is accessed via the femoral vein for venous drainage and oxygenated blood is returned via the contralateral femoral artery. The advantage of using femoral access points is that they can usually be achieved percutaneously; a potential disadvantage is of precipitating ischaemia due to disruption of blood flow down the femoral artery, though this risk can be mitigated by placing an additional cannula supplying oxygenated blood into the ipsilateral profunda femoris artery. *Venovenous* access is the more usual route for isolated respiratory failure in adults, the right atrium and inferior vena cava being accessed by the internal jugular and femoral vein respectively. Venovenous support has several advantages over arteriovenous support when additional haemodynamic support is not required, the risk of cerebrovascular accident is significantly reduced, relatively normal haemodynamics are maintained and the risk of ischaemia to the lower extremity is very small indeed. In both techniques, the cannulae involved are of considerable diameter (19 to 29 Fr) and placement should only be considered by experienced operators (Fig. 32.1).

When bypass is initiated, the circuit provides the majority of support and the ventilator settings can be minimized to reduce ongoing ventilator induced lung damage. Systemic heparin administration is required throughout, with target activated partial thromboplastin times (APTTs) of between 2.5 and 3.5, and maintaining bronchial toilet is also of great importance. Significant complications are relatively frequent, the most common being bleeding; mechanical

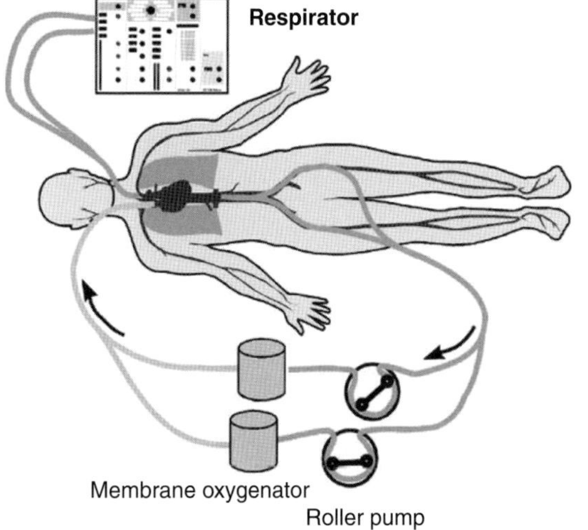

Fig. 32.1 Schematic diagram illustrating extracorporeal membrane oxygenation (ECMO).

complications include oxygenator failure, pump head failure, clotting and rupture of the circuit. In experienced hands, ECMO can be maintained for some weeks without major difficulties.

Current criteria used for determining if ECMO might be indicated in ARDS include a predicted mortality >80% within 5 days of intubation. This usually equates to a severe alveolar–arterial oxygen gradient (>600 mmHg) on the second to fourth day following intubation. As ECMO is currently of limited geographical availability in the UK, the transport of gravely ill and inherently unstable patients to a centre capable of providing it poses an important limitation to this form of support.

Currently whether ECMO offers improved outcomes from severe ARDS-related respiratory failure is uncertain. The CESAR trial, a UK single-centre, randomized controlled trial, has recently closed and its results are much anticipated, but it is unlikely to completely answer this question.

Extracorporeal carbon dioxide removal

Extracorporeal carbon dioxide removal ($ECCO_2R$) is a form of extracorporeal support that focusses on removal of carbon dioxide rather than improving oxygenation. Extracorporeal CO_2 removal potentially offers not only a rescue intervention in patients with severe hypercarbic respiratory failure, but also the possibility of allowing lung rest (through applying apnoeic oxygenation) to those with less severe disease; whether either approach offers improved clinical outcomes is yet to be determined.

In stark contrast to ECMO, effective CO_2 removal can be achieved with very modest flows through an extracorporeal circuit, and this is one of its key attractions. Initially $ECCO_2R$ was usually achieved through a pumped venovenous circuit and this is still widely practised. In this form it remains a complex procedure, however, differing only marginally from venovenous ECMO, and is only really possible in centres with adequate experience of extracorporeal support. More recently the development of very low resistance membrane lungs has allowed the development of pumpless arteriovenous CO_2 removal ($AVCO_2R$, also termed ECLA – extracorporeal lung assist, or PECLA – pumpless extracorporeal lung assist), relying on the patient's own cardiac output to drive the extracorporeal circuit, and hence potentially broadening the application of this technique.

Arteriovenous CO_2 removal is generally achieved via bi-femoral cannulation, employing 17–21 Fr arterial cannulae and 19–21 Fr venous cannulae. Its application is limited to patients whose cardiovascular system can tolerate an increased cardiac output and whose arterial pressure can achieve sufficient flows through the circuit to achieve sufficient CO_2 removal (shunt flows of 1 to 2.5 litres/min). Vasopressors can be added to increase shunt flow, but no direct intervention can otherwise regulate it. Except in severe hypoxaemia, the amount of oxygen that can be transferred to the arterial blood can only marginally influence systemic oxygenation. In contrast to venovenous $ECCO_2R$, no simple conversion to ECMO is possible. Systemic anticoagulation is required.

Complications of $AVCO_2R$ remain a significant problem, with bleeding and limb ischaemia (up to 20%) being relatively frequent, while evidence of its efficacy in terms of improving clinical outcomes is limited. Current UK guidance suggests this procedure should only be used with special arrangements for clinical governance, consent and for audit or research.

Liquid ventilation

Liquid ventilation (LV) is an experimental technique that involves the instillation of fluorinated organic liquids into the lungs. It can be performed by two methods, *total liquid ventilation* (TLV) and *partial liquid ventilation* (PLV). In TLV the lungs are filled with perfluorocarbon to a volume equivalent to functional residual capacity (FRC) and a specialized mechanical liquid ventilator delivers and removes perfluorocarbon tidal volumes to and from the lungs. In PLV, a conventional mechanical ventilator delivers gas tidal volumes to lungs filled with perfluorocarbons, again usually to a volume equivalent to FRC (Fig. 32.2).

Perfluorocarbons are clear, odourless, inert liquids with unique physical properties. They have a density about twice that of water, but a remarkably low surface tension. In addition, they have excellent oxygen and carbon dioxide carrying capacities – the oxygen content of perflourocarbons at 1 atm of oxygen is approximately 20 times that of water and about twice that of blood. Together this means that they have the potential to support gas exchange under normobaric conditions. The high density of perfluorocarbons means that when they are introduced into the airway, they distribute preferentially to dependent lung regions, which leads to recruitment of alveoli that would otherwise tend to be collapsed or filled with inflammatory exudates in the setting of ARDS. Perfluorocarbons also, through their physical and surface tension properties, tend to increase alveolar stability by acting as an artificial surfactant, while not apparently interfering with endogenous surfactant production or function.

There is very little experience of liquid ventilation in adults; the first clinical study of LV for respiratory failure was reported in 1995. In the study, PLV was used as an adjunctive therapy to extracorporeal lung support (ECLS) in 18 subjects; 10 of them were adults. Patients receiving PLV demonstrated a significant decrease in their alveolar–arterial oxygen gradients and an increase in their pulmonary compliance when

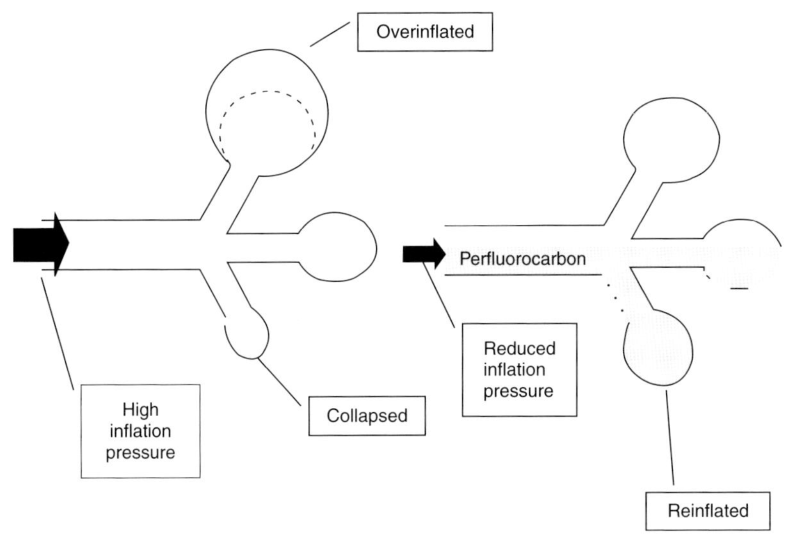

Fig. 32.2 Liquid ventilation.

ECLS was discontinued for short periods. The overall survival was 58%.

Liquid ventilation is in the early stages of its development; whether it might in the future offer clinical advantages either alone or as part of a raft of lung protective strategies in severe respiratory failure is uncertain.

Transtracheal gas insufflation

Transtracheal gas insufflation (TGI) consists of the continuous or phased injection of fresh gas into the central airways for the purpose of improving the efficiency of alveolar ventilation and/or minimizing the ventilator pressure requirements. As such it may have a role as an adjunct to conventional mechanical ventilation in patients with ventilatory failure.

This technique attempts to minimize dead space effects by delivering fresh gas, through an intratracheal catheter, to flush CO_2 out of the anatomical dead space. As gas flow during exhalation washes CO_2 out of the dead space, less is available to be re-inhaled during inspiration; in addition, gas flow during inhalation contributes to inspired tidal volumes, but this component of the tidal volume has avoided the dead space proximal to the catheter tip, again reducing the recycling of CO_2. At higher catheter flows, turbulence generated at the catheter tip can also enhance gas mixing in regions distal to the catheter, again potentially enhancing CO_2 removal.

Studies of TGI in acute lung injury and ARDS have focussed on demonstrating its ability to allow a reduced tidal volume to be delivered while maintaining a constant $PaCO_2$, or on achieving reductions in $PaCO_2$ thus allowing greater degrees of permissive hypercapnia. Unfortunately, despite TGI being first tested in humans receiving mechanical ventilation some 40 years ago, randomized clinical trials exploring clinical end-points are still lacking.

There is currently no standard method of introducing a TGI catheter into the trachea for use during mechanical ventilation. Some have used an intraluminal approach, passing the catheter through a standard endotracheal tube, while others have placed the catheter alongside the endotracheal tube. Both approaches have their own problems, but with each technique the catheter can interfere with suctioning and can cause trauma to the lumen of the trachea. New designs that incorporate channels within the endotracheal tube wall would solve some of these problems and simplify the process.

Transtracheal gas insufflation can 'interfere' with mechanical ventilation through other mechanisms; during volume control ventilation when ventilator-applied PEEP is kept constant, TGI can result in increased end-expiratory pressures and auto PEEP. During pressure control ventilation when ventilator-applied PEEP and inspiratory airway pressures are left unchanged, delivered tidal volumes may fall through a similar mechanism. Probably of more importance is the potential for TGI to interfere with ventilator triggering at low peak inspiratory flows in patients receiving CPAP via a mechanical ventilator; weak patients may fail to open the demand valve at high catheter flow rates which, in turn, may significantly increase their work of breathing.

Nevertheless, TGI appears a promising complementary technique to mechanical ventilation; its clinical role is yet to be determined and may need to await further technological developments not only in catheter design, but also to allow close co-ordination between TGI delivery and the functioning of standard mechanical ventilators.

Key points

- There is a range of alternative ventilator strategies which are mostly used when conventional ventilation has failed to improve gaseous exchange in patients.
- These interventions also involve high risks and have limited clinical evidence.

Further reading

- National Institute for Clinical Excellence (2004) *Extracorporeal Membrane Oxygenation (ECMO) in Adults*, Interventional Procedures Guidance No.39. London: NICE. www.nice.org.uk/pdf/ip/029overview. pdf
- National Institute for Clinical Excellence (2008) *Arteriovenous Extracorporeal Membrane Carbon Dioxide Removal*. Interventional Procedures Guidance No. 250. London: NICE. www.nice.org.uk
- Tobin MJ (ed.) (2006) *Principles and Practice of Mechanical Ventilation*. New York: McGraw Hill.

Acute gastrointestinal bleeding and perforation

Mamta Patel and Richard Skone

Introduction

Acute gastrointestinal bleeding can be a reason for admission to the intensive care unit (ICU) as well as arising as a consequence of being critically ill. It is associated with considerable morbidity and mortality.

The gastrointestinal (GI) tract receives approximately 1400 ml/min of blood at rest, the majority of which supplies the mucosa. It is capable of extensive autoregulation and can decrease its flow to 600 ml/min during exercise.

Three common forms of presentation for acute GI bleeds are:

(1) Haematemesis – vomiting fresh blood that is upper GI in origin and can mimic haemoptysis.

(2) Melaena – this appears as black tarry stools, caused by partly digested blood. It is upper GI in origin.

(3) Haematochezia – this is bright red or maroon blood passed per rectum. It is usually caused by lower GI bleeding but may also occur with massive upper GI blood loss.

Complications associated with GI bleeding

- Cardiovascular collapse.
- Consequences of hypotension – arrhythmias, myocardial ischaemia/infarction and end organ failure.
- Aspiration pneumonia.
- Sepsis.
- Spontaneous bacterial peritonitis.
- Over transfusion.
- Rebound rebleeding.
- Encephalopathy.

Management of a large GI bleed

- Rapid resuscitation.
- Haemodynamic stabilization.
- Early endoscopy to aid diagnosis, risk stratification and treatment.
- Multi-disciplinary approach including gastrointestinal, surgical and radiological consultation.

Resuscitation

Initial resuscitation of a patient with a large GI bleed, as with any medical emergency, centres around the ABC approach of resuscitation.

Airway

Haematemesis can lead to aspiration of blood, with severe consequences. The assessment of the airway therefore must take into account:

(1) Consciousness level of the patient

(2) Risk of aspiration

(3) Cardiovascular status

(4) Further management and procedures.

If there is any doubt as to the patient's consciousness level or risk of aspiration then the patient should be intubated. Intubation should be carried out using a rapid sequence induction (taking care to manage the cricoid pressure appropriately in the face of active vomiting). A difficult airway should be anticipated as blood may obscure the view of the larynx. Adequate suction, assistance, airway aids and a tilting trolley should be available. The endotracheal tube should be secured appropriately as it can become dislodged during endoscopy.

Core Topics in Critical Care Medicine, eds. Fang Gao Smith and Joyce Yeung. Published by Cambridge University Press.

Breathing and oxygenation

Ventilation of a patient with upper GI bleeding may become difficult if significant aspiration of blood has occurred. An initial chemical pneumonitis may be followed by a lower respiratory tract infection. Patients with large GI bleeds may also develop acute respiratory distress syndrome (ARDS) from the above or from large blood transfusions. They should be managed according to the open lung strategy advocated by the ARDSnet study group.

Circulation

In the case of large GI bleeds it is important to start fluid resuscitation urgently, being guided by measurable parameters. The aim of resuscitation is to re-establish organ perfusion and oxygen delivery. This is achieved by:

- Siting two 14–16 g intravenous cannulae.
- Immediate fluid resuscitation.
- Urgent cross-matching of blood (O negative type may be needed until cross-matched, or group-specific blood is available).
- Alerting the Blood Bank to the potential need for large quantities of blood products.
- Using invasive monitoring, i.e. arterial line and central line, although these should not delay resuscitation and treatment of the cause of bleeding.

A Cochrane Review in 2003 of fluid replacement strategy in uncontrolled haemorrhage found no benefit from one particular regime with regards to either the type of fluid or rate of infusion, i.e. aggressive fluid replacement versus conservative titration. A further review in 2007 of patients requiring replacement of circulating volume found no benefit in the use of colloid versus crystalloid fluids.

The ideal ratio of blood to clotting products (such as fresh frozen plasma) is unclear. Each hospital should have guidelines for the management of major haemorrhage. This should involve consultation with the haematology team to guide the replacement of blood products and frequency of blood tests.

Coagulation

A coagulopathy may develop secondary to the patient's underlying pathology, hypothermia or due to a large blood transfusion. Therefore close monitoring is essential.

Antifibrinolytics

Aprotinin and tranexamic acid are used to promote clotting in patients and decrease fibrinolysis.

Tranexamic acid (a lysine analogue) has been shown to decrease the need for surgery in patients with upper GI bleed as well as decreasing mortality and risk of rebleeding.

Aprotinin (a serine protease inhibitor) has been studied in detail as a pre-emptive drug to minimize blood loss in surgery where a large amount of blood loss is expected. However concerns have been raised about its safety profile. Therefore it should only be used when the risk of renal, cardiac or neurological damage is outweighed by the need for haemostasis.

Recombinant activated factor VII

In cases of uncontrollable bleeding case reports have been published citing the use of recombinant activated factor VII (rFVIIa) to promote clot formation. Evidence of benefit for rFVIIa is largely limited to case reports, although one trial has shown some benefit in a subgroup of patients with severe cirrhosis (Child classification B or C). None of the patients that received rFVIIa in this group re-bled within the first 24 hours (compared to 11% in the control group).

The use of rFVIIa carries a risk of unwanted thrombogenesis within vessels; the magnitude of this risk may vary with the presenting pathology and presence or absence of a coagulopathy. Therefore, as with aprotinin, care should be taken to only use this drug when the risk of uncontrolled bleeding exceeds that of thrombosis.

Monitoring

The potential for massive blood loss and haemodynamic instability means that close monitoring of all patients is essential. Results should be interpreted in conjunction with the patient's clinical state. Suggested types of monitoring are given in Table 33.1.

Investigations

Investigations should be dictated by the clinical scenario. In addition to the warranted specific investigations, they should include those listed in Table 33.2.

Table 33.1 Suggested monitoring for a patient with GI bleeding

ECG monitoring
Oxygen saturation probe
Invasive blood pressure monitoring
Capnograph
Urinary catheter (hourly urine output)
Central venous pressure
Regular arterial blood gas analysis
Temperature
Nasogastric tube (may give an early sign of rebleeding)
Cardiac output monitoring

Table 33.2 Suggested investigations

Assessing oxygen delivery
Full blood count
Arterial blood gases
Serum lactate
Mixed venous saturations/central venous saturations

Assessing coagulation
Clotting studies (INR/APTT)
Platelets
Fibrinogen
Calcium

Other
Urea and electrolytes
Blood glucose
Liver function tests
Chest X-ray (to assess for perforation or extent of aspiration)

Upper GI bleeding

Incidence

Acute upper GI bleeding has an incidence of 50 to 150 per 10 000 per year which is approximately four times more common than lower GI bleeding.

Aetiology

On investigation a cause of bleeding is found in 80% of cases. The commonest causes are shown in Table 33.3.

Mortality

The mortality rate for patients admitted to hospital because of GI bleeding is 11%. Patients who develop GI bleeds in hospital have a mortality rate of 33%.

Table 33.3 Common causes of upper GI bleeding

Causes	%
Duodenal ulcers	35
Gastric ulcers	20
Gastric erosions/haemorrhagic gastritis	15
Gastro-oesophageal varices	5–11
Mallory–Weiss tear	10
Gastric carcinoma	6
Other	3–9

Predicting outcome in upper GI bleeding

Scoring systems such as the Rockall Score can be used to guide management of upper GI bleeds. This is calculated for patients post endoscopy and comprises five categories. The maximum total score achievable is 11. A total of less than 3 is taken as low risk of rebleeding (4.3%) or death (0.1%), while scores greater or equal to 8 have a high risk (37% rebleed and 40% mortality) (Table 33.4).

Management of non-variceal upper GI bleeding

Initial management

As for management of a large GI bleed.

- Rapid resuscitation and haemodynamic stabilization.
- Early endoscopy to risk stratify, diagnose and aid treatment.
- Multi-disciplinary involvement including gastroenterology, surgical and radiological consultation.

Specific management

Several other treatment modalities can be employed to stop bleeding and prevent rebleeding.

Pharmacotherapy

Proton pump inhibitors (PPI) – Administered in high doses PPIs reduce the incidence of rebleeding, blood transfusion requirement and duration of hospital stay in patients with upper GI bleed. A typical regime

Table 33.4 Rockall Score

	0	1	2	3
Age	<60	60–79	>80	
Shock	Heart rate <100 SBP >100	Heart rate >100 SBP >100 mmHg	Systolic BP <100 mmHg	
Co-morbidities	None		CCF, IHD, major co-morbidities	Metastatic malignancy, renal failure, liver failure
Endoscopic stigmata	Mallory–Weiss tear	All other diagnoses	Gastric malignancy	
Evidence of bleeding	None		Adherent clot, spurting vessel	

Source: Adapted from Rockall *et al.* (1996) *Gut* **38**: 316–21.

involves an intravenous bolus dose of 80 mg of omeprazole followed by an infusion of 8 mg/hour for 72 hours. The mechanism of action is to raise the intragastric pH (a pH of lower than 6 has been shown to inhibit platelet aggregation and promote clot lysis).

Endoscopy

Endoscopy is used to:

(1) Diagnose the cause of bleeding
(2) Assess the risk of rebleeding
(3) Act as a treatment modality.

Endoscopic treatment achieves haemostasis in the majority of bleeding patients.

After this, the concern becomes the prevention of rebleeding: 20% of patients with upper GI bleeds and 70% of those with varices rebleed.

Resuscitation of the patient usually takes precedence over the timing of endoscopy but, obviously, some judgement must be exercised as stopping the bleeding may become the overriding concern in catastrophic bleeding. In the case of large GI bleeds endoscopy may have to be performed in theatre with the airway secured and the surgical team standing by.

The treatment options available to the endoscopist are:

(1) Injection of 1: 10 000 adrenaline around the bleeding point – this arrests bleeding in up to 95% of patients (rebleeding rate 15–20%).
(2) Thermocoagulation – this may be beneficial in conjunction with adrenaline when treating active arterial bleeding.
(3) Laser phototherapy – using a Nd-YAG laser to thermocoagulate.
(4) Mechanical clips – these may be useful for actively bleeding large vessels, but can be difficult to apply.

Further management

Rebleeding after initial successful treatment

A second endoscopic procedure may be appropriate as it has been shown that these patients have similar outcomes to those who proceed to surgery at first rebleed.

Persistent bleeding not amenable to endoscopic treatment

Surgical options should be considered.

Upper GI bleeding indications for surgery

- Failure of medical therapy/endoscopy.
- Coexisting reason for surgery, e.g. perforation or malignancy.
- Prolonged bleeding with loss of 50% circulating volume.
- Second hospitalization for peptic ulcer haemorrhage.

Variceal bleeding

Gastro-oesophageal varices are dilated submucosal veins which occur in approximately 40–60% of patients with cirrhosis. They are caused by obstruction to blood flow within the portal venous system, leading to increased portal pressure which is transmitted retrogradely through the valveless system. The presence and size of varices depends on the underlying cause, duration and severity of the cirrhosis.

Varices can occur at:

(1) the cardia of the stomach
(2) the distal 2–5 cm of the oesophagus
(3) the anal canal
(4) the abdominal wall
(5) para-umbilical veins
(6) abdominal viscera and into the left renal vein.

Variceal hemorrhage occurs in 25–35% of patients with cirrhosis and accounts for 80–90% of bleeding episodes in these patients. Up to 30% of these are fatal on initial presentation.

Management of variceal bleeding

Initial management

As for initial management of a large GI bleed or of non-variceal upper GI bleeding.

Specific management

Control of the bleeding can be attempted using several different treatment modalities.

Endoscopy

Control of active variceal bleeding has been shown to be achievable with sclerotherapy (80%) or band ligation (94%). Although previous studies had shown very little difference between both modalities, band ligation has been shown to have fewer complications.

Pharmacological treatment

Terlipressin (a vasopressin analogue) and octreotide (a somatostatin analogue) both cause splanchnic vasoconstriction, thereby lowering portal venous pressure and hence variceal wall tension. Evidence for the beneficial effect of both drugs has been conflicting. However both may be of advantage in conjunction with endoscopic therapy by decreasing the incidence of uncontrollable hemorrhage.

Beta-blockers such as propranolol can also be used long term to reduce portal pressure.

Balloon tamponade

Balloon devices have been shown to control acute bleeding in up to 90% of cases, although 50% rebleed on removal of the balloon. The Sengstaken–Blakemore tube is an orogastric tube with two balloons (one gastric and one oesophageal) and ports for aspirating stomach and proximal oesophageal content (Fig. 33.1). It compresses the varices to tamponade bleeding.

Complications of balloon tamponade include:

- Aspiration and airway distortion
- Oesophageal perforation or rupture
- Gastro-oesophageal erosions and ulcers.

Transjugular intrahepatic portosystemic shunt

Transjugular intrahepatic portosystemic shunt (TIPS) is used in major centres and requires considerable expertise. Under fluoroscopic guidance a catheter is passed via the hepatic vein into a branch of the portal vein (Fig. 33.2). A metal stent is then introduced to create an intrahepatic portosystemic shunt. It can dramatically control variceal bleeding.

Risks of TIPS include:

- Hepatic encephalopathy (in 25–60% of patients)
- Shunt dysfunction (50–60% of patients at 6 months)
- Intra-abdominal bleeding.

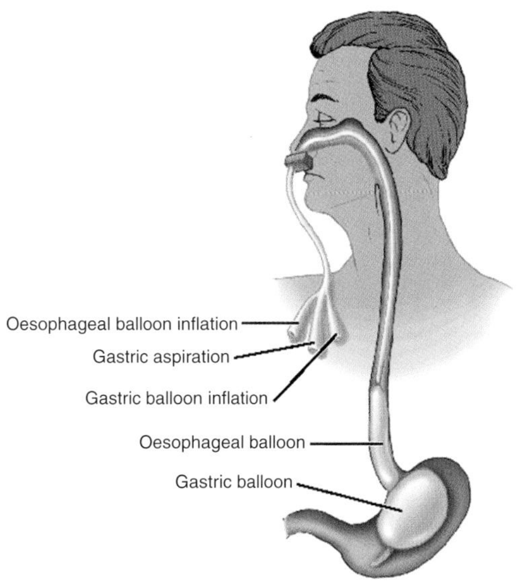

Fig. 33.1 Sengstaken–Blakemore tube.

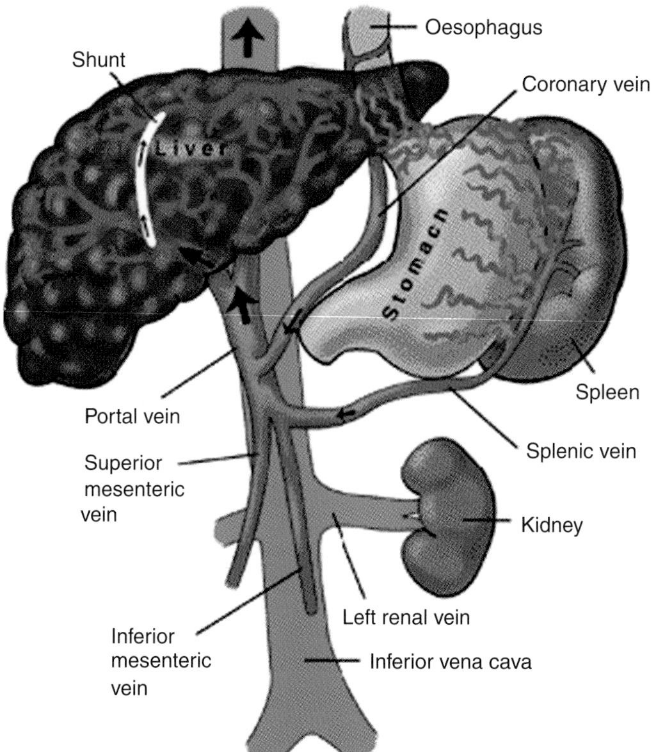

Fig. 33.2 Transjugular intrahepatic portosystemic shunt (TIPS). A radiologist tunnels through the liver with a needle and inserts a stent connecting the portal vein to one of the hepatic veins. The shunt allows the blood to flow normally through the liver to the hepatic vein. This reduces portal hypertension, and allows the veins to shrink in size and stop variceal bleeding.

Other supportive management of varices

- Blood and clotting products
- Lactulose to reduce nitrogen load
- Nutrition, vitamin K, folic acid and thiamine.

Prevention of upper GI bleeding on ICU

The incidence of clinically important upper GI bleeding in ICU is 1.5%, with an overall mortality of 9.7%. The main risk factors for clinically important bleeding amongst ICU patients are respiratory failure, head injury, burns and coagulopathy.

Methods used to decrease the incidence of upper GI bleeding on ICU include:

- Early enteral feeding
- The use of acid prophylaxis.

H_2 antagonists or proton pump inhibitors may be associated with an increase risk of ventilator associated pneumonia.

Lower GI bleeding

Lower GI bleeds account for only 18% of episodes of acute GI bleeding.

Of these, half will be caused by diverticular bleeding, while a significant proportion is accounted for by colonic angiomata. Other causes include inflammatory bowel disease, Meckel's diverticulum, polyps and carcinomata.

Management of lower GI bleeding

Initial management

As for initial management of a large GI bleed non-variceal upper GI bleeding and variceal bleeding.

Specific management

Endoscopy

Endoscopic (colonoscopy and sigmoidoscopy) treatment modalities are similar to those for upper GI bleeds. However, these are only indicated if a discrete source of bleeding is detected, which may only occur in 20% of patients with a lower GI bleed.

Patients with known risk factors for upper GI bleeding should undergo upper GI endoscopy first to exclude upper GI pathology as a cause of haemorrhage. About 10–15% of patients with rectal bleeding have a cause located proximal to the ligament of Treitz, i.e. upper GI bleeding.

Radiology

Isotope scan

If the bleeding is less than 0.5 ml/min, ^{99M}Tc radio-labelled red blood cells can isolate the bleeding vessel.

Angiography

When bleeding exceeds 0.5 ml/min angiography may help isolate and treat bleeding sites by embolization or infusion of vasopressin via the angiography catheter.

Radiological therapy poses logistical problems, including:

- remote location
- limited space in the angiography suite
- lack of appropriate equipment
- difficulty monitoring patients.

Therefore a decision has to be made as to whether a patient is stable enough to be subjected to this environment.

Consideration for surgery

- If medical therapy has failed.
- Segmental colectomy if bleeding point has been identified, otherwise a sub-total colectomy should be considered.

GI perforation

As with GI bleeding, the presentation of this pathology may vary with the site of the lesion.

Causes

The possible causes of GI perforation include:

- malignancy
- ulceration
- diverticular disease
- appendicitis
- foreign body ingestion, infection
- iatrogenic causes, e.g. perforation due to endoscopy.

Upper GI Perforation

Incidence

The incidence of peptic ulcer perforation has decreased in recent years, due to improved treatment of peptic ulcer disease.

- Duodenal ulcers are 2–3 times more likely to perforate than gastric ulcers.
- Approximately one-third of gastric perforations are due to gastric carcinoma.

Oesophageal perforation is rare but carries a high mortality rate.

- Only 15% are due to Boerhaave syndrome (rupture due to vomiting).
- Iatrogenic causes make up to 75% of cases.

Upper GI perforations can be classified as either free perforations or contained:

Free perforation – occurs when connection between the GI lumen and abdominal cavity allows the drainage of the former into the latter. It causes severe abdominal pain, nausea, vomiting and pyrexia.

Contained perforation – occurs when adjacent viscera directly prevent the leakage of GI content into the abdominal cavity.

Because of the sterile nature of the upper GI tract the patient may present initially with a chemical peritonitis. Bacterial colonization may however occur in the presence of other gastric pathology or if food enters the abdominal cavity. Bacterial contamination of the peritoneal cavity is rare when the perforation is treated promptly.

Surgery forms the mainstay of management of peptic ulcer perforation. This is usually performed as an open procedure, although laparoscopic techniques are becoming increasingly popular.

Lower GI perforation

Incidence

Approximately 15% of patients with diverticulitis will develop bowel perforation. The mortality rate is high (20–40%) as patients may suffer from sepsis and multi-organ failure.

The perioperative mortality rate for perforation in the presence of an adenocarcinoma of the colon is around 30%, with the one year survival being considerably worse.

Management of bowel perforation

If bowel perforation is suspected, the diagnosis can be aided by the use of imaging. An erect chest radiograph will show air under the diaphragm in 60% of cases (Fig. 33.3); similarly gas and fluid can be visualized on computed tomography of the abdominal cavity.

Initial management

This follows the ABC approach to resuscitation of critically ill patients.

Specific management

(1) Fluid balance – large fluid losses can occur into the abdominal cavity or into the bowel itself.

(2) Co-morbidities – mortality from bowel perforation increases with age and the presence of significant co-morbidities.

(3) Antibiotics – these need to cover gram-negative organisms and anaerobic bacteria.

(4) Surgery – although surgery forms the mainstay of treatment, in the absence of peritonitis or infection conservative management may be undertaken. Where indicated, surgery is undertaken to:

- remove bowel content
- remove devitalized tissue
- drain abscesses and collections
- defunction the bowel to prevent further contamination.

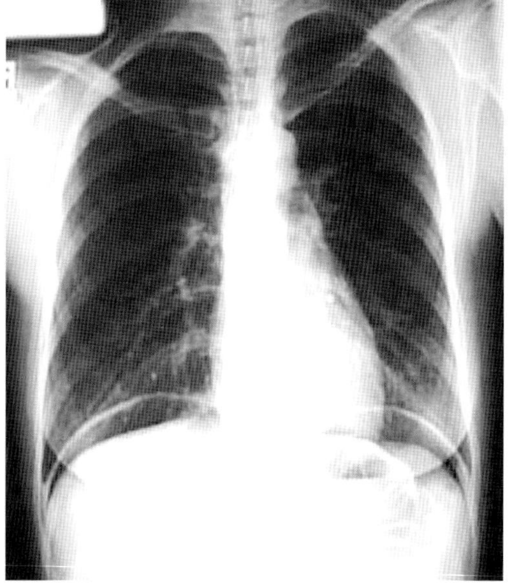

Fig. 33.3 Chest X-ray showing air under the diaphragm.

Post-operative complications

The bowel distal to the terminal ileum is colonized by bacteria including aerobic organisms such as *E. coli* and anaerobic organisms such as *B. fragilis*. Untreated these can form abscesses or cause overwhelming abdominal sepsis.

Invasive monitoring may become essential on the ITU as patients have the potential to develop:

- Overwhelming infection secondary to faecal contamination.
- ARDS.
- Abdominal compartment syndrome (damage occurs at abdominal pressures greater than 20 cmH_2O).
- Multi-organ failure.

Key points

- Management of significant GI bleed starts with the ABC approach. It requires an early multi-disciplinary approach involving gastrointestinal, surgical and radiological consultation.
- High doses of proton pump inhibitors reduce the incidence of rebleeding, blood transfusion requirement and duration of hospital stay in patients with upper GI bleed.
- Endoscopic treatment achieves haemostasis in the majority of patients with non-variceal bleeding.
- Balloon tamponade has been shown to control acute bleeding in up to 90% of variceal bleeding.
- Patients with bowel perforation will need resuscitation using the ABC approach and surgery if signs of peritonitis are present.

Further reading

- Acute Respiratory Distress Syndrome Network (2000) Ventilation with lower tidal volumes as compared with traditional tidal volumes for acute lung injury and the acute respiratory distress syndrome. *N. Engl. J. Med.* **342**: 1301–8.
- Cook DJ, Fuller HD, Guyatt GH *et al.* (1994) Risk factors for gastrointestinal bleeding in critically ill patients. *N. Engl. J. Med.* **330**: 377–81.
- Kwan I, Bunn F, Roberts I (2001) Timing and volume of fluid administration for patients with bleeding following trauma. *Cochrane Database Syst. Rev.* CD002245.

- Lo GH, Lai KH, Cheng JS *et al.* (1995) A prospective, randomized trial of sclerotherapy versus ligation in the management of bleeding esophageal varices. *Hepatology* **22**: 466–71.
- Palmer K (2002) British Society of Gastroenterology Endoscopy Committee: Non-variceal upper gastrointestinal haemorrhage – guidelines. *Gut* **51** (Suppl. 4): iv1–iv6.
- Papatheodoridis GV, Goulis J, Leandro G, Patch D, Burroughs AK (1999) Transjugular intrahepatic portosystemic shunt compared with endoscopic treatment for prevention of variceal rebleeding: a meta-analysis. *Hepatology* **30**: 612–22.
- Rockall TA, Logan RF, Devlin HB, Northfield TC (1995) Incidence of and mortality from acute upper gastrointestinal haemorrhage in the United Kingdom: Steering Committee and members of the National Audit of Acute Upper Gastrointestinal Haemorrhage. *Br. Med. J.* **311**: 222–6.
- Sharara AI, Rockey DC (2001) Gastroesophageal variceal hemorrhage. *N. Engl. J. Med.* **345**: 669–81.
- Stiegmann GV, Goff JS, Michaletz-Onody PA *et al.* (1992) Endoscopic sclerotherapy as compared with endoscopic ligation for bleeding esophageal varices. *N. Engl. J. Med.* **326**: 1527–32.

Severe acute pancreatitis

Andrew Burtenshaw and Neil Crooks

Introduction

Acute pancreatitis is one of the most common abdominal conditions necessitating hospital admission in the UK, with an annual incidence of 150–420 per million. Despite advances in organ support, the mortality rate from the disease has remained relatively constant since the 1970s, and the incidence appears to be rising. Of the cases diagnosed, approximately 20% are classified as severe and are associated with a high rate of morbidity and mortality. Severe acute pancreatitis (SAP) is addressed in this chapter, as this is most likely to require critical care support.

The multiple aetiologies for the initial acute inflammation of the pancreas are discussed later in the chapter. The natural progression of the disease is related to the intrapancreatic activation of proteolytic enzymes, which occurs when the protective physiological mechanisms are disrupted. This has been described as an 'autodigestive' state.

From the critical care perspective, SAP may be defined as acute pancreatitis accompanied by systemic organ dysfunction. Two distinct phases of mortality in SAP are described – early (due to the systemic inflammatory response syndrome) and late (due to secondary infection of necrotic pancreatic tissue).

Other common complications of SAP include peri-pancreatic fluid collections, tissue necrosis, haemorrhage and abscess or pseudocyst formation. With or without these features, SAP is a potent cause of systemic inflammatory response syndrome (SIRS), severe sepsis and multiple organ dysfunction syndrome (MODS).

Aetiology

Regardless of the underlying aetiology, a common pathophysiological mechanism is proposed in acute pancreatitis. Within the pancreatic acinar cells there is regulatory failure of trypsinogen activation to trypsin. This, together with the generation and release of pro-inflammatory mediators, leads to inflammation and necrosis of acinar cells and activates systemic inflammatory processes. These pro-inflammatory agents include IL-1, IL-6, IL-8, phospholipase A_2 and oxygen free radicals.

Although there are a multitude of potential triggers for this mechanism, alcohol and biliary obstruction due to gallstones are implicated in the majority (approximately 80%) of cases in the developed world. A more complete summary of causes can be divided as follows.

Obstructive causes

With a peak incidence in the sixth and seventh decades, gallstone disease (choledocolithiasis) affects women more commonly than men. In series examining patients from the USA, Asia and Western Europe gallstones were found to account for approximately 45% of cases of acute pancreatitis. However, there are large variations in published figures depending upon the population being studied.

Other causes of obstructive acute pancreatitis are uncommon. They include:

- Pancreatic carcinoma – acute pancreatitis may be the presenting feature in approximately 3% of cases of carcinoma of the head of pancreas.
- Anatomical obstruction – duodenal diverticula and choledochal cysts may obstruct the pancreatic duct.
- Pancreas divisum – approximately 5–7% of the population possess a congenital variation in the anatomical arrangement of ducts draining the pancreas. In this situation the duct of Santorini (which drains the posterior pancreas) does not fuse

Core Topics in Critical Care Medicine, eds. Fang Gao Smith and Joyce Yeung. Published by Cambridge University Press.

with the duct of Wirsung (which drains the anterior pancreas), and enters the duodenum via a separate papilla. This duct is thought to be at increased risk of stenosis and explains the increased incidence of acute pancreatitis in patients with this congenital variation.

- Ascariasis – migration of helminths via the biliary and pancreatic ducts may result in obstruction. Although rare in developed countries, this is particularly common in India.
- Hypertensive sphincter of Oddi – a sphincter pressure of 40 mmHg or greater, measured endoscopically, may account for up to 15% of cases of acute pancreatitis where no other cause has been identified.
- Any other lesion obstructing the pancreatic duct, such as metastatic deposits, has the potential to precipitate acute pancreatitis.

Toxins and drugs

After gallstones, alcohol is the second most common cause of acute pancreatitis. The incidence of alcohol-related acute pancreatitis in the developed world is reported to have markedly increased over the last 40 years. The mechanism of alcohol-induced acute pancreatitis is incompletely understood, although some evidence points to increased sensitivity of acinar cell cholecystokinin receptors leading to increased release of trypsin.

A significant number of other drugs and toxins are also implicated in the aetiology of acute pancreatitis, including:

- azathioprine
- cimetidine
- didanosine
- erythromycin
- frusemide
- mercaptopurine
- methanol
- methyldopa
- metronidazole
- nitrofurantoin
- organosphosphorus insecticides
- pentamidine
- ranitidine
- salicylates
- steroids
- sulphonamides
- tetracycline
- valproic acid.

Metabolic causes

Hyperlipidaemias (particularly types I, IV and V) are associated with acute pancreatitis. Hypercalcaemia is a very rare cause.

Trauma and surgery

This includes either blunt abdominal trauma or iatrogenic trauma resulting from instrumentation of the pancreatic ductal system, e.g. during endoscopic retrograde cholangiopancreatography (ERCP) and endoscopic sphincterotomy. Acute pancreatitis has been described as a post-operative complication of thoracic and abdominal surgery, and has also been associated with cardiopulmonary bypass.

Infection

Viral infection is an uncommon cause of acute pancreatitis. Known precipitants include mumps, coxsackievirus, cytomegalovirus, hepatitis A, hepatitis B and non-A, non-B hepatitis.

Immunocompromised patients, including those with AIDS, are at significantly increased risk of acute pancreatitis of infective aetiology resulting from opportunistic infection. The organisms implicated include cytomegalovirus, *Toxoplasma gondii*, *Cryptococcus neoformans* and *Mycobacterium tuberculosis*. As discussed above, some antiviral agents and antiretrovirals are independently associated with pancreatitis.

Miscellaneous

Other unusual causes of pancreatitis include hypothermia, autoimmune pancreatitis and scorpion venom.

Idiopathic pancreatitis

Idiopathic pancreatitis is a diagnosis of exclusion, and typically accounts for approximately 10% of cases. Recent evidence involving biliary drainage studies, evaluation of subsequent cholecystectomy specimens and ERCP with sphincterotomy suggests that many of these cases may be caused by microlithiasis.

Diagnosis

The diagnosis of acute pancreatitis relies upon the combination of history, clinical examination, laboratory investigations and imaging.

The clinical picture may vary but patients typically present with epigastric pain, often radiating to the back, accompanied by nausea and vomiting. Examination findings may reveal signs of peritonitism and occasionally periumbilical discoloration (Cullen's sign: Fig. 34.1) or bruising of the flanks (Grey-Turner's sign: Fig. 34.2), both of which are suggestive of retroperitoneal haemorrhage and typically take 24–48 hours to develop.

The clinical findings are not pathognomonic and may be associated with other pathologies such as ruptured or leaking aortic aneurysm, ruptured ectopic pregnancy, perforated viscus or blunt abdominal trauma.

Serum amylase level is a sensitive diagnostic marker only if the patient presents within hours of the onset of abdominal pain as the level may subsequently return to normal. The extent of hyperamylasaemia is a poor indicator of illness severity and is believed to be lower in alcoholic than non-alcoholic pancreatitis. Serum amylase rise is also well documented in other intra-abdominal inflammatory processes and therefore the specificity of this test is poor.

Serum lipase assays offer a higher sensitivity and specificity than amylase and return to baseline levels less rapidly, making this a more useful diagnostic tool for late presentation of suspected acute pancreatitis. This assay, however, is not universally available.

Elevation of serum alanine aminotransferase to three or more times the upper limit of normal is particularly suggestive of gallstone pancreatitis. Other laboratory tests include serum trypsinogen, immunolipase and fractionation of pancreatic isoamylase. None of these tests is currently believed to offer diagnostic superiority compared to amylase or lipase when used in combination with clinical and radiological findings.

An abdominal X-ray may demonstrate local ileus in the presence of severe acute pancreatitis, and is referred to as a 'sentinel loop' (Fig. 34.3). Contrast enhanced computed tomography (CT) has a very high sensitivity and specificity in the context of severe acute pancreatitis, but may miss mild disease (Fig. 34.4). CT will demonstrate the extent of pancreatic damage and identify many of the associated complications of SAP, such as haemorrhage or cyst formation (Fig. 34.5). It may also identify some obstructive causes. However, ultrasonography remains a superior means of examining the integrity and patency of the biliary tract, frequently identifying gallstones not represented on CT scan (Fig. 34.6 and Fig. 34.7). One disadvantage of ultrasound is that overlying bowel gas may obscure the view.

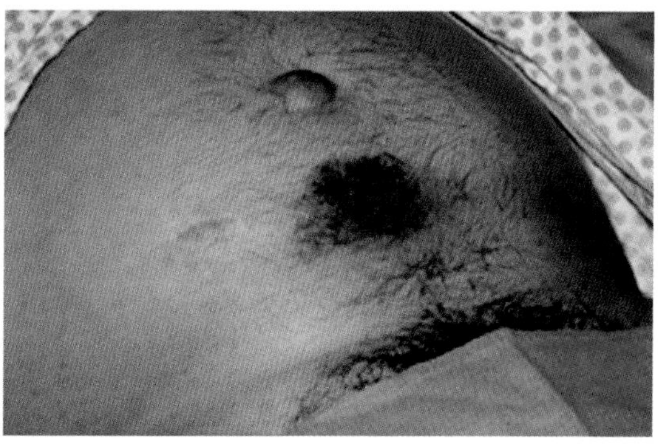

Fig. 34.1 Cullen's sign.

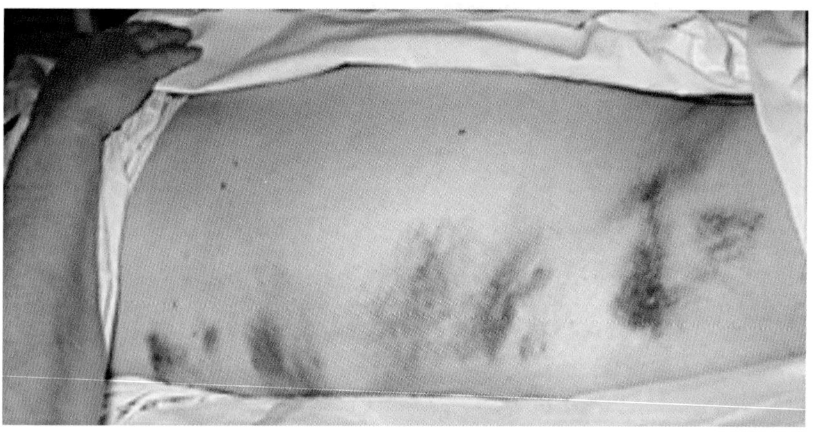

Fig. 34.2 Grey-Turner's sign.

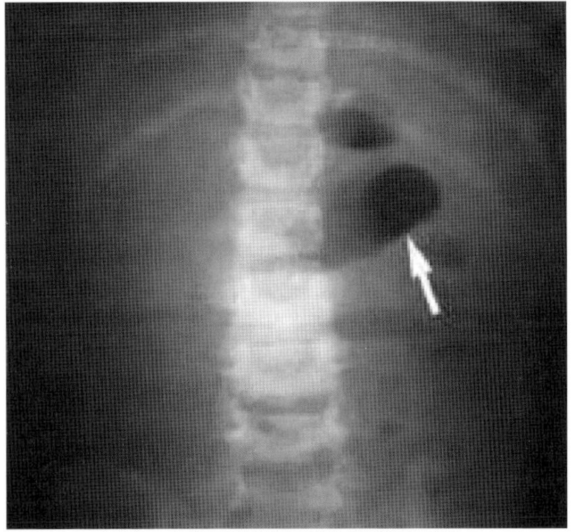

Fig. 34.3 Abdominal X-ray showing sentinel loop (arrow) associated with acute pancreatitis.

Finally, ERCP with manometry may be used as a diagnostic tool if the history, clinical examination and imaging have failed to identify a cause. ERCP typically demonstrates a cause in up to 50% of cases, and enables identification of pathologies such as pancreatic ductal strictures, microlithiasis, small pancreatic tumours, hypertensive sphincter of Oddi, pancreas divisum and choledochocoele.

Prognostic factors

On account of the wide spectrum of disease severity in acute pancreatitis there is particular interest in prognostic indicators that may help to determine the requirement for therapeutic interventions.

The overall mortality associated with SAP is approximately 30% with deaths occurring predominantly at two distinct time intervals. In the early phase

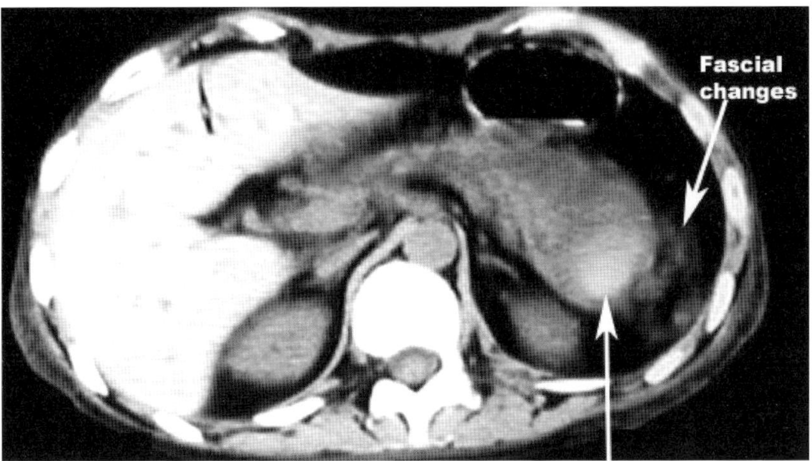

Fig. 34.4 CT scan showing haemorrhagic pancreas.

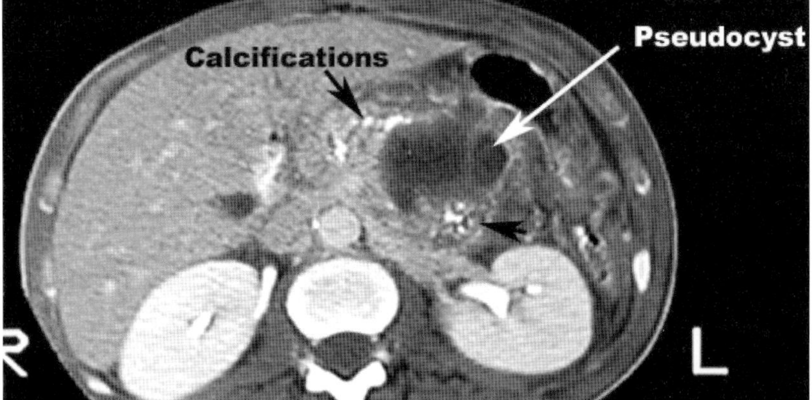

Fig. 34.5 CT scan showing a pseudocyst and calcification.

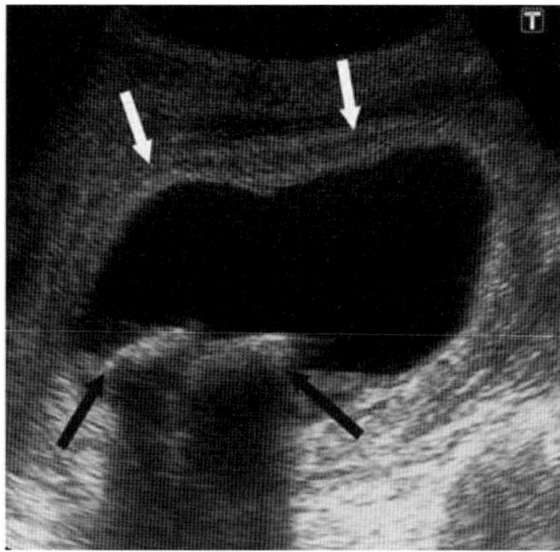

Fig. 34.6 Ultrasound image showing gallbladder with thickened walls (white arrows) and calcified gallstones at the bladder neck (black arrows), consistent with acute cholecystitis.

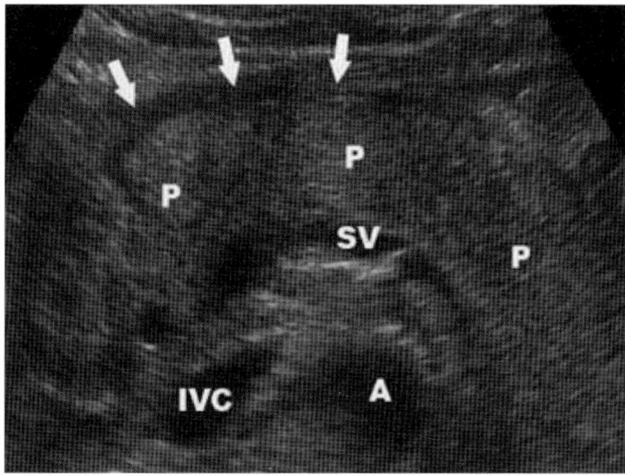

Fig. 34.7 Axial ultrasound image showing pancreatitis. The pancreas (P) is draped over the splenic vein (SV), which is hypoechoic and swollen, with a rim of fluid around its edge (white arrows). A is the aorta and IVC the inferior vena cava.

(up to 14 days) massive cytokine release precipitates a systemic inflammatory response causing death from multiple organ failure. The late phase of mortality occurs as a result of local and systemic infection. The presence of necrosis is almost universal in those described as having SAP. If this becomes infected, the mortality rate rises dramatically from approximately 10% to as much as 60%. However, patients with sterile pancreatic necrosis but high illness severity scores also demonstrate significantly elevated mortality rates.

The key features likely to have an adverse impact upon morbidity and mortality in acute pancreatitis include the development of pancreatic and peripancreatic necrosis, retroperitoneal fat necrosis, presence of biologically active compounds in pancreatic ascites, infection of necrotic tissue and pancreatic pseudocyst or abscess formation. These features will each have an independent effect on the risk of death from sepsis and multiple organ failure.

The use of the biochemical markers procalcitonin and IL-6 is gaining importance as they may give an earlier prediction of severity in acute pancreatitis.

Severity of illness scores

A number of scoring systems have been developed to attempt risk stratification in acute pancreatitis. Some of these were developed prior to the widespread availability of CT scanning, and therefore do not take into account radiological findings, instead focusing on biological and biochemical markers.

Ranson criteria

In 1974 Ranson published criteria which were developed following the evaluation of 100 patients with predominantly alcohol-related pancreatitis. These criteria were based on clinical and laboratory data obtained at the time of admission and at 48 hours afterwards (Table 34.1). The number of positive criteria was summated to produce a predicted mortality rate.

This scoring system requires 48 hours to complete and as a result relates poorly to the requirements of modern critical care medicine which is characterized by rapid and ongoing evaluation and early goal-directed therapy. Equally, the modern emphasis on early resuscitation and advances in therapeutic options mean that a Ranson score exceeding 6 is no longer associated with a mortality rate of 100%, as originally published.

Glasgow score

Blamey *et al.* reviewed Ranson's criteria and identified LDH, base deficit and fluid sequestration volume as poor predictors of outcome. The revised system excluded these and became known as the Glasgow or Imrie score.

APACHE II score

The Acute Physiology and Chronic Health Evaluation (APACHE) II score can produce serial data to delineate deterioration or improvement rather than being restricted to use within the first 48 hours of admission, although prospective use of this as a predictive tool has

Table 34.1 Ranson score

On admission	Age >55 years White cell count >16 000/mm^3 Glucose >11 mmol/l LDH >400 IU/l AST >250 IU/l
Within 48 hours of hospitalization	Decrease in haematocrit >10% Increase in blood urea >1.8 mmol/l Calcium <2 mmol/l PaO_2 <8 kPa Base deficit >4 mmol/l Fluid requirement >6 l
Risk factors	**Mortality rate**
0–2	<1%
3–4	>15%
5–6	>40%
>6	>100%

only been evaluated for the first 24–48 hours after onset of pancreatitis. Although complex to calculate, most units undertake initial APACHE II scoring as part of the Intensive Care National Audit and Research Centre (ICNARC) audit process. This scoring system is covered in more detail in Chapter 5.

Pancreatitis outcome prediction (POP) score

In 2007, Harrison *et al.* published a scoring system based upon the retrospective study of 2462 SAP patients from 159 intensive care units in the UK. SAP was defined as pancreatitis with distant organ dysfunction. Six parameters were identified as being closely linked to outcome and were weighted to produce a prognostic score ranging from 0 to 40 points. These six factors in order of decreasing impact were:

- arterial pH
- age
- serum urea
- mean arterial pressure
- PaO_2/F_iO_2 ratio
- total serum calcium.

Treatments

The mainstay of treatment in SAP is supportive care. The mortality associated with the first peak in the biphasic mortality curve is attributable to systemic inflammatory response and multiple organ failure. Full intensive care support may be necessary including ventilatory, cardiovascular and renal support.

Once the precipitating cause of pancreatitis has, where possible, been eliminated the specific treatment options available in SAP include the following.

Analgesia

Acute pancreatitis typically causes severe abdominal pain which may require aggressive analgesia. Failure to provide adequate pain relief may adversely affect respiratory function, increasing the risk of basal atelectasis and subsequent healthcare associated pneumonia (HCAP).

Traditionally pethidine has been used in preference to morphine due to fears that morphine may cause greater constriction of the sphincter of Oddi. Non-steroidal anti-inflammatory drugs are best avoided due to the risk of contributing to renal dysfunction.

Fluid replacement

Large volumes of fluid are usually sequestered as inflammatory exudate in the region of the pancreas in the retroperitoneum and as reactive ascites. In addition, low colloid oncotic pressure and capillary leak contribute to substantial fluid losses and maldistribution throughout the body tissues producing significant intravascular fluid depletion.

This may be exacerbated by relative hypovolaemia due to a low systemic vascular resistance as a result of SIRS and sepsis. Haemorrhage into necrotic pancreatic tissue is common, contributing further to intravascular depletion.

Consequently, large volumes of fluid are almost invariably required, necessitating central venous pressure measurement and cardiac output studies in the majority of cases. The choice of fluid remains controversial, as does the extent of fluid replacement.

Electrolyte management

Sequestration of calcium frequently results in hypocalcaemia requiring replacement therapy. In addition, magnesium and phosphate plasma levels are often diminished.

Insulin requirements

To compound the loss of endocrine function of the pancreas, the systemic inflammatory response and sepsis associated with SAP contribute to hyperglycaemia. Therefore, hyperglycaemia is a common feature and requires correction with insulin replacement.

Depending on the degree of pancreatic damage, survivors of SAP may exhibit endocrine and exocrine insufficiency, requiring long-term insulin therapy.

Prophylactic antibiotic agents

As alluded to earlier, infection is an important aspect of SAP contributing to 80% of deaths. Infectious complications may be intra- or extrapancreatic and account for the majority of cases of late-phase mortality.

Early studies using ampicillin in patients with alcoholic pancreatitis showed no change in the clinical course of those treated compared to those given placebo. However, ampicillin is known to have poor penetration into pancreatic tissue.

Subsequent studies have examined the use of other agents, particularly the carbapenems (e.g. imipenem and meropenem), which are known to have excellent pancreatic penetration. Studies using prophylactic carbapenems in SAP have yielded conflicting results with some studies showing a reduction in infectious complications and improvement in mortality rates. Therefore two recent meta-analyses failed to demonstrate a reduction in the rate of infected necrosis, extrapancreatic infection, need for surgical intervention or mortality.

A Cochrane Review examining the role of prophylactic antibiotics in acute pancreatitis also failed to identify sufficient conclusive data upon which to base a recommendation. Similarly, there is divided opinion on the role of prophylactic antifungal agents in SAP. Therefore the use of prophylactic antimicrobial therapy varies between centres.

Nutritional support

Although it is clear that nutrition is an essential component of supportive treatment in SAP, the optimum route of administration has been debated over the years. The consensus of opinion now appears to be that enteral nutritional support should be commenced as early as possible.

If absorption of enteral nutrition (EN) is impaired for 5 days or more due to ileus, total parenteral nutrition (TPN) is often commenced. However, the use of TPN in critical care patients has declined considerably over the last decade following observations of increased catheter-related sepsis and other septic complications, increased permeability of the gut wall and financial considerations. Meanwhile, a lack of evidence to support the use of TPN in acute pancreatitis together with increased evidence of adverse effects has resulted in a move away from TPN towards EN.

In health, intragastric feeding promotes the release of secretions from the pancreatic gland, although the response in SAP is unknown. As a consequence it has been suggested that provision of nutrients beyond the ligament of Treitz, which indicates a point below the cholecystokinin (CCK) cells, will not have a deleterious effect on the natural progression and resolution of the disease process as pancreatic exocrine function will not be stimulated. This necessitates a jejunal feeding tube, which can either be placed endoscopically, surgically or by means of a self-propelling nasojejunal feeding tube. Despite this speculation, the current British Society of Gastroenterologists guidelines state that the nasogastric route may be effective in up to 80% of cases and recommend this route in the first instance.

Surgical debridement

Early surgery (<48 hours) in patients with gallstone pancreatitis was found in early studies to dramatically increase mortality as compared to delayed surgery (>48 hours), particularly in a subset of patients with severe pancreatitis. Despite later studies which have failed to support this, many surgeons are reluctant to operate unless strictly necessary. Which factors constitute 'necessity' remains controversial.

Potential surgical interventions include pancreatic resection, necrosectomy (excision of necrotic tissue) and local drainage, necrosectomy and lavage of the lesser sac, or necrosectomy with open packing and planned re-exploration. In deciding which patients are appropriate for surgical intervention, it is important to separate those with *infected* pancreatic necrosis from those with *sterile* pancreatic necrosis. The evidence suggests that patients with sterile necrosis who are managed surgically have a worse outcome than those managed conservatively.

It is generally agreed that the following are indications for surgical intervention:

- Where there is doubt as to the correct diagnosis explorative laparotomy is unlikely to exacerbate the situation but may confirm an alternative diagnosis allowing appropriate management.

- Persistent biliary pancreatitis. Biliary washout and insertion of a T-tube into the common bile duct together with placement of a feeding jejunostomy tube is often advocated, although ERCP may represent a safer option.
- Infected necrotic pancreatic tissue is generally accepted as an indication for surgical debridement. The ideal surgical procedure remains uncertain.
- The presence of a pancreatic abscess necessitates drainage. A high failure rate with radiologically placed percutaneous drainage brings surgical drainage into consideration.

In terms of the surgical approach itself, there is now some evidence to suggest that a minimally invasive (retroperitoneal) approach may offer advantages, in terms of improved outcome, compared to open laparotomy.

ERCP

In contrast to disappointing results following early surgical intervention in SAP, emergency intervention by ERCP has produced more satisfactory results. However, the studies to date have been small and, although they have indicated a significantly lower morbidity in SAP secondary to gallstones, they have been underpowered and have only demonstrated a trend towards reduced mortality.

Percutaneous drainage

Percutaneous drainage of necrotic pancreatic tissue has been attempted, but has been largely unsuccessful due to the propensity for drain blockage. However, drainage of pancreatic abscesses under radiological guidance may be considerably more successful due to the lack of necrotic tissue within, potentially obviating the need for open surgery.

Selective digestive decontamination (SDD) of the gut

It has been proposed that the presence of pancreatitis encourages bacterial translocation across the gut wall precipitating infection within the pancreatic and peripancreatic tissues. Therefore, it is thought that elimination of gram-negative bacteria within the gut may reduce the incidence of septic complications. Whilst there is limited evidence to support this, it is rarely performed in practice because of the difficulties associated with its administration and assessment of effective decontamination. In addition, there are concerns that resistant gram-positive cocci such as methicillin-resistant *Staphylococcus aureus* (MRSA) may benefit from a positive selection bias.

Other specific interventions

Other treatment modalities have been aimed at reducing pancreatic exocrine secretion in an attempt to interrupt the autodigestive cycle. Compounds examined to date include glucagon, somatostatin, octreotide, cimetidine, atropine, calcitonin and fluorouracil. None of these has been shown to confer significant benefit.

The autodigestive process that occurs in acute pancreatitis is due to an imbalance between proteases and antiproteases. Therefore, it has been suggested that intravenously administered proteolytic enzyme inhibitors, such as aprotinin and gabexate mesilate, may reduce the severity of the pathological process. Two randomized, controlled, double-blind studies have shown no difference in mortality, complication rate or the need for surgery between treatment and placebo groups. Studies using intraperitoneal aprotinin also failed to demonstrate an outcome benefit.

Two controlled studies have also examined peritoneal lavage and failed to demonstrate a survival benefit. It is therefore rarely performed.

Key points

- Severe acute pancreatitis (SAP) carries a high morbidity and mortality rate.
- Effective management involves a multidisciplinary team approach comprising intensivists, gastroenterologists, surgeons and interventional radiologists.
- Severity of illness scores may offer prognostic information, which may in turn affect the selection of therapies and interventions.
- Aggressive resuscitation with continuing supportive care is the mainstay of treatment.
- The consensus of opinion supports early nutritional support, whilst the ideal route remains controversial.
- The benefits of most other specific treatments, including prophylactic antibiotic therapy, remain unclear.

Further reading

- Baron TH, Desiree EM (1999) Acute necrotizing pancreatitis: Review. *N. Engl. J. Med.* **340**: 1412–17.
- Frossard J-L, Steer ML, Pastor CM (2008) Acute pancreatitis. *Lancet* **371**: 143–52.
- Harrison DA, D'Amico G, Singer M (2007) The Pancreatitis Outcome Prediction (POP) score: a new prognostic index for patients with severe acute pancreatitis. *Crit. Care Med.* **35** (7): 1703–8.
- Nathens AB, Curtis JR, Beale RJ *et al.* (2004) Management of the critically ill patient with severe acute pancreatitis. *Crit. Care Med.* **32**: 2524–36.
- Steinberg W, Tenner S (1994) Acute pancreatitis: Review. *N. Engl. J. Med.* **330**: 1198–1210.
- UK Working Party on Acute Pancreatitis (2005) UK guidelines for the management of acute pancreatitis. *Gut* **54**: 1–9
- Wyncoll D (1999) The management of acute severe necrotising pancreatitis: an evidence-based review of the literature. *Intens. Care Med.* **25**: 146–56.

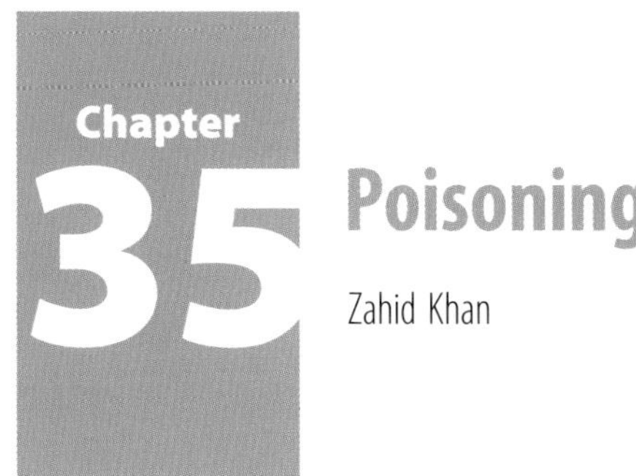

Poisoning

Zahid Khan

Introduction

Acute poisoning is a common emergency making up to 10–20% of hospital medical admissions. Deliberate self-poisoning is usually an intentional oral ingestion of a variety of drugs by previously well adults and makes up 95% of cases. Only a few drugs make up of 90% of overdoses. The most frequent compounds involved in the United Kingdom are aspirin, paracetamol, benzodiazepines, tricyclic antidepressants, carbon monoxide and alcohol. Poisoning is the most common cause of non-traumatic coma in under 35-year-olds. Although the majority of patients with poisoning and drug overdose do not require access to an intensive care unit, they account for approximately 15% of the intensive care unit admissions. The mortality remains low at around 1% with anoxic brain injury, cardiac arrhythmias and seizures being the common causes. The evidence for treatment is limited and recommendations are based on clinical experience. In only a small number of cases are specific antidotes available, but fortunately in most cases good basic supportive care is all that is required.

The general principles of care are diagnosis, resuscitation, clinical examination, investigation, drug manipulation, continued supportive care and specific measures. In acute cases all will be carried out simultaneously. It must also be remembered that deliberate self-poisoning may be a presenting symptom of underlying psychosocial problems and the patient may be at significant suicide risk.

History and diagnosis

It is important for diagnosis and management to take a detailed history of the overdose. The type, quantity and time elapsed since drug consumption, initial symptoms especially vomiting and diarrhoea and any co-morbidity should be sought. The information from the patient and family may be inaccurate and unreliable because overdose may be a suicide attempt or for fear of prosecution if illegal drugs are involved. In the United Kingdom a visual drug identification database is available called TICTAC.

Initial assessment and resuscitation

Airway and breathing

The patients with suspected overdose should have their vital signs assessed and a patent airway with adequate ventilation and perfusion should be secured (ABCs). The airway is at risk of obstruction in patients in a coma, particularly if narcotics or sedatives have been ingested; the patient should be placed in the recovery position and high-flow oxygen administered (except in paraquat poisoning). Patients who exhibit signs of partial airway obstruction such as noisy respiration should have dentures removed, the oropharynx cleared and an oral or nasal airway inserted; anaesthetic help should be sought early. Those patients who have a Glasgow Coma Score <8 and do not possess a gag reflex should be intubated to protect their airway with an endotracheal tube. Intubation and controlled ventilation may also be necessary in those patients who are hypoventilating due to severe central nervous system depression. Central nervous system stimulation or metabolic acidosis can result in hyperventilation; this suggests ingestion of salicylates, theophyllines, amphetamines, cocaine, methanol, phencyclidine, cyanide or carbon monoxide.

Circulation

Resuscitation of the circulation should be promptly carried out in those patients who are hypotensive or showing signs of hypoperfusion by the securing of intravenous access and the administration of

Core Topics in Critical Care Medicine, eds. Fang Gao Smith and Joyce Yeung. Published by Cambridge University Press.

crystalloid fluids. An evident tachycardia is a sign of anticholinergic, amphetamine, cocaine or cyclic antidepressant overdose. Digitalis, clonidine, beta-blocker and calcium channel blocker overdoses can cause sinus bradycardia or heart block. Marked hypertension may indicate amphetamine, cocaine, thyroid hormone or catecholamine toxicity. Hyperthermia may suggest the presence of anticholinergic, amphetamine or cyclic antidepressant drugs and is also seen in alcohol withdrawal. Hypothermia can be seen with alcohol and sedative overdoses often due to prolonged cold environmental exposure.

Many doctors support the early administration of intravenous thiamine to prevent Wernicke's encephalopathy, glucose if hypoglycaemic as this can imitate several drug overdoses and is easily corrected, and the narcotic antagonist naloxone. It is important not to neglect coexisting trauma and medical illness. Patients with altered mental status may have suffered a head injury or be suffering from meningitis/encephalitis or hypoglycaemia; other causes of coma should be considered if there are lateralizing signs or no recovery within 18 hrs of ingestion. The computed tomographic scan of head and neck can be used to rule out significant cervical or intracranial injury. Examination of the mouth may reveal undigested tablets or evidence of caustic injury. The ingestion of certain substances has a characteristic breath odour, e.g. sweet smell of ketones, almond smell of cyanide, garlic smell of organophosphates; chloral hydrate smells of pear. Miosis is caused by narcotics, barbiturates, organophosphates and phenothiazines. Drugs with anticholinergic properties such as amphetamines, antihistamines, cocaine and cyclic antidepressants cause mydriasis. Ethanol, carbamezapine, phenytoin, lithium and phenycyclidine overdoses often cause nystagmus. Reactive dilated pupils suggest anticholinergic or sympathomimetic overdose whilst fixed dilated pupils are a feature of mushroom or glutethimide poisoning.

Clinical examination

The patient's symptoms and signs elicited on physical examination will provide clues to the most likely drugs involved and guide early therapy especially when the cause is unidentified (Table 35.1). Many poisons affect several organ systems with non-specific signs and symptoms that appear in clusters that can be categorized into classic 'toxic syndromes' (Table 35.2).

Table 35.1 Symptoms and signs related to common poisons

Clinical effects	Possible poisons
Coma, lethargy	Alcohols, barbiturates, benzodiazepines, opiates, lithium, salicylates
Miosis	Opioids, organophosphates
Mydriasis	Hypothermia, hypoxia, tricyclics, phenothiazines, anticholinergics
Nystagmus	Alcohols, carbamazepine, phenytoin, phencyclidine, sedatives
Seizures	Tricyclics, isoniazid, lithium, amphetamines, carbon monoxide, phenothiazines, cocaine
Agitation, confusion	Cocaine, amphetamines, phencyclidine, hallucinogens, antidepressants
Respiratory depression	Opiates, alcohols, antidepressants, barbiturates, benzodiazepines
Bradycardia	Digoxin, beta-blockers, organophosphates, sedatives
Tachycardia	Anticholinergics, salicylates, theophylline, amphetamines, digoxin, cocaine
Arrhythmias	Digoxin, phenothiazines
Hypotension	Tricyclics, antihypertensives, calcium channel blockers
Nausea, vomiting	Acetaminophen, alcohols, iron, salicylates, theophylline
Hyperthermia	Anticholinergics, tricyclics, amphetamines, cocaine, theophylline
Hypothermia	Barbiturates, alcohol, opiates, sedatives
Rhabdomyolysis	Amphetamines, cocaine, phencyclidine
Metabolic acidosis	Salicylates, methanol, ethylene glycol, iron, isoniazid, cyanide, carbon monoxide
Diaphoresis	Salicylates, organophosphates, amphetamines, cocaine
Bullae	Barbiturates, tricyclics

Investigations

Electrocardiogram

The ECG is a useful investigation in drug overdoses. Arrhythmias are common with tricyclic antidepressant and sympathomimetic overdoses especially ectopics. Digoxin, beta-blockers, calcium channel blockers, cholinergic drugs, cyanide and phenytoin can cause atrioventricular block. Widening of the QRS complex and prolonged QT interval suggests tricyclic antidepressant, quinidine or procainamide poisoning.

Table 35.2 Common toxic syndromes

Syndrome	Common signs	Common causes
Narcotic (opiates)	Coma, respiratory depression, miosis, bradycardia, hypotension, hypothermia, hypothemia, hyporeflexia	All types of narcotics
Sedatives/ hypnotics	Coma, respiratory depression, hypotension, hypothermia, hyporeflexia	Benzodiazepines, barbiturates, ethanol
Sympathomimetic	Delusions, paranoia, mydriasis, hypertension, tachycardia, hypertension, diaphoresis, hyperpyrexia, hypereflexia. Severe cases – seizures, hypotension, dysrhythmias	Amphetamines, cocaine, caffeine, ephedrine, theophylline
Anticholinergic	Delirium, mydriasis, flushed dry skin, tachycardia, hyperpyrexia, urinary retention. Severe cases – seizures, dysrhythmias	Antihistamines, antipsychotics, antiparkinson's drugs, antidepressants
Cholinergic	Confusion, miosis, bradycardia, seizures, weakness, salivation, lacrimation, urinary incontinence, emesis	Physostigmine, edrophonium, organophosphate insecticides
Serotoninergic	Confusion, weakness, tachycardia, agitation, tremor, extrapyramidal symptoms, hyperpyrexia,	Selective serotonin reuptake blocking agents

Arterial blood gases

Gas exchange and acid–base status can be assessed by arterial blood gases (ABGs). A mixed metabolic acidosis and respiratory alkalosis is evidence of possible salicylate poisoning. Cyanide and carbon monoxide poisoning commonly feature a severe metabolic acidosis and compensatory hyperventilation. It is useful to measure the haemoglobin saturation and the oxygen content of arterial blood by co-oximetry. Carboxyhaemoglobin concentrations are elevated in carbon monoxide poisoning and a number of drugs can oxidize haemoglobin to methaemoglobin. In both cases there is a disparity between the measured oxygen content or haemoglobin saturations and that calculated from the arterial oxygen tension. The normal anion gap is between 10 and 14 mmol/l and it is the difference between the serum sodium and the sum of the chloride and bicarbonate; an important point is that it is reduced by 2.5 mmol/l for each 1 mg/l fall in albumin. The anion gap is elevated in salicylate, methanol, ethanol, ethylene glycol, isoniazid, metformin, cyanide and carbon monoxide poisoning. Because these are relatively common poisons it is essential to calculate the anion gap in cases of suspected poisonings. The osmolar gap is the difference between the calculated osmolarity (2(Na + K) + urea + glucose) and the measured; when it is greater than 10 mOsm ethanol, ethylene glycol and methanol are likely culprits. The presence of ketoacidosis suggests diabetes, or paraldehyde or ethanol as causes. Isopropyl alcohol toxicity causes no systemic acidosis but elevated ketones.

Radiology

Ethylene glycol, oxalate and barium toxicity can cause hypocalcaemia. Rarely, radiopaque tablets are seen on chest or abdominal radiographs. The chest X-ray may provide evidence of aspiration.

Drug screening

Thin-layer chromatography is used to assay blood or urine for qualitative drug screening. The drug screen has limited usefulness; there is no identified standard for which drugs are assayed, in fact many common drugs are omitted from routine screens, results are often delayed, some toxins are not identified and they seldom change empirical management. Therefore a specific assay request for a suspected drug may provide rapid quantitative results. Clinical judgement should always overcome a negative drug screen because of the problems of timing and sensitivity. A quantitative analysis is particularly useful for drugs with specific therapies such as paracetamol (acetaminophen), salicylates (aspirin), ethanol, methanol, ethylene glycol, digoxin, theophylline, iron, lithium, phenobarbital and carbon monoxide.

Regional poisons centres have the most up to date recommendations available and phoning for advice should be considered (UK NPIS tel 0844 892 0111, Ireland NPIC tel (01) 809 2566). The national poisons information service also provides an online database called TOXBASE.

Drug manipulation

The importance of maintaining physiological stability whilst minimizing the toxic effects of drug ingestion is paramount. The toxicity can be diminished by preventing drug absorption, inhibition of toxic metabolite formation and augmentation of drug elimination. Where possible an antidote should be given and the toxin removed.

Preventing drug absorption

Removal of contaminated clothing and washing of skin will prevent cutaneous absorption of toxins such as organophosphates. The use of induced emesis is not effective or safe in most cases of oral ingestion of drugs and is not recommended.

Gastric lavage may be useful if carried out within 1 hour of ingestion, but this rarely possible. It has been suggested that gastric lavage may be effective for up to 12 hours after ingestion of drugs that delay gastric emptying, e.g. opiates and tricyclic antidepressants, or drugs that form concretions, e.g. salicylates. Its use is contraindicated if corrosive, acidic or caustic substances have been ingested. Patients with reduced consciousness should have their airway secured with an endotracheal tube and be placed in the lateral decubitus position prior to insertion of a large-bore orogastric tube for gastric lavage. The complications of gastric lavage include aspiration and oesophageal or gastric perforation.

Activated charcoal 1 mg/kg can be given to bind toxins and limits their absorption. It should be used within 1 hour of ingestion except suspected opioids and tricyclic antidepressants that delay gastric emptying. A number of common drugs are not absorbed by activated charcoal, e.g. alcohols, ethylene glycol, acids and iron, therefore the routine use for all poisonings is not recommended. The complications include vomiting, constipation and aspiration leading to pneumonitis and bowel obstruction. Cholestyramine has also been used to specifically bind thyroid hormone.

Whole bowel irrigation with non-absorbable polyethylene glycol solution is used to produce brisk catharsis until rectal effluent is clear of pills. This technique is useful to limit the absorption of sustained release drugs; iron, lithium and illicit drugs are packed in the bowel.

Inhibition of toxic metabolite formation

The formation of toxic metabolites from relatively passive drugs such as acetaminophen, methanol and ethylene glycol through metabolism can lead to organ failure. Therefore specific therapies are used to limit the formation of toxin formation and will be discussed in the relevant sessions in this chapter.

Augmentation of drug elimination

A process known as gut dialysis has been used to eliminate drugs undergoing enterohepatic circulation. Repeated (3–4) doses of activated charcoal (0.5–1 mg/kg every 2–4 hours) are given to bind drugs excreted by bile, e.g. theophylline, digoxin, carbamazepine, quinine, phenobarbitone. Alkalinization of the serum and urine can be achieved by the administration of 2 mmol/kg of sodium bicarbonate intravenously every 3–4 hours; urine output is maintained at 2–3 ml/kg per hour. The blood pH should be >7.45 and urine pH 7–8; hypokalaemia should be avoided. This may limit the transfer of weak acids, e.g. saliyclates, tricyclic antidepressants, chlorpropamide or phenobarbitone, across the blood–brain barrier and enhance their elimination by the kidneys by ‘ion trapping’. The urine can be acidified using ammonium chloride to increase the excretion of weak bases, e.g. amphetamines or quinidine, although the risk/benefit ratio for this is questionable.

Haemodialysis is effective at clearing methanol, ethylene glycol, salicylates and lithium. Charcoal haemoperfusion clears theophylline, phenytoin and carbamazepine but has increased risk of complications.

General supportive care

The general care of the unconscious patient includes regular monitoring of vital signs and organ support. Special attention is needed to monitor the patient's fluid balance, correct electrolyte imbalance and provide early nutritional support. These patients are at risk of nosocomial infections including ventilator-associated pneumonias and these should be suspected and treated.

Specific drug management

Salicylates (aspirin)

A third of the patients with salicylate overdose die soon after admission, with a lethal dose range of 250–500 mg/kg. Moderate toxicity is seen with serum levels between 500 and 700 mg/l. Severe toxicity is associated with serum levels >700 mg/l and an initial serum level exceeding 1200 mg/l. Severe salicylate poisoning has a high mortality because salicylates uncouple oxidative phosphorylation and inhibit cellular enzymes at high doses.

Patients can present with a range of symptoms including altered mental status, tinnitus, deafness, diaphoresis, hypoxia, hyperthermia, hypoglycaemia, pulmonary oedema and seizures. Arterial blood gases reveal a compensated respiratory alkalosis due to direct CNS stimulation and later metabolic acidosis. An increased anion gap (see Fig. 35.1) is due to increased pyruvate, lactate and ketone production. There is also an increased risk of haemorrhage due to inhibition of prothrombin, platelet function impairment and direct gastric irritation.

Multiple doses of activated charcoal can be given, as well as glucose and vitamin K to counteract the effects. The urine and serum should be kept alkaline to promote ion trapping and excretion and limiting transfer across the blood–brain barrier. Haemodialysis should be considered if serum levels exceed 500 mg/l or in the presence of coma, seizures, pulmonary oedema or renal failure.

Acetaminophen (paracetamol)

Paracetamol overdoses are very common but luckily most patients who present after ingesting paracetamol do not have severe or life-threatening poisoning and do not require specific treatment. However, paracetamol poisoning at a dose exceeding 7 g in an adult or 150 mg/kg is normally fatal.

The ingested paracetamol is normally absorbed within 1 hour, with the most of it undergoing liver metabolism to non-toxic compounds with glucuronide and sulphates. About 5% is metabolized via hepatic cytochrome P450 system to reactive metabolites such *N*-acetyl-p-benzoquinone-imine (NAPQI) which are detoxified by conjugation with hepatic glutathione under normal circumstances. During substantial overdose, the glutathione supply is overwhelmed and NAPQI accumulates to cause liver damage. Nausea and vomiting may be the only symptoms in the first 24 hours, followed by right upper quadrant pain, oliguria and decline in liver function. Hepatic necrosis and failure develop over the next 3 days. Late presentation, coagulopathy, metabolic acidosis, renal failure and cerebral oedema are all poor prognostic factors. Mortality is around 10%.

If the presentation is within 1 hour of ingestion then gastric lavage and activated charcoal are indicated. Serum level should be assayed and the need for antidote is estimated according to normogram. If there is any doubt about the level of toxicity or late presentation, the patient should be treated before the

Anion gap = $[Na^+] - [Cl^-] - [HCO_3^-]$

Reference range is 8 to 16 mmol/l.

Anion gap represents the concentration of all the unmeasured anions in the plasma. Under normal circumstances, the negatively charged proteins account for 10% of plasma anions and the majority of the unmeasured anions. The acid anions (e.g. lactate) produced during a metabolic acidosis are not measured as part of the usual laboratory biochemical profile. The H^+ produced reacts with bicarbonate buffers and the CO_2 produced is excreted via the lungs. The net effect is a decrease in the concentration of measured HCO_3 anions and an increase in the concentration of unmeasured anions so the anion gap increases.

Fig. 35.1 Formula for calculating the anion gap.

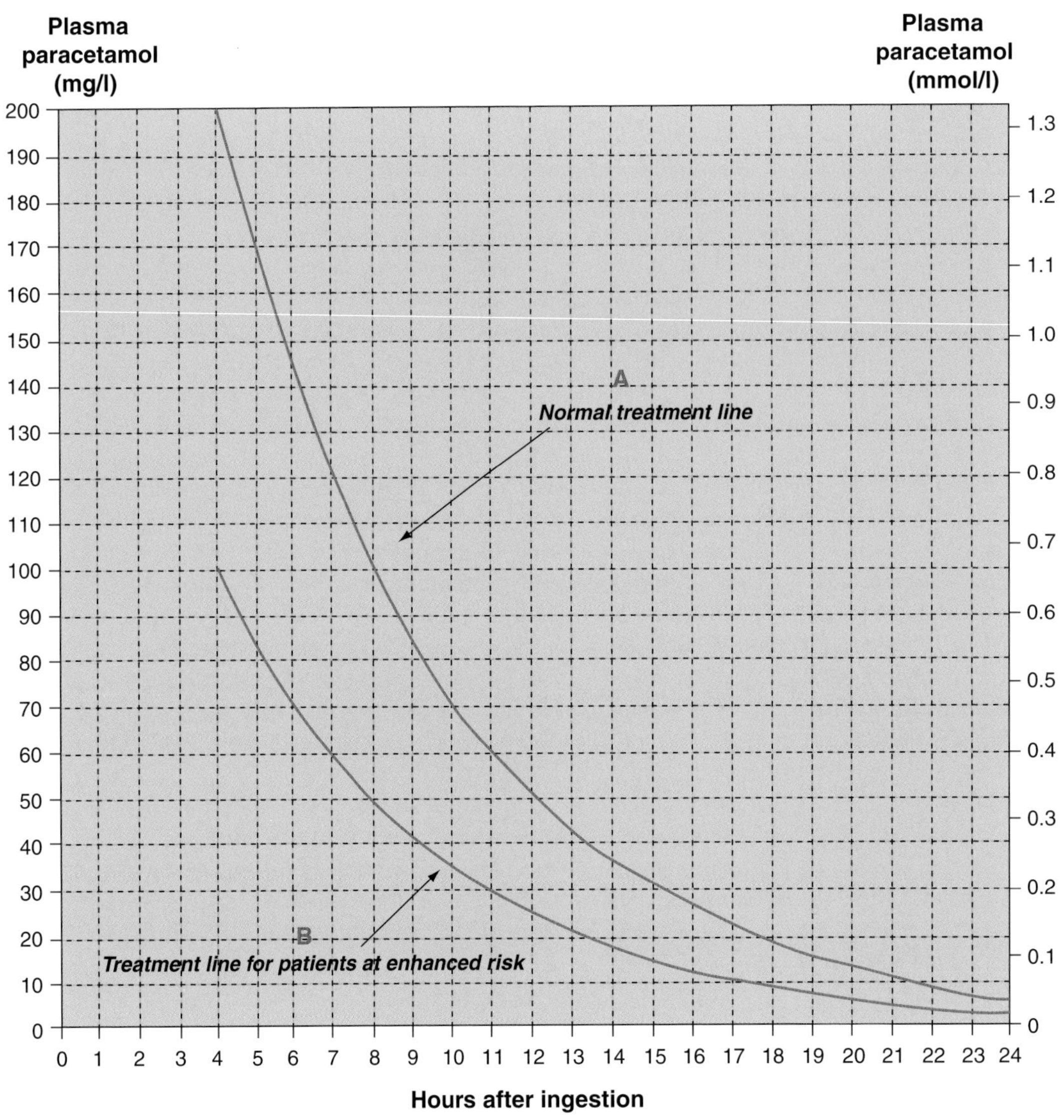

Fig. 35.2 Nomogram for treatment of paracetamol overdose.

drug level is known. Serum concentrations of greater than 140 mg/l are predictive of serious toxicity, while serum concentrations at 4 hours of >200 mg/l or >50 mg/l at 12 hours suggest high risk of hepatic damage and require treatment with specific antidote *N*-acetylcysteine. *N*-acetylcysteine is given intravenously at 150 mg/kg in 200 ml of 5% dextrose over 15 mins plus 50 mg/kg in 500 ml of 5% dextrose over 4 hours plus 100 mg/kg in 1000 ml of 5% dextrose over 16 hours. *N*-acetylcysteine works by binding toxic metabolites and replenishing glutathione stores (Fig. 35.2). Late doses commenced after 16 hours post ingestion may not prevent fulminant hepatic failure but may improve patient outcome. Patients who are malnourished or have a high alcohol intake are particularly at risk of hepatic injury. Hypoglycaemia should be treated and expert opinion regarding liver transplantation should be considered in those with hepatic necrosis (see Chapter 36: Liver failure).

Tricyclic antidepressants

Tricyclic antidepressants (TCAs) are commonly used for depression so are frequently seen in overdoses and are a leading cause of death. TCAs block the uptake of noradrenaline by adrenergic nerve fibres and signs of toxicity are predominantly anticholinergic

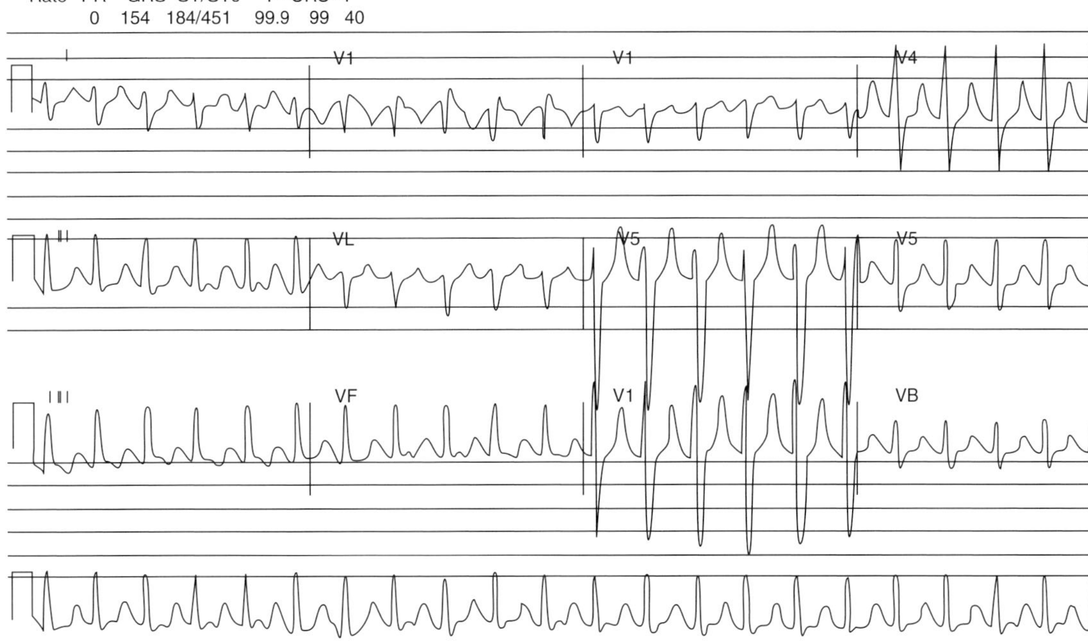

Fig. 35.3 ECG showing some classic changes after TCA overdose. Features include: sinus tachycardia, QRS duration greater than 100 ms, right axis shift seen as an R-wave deflection in aVR (or S wave in I or aVL).

(antimuscarinic) effects and include warm dry skin, dry mouth, and fixed dilated pupils with blurred vision, confusion, hyperthermia, ileus, urinary retention, psychosis and hallucinations.

Gastric lavage and oral charcoal may be useful; widening of QRS >160 ms is a sign of impending cardiac toxicity and seizures. Toxicity is worsened by acidosis, hypotension and pyrexia. Tachycardia, right bundle branch block and ventricular arrhythmias are common (Fig. 35.3). Arrhythmias respond to sodium bicarbonate 1–2 mmol/kg up to pH of 7.5 and lignocaine can also be useful. Electrical cardioversion is best avoided because of risk of asystole. Intravenous fluids and noradrenaline maybe required for treatment of hypotension. Diazepam and lorazepam are used to control seizures.

Sedatives

In large overdose sedative drugs depress consciousness and respiration, reduce cardiac output and cause vasodilatation. Benzodiazepines have a wide therapeutic range and can be reversed by flumazenil in most cases: relapse in 10% due to short duration of action, 0.2 mg every 2 minutes up to 3 mg. However, repeated doses of flumazenil should be given cautiously and it has been known to cause seizures particularly if tricyclics are also ingested.

Barbiturates can cause profound CNS depression and an isoelectric EEG. Activated charcoal and gastric lavage are potentially useful treatments.

Opioids can cause sedation, respiratory depression with increased risk of aspiration, hypotension and pinpoint pupils. They can lead to hypothermia, decreased gut motility, pulmonary oedema and seizures. Supportive treatment and gastric lavage may be useful because of delayed gastric emptying. Naloxone, a competitive antagonist at opiate receptors, is the specific antidote, 0.2–0.4 mg intravenously up to 10 mg. There is the risk of resedation due to shorter action of naloxone than most opioids and repeated doses may be necessary.

Carbon monoxide

Carbon monoxide has a far higher affinity for haemoglobin than oxygen and can lead to cellular anoxia. The PaO_2 levels may be normal and the carboxyhaemoglobin levels need to be measured by direct co-oximeter; levels >40% can lead to seizures and coma. Treatment is the administration of 100% oxygen, the half-life of carbon monoxide being 59 minutes. The use of hyperbaric oxygen is contentious.

Alcohols

Ethanol is often involved in drug overdoses, and levels of greater than 3000 mg/l will cause coma. Acute intoxication requires supportive treatment with administration of glucose and thiamine and potassium and magnesium correction. Patients may experience acute withdrawal with delirium tremens being the worse form; this can be managed with benzodiazepines such as lorazepam.

Ethylene glycol forms the toxic metabolites oxalic and glycolic acids, methanol forms formic acid and formaldehyde. The formation of toxic metabolites can be delayed by administration of ethanol. Both toxins can cause coma, hyporeflexia, nystagmus and seizures with ingestion of less than 100 ml. Patients may develop a tachycardia, hypertension, pulmonary oedema, acidosis with an increased anion gap. Ethylene glycol poisoning is more likely to present with renal failure, whereas methanol toxicity can result in blindness due to optic neuritis. Ethanol fomepizole can be given intravenously to compete for alcohol dehydrogenase and limit metabolite formation; levels of 100 mg/dl are required to be maintained. 4-Methylpyrazole is an alternative to ethanol. If serum levels are above 50 mg/dl then dialysis is indicated. Calcium replacement is often required.

Stimulants

Patients who have overdosed on amphetamines, methylenedioxymethamphetamine (MDMA: ecstasy), cocaine or phencyclidine may present with agitation, hypertension, tachycardia, dry mouth, sweating, mydriasis and less commonly rhabdomyolysis, metabolic acidosis, hyperkalaemia, seizures, acute renal failure, disseminated intravascular coagulation (DIC) and multiple organ failure. Ecstasy can cause dehydration, hyperthermia and hyponatraemia from excessive water intake. Phencyclidine can cause nystagmus. Cocaine can cause myocardial ischaemia and pulmonary haemorrhage; a dose as small as 1 g can be fatal. If presenting within 1 hour then activated charcoal can be used. The agitation, hypertension and tachycardia can be controlled with benzodiazepines and direct vasodilators with or without beta-blockers. If patients present with a hyperthermic syndrome, then cold intravenous fluids, dantrolene or ketanserin may be used.

Organophosphates

Organophosphates inhibit acetylcholinesterase which leads to the accumulation of acetylcholine at neuromuscular junctions. The clinical presentation is one of cholinergic excess with tremor, salivation, miosis, bradycardia, lacrimation, bronchconstriction, urination, emesis, diarrhoea (the muscarinic effects), and fasciculation, muscle weakness, skeletal cramping, tachycardia and hypertension (the nicotinic effects). Respiratory support and atropine 2–4 mg reverses muscarinic effects only. Pralidoxime reverses nicotinic effects; 1–2 g is effective for up to 24 hours.

Theophylline

Theophylline toxicity is very serious because of the high mortality. Toxicity can occur due to impaired clearance caused by drug interactions, e.g. erythromycin in patients with liver or heart failure. Agitation, tremor, arrhythmias and gastrointestinal symptoms can occur at therapeutic serum levels of 10–20 μg/ml, levels between 20 and 40 μg/l are required before serious cardiac arrhythmias occur, and seizures are a high risk with levels above 40 μg/l. Gastric lavage, repeated activated charcoal, whole bowel irrigation, haemoperfusion or haemodialysis may be indicated especially if sustained release drug taken. Lignocaine is recommended for ventricular arrhythmias and benzodiazepines for seizures.

Digitalis (digoxin)

Renal impairment, hypothyroidism, heart failure, hypokalaemia, hypomagnesaemia and amiodarone use can all predispose to digoxin toxicity. The clinical presentation is fatigue, weakness, nausea and visual disturbances. Toxicity can present as any arrhythmias but commonly seen as AV nodal block and hyperkalaemia due to inhibition of the sodium–potassium pump. Electrolyte abnormalities need to be corrected and activated charcoal can be given to decrease absorption. Bradycardia should be treated with atropine and pacing, lignocaine can be used for ventricular arrhythmias. Specific antidote is IgG Fab antibody fragments if digoxin levels greater than 6 mg/l.

Serotonin reuptake inhibitors (SSRIs)

Selective serotonin reuptake inhibitors (SSRIs) including citalopram, fluoxetine, sertraline and paroxetine are popular choices for treatment of depression. They act by increasing brain serotonin levels and can interact with other drugs that affect serotonin levels. Lithium is a serotonin agonist, amphetamines increase serotonin release and monoamine oxidase inhibitors decrease its breakdown. Patients with SSRI overdoses can present with fever, confusion, restlessness, hyperreflexia, shivering and nausea. Severe cases lead to seizures, coma, myoclonus, muscle rigidity or rhabdomyolysis. Treatment is with benzodiazepines for agitation and rigidity. Lithium can cause neurological damage and nephrogenic diabetes inspidus; serum levels >3.5 mmol/l need extracorporeal methods of clearance.

Calcium channel and beta-blockers

Both groups can cause bradycardia, conduction defects and hypotension due to impaired cardiac contractility and peripheral vasodilatation. Beta-blockers cause hypoglycaemia, calcium channel blockers cause hyperglycaemia. Gastric lavage and whole bowel irrigation is indicated if sustained release preparation ingested. Treatment with intravenous fluids, atropine 0.6 mg, inotropes such as adrenaline and noradrenaline, calcium 1 mg, glucagon 5 mg and pacing will result in immediate correction of bradycardia and hypotension. Insulin administration at 0.5 U/kg per hour should also be started to control blood sugar level. Bronchospasm can also be a rare complication.

Useful toxicology search engines and databases

http://www.tictac.org.uk
http://www.toxbase.co.uk
http://www.intox.org
http://www.micromedex.com
http://www.toxnet.nim.nih.gov

Key points

- Adult cases often involve multiple substances with an inaccurate and incomplete history of types or quantity of drugs taken.
- Immediate assessment of an adequate airway, breathing and circulation is paramount.
- Management includes limiting absorption of toxin, preventing toxic metabolite formation and enhancing drug elimination.
- Patients will need continuous monitoring, reassessment and organ support.
- Treat with specific antidotes where available.

Further reading

- Ellenhorn MJ, Barceloux DG (1997) *Ellenhorn's Medical Toxicology: Diagnosis and Treatment of Human Poisoning*. Baltimore, MD: Lippincott Williams & Wilkins.
- Goldfrank LR, Flomenhaum NE, Lewin NA (2002) *Goldfrank's Toxicological Emergencies*, 7th edn. New York: McGraw-Hill.
- Mokhlesi B, Leiken JB, Murray P, Corbridge TC (2003) Adult toxicology in critical care. I: General approach to the intoxicated patient. *Chest* **123**(2): 577–92.
- Mokhlesi B, Leiken JB, Murray P, Corbridge TC (2003) Adult toxicology in critical care. II: Specific poisonings. *Chest* **123**(3): 897–922.

Liver failure

Nick Murphy and Joyce Yeung

Introduction

Liver failure is most often encountered following decompensation in a patient with chronic liver disease. It is characterized by a constellation of clinical signs and symptoms including hepatic encephalopathy, jaundice and other biochemical abnormalities such as coagulopathy. Much more rarely it can occur de novo in someone without evidence of previous liver disease. In fulminant or acute liver failure (ALF) the time from the onset of first symptoms to the first signs of hepatic encephalopathy is often used to predict the likely prognosis and clinical manifestations.

The first part of the chapter will focus on acute liver failure and the second part will look at acute on chronic liver failure.

Presentation of acute liver failure

Liver failure is not a disease in itself but the result of some other underlying aetiology. The balance between liver injury and regeneration provides a useful paradigm through which to conceptualize presenting symptoms and signs. The rate of progression of the syndrome and the aetiology dictate the presentation:

- Hyperacute presentations are due to the overwhelming effect of toxin, ischaemic or immunological injury. Little regeneration can occur in time to prevent the sequelae of the abrupt cessation of liver function. In addition the toxins associated with the injured liver provide another probable mechanism for the profound secondary organ dysfunction seen.
- In subacute liver failure, early symptoms can often be traced back weeks or months before the diagnosis is made. Jaundice is the usual presenting feature but some patients can present with non-specific general malaise. Ascites will develop in many cases followed by eventual encephalopathy.

Cerebral oedema and renal failure are more common in hyperacute and acute liver failure when compared to subacute. The circulatory changes are much more profound, often requiring large volume resuscitation and vasopressor support. Interestingly overall survival, with supportive care, is better with paracetamol toxicity and viral-induced liver failure when compared to sero-negative hepatitis. This is due to the severely disrupted architecture of the liver and patchy liver regeneration seen in sero-negative liver failure. Survival without transplantation is very poor.

The course of liver failure is inextricably linked to that of infection and sepsis. Acute liver failure is associated with immune dysfunction. Infection is common and deterioration in organ function and cerebral herniation are associated with the onset of sepsis. The major cause of death in recent series of ALF has been sepsis and multiple organ failure.

Management of acute liver failure

The management of acute liver failure can be split into:

- Treatment of the underlying cause.
- General supportive care.
- Management of the complications of liver failure.
- Early prognostication and liver transplantation in selective cases.

Causes of liver failure

Paracetamol poisoning

Epidemiology

Acute liver failure is rare, with a reported incidence of about 2000 cases per year in the USA. The most common cause in Western Europe, Australia and the

Core Topics in Critical Care Medicine, eds. Fang Gao Smith and Joyce Yeung. Published by Cambridge University Press.

USA is acute paracetamol poisoning. This is most often due to intentional overdose in the UK but can also be due to therapeutic misadventure, more commonly seen in the USA. Unintentional overdose is often associated with the ingestion of multiple paracetamol-containing preparations. These are staggered by nature and patients tend to present late with low serum paracetamol levels making the commonly used nomograms for the assessment of toxicity uninterpretable. After paracetamol poisoning, the case related incidence of ALF is very low. Approximately 0.6% of patients will progress to ALF.

Legislation was introduced in 1998 in the UK to reduce pack size and presentation in an attempt to reduce the increasing problem of paracetamol overdose over the previous 20 years. Since then there has been a steady reduction in the incidence of both overdose and liver failure. Others have questioned the causal link between the two because of the fall in overdose due to other drugs and suicide in general over the same time period.

Presentation

Paracetamol-induced liver failure is the archetype for a hyperacute presentation in which hepatic encephalopathy develops within 1 week of the first symptoms. Nausea and vomiting are often the initial symptoms within the first 24 hours following ingestion. Over the next couple of days symptoms often subside before the onset of liver failure. In its most severe form it is often associated with a rapid progression to multiple organ failure. Renal failure is prominent and cerebral oedema is common, reported in up to 80% of patients that progress to grade 4 encephalopathy.

Treatment

(1) *N*-acetylcysteine

The vast majority of paracetamol is metabolized in the liver via a single step conjugation. A small proportion is excreted unchanged in the urine and a small amount is metabolized via a mixed function oxidase. During overdose the half-life is greatly prolonged because the conjugation pathways become saturated. As a result, phase I metabolism increases resulting in the increased production of a reactive intermediary, *N*-acetyl-p-benzoquinine-imine (NAPQI). NAPQI is normally conjugated via glutathione and excreted in the urine. Glutathione stores become rapidly exhausted during the early stages of overdose resulting in an build up in NAPQI within hepatocytes. NAPQI toxicity results from the covalent bonding of NAPQI to protein adducts within hepatocytes. The proteins affected include those responsible for intracellular signalling and energy production. A cascade of actions follows resulting in hepatocyte necrosis, apoptosis and secondary inflammatory infiltration of the liver (Fig. 36.1).

The *N*-acetyl derivative of the amino acid cysteine (NAC) serves as a precursor to the production of glutathione and is the treatment of choice in early paracetamol toxicity. NAC greatly enhances glutathione production. If given within 8 hours of a non-staggered overdose if provides complete protection. If given after this, *N*-acetylcysteine provides partial protection and has been shown to reduce mortality even if given up to 72 hours following overdose, although the mechanism of action at this stage is unknown.

(2) Referral to liver transplant centre

The case progression to liver failure is very low in paracetamol toxicity and so most cases of severe liver injury can be managed over the phone from a liver transplant centre. Early referral should be made in any patient with a coagulopathy and a significant liver enzyme rise. Blood tests should be repeated twice daily

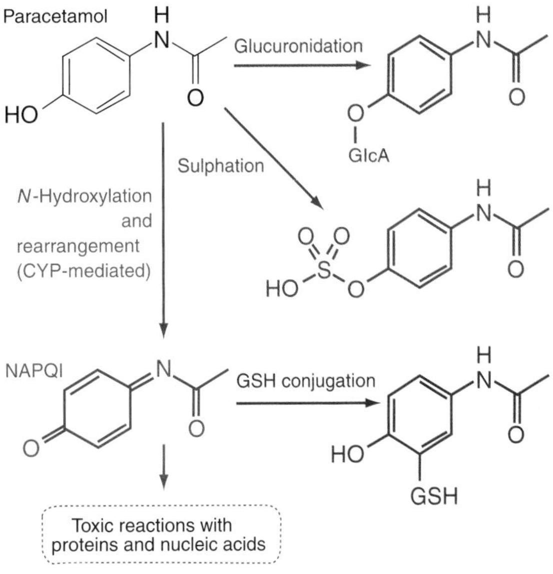

Paracetamol
Glucuronidation
GlcA
Sulphation
N-Hydroxylation and rearrangement (CYP-mediated)
NAPQI
GSH conjugation
GSH
Toxic reactions with proteins and nucleic acids

Fig. 36.1 Metabolism of paracetamol.

in the initial stages. Poor prognostic signs include evidence of a metabolic acidosis, renal dysfunction, a steadily rising international normalized ratio (INR) and any signs of encephalopathy. In patients with these signs transfer should be considered. Locally, patients should be moved to a high dependency or critical care area to enable close monitoring and adequate fluid resuscitation.

(3) General

Prophylactic antibiotics and upper gastrointestinal (GI) prophylaxis should be started.

Hepatitis

Epidemiology

The largest cause of acute liver failure worldwide is probably hepatitis E. This is an epidemic, enterally transmitted, virus seen commonly in young adults in India and sub-Saharan Africa. Hepatitis E is similar to hepatitis A in that it is associated with poor sanitation although hepatitis A tends to affect children to a greater extent. Again, the case progression to ALF following acute viral hepatitis is very low with a quoted incidence of 0.2–4%.

Hepatitis B can lead to ALF via a number of circumstances including acute infection, but also due to an enhanced immune response following the withdrawal of immunosupressive therapy in a patient with previous hepatitis B exposure indicating the immunologically induced pathophysiology of the syndrome.

Presentation

ALF following acute hepatitis E infection is higher in the immunosuppressed. This is seen most often during pregnancy when rates of ALF can reach 20% in the third trimester. Viral causes of ALF tend to run an acute course with the onset of encephalopathy within a month of the first symptoms.

Treatment

Following acute viral hepatitis there is little controlled evidence that the initiation of antiviral therapy, once there are signs of liver failure, has any benefit. Other specific therapies such as copper chelation in acute Wilson's disease and silymarin in acute mushroom poisoning are of unproven benefit.

General supportive care

Fluid resuscitation

Patients with hyperacute or acute liver failure often require significant volumes of fluid resuscitation. Salt-poor solutions such as 5% glucose should be avoided as they tend to exacerbate hyponatraemia which can contribute to later complications such as cerebral oedema.

Blood sugar monitoring

Patients with liver failure are prone to hypoglycaemia. Regular blood sugar monitoring will alert to the need for a 50% glucose infusion.

Coagulation

Liver failure leads to a loss of synthetic function of hepatocytes and reduction of coagulation factors and INR is a very important prognostic factor. Despite a worsening INR, the use of fresh frozen plasma should be avoided before line insertion. Bleeding from line insertion is rarely a problem.

Complications of liver failure

Hepatic encephalopathy

The time from the first symptoms to the onset of hepatic encephalopathy (HE) helps predict the likely aetiology, course and prognosis of acute liver failure. The cause of encephalopathy in ALF is not completely clear but ammonia toxicity within the brain leading to the swelling of astrocytes undoubtedly occurs. The West Haven criteria designed to describe the severity of HE in patients with cirrhosis are often used in the context of ALF (Fig. 36.2). The clinical manifestations are subtly different. In particular, the agitation commonly seen in the early stages in ALF is rarely seen in cirrhosis. Despite this, the grading provides a rough description of the severity and indicates the likelihood of developing cerebral oedema. In patients with ALF, progression of coma grade can be very rapid, often over a few hours. Those with the early manifestations of HE should be managed within an intensive care unit. Once patients reach grade 2 encephalopathy preparations should be made to intubate and ventilate the patient. This provides control, permits the safe use of sedation, protects the airway and enables monitoring for signs of raised intracranial pressure.

West Haven Criteria of Altered Mental Status in Hepatic Encephalopthy			
Stage	Consciousness	Intellect and Behavior	Neurologic Findings
0	Normal	Normal	Normal examination; impaired pyschomotor testing
1	Mild lack of awareness	Shortened attention span; impaired addition or subtraction	Mild asterixis or tremor
2	Lethargic	Disoriented; inappropriate behavior	Obvious asterixis; slurred speech
3	Somnolent but arousable	Gross disorientation; bizarre behavior	Muscular rigidity and clonus; hyperrflexia
4	Coma	Coma	Decerebrate posturing

Fig. 36.2 West Haven Criteria. (With permission from Ferenci P, Lockwood A, Mullen K, Tarter R, Weissenborn K, Blei A (2002). Hepatic encephalopathy: definition, nomenclature, diagnosis, and quantification: final report of the working party at the 11th World Congresses of Gastroenterology, Vienna, 1998. *Hepatology* **35**(3): 716–21.)

Treatment

(1) Reduce protein intake

Traditionally, it has been assumed that excessive protein intake leads to increased generation of ammonia, which will accumulate and worsen the hepatic encephalopathy. While very large protein loads are known to precipitate encephalopathy (e.g. gastrointestinal haemorrhage), there is no evidence to support the need for patients with chronic liver disease to be protein restricted. As chronic liver disease is a catabolic state, a protein-restricted diet could potentially lead to protein malnutrition and a negative nitrogen balance. Advice should be sought from dietician regarding a suitable caloric intake for each patient.

(2) Correction of electrolyte imbalance

Any hypokalaemia should be corrected, as hypokalaemia increases renal ammonia production and may promote conversion of ammonium into ammonia, which can cross the blood–brain barrier.

(3) Lactulose

Lactulose causes osmotic diarrhoea and reduces the time available for intestinal bacteria to metabolize protein into ammonia within the bowel. Lactulose also acidifies the environment in the lumen of the bowel and promotes the conversion of luminal ammonia to ammonium ions, which are less likely to cross lipid membrane due to their positive charge and less readily absorbed into the bloodstream from the bowel. Despite these theoretical advantages, a recent Cochrane Review has failed to find evidence to support the use of lactulose in hepatic encephalopathy.

(4) Antibiotics

Research has examined the potential role of antibiotics in reducing ammonia-producing bacteria in the gastrointestinal tract. Clinical trials have demonstrated that rifaximin at a dose of 400 mg orally 3 times a day was as effective as lactulose at improving hepatic encephalopathy symptoms. It remains to be determined whether rifaximin can improve severe encephalopathy symptoms as rapidly as lactulose.

(5) Flumazenil

A meta-analysis by the Cochrane Collaboration found potential benefit from flumazenil. However, the doses of flumazenil given were variable and some trials used bolus injections while others used continuous infusions. The median duration of treatment was 10 min (range 1 min to 72 hours). However, the benefit was short-lived.

(6) L-Ornithine-L-aspartate

L-Ornithine-L-aspartate stimulates the urea cycle which is a major route for removal of the ammonia produced in the metabolism of amino acids in the liver and kidney (Fig. 36.3). It has shown some encouraging results in recent randomized controlled trials.

Intracranial hypertension

Intracranial hypertension (ICH) is common in ALF, occurring in about 20–30% of all patients. The rapid

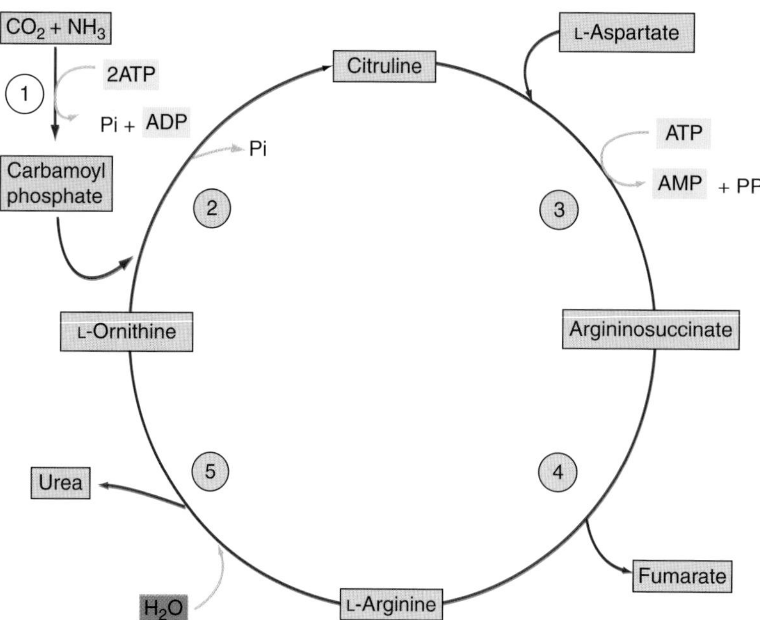

Fig. 36.3 The urea cycle.

KEY TO ENZYMES (circled numbers)
1. Carbamoyl-phosphate synthase (ammonia)
2. Ornithine carbamoyltransferase
3. Argininosuccinate synthase
4. Argininosuccinate lyase
5. Arginase

onset and burden of necrotic liver in hyperacute liver failure increases the risk of ICH. Other risk factors include younger age, hyperglycaemia, hyponatraemia, severity of systemic inflammatory response and plasma ammonia concentration. ICH has been reported in up to 80% of patients with hyperacute liver failure with grade 4 encephalopathy.

Management

(1) Intracranial pressure monitoring

Intracranial pressure monitoring in ALF is controversial as there are significant potential risks. There is a higher risk of intracranial bleeding than seen in other settings such as traumatic brain injury. Without intracranial pressure monitoring the indications for intervention rely on clinical signs such as dilated pupils or seizure activity. The signs can occur late as a result of established ICH. Without monitoring, the use of protocols will be problematic and the effect of intervention will be difficult to determine.

(2) Treatment of ICH

ICH seen in ALF is due to cerebral swelling for the most part. Additionally there is a loss of cerebral vascular autoregulation with a resulting increase in cerebral blood volume, often seen later in the course. The cause of cerebral swelling is incompletely understood but it occurs within the astrocytes and is related to ammonia toxicity either due to the production of glutamine or via the direct effects of ammonia or both. The blood–brain barrier remains intact and initial osmotic therapy with mannitol and hypertonic saline in an attempt to reduce brain water is often used. Additional therapy can be directed to reduce cerebral blood volume with sedatives, such as propofol, and direct cerebral vasoconstrictors such as hyperventilation and indomethacin.

Renal failure

Renal failure is common in ALF. Early extracorporeal support is indicated to facilitate fluid balance and may provide some increase in cardiovascular stability.

Adrenal dysfunction

Adrenal dysfunction has been shown to occur commonly in patients with ALF and is related to the severity of liver failure. The use of corticosteroids has not been shown to improve outcome but can lead to earlier shock reversal and a reduction in vasopressor use.

Prognostication and liver transplantation

In a selected group of patients liver transplantation is the treatment of choice. Overall survival, without transplantation, is about 40% following the onset of ALF. Liver transplantation in ALF has been used since the late 1980s and is now a standard form of therapy. The use of validated prognostic markers early in the course of the illness enables the intervention to be performed before catastrophic organ failure precludes a successful outcome. Prognostic criteria are based on the aetiology of liver disease, biochemical markers of liver function and markers of other organ failure. An example is the King's College Criteria, shown in Fig. 36.4. The majority of patients with sero-negative hepatitis or acute Wilson's disease will be offered a liver transplant, while only a small proportion of patients with paracetamol toxicity will be.

In some countries where the lack of cadavaric donation means a reduced availability of livers for transplantation, living related lobe donation is sometimes used. In small children an adult left lode can be sufficient to provide adequate function. In adults, however, a right lobe is needed to provide the necessary function for the recipient. Donation of a right lobe is associated with significant morbidity and a small mortality for the donor. The ethical issues surrounding living donation should not be underestimated. There is often little time for adequate counselling and the pressure to 'do the right thing' can be overwhelming.

Following ALF in paracetamol toxicity and some cases of viral hepatitis recovery is associated with normal or near-normal liver morphology and function. The liver has astonishing powers of regeneration following injury and if the patient can be supported through the acute stages of liver failure a normal life expectancy can be expected. This has led to the concept of auxiliary or partial liver transplantation. In these cases, a right lobe is transplanted into the recipient and after 1 year, immunosuppression is gradually withdrawn to allow native liver regeneration. The

King's College Hospital Criteria for Liver Transplantation in Fulminant Hepatic Failure
Paracetamol-induced disease Arterial pH <7.3 (irrespective of the grade of encephalopathy) or Grade 3 or 4 encephalopathy, and Prothrombin time >100 s, and Serum creatinine >3.4 mg/dl (301 μmol/l) **All other causes of fulminant hepatic failure** Prothrombin time >100 s (irrespective of the grade of encephalopathy) Or Any three of the following variables (irrespective of the grade of encephalopathy) Age <10 years or >40 years Aetiology: non-A, non-B hepatitis, halothane hepatitis, idiosyncratic drug reactions Duration of jaundice before onset of encephalopathy >7 days Prothrombin time >50 s Serum bilirrubin >18 mg/dl (308 μmol/l)

Fig. 36.4 King's College Criteria. The positive predictive value of the criteria in predicting death from ALF has ranged from 70% to 100%. A meta-analysis assessing various prognostic indices found that the specificity of the King's College Criteria in predicting mortality exceeded 90%, with a sensitivity of 69%. As a result, the American Society for Study of Liver Diseases has recommended the King's College Criteria as being helpful early parameters in ascertaining the need for liver transplantation in patients with acute liver failure. (Adapted from O'Grady J, Alexander G, Hayllar K, Williams R (1989) Early indicators of prognosis in fulminant hepatic failure. *Gastroenterology* **97**(2): 439–45.)

transplanted lobe will eventually wither and die. Occasionally it has to be removed surgically.

Acute on chronic liver disease

Pathophysiology

Acute on chronic liver failure represents the decompensation of otherwise stable chronic liver disease. It usually occurs following a precipitating event such as a significant insult associated with systemic inflammation and the release of pro-inflammatory cytokines. These can be split into two types: those due to a direct insult to the liver such as an alcoholic binge resulting in alcoholic hepatitis or a low cardiac output state resulting in liver ischaemia such as in gastrointestinal haemorrhage or an unrelated infection.

Most, if not all, of the pathophysiological changes associated with decompensation in chronic liver disease are due to the associated circulatory effects. Splanchnic circulatory vasodilatation seen in patients with severe chronic liver disease is exacerbated. This results in effective systemic arterial underfilling. Compensatory mechanisms are induced, resulting in sodium and water retention and vasoconstriction in many organ beds. Due to arterial underfilling cardiac output may be decreased in the late stages of the syndrome prior to resuscitation and vasoconstriction within organ beds aggravates organ dysfunction. In particular, renal vasoconstriction leads to a reduced urine output and, ultimately, renal failure. This is often reversible in the early stages with therapy focused on restoring arterial vascular volume and reducing the compensatory vasoconstriction. Acute on chronic liver disease (AoCLD) usually leads on to multiple organ dysfunction with the respiratory system, cardiovascular system, the kidneys, adrenal glands and the brain all being affected.

Presentation

In AoCLD synthetic liver function is deranged and significant jaundice is invariable. Impaired production of liver derived clotting factors results in a prolonged INR and hypoalbuminaemia can be profound. Portal venous pressure often increases leading to exacerbation of ascites and the precipitation of variceal bleeding or portal gastropathy. Disseminated intravascular coagulation (DIC) often accompanies AoCLD as a result of sepsis or systemic inflammation.

Patients with AoCLD have an increased risk of infection because of a relatively immunosuppressed state. Loss of portal venous filtering and Kupffer cell dysfunction contribute to this but there are many noted abnormalities. Patients with AoCLD tend to have a somewhat blunted response to infection when compared to patients without chronic liver disease. This often makes the diagnosis more difficult in the early stages.

Management

Prevention is the best cure. This is never truer than in patients with AoCLD. The prognosis following decompensation is poor and so preventing it happening in the first place is important. AoCLD is usually precipitated by sepsis or GI bleed. Prophylactic antibiotics improve the prognosis in patients following an upper GI bleed and an episode of bacterial peritonitis. Other secondary preventative measures include the use of beta-blockers and transjugular intrahepatic portosystemic shunt (TIPS) in the prevention of a second variceal bleed.

In general, aggressive cardiovascular support and antibiotics are the main focus of supportive care. The maintenance of intravascular volume and blood pressure with fluids and vasopressor help to reduce the intensity of reflex sympathetic and hormonal changes associated with decompensation. Terlipressin, an analogue of the vasoactive hormone vasopressin, is active at the V1 receptor and is a potent vasoconstrictor. It is a pro-drug and can be given in bolus form which increases its use outside of a critical care area. Vasoconstrictor therapy works by reducing intrinsic compensatory mechanisms encouraging intra-organ vasodilatation although it is not clear if terlipressin is any better than noradrenaline in this setting. Vasoconstrictor therapy is often accompanied by volume replacement and there is some evidence that albumin is better than artificial colloids.

Decompensated chronic liver disease has a relatively poor prognosis if established organ failure sets in. Organ failure scores such as the Sepsis-related Organ Failure Assessment (SOFA) are useful in describing the severity and have been shown to predict outcome in this group of patients.

Key points

- Paracetamol poisoning is the most common cause of acute liver failure in Western Europe, Australia and USA.

- *N*-acetylcysteine (NAC) is a precursor to the production of glutathione and is the treatment of choice in paracetamol toxicity. If given within 8 hours of a non-staggered overdose it provides complete protection but it has been shown to provide partial protection and reduce mortality even if given up to 72 hours.
- Fluid resuscitation with salt poor solutions such as 5% glucose should be avoided as they tend to exacerbate hyponatraemia and cerebral oedema.
- Hepatic encephalopathy is a common complication of liver failure and is probably caused by accumulated ammonia. Management includes ventilator support in patients with grade 2 encephalopathy and above, careful protein intake, correction of hypokalaemia, and lactulose.
- It is important to use prognostic criteria to assess patients early in their disease so early transplantation can be offered if appropriate.

Further reading

- Als-Nielsen B, Gluud LL, Gluud C (2004) Benzodiazepine receptor antagonists for hepatic encephalopathy. *Cochrane Database Syst. Rev.* CD002798.
- Als-Nielsen B, Gluud LL, Gluud C (2004) Nonabsorbable disaccharides for hepatic encephalopathy. *Cochrane Database Syst. Rev.* CD003044.
- Larson AM, Polson J, Fontana RJ *et al.* (2005) Acetaminophen-induced acute liver failure: results of a US multicenter, prospective study. *Hepatology* **42**: 1364–72.
- Ostapowicz G, Fontana RJ, Schiodt FV *et al.* (2002) Results of a prospective study of acute liver failure at 17 tertiary care centers in the United States. *Ann. Intern. Med.* **137**: 947–54
- Williams R, James OF, Warnes TW, Morgan MY (2000) Evaluation of the efficacy and safety of rifaximin in the treatment of hepatic encephalopathy: a double-blind, randomized, dose-finding multi-centre study. *Eur. J. Gastroent. Hepatol.* **12**(2): 203–8.

Acute renal failure

Andrew Burtenshaw

Introduction

Acute renal failure (ARF) may be defined as a rapid loss (days to weeks) of the functional ability of the kidneys to excrete the waste products of metabolism and to maintain fluid, electrolyte and acid–base homeostasis. It is a common condition, which contributes significantly to the morbidity and mortality of critically ill patients.

There is great disparity between the many published definitions of ARF. In the absence of a consensus the published literature describing its epidemiology is often discordant.

Although acute renal failure may occur as a single organ phenomenon, it is frequently seen in the critical care environment as part of a multiple organ failure syndrome. In this setting, multiple factors must be taken into account when considering precipitating causes and appropriate management. ARF may complicate up to 5% of hospital admissions and 30% of emergency admissions to critical care.

Physiological considerations

Although the kidneys constitute approximately 0.5% of the total body weight of an adult patient, they receive in the region of 20–25% of the cardiac output. This is necessary to provide a sufficient glomerular filtration rate (GFR) to permit renal excretion of waste products, in addition to maintaining the very high oxygen and metabolic demands of the renal tissues themselves. The vast majority of blood flow to the renal tissues perfuses the cortex, whilst the inner medulla – the region responsible for the most intense water reabsorption and concentrating activity – receives the least blood flow.

The requirement for a high renal blood flow (RBF), together with considerable metabolic demands and the tendency for afferent vessel vasoconstriction in the event of hypotension or low flow states to preserve perfusion of less tolerant organs (brain, heart), results in the kidneys often acting as an early marker of global tissue hypoperfusion which also makes them highly susceptible to failure.

Classification

The aetiology of ARF is classically divided into prerenal, renal (intrinsic) and postrenal causes. Whilst pre-renal causes are overall the most common precipitants for hospital admissions with ARF, acute tubular necrosis (ATN) from ischaemic and nephrotoxic insults is the most common reason for ARF developing in established critical care patients.

The term acute kidney injury (AKI) has been recently suggested to replace the term acute renal failure. The RIFLE criteria here recently emerged as an international consensus classification for AKI (see Further reading).

Prerenal causes

Prerenal ARF typically results from hypotension leading to a reduction in renal perfusion below a threshold necessary to maintain adequate function. This is most commonly due to blood loss, dehydration (e.g. due to diarrhoea or vomiting), or causes of low vascular resistance states such as septic, spinal or anaphylactic shock, which result in hypotension due to actual or relative hypovolaemia. Prerenal causes account for up to 60% of ARF seen in the hospital environment.

Prerenal causes of acute renal failure are almost always preceded by a period of oliguria in which there is maximal fluid reabsorption by the kidney. This effort to maintain homeostasis may impair optimal waste product elimination. This 'prerenal uraemia' is an appropriate functional response to inadequate renal perfusion and usually responds to fluid resuscitation

Core Topics in Critical Care Medicine, eds. Fang Gao Smith and Joyce Yeung. Published by Cambridge University Press.

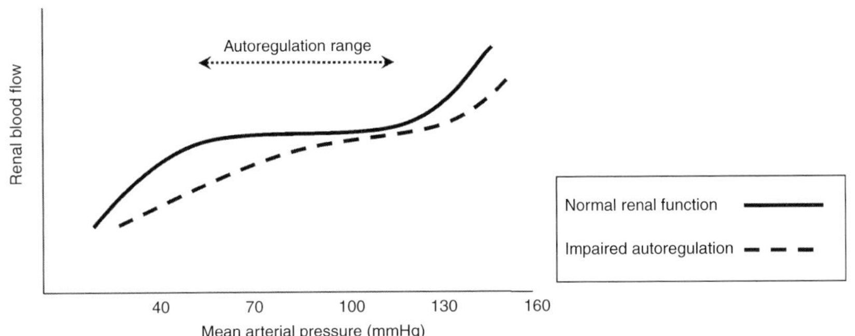

Fig. 37.1 Renal autoregulation in normal and impaired renal function.

as a means of preventing progression to established ARF. In prerenal uraemia there is preservation of the normal parenchymal structure.

Autoregulation describes the normal response to a change in renal arterial perfusion pressure to preserve RBF and GFR. This occurs throughout a range of blood pressures and is determined by a combination of myogenic theory (elevated pressure in the afferent arteriole stimulates greater smooth muscle constriction and increased resistance to flow) and variable relative resistances of the afferent and efferent arterioles in response to a variety of vasoconstrictor and vasodilatory factors. The resultant filtration fraction is determined by the balance of hydrostatic and oncotic pressures acting across the capillary endothelium and the glomerular basement membrane. Normal adult GFR is approximately 125 ml/min. The autoregulatory range is thought to occur between renal arterial pressures of 70 and 170 mmHg, such that when the pressure falls below 70 mmHg there is a direct relationship between filtration and renal artery pressure. A renal insult may cause disruption of this autoregulatory relationship such that the same RBF and GFR may require a significantly higher mean arterial pressure (MAP) than in health. As a result perfusion pressures normally considered adequate may be insufficient to produce adequate glomerular filtration (see Fig. 37.1).

However, if the MAP drops below the autoregulatory range further vasoconstriction of the efferent arterioles occurs in an attempt to maintain the hydrostatic pressure necessary for glomerular filtration. This leads to a reduction in the total RBF and, as a consequence, the GFR. If the volume of glomerular filtrate is insufficient to carry the quantity of waste products required despite the kidneys maximal medullary concentrating ability, serum urea and creatinine levels will rise. This will result in prerenal uraemia.

Progression from prerenal uraemia occurs when persistent ischaemia results in inadequate perfusion of the postglomerular capillary bed. This is the source of the blood supply to the renal tubules. The metabolic requirements of the tubules, including the thick ascending loop of Henle, cannot be met and cellular death ensues. Sloughing of tubular epithelial cells, accumulation of brush border membranous debris and cast formation cause obstruction of the tubules.

However, prerenal ARF may also occur in the presence of normal blood pressure. In this case it can be termed 'normotensive ischaemic acute renal failure'. This represents impairment of the normal autoregulatory processes, which results in failure to produce an adequate GFR despite a measured blood pressure within the normal range.

Some patients can be recognized as having a predisposition to normotensive ischaemic ARF. This is most likely in patients with hypertension, chronic renal failure (CRF), atherosclerosis or those receiving non-steroidal anti-inflammatory drugs (NSAIDs), cyclooxygenase (COX-2) inhibitors, angiotensin-converting enzyme (ACE) inhibitors or an angiotensin II receptor antagonist (ARB). Hypertension, malignant hypertension, CRF, renal artery stenosis and atherosclerosis may all result in changes to the afferent arteries or arterioles which limit appropriate vasodilatation and prevent the normal maintenance of RBF. CRF may also be associated with chronic compensatory arteriolar vasodilatation which maximizes the RBF within the remaining functioning glomeruli but which depletes any vasodilatory reserve in the event of hypoperfusion and therefore increases susceptibility to ischaemia. NSAIDs and COX inhibitors can attenuate the vasodilatory response of the afferent arteriole by inhibiting the production of prostaglandins responsible for arteriolar vasodilatation with consequent reductions in both RBF and GFR. ACE inhibitors and ARBs may prevent efferent arteriolar vasoconstriction resulting in a reduction in GFR despite an adequate RBF.

Normotensive ischaemic ARF requires a precipitant which results in ARF in susceptible patients. Hypoperfusion in the presence of high levels of vasoconstricting substances results in a low flow, high resistance state. In this situation susceptible patients experience a significant reduction in renal blood flow and function despite compensatory maintenance of blood pressure. This may include compensated hypovolaemia due to fluid and blood loss or cardiac failure (e.g. ischaemic or other cardiomyopathy, cardiac tamponade, pulmonary embolism, valvular disease, etc.). Abnormal blood distribution may be the precipitating cause, as in (normotensive) sepsis or the hepatorenal syndrome.

Intrinsic causes

These can be grouped into an anatomical classification of abnormalities of the glomerulus, renal vasculature, interstitium and renal tubules.

Glomerulus

There are many causes of glomerulonephritis including:

- IgA nephropathy
- Henoch–Schönlein purpura
- minimal change glomerulonephritis
- focal segmental glomerulosclerosis
- thin basement membrane nephropathy
- mesangiocapillary glomerulonephritis
- membranous nephropathy
- proliferative glomerulonephritis.

These seldom occur within the critical care environment because they are usually isolated pathologies frequently presenting as chronic renal failure. Therefore they will have been managed by a nephrologist and their dialysis requirements may be anticipated and accommodated within an independent dialysis programme.

However, rapidly progressive glomerulonephritis (RPGN) can present within weeks and may therefore require renal replacement therapy within a critical care environment prior to transfer to an appropriate dialysis facility for ongoing care. Examples of this include anti-glomerular basement membrane disease (Goodpasture's disease), post-streptococcal glomerulonephritis and RPGN due to drugs (rifampicin, penicillamine, hydralazine). In unusual circumstances these may present as multi-organ disease requiring support, such as in the case of pulmonary haemorrhage associated with Goodpasture's disease.

Renal vasculature

Examples of renovascular disease include hypertension (including malignant hypertension, pre-eclampsia and the haemolysis–elevated liver enzymes–low platelets (HELLP) syndrome), diabetes, atherosclerosis, renal artery stenosis, thrombotic thrombocytopenic purpura, haemolytic uraemic syndrome and cholesterol emboli.

Of these, atherosclerosis and diabetic nephropathy are the most common causes of borderline renal function seen in the critical care unit, which may predispose to development of established acute renal failure in response to minimal insult.

Interstitium

Acute interstitial nephritis due to drugs (e.g. NSAIDs, penicillin, amphotericin, gentamicin, vancomycin, frusemide and radiocontrast) or following infection accounts for the majority of interstitial nephritides presenting with ARF to the critical care unit. Urate nephropathy, Balkan nephropathy, radiation nephritis and hypercalcaemic nephropathy are rare presentations.

Tubules

Acute tubular necrosis accounts for the majority of tubular causes of ARF, and is usually the direct consequence of inadequately treated prerenal uraemia. The ischaemic insult results in intense afferent arteriolar vasoconstriction and loss of the normal renal vasodilatory mechanisms (prostaglandin I_2 and nitric oxide). This leads to redistribution of blood flow within the kidney and a diminished GFR. Energy-dependent cells within the proximal tubule and the ascending loop of Henle sustain hypoxic injury and cell necrosis, mediated by oxygen free radicals. Casts are formed as the tubular cells break away from the basement membrane blocking any remaining urinary flow.

Rhabdomyolysis is a relatively frequently encountered cause of tubular ARF in which the pathophysiology is multifactorial. Initially there is an enormous release of lactic acid producing a high anion gap acidosis, together with release of intracellular potassium. Muscle necrosis together with cellular inflammation results in a large accumulation of fluid within

Table 37.1 Known causes of postrenal ARF

Luminal	Blood clots Renal stones Sloughed papilla Tumour (renal, ureteric or bladder) Ureteric trauma
Mural	Strictures Ureteric oedema (e.g. following instrumentation) Schistosomiasis
Extra-mural	Enlarged prostate Abdominal mass Pelvic mass Retroperitoneal fibrosis

the muscle which can render the patient intravascularly fluid deplete. This relative hypovolaemia reduces organ perfusion. Hepatic hypoperfusion limits the metabolism of lactate exacerbating the acidosis, whilst renal hypoperfusion promotes renal failure. Myoglobin has a molecular weight of 18 000 daltons and is therefore freely permeable through the glomerular membrane. As water is reabsorbed the concentration of myoglobin within the nephron increases dramatically, causing it to precipitate within the tubules resulting in cast formation and tubular obstruction. The relative hypovolaemia enhances this precipitation by both reducing glomerular filtration and increasing water reabsorption. In addition to this there is an increased production of uric acid which also precipitates within the tubules. Urinary acidosis results from systemic acidosis enhancing deposition of cast and crystal precipitants further. Finally, free iron, which is released from the degradation of intraluminal myoglobin, catalyses the production of free radicals which are an independent cause of ischaemic tubular cellular damage.

Other causes of renotubular ARF include distal (Type I) renal tubular acidosis, proximal (Type II) renal tubular acidosis, hyperkalaemic (Type IV) renal tubular acidosis, Bartter's syndrome and light chain deposition (myeloma). These are uncommon within the critical care unit.

Postrenal causes

In postrenal uraemia there are initially minimal changes to the parenchymal structure, usually characterized by hydronephrosis and blunting of the renal papilla (Table 37.1). Resumption of normal renal function is possible if the obstructing lesion can be removed or bypassed before more significant structural changes occur.

This is the least common cause of ARF to be found within the critical care environment and, although more common in the overall hospital patient population, still accounts for less than 10% of all causes of ARF.

These require rapid, appropriate investigation and are frequently amenable to expedient surgical or radiological intervention.

Diagnosis and assessment of acute renal failure

A detailed history will often identify the likely cause of ARF. Events predisposing to impaired renal perfusion are usually evident and in the case of renal and postrenal causes, previous medical history, family history and a list of medications will frequently lead to the likely diagnosis. Similarly a full examination may be of benefit and particularly in the case of renal causes of ARF may reveal evidence of multisystem disease.

In the critical care environment, oliguria is usually the first indicator of impending renal failure. Urine output less than 0.5 ml/kg per hour is usually regarded as a threshold for acceptable urine output because this is the minimum volume of urine capable of carrying the body's waste products provided the urine is maximally concentrated. This applies particularly to the case of elderly patients or those with coexistent renal pathologies in whom the maximal concentrating ability is reduced, whilst younger patients may be able to cope with a marginally lower minimum urine output due to better inner medullary concentrating capabilities. However, up to 10% of cases of ARF may present without oliguria, as is commonly seen with drug- or radiocontrast-induced ARF.

Subsequent rises in blood urea, creatinine and potassium concentrations occur together with sodium and water retention and the development of a metabolic acidosis. Whilst all these findings commonly coexist, they are not all required in order to make the diagnosis of acute renal failure.

There are two main elements important in the early assessment of ARF. These are the identification of the cause of ARF and evaluation of the requirement to initiate appropriate treatment, including renal replacement therapy.

Effective management of early ARF invariably depends upon identification of the causative pathology. The cause may be obvious, such as a prolonged period of hypotension or a known obstructive lesion. Early identification of reversible causes of renal

Table 37.2 Laboratory results that may be used to assist in the distinction between prerenal uraemia and acute tubular necrosis

	Prerenal uraemia	Acute tubular necrosis
Urinary [Na] (mmol/l)	<20	>40
Urine/plasma osmolality	>1.5 : 1	<1.1 : 1
Urine/plasma urea	>10	<7
Urine/plasma creatinine	>40	<20

impairment with expedient intervention may prevent progression to established ARF.

In the first instance, the history (including drug administration) and examination findings may suggest the likely cause. Prerenal uraemia must be distinguished from established renal failure as aggressive fluid resuscitation and restoration of renal perfusion may be effective, providing ATN has not yet occurred. In prerenal uraemia there is aggressive reabsorption of sodium and water resulting in low sodium concentration, high osmolality urine samples with high urea and creatinine concentrations relative to the plasma concentrations (Table 37.2).

The possibility of postrenal obstruction should be considered in all cases, and an urgent ultrasound scan of the renal tract organized when indicated. Early relief of urinary obstruction, either by removal of the cause or provision of an alternative path for urine drainage (e.g. nephrostomy), may prevent progression to established renal failure and obviate the requirement for renal replacement therapy.

If the renal failure cannot be explained by prerenal causes or postrenal obstruction, other causes such as glomerular disease must be considered and a renal biopsy may be indicated. A nephrology opinion should be sought at this stage.

There may be indicators available to help distinguish between acute and chronic renal failure. In particular, one should consider the potential association of co-morbidities with renal failure (e.g. diabetes mellitus), evidence of previously deranged renal function tests, associated blood test abnormalities consistent with chronic renal failure (anaemia, hypocalcaemia and hyperphosphataemia) and the presence of atrophic kidneys on ultrasound scan.

Where obvious causes cannot be established, factors predisposing to normotensive ischaemic ARF should be sought together with potential precipitating events (e.g. undiagnosed acute myocardial infarction). The patency of the renal vessels and of the aorta should also be considered as possible causes of renal failure.

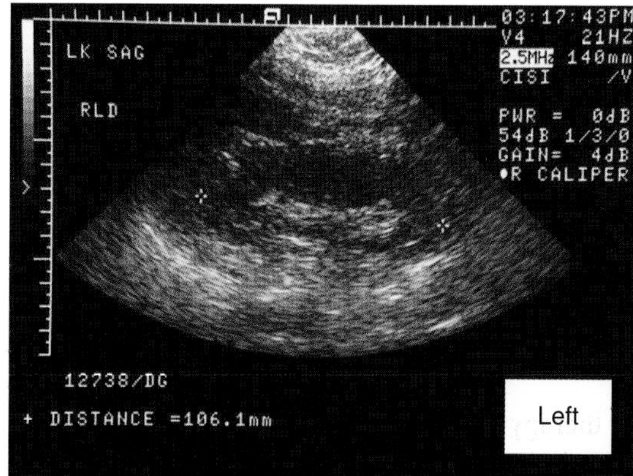

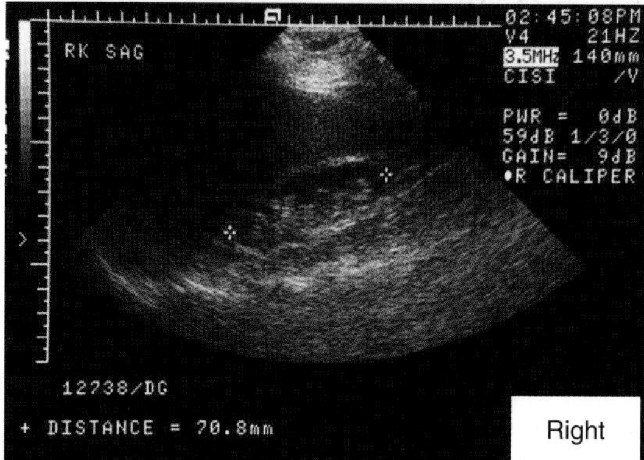

Fig. 37.2 Ultrasound of kidneys. The left kidney demonstrates normal echotexture. No hydronephrosis, nephrolithiasis, perinephric fluid collection or abnormal renal mass is identified. The left kidney measures 10.6 cm in length. The right kidney is small, measuring 7.1 cm in length. Cortical atrophy is identified.

The most common indications for commencing renal replacement therapy are:

- hyperkalaemia ([K^+] >6.5 mmol/l)
- progressive metabolic acidosis (pH <7.1)
- symptomatic uraemia (vomiting, encephalopathy, pericarditis)
- fluid overload (pulmonary oedema).

Management

Prerenal uraemia should be treated by urgent restoration of circulating volume and renal perfusion pressure and by correction of electrolyte deficits. Whilst

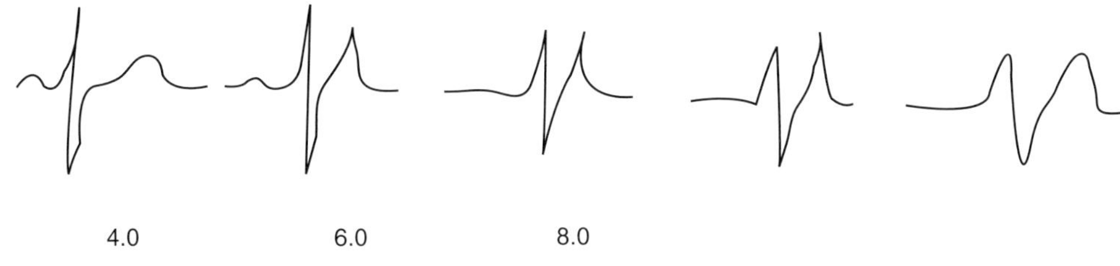

Fig. 37.3 ECG changes in hyperkalaemia: tall T waves, absent P wave, widening of QRS complexes.

fluid therapy alone may be sufficient to achieve this, appropriate use of inotropic and/or vasopressor agents may be indicated as guided by the clinical circumstances and haemodynamic monitoring.

Cases of renal outflow obstruction should be considered a surgical emergency and a means of relieving the obstruction should be sought immediately. This should include the assessment and timely relief of abdominal tamponade.

Multiple therapeutic options have been employed in early renal failure in an attempt to reverse the progression of ATN. Despite many trials in this area there remains little evidence to support the notion that renal function can be affected by these interventions. Drugs that have been employed include dopamine, mannitol, loop diuretics and calcium channel blockers. Of these, frusemide remains the most frequently employed therapy. Whilst there is little evidence that the use of frusemide can improve renal outcome or halt progression of incipient renal failure, its use can increase the volume of urine produced and may therefore offer benefit in limiting fluid overload and potentially avoiding or delaying the necessity for renal replacement therapy. The suggestion that furosemide can protect the kidneys from hypoxic or ischaemic insult by reducing the metabolic requirements of the thick ascending loop of Henle remains unsupported by outcome data.

Once it is certain that progression to established renal failure is unavoidable, the rationale for fluid management changes from fluid challenges in the hope of restoring glomerular filtration to fluid restriction to limit fluid overload and pulmonary oedema. Fluid therapy should replace insensible loss and sodium or potassium administration should be avoided in most situations. Hyponatraemia is a common finding in the early oliguric phase of renal failure and is usually due to relative volume overload as opposed to abnormalities of total body sodium content, which is usually normal or increased.

- antibiotics:
  - penicillins
  - cephalosporins
  - aminoglycosides
  - tetracycline
- beta-blockers
- diuretics
- lithium
- digoxin
- procainamide
- cimetidine
- ranitidine

Fig. 37.4 Common examples of drugs excreted by the kidney, which should be given with caution in renal failure.

The development of hyperkalaemia may be rapid, particularly if the failure of renal potassium excretion is exacerbated by increased intracellular potassium release. This may occur as a result of trauma, crush injuries, rhabdomyolysis, haemolysis, sepsis or acidaemia. Dangerous hyperkalaemia produces characteristic ECG changes (flat or absent P waves, widened QRS complexes, 'tented' T waves), which precede cardiac arrest and should provoke urgent intervention (Fig. 37.3).

Renal replacement therapy is likely to be required but a number of temporizing measures may be employed initially. These include insulin and dextrose solutions (e.g. 20 units insulin in 50 ml 50% dextrose), nebulized β-agonists (salbutamol) and intravenous sodium bicarbonate, all of which promote intracellular passage of potassium ions. Calcium exchange resins (calcium resonium) and cardiac protection with 10% calcium chloride solution should also be considered.

Renal replacement therapy (RRT) is the mainstay of treatment for established acute renal failure and is the subject of Chapter 38.

Care should be taken with drugs that undergo renal excretion (Fig. 37.4). Dosages should be changed appropriately and certain drugs (e.g. gentamicin, digoxin) may require plasma level assays. Nephrotoxic agents should be discontinued unless essential. Radio-opaque contrast agents should only be used when the benefit of potential diagnosis is considered to outweigh the risk of nephrotoxicity. Patients at particular risk of contrast-induced renal failure include those with diabetes, myeloma and other causes of paraproteinaemia and those who are inadequately hydrated. Preloading the patient with fluid prior to contrast injection may reduce the potential nephrotoxic effect, as may concurrent administration of *N*-acetyl cysteine or sodium bicarbonate solution.

Outcome

Survival following an episode of ARF is variable and, within the critical care environment, is largely dependent upon the accompanying pathological conditions, e.g. severe sepsis. In those who survive the initial illness, ARF frequently persists beyond the resolution of the precipitating disease process, although evidence suggests that the majority achieve independence from RRT by 90 days. There is insufficient evidence at present to prognosticate the quality of renal recovery and whether this may be modifiable by interventions during the critically ill period.

Key points

- ARF is a common condition which is a major contributor to morbidity and mortality amongst critical care patients.
- Because renal function is highly dependent upon adequate renal blood flow and glomerular filtration pressure, oliguria is an early marker of an inadequate haemodynamic status.
- Early reversible causes of renal failure must be considered and treated expediently to limit progression to established renal failure.
- The duration of renal failure is frequently longer than the duration of the precipitating illness, but restoration of sufficient renal function to discontinue RRT usually occurs within 90 days.
- Whilst RRT allows effective treatment for renal failure, the coexistence of ARF with other pathologies (e.g. sepsis) significantly worsens prognosis.

Further reading

- Abuelo JG (2007) Normotensive ischemic acute renal failure. *N. Engl. J. Med.* **357**: 797–805.
- Bagshaw SM (2006) The long-term outcome after acute renal failure. *Curr. Opin. Crit. Care* **12**(6): 561–6.
- Hoste EAJ *et al.* (2006) RIFLE criteria for acute kidney injury are associated with hospital mortality in critically ill patients: a cohort analysis. *Crit. Care* **10**: R73.
- Schrier RW, Wang W (2004) Acute renal failure and sepsis. *N. Engl. J. Med.* **351**: 159–69.

Renal replacement therapy

Andrew Burtenshaw

Introduction

Acute renal failure occurs in up to 30% of emergency admissions to intensive care. Consequently, renal replacement therapy (RRT) has become a fundamental element of critical care management. Advances in membrane and machine technology have improved the efficacy of RRT, provided new modes of delivering RRT and reduced the associated adverse effects. Recently there has been increasing interest in the role of RRT in sepsis and the systemic inflammatory response and multiple organ dysfunction syndromes.

Principles of renal replacement therapy

The functions of the kidney that RRT aims to replicate are removal of water and waste products from the circulation and maintenance of electrolyte and acid–base homeostasis. These are achieved by transport of water and solute molecules across a semipermeable membrane via the mechanisms of *ultrafiltration, diffusion* and *convection*. The semipermeable membrane may be synthetic, as in the case of intermittent haemodialysis (IHD), or autologous, as in the case of peritoneal dialysis. Although utilized in the early development of RRT for critical care, peritoneal dialysis is now rarely used within the critical care environment and will not be discussed further. Whilst early RRT machines utilized arterial pressure to drive blood flow using an arterio-venous circulation, veno-venous blood circulation has superseded this as it enables better regulation of blood flow and is associated with fewer adverse events.

Ultrafiltration

Ultrafiltration refers to the flow of small molecules (in this case water, electrolytes and low molecular weight substances) through a semipermeable membrane whilst larger molecular weight compounds are held back. The rate of ultrafiltration is dependent upon the pressure difference between each side of the semipermeable membrane and the pore size.

Diffusion

Diffusion describes the spontaneous migration of substances from a region of high concentration to one of low concentration as a result of random molecular movement. This tendency ultimately leads to the development of an equal concentration on either side of a semipermeable membrane. Diffusion is the underlying principle of dialysis.

When two volumes of fluid are separated by a semipermeable membrane, the rate of diffusion is dependent upon the following factors: solute characteristics and concentration, permeability and properties of the membrane and fluid movement either side of the membrane.

Solute

- Size – smaller molecules tend to migrate more rapidly across a semipermeable membrane.
- Charge – electrical charge may exert a force which will influence transmembrane transport.
- Protein binding – molecules bound to proteins, which are too large to travel across the membrane, will not diffuse across unless they become dissociated from the protein. Their diffusion rate is therefore substantially reduced.

Solute concentrations

Diffusion will continue to occur randomly but will tend towards a state of equilibrium with equal

Core Topics in Critical Care Medicine, eds. Fang Gao Smith and Joyce Yeung. Published by Cambridge University Press.

concentrations of a substance on either side of a membrane. The quantity of a substance that traverses a membrane can therefore be influenced by the concentration of that substance on the dialysate side of a semipermeable membrane. For example, in order not to excessively diminish plasma potassium levels, most dialysate fluids contain potassium in a low concentration such that equilibrium is achieved with only moderate diffusion of potassium across the membrane.

Semipermeable membrane

- Type – early cellulose-based membranes had a low permeability coefficient to water and tended to activate inflammatory cascades. Modern filters predominantly use synthetic membranes which are far more water permeable, have high sieving coefficients for a wide range of molecular weight solutes and cause less damage to platelets and white cells passing through the filter.
- Porosity – when more pores are available within a semipermeable membrane, the number of molecules per unit time migrating across the membrane will be increased and diffusion will be more rapid.
- Thickness – random migration of molecules is less likely across thicker membranes and the rate of diffusion is therefore correspondingly reduced. Thin membranes encourage rapid diffusion.
- Surface area – the greater the surface area, the greater number of pores available at any one time through which random migration can occur. Diffusion rate is increased with increased surface area.

Fluid movement

- Continuous movement of the filtrate and dialysate fluids prevents equilibrium from being achieved and therefore promotes continuing diffusion. Faster fluid movement on either side of the membrane helps to optimize the concentration gradient, preventing the rate of diffusion from becoming significantly diminished.
- Placing the flow of filtrate and dialysate in opposite directions is known as *counter-current exchange*. This allows a concentration gradient to be maintained down which diffusion can continue to occur for a much longer period of contact. The result is significantly greater total solute diffusion than would occur if the flows of filtrate and dialysate were in the same direction. This is a fundamental principle of dialysis.

Convection

Convection describes the movement of a solute across a membrane in a moving stream of ultrafiltrate. Convection may also be referred to as 'solvent drag' and is the underlying principle of haemofiltration.

The rate of convection is dependent upon:

- Pore size – this determines which solutes can be transported by the convective flow.
- Direction and force of fluid flux – this determines the convective current, which directly relates to the rate of convection.

Convective flow from the blood compartment of an RRT machine is dependent upon the rate of blood flow to the membrane. This produces a transmembrane pressure which in turn determines the rate of ultrafiltration.

In terms of renal replacement, solute transport predominantly relies upon diffusion during haemodialysis techniques and convection during haemofiltration. These processes may occur simultaneously (haemodiafiltration) in which case ultrafiltration, convection and diffusion are all playing a part in water and solute transport across the membrane.

Indications for renal replacement therapy

RRT is utilized when medical management of renal dysfunction has failed to prevent the development of established renal failure. Although critical care units vary, commonly used triggers for commencing RRT are:

- Metabolic acidosis pH <7.1
- Hyperkalaemia [K^+] >6.5 mmol/l
- Severe fluid overload adversely affecting organ function (e.g. pulmonary oedema)
- Symptomatic uraemia (e.g. vomiting, seizures, pericarditis)

Other factors that may provoke consideration of RRT but are not absolute indications include:

- Drug intoxication amenable to RRT
- Severe hyperthermia refractory to other methods of treatment
- Severe hypothermia refractory to other methods of treatment
- Anuria/oliguria anticipated to progress to established acute renal failiure (ARF) and not responding to medical management

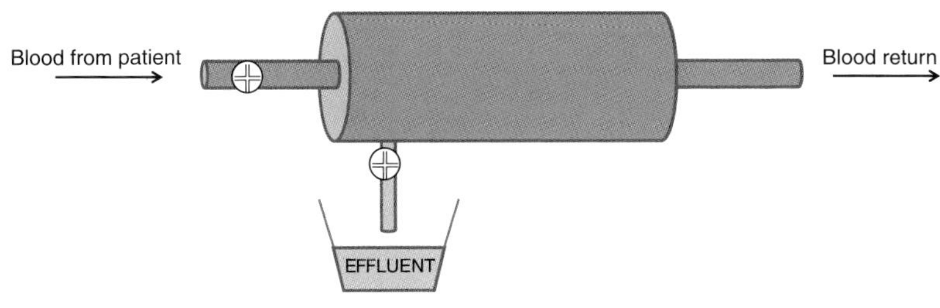

Fig. 38.1 Slow continuous ultrafiltration (SCUF).

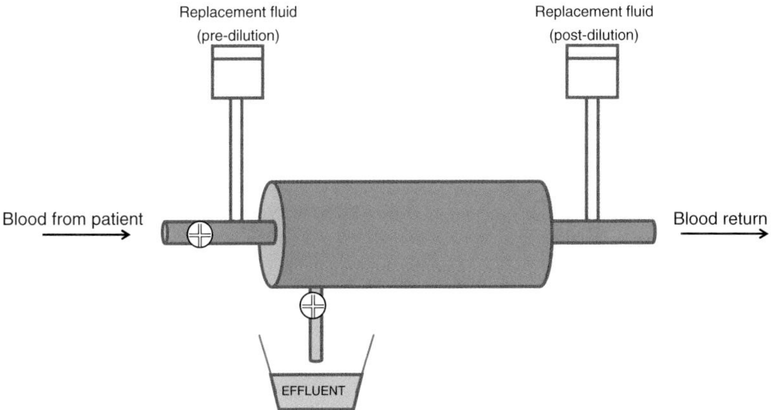

Fig. 38.2 Continuous veno-venous haemofiltration (CVVH).

- Severe dysnatraemia ($[Na^+]$ <115 mmol/l or $[Na^+]$ >160 mmol/l)
- Multiple organ dysfunction syndrome (MODS), systemic inflammatory response syndrom (SIRS) or severe sepsis/septic shock.

Modes of renal replacement therapy

Slow continuous ultrafiltration

Slow continuous ultrafiltration (SCUF) is highly efficient where fluid removal is required without manipulation of solute concentration (Fig. 38.1). As volume overload in the absence of renal failure is rare, SCUF is seldom used within critical care. The technique does, however, demonstrate the principle of ultrafiltration in which water is driven through a semipermeable membrane under the influence of hydrostatic pressure. Ultrafiltration rate is set low at approximately 5–15 ml/min, with a circuit blood flow usually set between 100 and 250 ml/min.

Continuous veno-venous haemofiltration

Continuous veno-venous haemofiltration (CVVH) is a commonly used technique that uses the same principle as SCUF except that because the aim is solute and water removal, the convective flow must be higher. Thus the ultrafiltration rate is between 15 and 60 ml/min which generates a sufficiently high filtrate flux to produce adequate solute removal (Fig. 38.2). Similar blood flow rates in the circuit to those of SCUF (100–250 ml/min) are sufficient.

The rate of fluid removal is much higher in order to facilitate adequate solute removal so fluid must be replaced into the circuit; the volume of the fluid can be altered to control overall fluid balance. This may be replaced before the blood flow enters the filter (pre-dilution) or after (post-dilution), or a combination of the two. Whilst pre-dilution lowers the concentration of solutes which are intended to be removed by convection (i.e. reduces filter efficiency), it also has the effect of reducing the haematocrit passing through the filter and therefore increasing filter life by diminishing the risk of blood clot formation within the filter.

CVVH is effective for both solute and water removal and is therefore useful for renal failure or fluid overload.

Continuous veno-venous haemodialysis

Continuous veno-venous haemodialysis (CVVHD) relies upon diffusion to facilitate solute clearance and whilst effective in the treatment of renal failure,

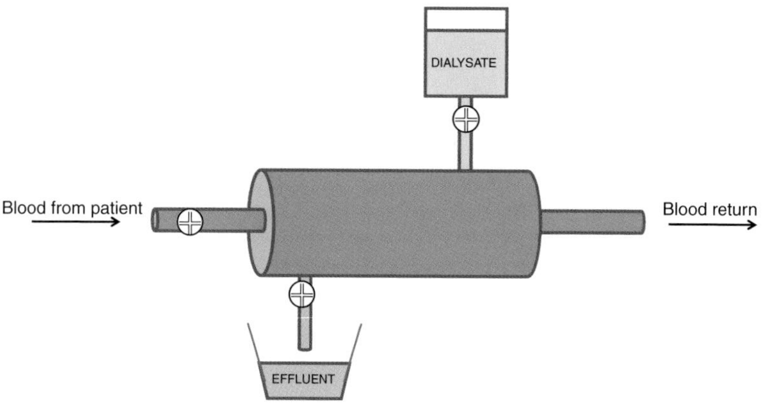

Fig. 38.3 Continuous veno-venous haemodialysis (CVVHD).

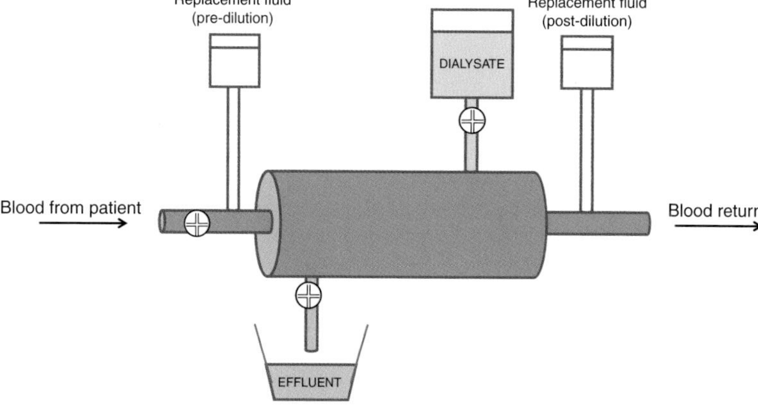

Fig. 38.4 Continuous veno-venous haemodiafiltration (CVVHDF).

electrolyte imbalance and metabolic acidosis, it is a poor means of treating fluid overload (Fig. 38.3).

Filter efficiency is optimized by passing high blood flow (up to 250 ml/min) and dialysate flow rates (15–60 ml/min) through a counter-current exchange circuit.

As the ultrafiltration rate is low, fluid replacement is not necessary.

Continuous veno-venous haemodiafiltration

Continuous veno-venous haemodiafiltration (CVVHDF) is a hybrid of CVVH and CVVHD in which hydrostatic pressure is exerted upon the blood compartment to produce an elevated ultrafiltration rate thus necessitating fluid replacement (Fig. 38.4). At the same time, a dialysate flow is simultaneously passed through the filter in a counter-current direction. Both diffusion and convection occur to maximize solute removal (blood flow rate 100–250 ml/min, ultrafiltrate rate 15 – 60 ml/min, dialysis flow rate 15–60 ml/min).

Intermittent vs. continuous

Continuous RRT carries a number of advantages over intermittent RRT for the critically ill patient.

Cardiovascular stability and volume fluctuation

Intermittent RRT requires high blood flow rates which may result in cardiovascular collapse due to a sudden fall in cardiac venous return, particularly when initiating filtration. Whilst this may also be a problem with continuous techniques, the blood flow rate is considerably lower and the cardiovascular effects correspondingly less severe. In addition, any fluid removal must be undertaken over a shorter period of time, providing less time for equilibration of fluid between body compartments, resulting in more profound fluctuations in venous pressure. Intermittent RRT necessitates relative hypovolaemia immediately post-dialysis and is associated with fluid overload prior to subsequent dialysis. Continuous RRT avoids these fluctuations and is thought to better support overall organ perfusion and function in critically ill patients.

Drug level stability

Maintenance of a relatively constant plasma volume together with a steady rate of drug clearance results in a much smoother plasma drug concentration during continuous RRT than compared to intermittent techniques. This may have a particular effect on drugs such as vasopressors and inotropes, but also affects the measurement of certain drug levels (e.g.antibiotics or anticonvulsants) and their corresponding management.

Minimization of electrolyte disturbance

Rapid changes in electrolyte concentrations may adversely affect cardiac function and have deleterious effects upon neurological function, as described by the dialysis disequilibrium syndrome. Continuous RRT provides more gradual changes in electrolyte concentrations, therefore minimizing these complications.

Less effective cytokine removal

RRT in critical care is frequently used for the treatment of ARF due to sepsis. Convective flow is more effective than diffusion in the removal of large molecular weight compounds such as the systemic inflammatory mediators and is therefore thought to have additional benefit in sepsis over and above the treatment of ARF. Likewise, continuous removal of these mediators is thought to be more effective than intermittent removal in terms of diminishing inflammatory response.

Outcome

Evidence supports the use of continuous RRT over intermittent techniques both in terms of mortality for critically ill patients with ARF and subsequent renal recovery in those who survive.

Problems

Unfortunately, continuous RRT is associated with substantially greater financial cost and staff requirements.

Associated therapeutic options

Plasmapheresis

Use of specific membranes which permit the ultrafiltration of plasma proteins up to a specified size, together with plasma replacement, is occasionally warranted within the ITU. These filters allow the passage of much larger molecules than conventional haemofilters (usually 100 000 to 1 000 000 kilodaltons as opposed to 20–50 kilodaltons). This method is in contrast to conventional centrifugal removal of plasma as commonly used in haematological practice, and has the advantage that it can usually be performed by standard RRT machines.

Examples of disease states that may be treated within critical care by this method include Guillain–Barré syndrome (acute inflammatory demyelinating polyneuropathy – AIDP), Goodpasture's syndrome, myasthenia gravis, Lambert–Eaton myasthenic syndrome and thrombotic thrombocytopenic purpura.

Haemoperfusion

Charcoal haemoperfusion involves passing the blood compartment over charcoal powder to permit removal of solute by adsorption to the charcoal molecules. This is of particular use in poisoning or accidental intoxication with lipid soluble drugs.

The use of other specific membranes for haemoperfusion has been investigated in the treatment of fulminant hepatitis with encephalopathy and sepsis, although convincing evidence to support this is currently lacking.

High-volume haemofiltration

High-volume haemofiltration (HVHF) utilizes high blood flow and ultrafiltration rates through highly permeable membranes with the aim of increasing the removal of systemic inflammatory mediators. This therapy is not yet commonplace in the treatment of sepsis.

Fluid prescriptions in renal replacement therapy

During haemofiltration, fluid removed by ultrafiltration must be replaced prior to delivery back to the patient. The exact volume of replacement fluid may be altered to produce the overall fluid balance required. 'One litre exchange' refers to the removal and simultaneous replacement of 1 litre of fluid per hour. One to three litre exchanges are commonly prescribed according to the degree of metabolic derangement.

Replacement fluid should contain electrolytes in a concentration similar to that of normal plasma, and must replace bicarbonate which is also lost in this process. During haemodialysis or haemodiafiltration, the dialysate concentration affects the rate and direction of solute diffusion across the membrane. The use of different dialysate fluids will therefore influence plasma solute transfer. Bicarbonate loss will also occur in this process if the dialysis fluid does not contain an appropriate concentration of bicarbonate.

Bicarbonate loss in ultrafiltrate or across a dialysis filter, together with plasma bicarbonate depletion as part of metabolic acidosis, means that bicarbonate replacement is necessary to prevent profound metabolic acidosis. Bicarbonate solutions have a short shelf-life and are both more expensive and more difficult to prepare. Bicarbonate cannot be put into solution with either calcium or magnesium as this will result in precipitation of their respective bicarbonate salts, and therefore these compounds must be administered separately. Alternatively, bicarbonate may be infused systemically as a separate infusion.

Lactate containing fluids are much more stable and may contain calcium and magnesium without the risk of crystal formation. Lactate is converted to bicarbonate by the tricarboxylic acid cycle within the liver. However, with impaired liver function or excessive lactate production, the enzymatic functional capacity may be fully saturated and bicarbonate solutions may be necessary to prevent excessive accumulation of lactate and associated metabolic acidosis.

Anticoagulation

Blood contact with the synthetic membrane surface stimulates the coagulation cascade resulting in a variable degree of blood clot formation. Fast blood flow rates, large-bore vascular access and avoidance of kinks in the system all prevent the development of stagnant areas of blood. Together with pre-dilution by replacement fluid in the case of haemofiltration these factors all contribute to a system with a low risk of clotting. In this way, RRT without anticoagulation is possible. However, blood clot formation not only has the financial implication of a new system and staff time to replace it, but also causes a period of time during which RRT is not taking place and increases blood transfusion requirements due to blood loss within the discarded system. For these reasons anticoagulation is standard.

Unfractionated heparin is the most common form of anticoagulation, where heparin is introduced by continuous infusion to the blood before it reaches the filter. This produces maximal effect at the filter itself, and results in less systemic anticoagulation than if the heparin is given intravenously. Because anticoagulation with unfractionated heparin is unpredictable, monitoring with activated clotting time (ACT) or activated partial thromboplastin time (APTT) is required. Heparinization of RRT systems is occasionally associated with heparin-induced thrombocytopenia (HIT).

Low molecular weight heparins are occasionally used as they provide a lower risk of HIT and have a more predictable clinical effect. However, monitoring of anticoagulant levels is more difficult (Factor Xa assays are not immediately available in most haematology laboratories) and anticoagulation has a longer clinical effect which cannot be easily reversed.

Prostacyclin may be used to provide anticoagulation within the RRT circuit by acting as an inhibitor of platelet aggregation. It has the advantage of being very short-acting which means that it produces very little, if any, systemic anticoagulant effect whilst providing good circuit anticoagulation. It is commonly used where HIT is thought to have occurred following heparin administration. In larger doses overspill beyond the filter circuit may occur, producing systemic hypotension. Use of prostacyclin also carries a cost implication as it is considerably more expensive than heparin.

Citrate infusion produces a localized anticoagulant effect by chelating calcium, thus preventing clot formation. Calcium chloride replacement is invariably necessary to prevent hypocalcaemia and it is also associated with the development of a metabolic alkalosis. However, this method does avoid the risks of HIT and systemic anticoagulation.

Future possibilities in renal replacement therapy for critical care

Extensive development and research is under way within the field of RRT for critical care and significant developments are likely to come into practice in the foreseeable future.

More widespread use of calcium chelation with citrate, the use of hirudin (a direct thrombin inhibitor) and argatroban (a synthetic arginine inhibitor) represent possible avenues for anticoagulation of filter systems.

The potential benefits of immunomodulation have been the subject of much research and debate over recent years. Some studies have demonstrated improved outcomes with high dose filtration (ultrafiltration rates >35 ml/hr per kg body weight) whilst there is increasing interest in the development of specific membranes capable of adsorbing inflammatory mediators. An example is coupled plasma filtration adsorption (CPFA) during which plasma is redirected via a plasma filter through a synthetic resin cartridge prior to returning it to the blood circulation.

Blood provides a common link to all organs within the body which means that manipulation of blood constituents within an extracorporeal circuit can be used for multiple functions. It is likely that our current concept of an extracorporeal RRT machine will diversify into a multi-organ support therapy (MOST) machine. This may incorporate extracorporeal lung support (ECLS) for use in acute lung injury (ALI), liver support (such as molecular adsorbent recirculating system – MARS) and sepsis immunomodulation, in addition to the rapidly developing possibilities within RRT.

Key points

- RRT relies upon the principles of diffusion and convection for solute removal.
- A number of modes of RRT are commonly available and can be tailored to the patient's medical requirements.
- Continuous RRT has a number of important advantages over intermittent RRT in the management of the critically ill patient.
- Other variations on RRT may be used to facilitate plasmapheresis, immunomodulation or influence other organ dysfunction.

Further reading

- Bellomo R, Ronco C (2000) Continuous haemofiltration in the intensive care unit. *Crit. Care* **4**:339–45.
- Kuhlen R, Moreno R, Ranieri M, Rhodes A (2007) *25 Years of Progress and Innovation in Intensive Care Medicine*. Brussols: European Society of Intensive Care Medicine.
- Schiffl H, Lang SM, Fischer R (2002) Daily haemodialysis and the outcome of acute renal failure. *N. Engl. J. Med.* **346**: 305–10.

Status epilepticus

Joyce Yeung

Introduction

Status epilepticus (SE) is defined as a continuous, generalized, convulsive seizure lasting longer than 5 minutes, or two or more seizures during which the patient does not return to baseline consciousness. It represents a failure of the natural homeostatic seizure-suppressing mechanism responsible for seizure termination. The condition is associated with significant morbidity and mortality and is a recognized medical and neurological emergency. Status epilepticus occurs on the intensive care unit, either because the patient has been admitted with refractory status epilepticus or as an incidental finding. Management of refractory status epilepticus in the critical care environment is warranted for adequate treatment of the physiological compromise that occurs in status epilepticus. Status epilepticus is also an under-recognized cause of persistent coma on the intensive care unit.

Population-based studies have found 18–28 cases per 100 000 people per year with 9000–14 000 new cases in the UK each year. About 5% of adults diagnosed with epilepsy have had at least one episode of status epilepticus, with children higher at 10–25%. Incidence of status epilepticus is U-shaped, with highest incidence in the very young, under 1 year old, and the elderly, over 60 years old.

Mortality has been reported to be 8% in children and 30% in adults. In addition, 5–10% of people with status epilepticus will be left with permanent disability such as permanent vegetative state or cognitive difficulties. It can occur de novo in approximately 60% of presentations or less commonly in a previously diagnosed epileptic. Status epilepticus can present as convulsive or non-convulsive; although convulsive status epilepticus has higher mortality and morbidity, both require prompt recognition and treatment. The primary predictors of poor outcome are identified as anoxia, duration of longer than 1 hour and old age.

Classification

Generalized convulsive status epilepticus (GCSE)

Generalized convulsive status epilepticus (GCSE) involves generalized convulsions with impaired consciousness which may progress to minimal or no apparent motor activity but still show seizure activity on EEG (Fig. 39.1). GCSE is diagnosed clinically by tonic–clonic seizures, loss of consciousness, urinary incontinence and tongue biting. Differential diagnosis includes myoclonic jerks, septic rigors, dystonia and pseudostatus epilepticus.

Non-convulsive status epilepticus

Non-convulsive status epilepticus (NCSE) can have a variety of presentations including coma, confusion, somnolence, aphasia, altered affect and also uncommon manifestations such as delusions, hallucinations and paranoia. This can be further divided into generalized, focal or other. NCSE should be an important differential diagnosis of coma as studies have found that up to 8% of patients in coma can be found to be in NCSE (Fig. 39.2).

Aetiology

In children 51% of status epilepticus cases are secondary to infections. In adults, the causes are more diverse and can include drug misuse and cerebral pathologies (Table 39.1).

Pathophysiology

GCSE causes a sympathetic overdrive which causes both systemic and cerebral effects, whereas systemic effects are more limited in NCSE (Table 39.2).

Core Topics in Critical Care Medicine, eds. Fang Gao Smith and Joyce Yeung. Published by Cambridge University Press.

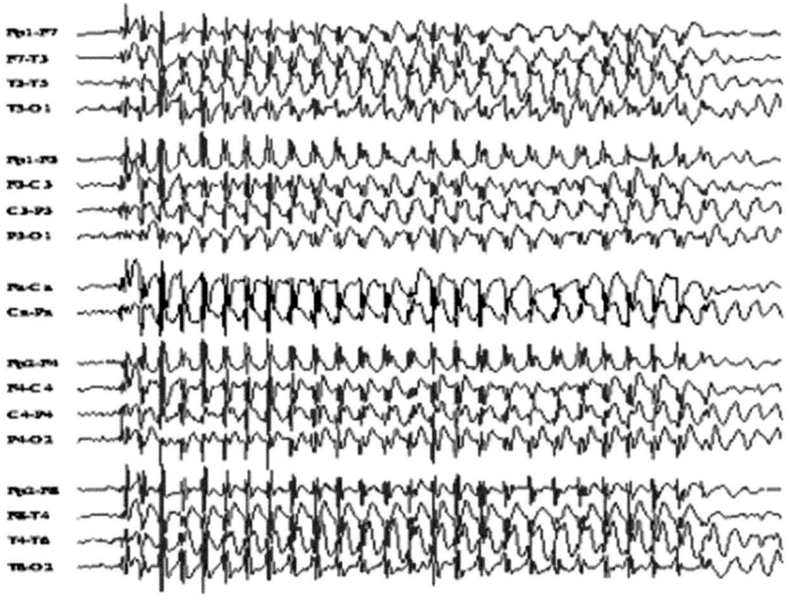

Fig. 39.1 Sample EEG of generalized convulsive status epilepticus (GCSE).

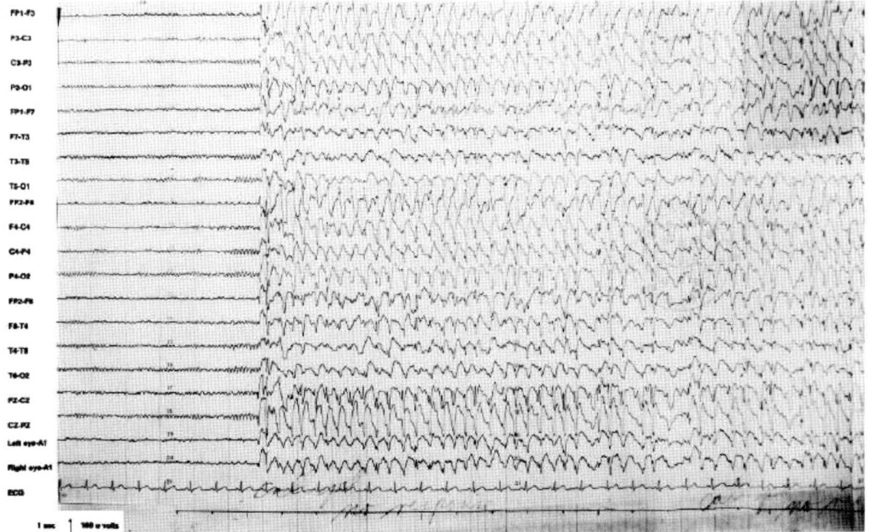

Fig. 39.2 Sample EEG of non-convulsive status epilepticus (NCSE). The first few seconds showed normal EEG waveform. Patient was awake but confused. No seizure activity seen.

In the early stages of established GCSE, there is an increase in blood pressure, glucose and lactate and a lower plasma pH. After 30 min and in the second phase, blood pressure and glucose will normalize or even decrease, lactate will normalize, respiratory compensation and hyperthermia will follow. The compensatory mechanisms will result in increased cerebral perfusion but these do not last. By 60–90 min these compensatory mechanisms will fail, hypotension and loss of cerebral autoregulation will ensue, leading to cerebral hypoperfusion and cerebral damage.

Neurons also suffer damage as a result of complex interplay of multiple factors termed excitotoxic neuronal injury. During this process, there is inhibition of the inhibitory neurotransmitter γ-aminobutyric acid (GABA) and excessive action of the excitatory neurotransmitter glutamate. High concentrations of excitatory neurotransmitter open *N*-methyl-D-aspartate

Table 39.1 Causes of convulsive status epilepticus

Previous history of epilepsy	Presenting for the first time with status
Withdrawal of anti-epileptic drug treatment	Cerebrovascular disease
Alcohol (or withdrawal of)	Cerebral tumour
Drug overdose	Intracranial infection
Cerebrovascular disease	Cerebral trauma
Cerebral trauma	Acute metabolic disturbances
Cerebral tumour	
Intracranial infection	
Acute metabolic disturbances	

Table 39.2 Systemic effects of status epilepticus

Cardiovascular system	Sympathetic overdrive
	Tachycardia, arrhythmias
	Initial increase in blood pressure and peripheral vascular resistance, followed by normalization and possible hypotension
Respiratory system	Increased respiratory rate and tidal volume
	Respiratory acidosis and when combined with metabolic acidosis leads to low pH on arterial blood gases
	Increased pulmonary vascular resistance and pulmonary oedema illustrated in animal studies
Musculoskelatal system	Anaerobic metabolism, lactic acidosis
Temperature	Increased core temperature

(NMDA) receptor-mediated calcium channels resulting in excessive intracellular calcium, leading to a sequence of events which results in neuronal damage and apoptosis.

Treatment of acute status epilepticus

The National Institute for Clinical Excellence has recommended the following strategy divided into different stages:

1st Stage (0–10 min) Early Status

- Secure airway and resuscitate
- Administer oxygen

Table 39.3 Emergency investigations

Arterial blood gases
Biochemistry – blood glucose, renal, liver function, calcium, magnesium
Haematology – full blood count, clotting profile
AED levels
Venous blood sample and urine sample for toxicology screen
Chest X-ray – aspiration
CT scan/ LP

- Assess cardiorespiratory function
- Establish intravenous access

2nd Stage (0–30 min)

- Institute regular monitoring
- Consider possibility of non-epileptic status
- Emergency anti-epileptic drug treatment (AED)
- Emergency investigations (see Table 39.3)
- Administer 50 ml of 50% dextrose and/or intravenous thiamine if there is history of alcohol abuse or poor nutrition
- Correct acidosis if severe with bicarbonate (not necessary in most cases)

3rd Stage (0–60 min) Established Status

- Establish aetiology
- Alert anaesthetist and ITU
- Identify and treat any medical complications
- Pressor therapy if required

4th Stage (30–90 min) Refractory Status

- Transfer to ITU
- Establish intensive care and EEG monitoring (see Table 39.4)
- Initiate intracranial pressure monitoring if there is persistent high intracranial pressure
- Initiate long-term maintenance AED therapy.

Terminating seizure activity

See Table 39.5 for a summary of emergency AED therapy.

Table 39.4 Monitoring

Regular neurological observations
Heart rate, ECG, blood pressure measurements
Temperature
Arterial blood gas
FBC, clotting, biochemistry
Drug levels
EEG required for refractory status epilepticus

Benzodiazepines

Benzodiazepines act by enhancing the neuroinhibitory effects of GABA. All patients given benzodiazepines should be monitored for side effects of respiratory depression and hypotension.

Diazepam

Diazepam can be given rectally (dose of 10–20 mg) in the premonitory stage or as first-line treatment intravenously (10–20 mg at 2 mg/min) during the established stage. Rectal diazepam will successfully terminate seizures in up to 70% of patients, with success by the intravenous route in 60–80% of patients. It is highly lipid soluble and has rapid CNS penetration, achieving sufficient levels at 1 min after intravenous administration and within 20 min by rectal route. Despite its long elimination half-life, when given intravenously diazepam is taken up by fat and muscle rapidly, leading to a redistribution half-life of only 30 min. This results in a rapid fall in plasma levels and the possibility of recurrence of seizures within 2 hours. Repeated boluses can lead to accumulation and sudden unexpected apnoea, cardio-respiratory collapse and CNS depression.

Lorazepam

Intravenous lorazepam (4 mg at 2 mg/min) is recommended as first-line treatment during the established stage and will terminate status epilepticus in 60–90% of patients. Lorazepam is less lipid soluble than diazepam and plasma levels rise at a slower rate after intravenous injection. In practice, however, diazepam and lorazepam are equally fast-acting. Lorazepam has the advantage of a longer redistribution half-life and a smaller chance of recurrent seizures when used alone. Cochrane Review in 2005 has found that lorazepam is better than diazepam or phenytoin alone for cessation of seizures and carries a lower risk of continued seizure needing another drug or general anaesthesia.

Table 39.5 Emergency AED therapy for convulsive status epilepticus

Premonitory stage	Diazepam 10–20 mg PR, repeat once 15 min later or midazolam 10 mg buccal
Early status	Lorazepam 0.1 mg/kg IV bolus, repeated once after 10–20 min Usual AED medication
Established status	One of the following: Phenytoin infusion 15–18 mg/kg at rate of 50 mg/min Fosphenytoin infusion 15–20 mg phenytoin equivalents (PE)/kg at rate of 50–100 mg PE/min Phenobarbitone bolus 10–15 mg/kg at rate of 100 mg/min
Refractory status	General anaesthesia with one of the following: Propofol 1–2 g/kg bolus, then 2–10 mg/kg per hour Midazolam 0.1–0.2 mg/kg bolus, then 0.05–0.5 mg/kg per hour Thiopentone 3–5 mg/kg bolus, then 3–5 mg/kg per hour (reduce rate after 2–3 days as fat stores deplete) Consider tapering dose after 12–24 hours after last known seizure

Midazolam

Midazolam can be given buccally (10 mg), sublingually or intranasally during the premonitory stage with a 75% chance of preventing further seizures. It also has the advantage that it can be given intramuscularly if intravenous access is difficult although absorption can be variable. Midazolam has a fast onset and hypotension is rare. Intravenous infusion of midazolam is also used in treating status epilepticus in the intensive care setting. Clinical studies have shown that midazolam bolus (0.1–0.3 mg/kg) followed by an infusion (0.05–2.0 mg/kg per hour) achieves rapid control of seizures that have been unresponsive to other agents. Prolonged usage is associated with tachyphylaxis and accumulation.

Phenytoin

Phenytoin is commonly used as a second-line treatment after benzodiazepines have failed or as a maintenance anti-seizure treatment after rapid control of seizures by benzodiazepines. About half of the patients who have not responded to initial benzodiazepines will respond to the addition of phenytoin. A loading dose of 15–20 mg/kg should be followed by infusion of 15–18 mg/kg per min. Potential side effects are respiratory depression, arrhythmias, hypotension, rash and purple glove syndrome on extravasation. Cardiac side effects are more common in older patients with history of cardiac disease. Blood pressure and ECG monitoring is mandatory in all patients and infusion should be slowed or stopped if cardiovascular complications occur. Phenytoin solutions have a pH of 12 and can result in precipitation if added to solutions of lower pH and should not be given with other infusions on the same line. Its high pH also causes thrombophlebitis. Purple glove syndrome describes the purple discoloration of the skin around the intravenous site, oedema and possibly necrosis, up to 12 hours after starting intravenous phenytoin. Due to its saturable pharmacokinetics, serum levels of phenytoin should be monitored regularly.

Fosphenytoin

Fosphenytoin is a water-soluble pro-drug of phenytoin and is converted to phenytoin by endogenous phosphatases. Doses are therefore expressed as phenytoin equivalents (PE). The preparation of fosphenytoin does not contain propylene glycol and as a result it can be given at a higher rate of 150 PE/min and it does not cause purple glove syndrome.

Barbiturates

Phenobarbitone

Phenobarbitone can be given intravenously (10–20 mg/kg at 100 mg/min) in established status and gives a 60–70% chance of success in terminating seizures. It is a potent anticonvulsant with a long duration of action, rendering ventilatory and resuscitative support mandatory for its use. Potential side effects are respiratory depression, hypotension and rash.

Thiopentone

Thiopentone is a general anaesthetic agent that has been successfully used to treat refractory status epilepticus. An induction dose of 3–5 mg/kg is used for intubation, followed by doses of 0.5–1 mg/kg until seizures are controlled. As thiopentone is rapidly redistributed to fat stores, an infusion of 1–5 mg/kg per hour should be started to maintain seizure control. Once fat stores are saturated, the duration of action will be prolonged due to subsequent plasma redistribution and recovery can take hours or even days. Potential side effects are hypotension, myocardial depression and immunosuppression.

Propofol

Many studies have demonstrated the efficacy of propofol in the treatment of refractory status epilepticus. Propofol has anticonvulsant properties due to its action in potentiating GABA receptors. It is a popular agent and has the ideal properties of being fast-acting and lipid soluble, and it has little tendency to accumulate. However, its use can still cause significant hypotension and if used long term it can cause hyperlipidaemia and metabolic acidosis, and rhabdomyolysis has been reported. Abrupt discontinuation of treatment can lead to recurrence of seizures and doses should be gradually tapered with caution. An initial bolus of 3–5 mg/kg is followed by infusion of 1–15 mg/kg per hour.

Refractory status epilepticus

Refractory status epilepticus is defined as continued seizures despite the use of two first-line agents. These patients will require intubation and ventilation and possibly pressor support in a critical care setting.

The traditional goal of burst suppression pattern on EEG for initial 12–24 hours has been challenged as there are no data to suggest that burst suppression is needed to control or prevent recurrent seizures. However, EEG monitoring is recommended in refractory status epilepticus to aid the titration of anticonvulsant drugs and ensure suppression of seizure activity. EEG can also provide prognostic information as continued electrographic activity is associated with a worse outcome. Mortality for refractory status epilepticus has been estimated to be as high as 48%, and only 29% of patients return to their premorbid functional status.

Long-term anti-epileptic drug therapy

Long-term and maintenance AED therapy must be given in tandem with emergency treatment. Choice of medication when commencing new maintenance therapy will depend on previous treatments, the type of epilepsy and clinical setting. Pre-existing AED therapy should be continued at full dose and any recent changes reversed. Maintenance AEDs should be started after oral loading dose. If phenytoin or phenobarbitone is started as emergency treatment and is to be continued, then it can be given orally or intravenously guided by serum level monitoring. Nasogastric feed can interfere with absorption of some drugs such

Table 39.6 Complications of status epilepticus

Central nervous system	Cerebral hypoxia Cerebral oedema Cerebral haemorrhage Cerebral venous thrombosis
Cardiovascular system	Myocardial infarction Hyper/hypotension Arrhythmias Cardiac arrest Cardiogenic shock
Respiratory system	Apnoea Respiratory failure Pneumonia Pulmonary oedema
Metabolic system	Hyponatraemia Hypoglycaemia Hyperkalaemia Metabolic acidosis Acute tubular necrosis Acute hepatic necrosis Acute pancreatitis
Miscellaneous	Disseminated intravascular coagulopathy Rhabdomyolysis Fractures

as phenytoin. Once the patient has been seizure-free for 12–24 hours and the plasma levels of AEDs are adequate, the general anaesthetic agent should be slowly decreased.

Outcome

The prognosis of patients with status epilepticus is related to the aetiology, age, duration of seizures and prompt initiation of treatment. Overall mortality is approximately 20–30% rising with age. The underlying cause is the most important factor influencing patient outcome. Young patients whose status epilepticus was caused by low AED levels or systemic infection have very low mortality. In contrast, status epilepticus caused by cerebrovascular accident in the elderly has mortality of 35% and that associated with anoxic injury is usually fatal. A normal EEG post event predicts a good outcome, while continued epileptiform abnormalities indicate risk of further seizures and necessitate the initiation of long-term AED treatment. Possible complications of status epilepticus are listed in Table 39.6.

Key points

- Status epilepticus (SE) is a recognized medical and neurological emergency and is associated with significant morbidity and mortality.
- SE is also an under-recognized cause of persistent coma on the intensive care unit.
- In children, most SEs are secondary to infections. In adults, the causes are more diverse and can include drug misuse and cerebral pathologies.
- Treatment starts with immediate resuscitation with ABC approach and referral to critical care team if in refractory status (more than 90 min of seizure activity).
- Benzodiazepines still remain the first-line treatment of SE with phenytoin as second-line treatment. Barbiturates and propofol have also been used to treat refractory SE successfully.

Further reading

- National Institute for Clinical Excellence (2004) *The Epilepsies: The Diagnosis and Management of the Epilepsies in Adults and Children in Primary and Secondary Care*, NICE Climical Guideline no. 20. London: NICE.
- Opdam H (2003) Status epilepticus. In *Oh's Intensive Care Manual*, 5th edn, eds. Bersten A, Soni N, Oh TE. New York: Elsevier, pp. 485–93.
- Sander JW, Walker MC, Smalls JE (2007) *Epilepsy 2007: From Cell to Community – A Practical Guide to Epilepsy*, 11th edn. Chalfont St Peter, UK: International League against Epilepsy (UK Chapter) and the National Society for Epilepsy.
- Walker MC (2003) Status epilepticus on the intensive care unit. *J. Neurol.* **250**(4): 401–6.
- Walker MC (2005) Status epilepticus: an evidence-based guide. *Br. Med. J.* **331**: 673–77.

Abnormal levels of consciousness

Anil Kumar

Introduction

Altered levels of consciousness and coma are among the most common problems encountered in critically ill patients. Consciousness is awareness of self and the environment. The normal state of consciousness can range from being alert and aware to a stage of sleep from which a person can be readily awakened. It is a result of complex interactions between reticular activating substance within the brainstem, cortex and the sensory stimuli.

Abnormal levels of consciousness represent a wide spectrum of conditions ranging from feeling lethargic on one end of the spectrum to coma on the other end. Any alteration in the complex interactions of ascending reticular activating system (RAS) and its numerous connections can lead to abnormal levels of consciousness (Fig. 40.1).

Spectrum of abnormal levels of consciousness

- **Consciousness** – awake and aware of self and the environment.
- **Sleep** – a natural state of bodily rest from which the patient is rousable.
- **Lethargy** – decrease in responsiveness in a rousable patient.
- **Clouding of consciousness** – very mild form of altered mental status in which reduced wakefulness may occasionally cause confusion.
- **Confusion** – a more serious alteration of the mental status in which patient may be disoriented, and may find it difficult to follow commands.
- **Delirium** – acute decline in attention, perception and cognition. It can be of a hyperactive or hypoactive variety.
- **Stupor** – an abnormal sleepy state from which the patient can be aroused by vigorous or repeated stimuli and when left undisturbed, the patient will immediately lapse back to the unresponsive state.
- **Coma** – a state of unrousable unresponsiveness.

Neurological conditions imitating coma

Vegetative state

As opposed to a conscious patient who is both awake and aware of self and the environment, in vegetative state the patient appears at times to be wakeful but has no sign of awareness or of a 'functioning mind'.

Minimally conscious state

Despite profound cognitive impairment patients show minimal signs of awareness. It is usually seen in patients emerging from vegetative state.

Locked-in syndrome

Patients are both awake and aware of the environment but as a result of brainstem pathology cannot move or communicate, but vertical eye movements and lid elevation remain unimpaired, thus allowing the patient to use this to communicate.

Brainstem death

This refers to a state of irreversible loss of brainstem function despite artificial maintenance of circulation and gas exchange.

Causes of unconsciousness

Unconsciousness can result from a wide variety of causes. It can broadly be categorized into (1) diffuse

Core Topics in Critical Care Medicine, eds. Fang Gao Smith and Joyce Yeung. Published by Cambridge University Press.

Table 40.1 Causes of unconsciousness

Diffuse cortical impairment	Direct injury to the brainstem and RAS	Brainstem injury due to pressure effect
Metabolic	Trauma	Bleeding and haematoma
Hypoglycaemia, diabetic ketoacidosis, hyperosmolar diabetic coma	Bleed	Ischaemia with surrounding oedema
Hyponatraemia, hypernatraemia	Ischaemia	Tumour
Hypocalcaemia, hypercalcaemia	Tumour	Infection with concomitant oedema
Hepatic encephalopathy	Infection	
Myxoedema coma, thyroid storm		
Uraemia		
Hypoxia		
Cardiac arrest		
Cerebrovascular accident (CVA)		
Drugs and toxins		
Alcohol abuse		
Barbiturates		
Benzodiazepines		
Antidepressants		
Recreational drugs		
Infection		
Encephalitis		
Meningitis		
Cerebral malaria		
Trauma		
Hypothermia and hyperpyrexia		

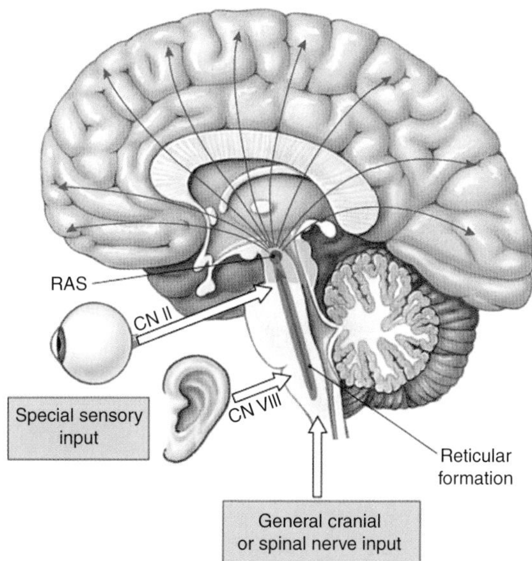

Fig. 40.1 The reticular activating system (RAS) and its association CN II 2nd cranial nerve/optic nerve; CN VIII 8th cranial nerve/vestibulocochlear nerve.

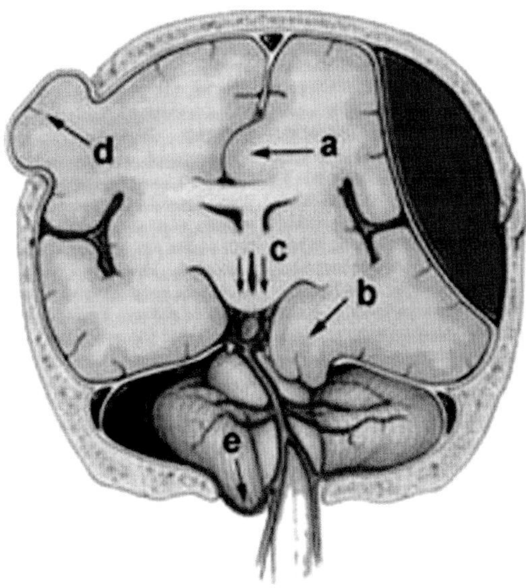

Fig. 40.2 Diagram illustrating different types of herniation. (a) Subfalcial (cingulate) herniation; (b) uncal herniation; (c) central herniation; (d) external herniation; (e) tonsillar herniation. Types (a), (b) and (e) are usually caused by focal, ipsilateral space-occupying lesions, such as tumour or extradural haemorrhage.

cortical impairment, (2) direct injury and (3) injury due to pressure effects (see Table 40.1).

Herniation

Displacement of brain tissue into a compartment that it normally does not occupy is called herniation (Fig. 40.2). The pressure effect may cause damage to the brainstem and the RAS and this in turn will cause unconsciousness and coma.

- Uncal herniation – displacement of uncus (anterior medial temporal gyrus) into the anterior portion of the tentorial opening. There may be ipsilateral papillary dilatation as a result of compression of the third cranial nerve.
- Central herniation – displacement of thalamus via the tentorial opening.
- Tonsillar herniation – displacement of cerebellar tonsils through the foramen magnum (Fig. 40.3).
- Subfalcial herniation – displacement of cingulate gyrus under the falx cerebri is one of the most common herniation patterns (Fig. 40.4). Complications are contralateral hydrocephalus (due to obstruction of the foramen of Monro) and anterior cerebral artery territory infarct (due to compression of anterior cerebral artery branches).

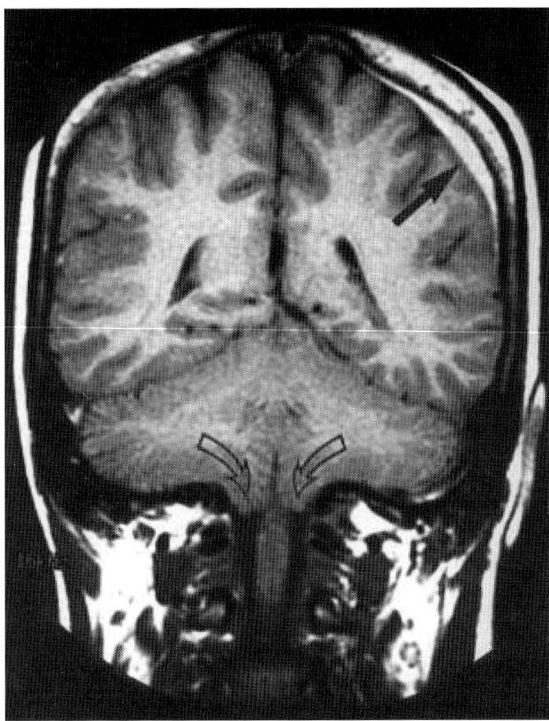

Fig. 40.3 MRI showing left-sided subdural haemorrhage (dark arrow) and tonsillar herniation (curved arrows).

Table 40.2 Glasgow Coma Scale

Best Eye Response (4)	Best Verbal Response (5)	Best Motor Response (6)
4 – Spontaneous eye opening	5 – Orientated	6 – Obeys commands
3 – Eye opening to verbal command	4 – Confused	5 – Localizing pain
2 – Eye opening to pain	3 – Inappropriate words	4 – Withdrawal from pain
1 – No eye opening	2 – Incomprehensible words	3 – Flexion to pain
	1 – No verbal response	2 – Extension to pain
		1 – No motor response

Assessment of unconscious patient

Immediate assessment

- Immediate assessment of airway patency, cervical spine stability (in cases of trauma), breathing and circulation should be performed and if compromised appropriate steps should be taken immediately to correct it.
- Assess the level of consciousness by using either Glasgow Coma Scale (GCS) or AVPU scoring system.
- Pupillary examination.

GCS scoring system

The GCS is scored between 3 and 15, 3 being coma and 15 fully awake. It is composed of three parameters: Best Eye Response, Best Verbal Response and Best Motor Response, as given in Table 40.2.

Individual elements as well as the sum of the score are important. Hence, it is good practice to express the score in the form 'GCS 7 = E1 V4 M3 at 09:00'. It is important to remember to regularly reassess the patient for a trend in GCS and a falling GCS will signal a worsening in patient's condition. A GCS ≤8 is the generally accepted definition of a coma and patients will require an airway assessment and securing of a definitive airway if needed.

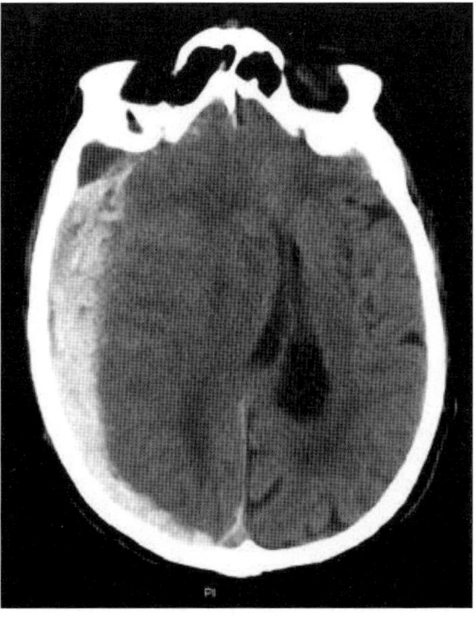

Fig. 40.4 CT showing subfalcial herniation.

Intubation and severe facial or eye swelling will make it impossible to test the verbal and eye responses. Under these circumstances, the score is given as 1 with a modifier attached e.g. 'E1c' where c = closed, or 'V1t' where t = tube.

AVPU score

AVPU is a quick and simple description of neurological state:

Alert	Patient is alert
Voice	Responding to voice
Pain	Responding to pain
Unresponsive	Unresponsive

'P' on the AVPU score approximates to a GCS of 8.

History

History should be obtained from paramedics, witnesses, police and relatives. In many cases, the cause of unconsciousness may be self-evident, e.g. drug overdosage. In other circumstances history should be obtained with specific emphasis on the circumstances, speed of onset, antecedent symptoms, drugs history and any past medical history.

Examination

- Temperature – hyper- and hypothermia.
- Skin – cyanosis, rash, pigmentation, injection marks.
- Respiratory rate and pattern.
  - Cheyne–Stokes respiration – sequential waxing and waning of tidal volume and periods of apnoea usually seen in bilateral cerebral dysfunction.
  - Kussmaul respiration – very deep and laboured breathing with normal or reduced frequency, found among people with severe acidosis usually due to diabetic ketoacidosis and uraemia.
  - Central neurogenic hyperventilation – also known as central reflex hyperpnoea. It is characterized by sustained deep hyperventilation usually due to pontine lesions.
  - Apneustic respiration – a series of slow, deep inspirations each one held for 30 to 60 s, after which the air is suddenly expelled. Usually as a result of lesion of mid to lower pons.
  - Cluster apnoea – it is characterized by groups of quick, shallow inspirations followed by regular or irregular periods of apnoea. It is caused by damage to the medulla oblongata.
  - Ataxic respiration – abnormal pattern of breathing characterized by complete irregularity of breathing, with irregular pauses and increasing periods of apnoea. Usually seen as a result of lesion of medulla oblongata.
- Pupils.
  - Unilateral fixed and dilated pupil – seen in uncal herniation due to compression of the third cranial nerve.
  - Bilateral fixed and dilated pupils – seen in severe barbiturate overdosage, brainstem death.
  - Unilateral papillary constriction and ptosis – Horner's syndrome. Seen in hypothalamic damage.
  - Bilateral pinpoint pupils – seen in opioid overdosage and in pontine lesions.
- Ocular movements.
  - Conjugate horizontal roving – usually the normal ocular axes in coma.
  - Conjugate horizontal ocular deviation to one side – indicates damage to the pons on the opposite side or frontal lobe lesion.
  - Ocular bobbing – brisk downward and slow upward movement with loss of horizontal eye movement. It is usually seen in bilateral pontine lesion.
  - Oculocephalic reflex – passive movement of head from side to side causes eye movements in opposite direction to the head movement (doll's eye reflex). It is abolished in brainstem lesions.
- Abnormal posturing (Fig. 40.5).
  - Decorticate rigidity – flexion of elbows and wrists and supination of the arm. Usually seen in lesions of cerebral hemispheres, the internal capsule and the thalamus.
  - Decerebrate rigidity – extension of elbows and wrists with pronation of the arm. Usually seen in brainstem lesions.

Investigations

Laboratory tests

Blood tests that should be carried out are listed in Table 40.3.

Radiological tests

CT scan of the head is indicated in unconscious patients especially in those with history of fall or trauma, or unclear history to rule out potential causes such as intracranial haemorrhage, space-occupying lesions or hydrocephalus. It is important to remember while a normal CT scan may mean that immediate surgical intervention is not indicated, some changes such as ischaemia may not be visible on early CT scans. More detailed MRI scan which will help delineate soft tissues maybe helpful in identifying the cause. Advice from the radiology department should be sought. Any patient with possible history of head trauma or fall should also have their cervical spine immobilized and have a lateral and AP plain radiograph or CT scan of their cervical spine (see Chapter 42).

Table 40.3 Blood tests

Blood test	Possible cause of unconsciousness
Toxicology screen	Paracetamol/salicylate levels if suspected drug overdose
	Blood alcohol level
Urea and electrolytes	Electrolyte disturbances, renal function: uraemia
Blood glucose	Hypoglycaemia
Liver function tests	Deranged liver function may be seen in hepatic encephalopathy
Arterial blood gas	Gas exchange: hypoxia and hypercarbia
	Acid–base abnormality: severe acidosis
Blood culture	If evidence of sepsis, possible source of infection

Electroencephalography

EEG can be useful as an adjunct in the diagnosis of the cause of coma. For example, α waves (8–12 Hz) are seen in coma but other wave forms such as θ waves (4–7 Hz) and δ waves (up to 4 Hz) are more specific to metabolic encephalopathy (Fig. 40.6). EEG is prone to artefacts and needs to be interpreted within its context. Both the performance and interpretation of EEG require expertise which limits its clinical use.

Lumbar puncture

This is usually done after radiological tests have proved inconclusive and there are no signs of raised intracranial pressure. It is helpful in the diagnosis of meningitis.

Management

The fundamental goal in management of unconscious patients should be to limit further damage to the brain and treat the underlying cause. Potentially reversible causes such as hypoxia, hypercarbia, hypotension, hyperthermia and electrolyte disturbances should be corrected immediately.

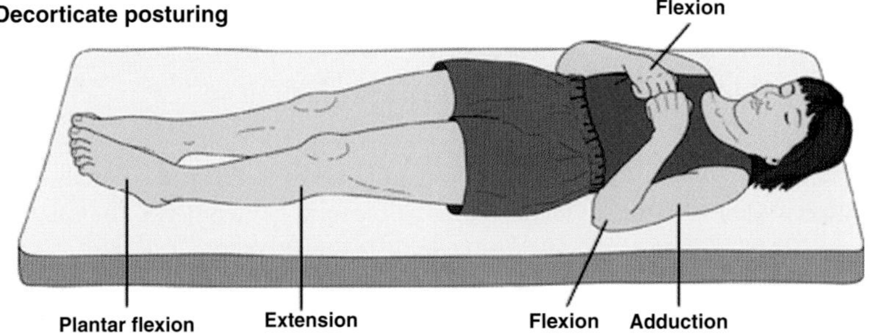

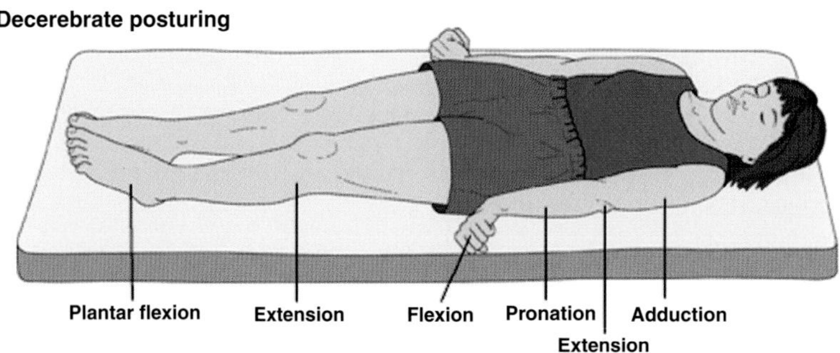

Fig. 40.5 Abnormal posturing.

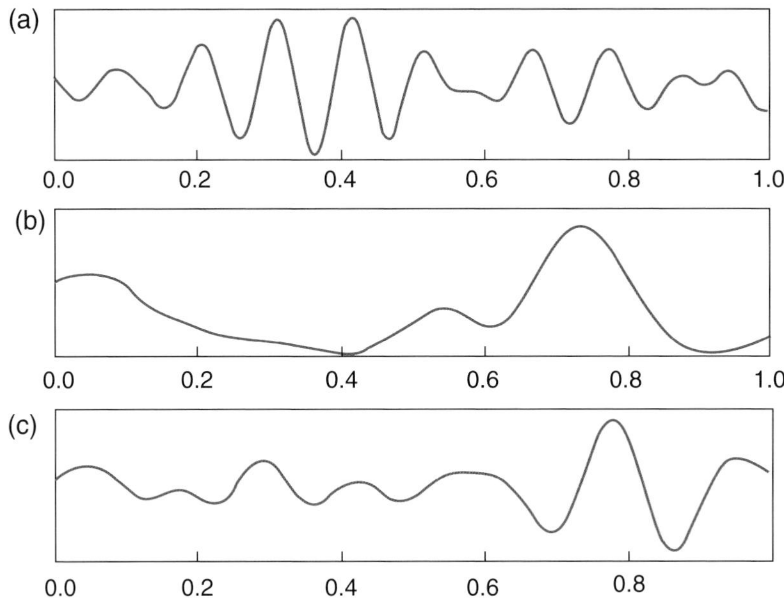

Fig. 40.6 EEG in abnormal consciousuess. (a) α waves; (b) δ waves; (c) θ waves.

Immediate management

Airway, breathing and cervical spine care

Airway should be maintained either by airway adjuncts like nasopharyngeal and oropharyngeal airways or by endotracheal intubation. High-flow oxygen should be administered. If the patient has been involved in trauma, cervical spine should be immobilized until cervical spine injuries are ruled out.

Circulation

Establish vascular access and administer intravenous fluids to maintain adequate blood pressure. Inotropic support may be needed to maintain adequate cerebral perfusion pressure.

Disability/exposure

Correct any electrolyte abnormalities and hypo- or hyperglycaemia. Measurement of body temperature should be taken to rule out hypothermia.

Expose the patient to look for possible signs of trauma or haemorrhage.

Definitive treatment

If neurosurgical intervention is possible then early involvement of the neurosurgeons is vital.

If appropriate level of care is not available at point of initial treatment then the patient may need to be transferred, once stabilized, to a more appropriate environment (e.g. neurosurgical centre).

Long-term management

Calories

Clinicians need to work closely with a dietician to ensure patients have adequate calorie intake either by enteral or parenteral route to improve wound healing and recovery. Nasogastric tube should be passed and gastric contents emptied regularly. Paralytic ileum occurs frequently in the unconscious patient and this may lead to aspiration of stomach contents.

Skin care

As the unconscious patient is unable to move appropriately, care should be taken to avoid pressure sores and infection. The patient should be turned on a regular basis and pressure areas checked to ensure skin integrity. Broken down areas should be dressed with hydrocolloid dressings.

Oral and eye care

It is important to maintain a clean moist mouth, to prevent the accumulation of oral and postnasal secretions and to prevent the development of mouth infections.

The blink reflex is absent in the unconscious patient and this may lead to corneal drying, irritation and ulceration.

Thromboprophylaxis

As the patient is unable to move, it is important to give thromboprophylaxis with low molecular weight heparins and use mechanical devices such as support stockings or calf compression devices to prevent deep vein thrombosis.

Bladder and bowel care

Regular catheter care is important to prevent urinary complication, infections and to prevent overdistending the balloon and damage to urethra. Bowel care should be carried out to prevent constipation and diarrhoea. Urine and faecal samples should be sent if infection is suspected.

Key points

- Abnormal levels of consciousness represent a wide spectrum of conditions in continuum.
- The fundamental goal in management of unconscious patients should be to limit further damage to the brain and treat the underlying cause.

Further reading

- Bates D (1991) Defining prognosis in medical coma. *J. Neurol. Neurosurg. Psychiatr.* **54**: 569-71.
- Bates D (1993) The management of medical coma. *J. Neurol. Neurosurg. Psychiatr.* **56**: 589–98.
- Clarke CRA (2005) Neurological diseases. In *Clinical Medicine*, 6th edn, eds. Kumar P and Clark M. New York: Elsevier Saunders, pp. 1173–272.
- Harper AH (2005) Acute confusional states and coma. In *Harrison's Principles of Internal Medicine*, 16th edn, eds. Kasper DL, Braunwald E, Fauci AS *et al.* New York: McGraw-Hill.
- Working Party of the Royal College of Physicians (2003) *The Vegetative State: Guidance on Diagnosis and Management*. London: RCP.

Meningitis and encephalitis

Nick Sherwood

Meningitis

Introduction

Meningitis is defined as inflammation of the brain meninges. It may be acute (hours to days) or chronic (days to months).

Aetiology

Meningitis can be classified according to aetiology:

- **Bacterial** – acute, often severe. This chapter will concentrate on bacterial meningitis.
- **Viral** – acute, less severe, usually self limiting and rarely leads to ICU admission.
- **Parasites and fungi** – Cryptococcus, histoplasmosis, amoeba, etc. Rare but can be seen in immunocompromised/suppressed individuals.
- **Aseptic** – similar clinical picture to bacterial meningitis but with no leucocyte response in the cerebrospinal fluid (CSF). Often due to partially treated bacterial causes or viruses.
- **Non-infectious** – including adverse drug reactions e.g. non-steroidal anti-inflammatory drugs, (NSAIDs), carcinomatosis and connective tissue disease.

Pathophysiology

All the infective causes of meningitis share common pathways in gaining access to the CNS. Initially there is colonization or localized infection of the skin, nasopharynx, and respiratory, gastrointestinal or genitourinary tracts. The majority of bacterial pathogens are transmitted through the respiratory route via droplet infection or infected saliva.

Once in the host the organism penetrates the submucosa and then gains access to the CNS via haematogenous spread (most bacteria and viruses), retrograde neuronal spread or direct penetration from adjacent structures (i.e. sinusitis, trauma, etc).

Once inside the CNS the organism survives the limited array of host defences in this body compartment and then replicates, producing meningeal inflammation. The cascade of inflammatory mediators producing meningeal inflammation is not unlike that producing severe sepsis and includes cytokines (TNF-alpha and IL-1) and secondary mediators (IL-6, IL-8). The net result is vascular endothelial injury and increased permeability of the blood–brain barrier which in turn leads to neutrophil penetration and interstitial oedema. Bacterial breakdown products and other cellular debris lead to cytotoxic oedema which, in combination with the interstitial oedema, leads to cerebral oedema. This in turn leads to intracranial hypertension and decreased cerebral perfusion. Cerebral tissue is forced to adopt anaerobic metabolic pathways leading to consumption of glucose in the CSF – this is compounded by decreased glucose transport in to the CSF.

If this process is not terminated or modified by effective treatment the result is transient neuronal dysfunction or even irreversible neuronal injury.

Incidence

Bacterial meningitis remains a serious disease with a high mortality. The US attack rate is reported as 0.6–4.0 cases per 100 000 population. Effective childhood vaccination programmes have resulted in meningitis moving from a disease of childhood to one that now occurs predominantly in adults. The median age of patients with bacterial meningitis has shifted from 15 months to 25 years.

Developments in vaccination have radically altered UK patterns of bacterial infection in the last decade.

Core Topics in Critical Care Medicine, eds. Fang Gao Smith and Joyce Yeung. Published by Cambridge University Press.

Haemophilus influenzae type B (Hib) was the most common form in children prior to the introduction of an effective vaccine in 1992; since then it has been virtually eliminated in children but can still affect unvaccinated adults. The meningococcal group comprises more than 13 known subtypes. Group C infection used to account for more than 30% of UK cases but introduction of vaccination in 1999 has again reduced the number of UK cases significantly. Group B has no effective vaccine and is now the commonest cause of bacterial meningitis in the UK. Pneumococcal meningitis is the second commonest form in the UK. Introduction of an effective childhood vaccine may well change this in the near future.

Mortality

Before the introduction of antibiotic therapy bacterial meningitis was uniformly fatal. Despite antimicrobial therapy and supportive care mortality rates remain high at approximately 25%. Mortality is highest with pneumococcal infection.

Clinical features

The history should identify any preceding trauma, respiratory tract and ear infection.
The classical features of meningism include:

- headache
- neck stiffness
- fever
- signs of cerebral dysfunction (lethargy, confusion and coma).

These features are less reliable in children and can be variable even in adults. Fever is the commonest sign while headache and neck stiffness are less common. However, absence of fever, neck stiffness and altered conscious level eliminates the diagnosis of meningitis in 99–100% of cases.

Atypical presentation may occur in the elderly (lethargy and no meningism), neutropenic or immunocompromised patient.

Physical signs include:

- Confusion, delirium, coma and photophobia
- Kernig sign (supine position: flex knee to 90°, flex hip to 90°, any further knee extension produces pain in hamstrings)
- Brudzinski sign (supine position: extend legs, passively flex neck, produces hip flexion)
- Nuchal rigidity (resistance to passive neck flexion)
- Cranial nerve palsies
- Focal neurological signs
- Seizures
- Papilloedema

Systemic signs include:

- Rash
  - Rapidly evolving non-blanching macules and petechiae suggest meningococcal septicaemia
  - Morbilliform rash with pharyngitis suggests viral meningitis
- Sinusitis, otitis or rhinorrhoea.

Systemic signs are most common with meningococcal disease (which may occur without meningitis) which may present with digital ischaemia and fulminant multi-organ failure. Seizures occur in 25–30% of cases of bacterial meningitis.

Investigations

As with any patient with an infectious process leading to critical illness antibiotic therapy needs to be commenced with a degree of urgency. The investigation of choice remains analysis of CSF obtained via lumbar puncture. However, if this is likely to lead to a significant delay in treatment it is acceptable to start empirical antibiotic therapy *after* taking venous blood cultures. (Even if an immediate lumbar puncture is possible blood cultures should still be obtained as the primary mode of spread is haematogenous.) A lumbar puncture must still be performed. CSF pressure should be measured.

Lumbar puncture in a patient with raised intracranial pressure (ICP) may lead to tentorial herniation. If the patient has recent onset seizures, papilloedema, moderate to severe impaired consciousness level or focal neurological signs a CT scan should be performed prior to lumbar puncture. If there is CT and/or clinical evidence of raised ICP then the benefits of lumbar puncture need to be balanced against the risks. In many centres it may be possible to obtain a diagnosis from blood DNA polymerase chain reaction (PCR) or rapid antigen testing.

CSF should also be sent for urgent gram stain and microbiological culture and is positive in approximately 50% of cases (Table 41.1). Other routine tests include full blood count, biochemistry (including glucose), chest X-ray and blood gases. Other sites of infection (sinuses and ears) should be investigated if appropriate.

Table 41.1 Typical CSF changes in meningitis

Cause	Pressure	White blood cells	Protein	Glucose
Bacterial	200–300 mm CSF	200–10 000/mm^3 polymorphs	>100 mg/dl	≤blood glucose
Viral	80–200 mm CSF	<500/mm^3 lymphocytes	15–50 mg/dl	=blood glucose
Tuberculous	160–300 mm CSF	100–500/mm^3 lymphocytes	>100 mg/dl	≤blood glucose
Aseptic	80–200 mm CSF	10–300/mm^3 lymphocytes	15–50 mg/dl	≥blood glucose (slight)
Normal	80–200 mm CSF	<5/mm^3	15–40 mg/dl	=blood glucose

Management

Raised intracranial pressure

Intracranial hypertension is a common complication of bacterial meningitis and can lead to altered consciousness level, airway compromise and seizures. The airway may need to be secured by endotracheal intubation and ICP reduced by controlled ventilation and 30° head-up posture. Cerebral perfusion pressure needs to be maintained at around 70 mmHg and in selected cases ICP monitoring and/or CSF drainage may be required.

Steroid therapy

Many of the detrimental pathophysiological effects of bacterial meningitis are due to the host defence response. This has led to efforts to modify host response while ensuring bacterial eradication.

Early steroid therapy has been shown to decrease the incidence of long term complications in children and mortality and morbidity in adults. This is particularly the case with Hib in children and pneumococcus in adults.

The timing of steroid administration is critical and if used it should be administered *before* thc first dose of antibiotic therapy.

Dexamethasone has been widely used. One possible dosing schedule is:

- Children – 0.15 mg/kg 6-hourly for 4 days
- Adults – 10 mg 6-hourly for 4 days.

Antibiotics

In common with management of other critical illnesses airway security is the primary objective (the ABC rule). However, 'A' also stands for antimicrobials – delaying administration of empirical antimicrobial therapy is a significant risk factor for adverse prognosis.

Table 41.2 Suggested empirical antibiotic therapy for bacterial meningitis

Patient group	Antibiotic	Suggested dose
<50 years	Ceftriaxone *or* cefotaxime	1 g 6-hourly (adult) 2 g 6-hourly (adult)
>50 years	Ceftriaxone *and* ampicillin	1 g 6-hourly 2 g 4-hourly
Immunocompromised (seek specialist advice)	Cefotaxime *and* Ampicillin *or* penicillin G	2 g 6-hourly 2 g 4-hourly 2.4 g 4-hourly
Surgery, shunts or trauma	Ceftazidime *and* vancomycin	2 g 8-hourly 1 g 12-hourly

The selected antibiotic needs to attain adequate therapeutic levels in the CSF and this depends on the agent's lipid solubility, molecular size, protein binding and degree of meningeal inflammation. Penicillins, third- and fourth-generation cephalosporins, carbapenems, fluoroquinolones and rifampacin all produce adequate CSF drug levels.

Empirical therapy needs to be guided by local incidence and resistance data and prompt communication with local microbiological services is essential. The likely infective organism changes with age and immune status and our empirical therapy needs to reflect these changes (Table 41.2).

Empirical therapy needs to be changed to targeted therapy as soon as CSF bacteriology results are available. Treatment courses are normally continued for 10–14 days. Patients with impaired cellular immunity must be discussed with local microbiological services as their treatment can be challenging. Repeat CSF samples may be needed at 48 hours after initiation of treatment in cases of resistance to ensure bacteriological improvement.

Public health

Prophylaxis is required for close contacts of patients with meningococcal disease. Medical staff who may have come into contact with infected saliva should also be treated. A 2-day course of oral rifampicin (600 mg 12-hourly) is commonly prescribed. Departments of Public Health should be contacted to co-ordinate contact tracing and treatment.

Viral encephalitis

Introduction

Encephalitis is a viral infection of brain tissue. It can be difficult to diagnose as the clinical picture and routine laboratory tests are frequently non-specific. The clinical picture can be very similar to viral meningitis, however encephalitis leads to *focal* neurological deficits.

Aetiology

Viral encephalitis can be either acute primary or post-infectious. Primary infection is associated with viral invasion of the CNS whereas in post-infectious disease the neurons are spared (but demyelination is common) and virus cannot be isolated.

A number of viral pathogens can cause encephalitis. Sporadic encephalitis is commonly caused by herpes simplex virus type 1. Geographical location can influence likely infections (i.e. St Louis or Japanese encephalitis and West Nile virus) as can history of exposure (i.e. rabies). Less commonly involved viruses include Epstein–Barr, HIV, *Herpes simplex* (HSV) and *Varicella zoster* (VZV).

Post-infectious encephalitis has been associated with many agents including mumps, measles, *Varicella zoster*, rubella and influenza viruses.

Clinical features

Encephalitis can produce a wide range of neurological deficits from the subtle neurological signs to coma. Meningeal irritation is classically absent but may be present in meningoencephalitis.

Seizures are common and focal deficits can include hemiparesis and cranial nerve palsies. More generalized signs include confusion and agitation.

Systemic examination can reveal clues to specific causes:

- Parotitis – mumps
- Flaccid paralysis – West Nile virus
- Tremors of extremeties, lips and eyelids – St Louis encephalitis
- Hydrophobia and pharyngeal spasm – rabies
- Grouped cutaneous vesicles – *Varicella zoster*.

Investigations

Imaging

CT or MRI scans are routinely performed (Fig. 41.1). CT has a limited role in diagnosing encephalitis but is useful to exclude space-occupying lesions or brain abscesses. Hydrocephalus can suggest a non-viral infection. MRI is useful for detecting demyelination or localizing the viral infection to a specific region – HSV frequently affects the temporal lobe.

Electroencephalogram

The EEG is frequently abnormal, and localization in the temporal lobe suggests HSV infection (Fig. 41.2).

Cerebrospinal fluid

A sample of CSF should be obtained unless ICP is raised. After measuring the opening pressure it should be analysed for:

- white cell count
- glucose
- protein
- DNA (polymerase chain reaction).

CSF examination will usually confirm an inflammatory disease process in the CNS. However the changes seen in meningoencephalitis and viral meningitis are often identical. In pure viral encephalitis there may be few, if any, changes. White blood cell count (WBC) is usually raised but $<250/mm^3$. There may be an increased neutrophil count initially but this soon shifts to a predominance of lymphocytes. If there is any doubt CSF should be reanalysed after 8 hours. Protein concentration is often slightly elevated (but <150 mg/dl) and glucose concentration is usually normal (but may be reduced in HSV). Red cells are usually absent but can be present in HSV-1 infection.

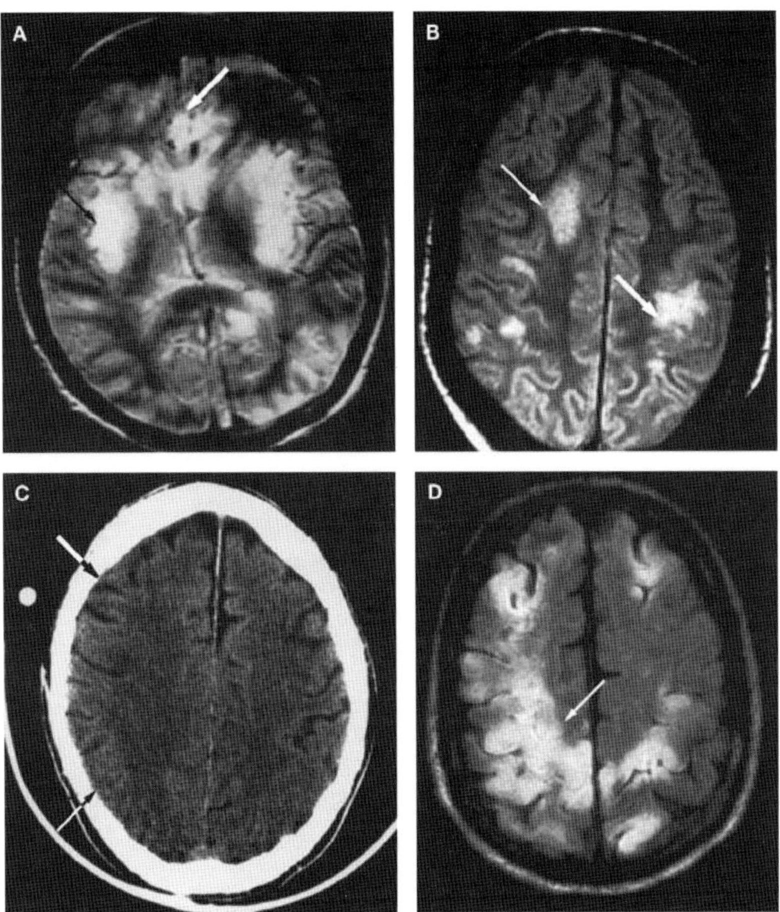

Fig. 41.1 Examples of MRI and CT scans in viral encephalitis. (A) *Herpes simplex* virus 1(HSV-1) encephalitis: T2-weighted MRI brain scan demonstrates bilateral involvement of temporal lobes. The exaggerated signal does not extend beyond the insular cortex (thin arrow), but does involve the cingulate gyrus (thick arrow). (B) *Varicella zoster* virus (VZV) vasculopathy: MRI scan shows multiple areas of infarction in both hemispheres, particularly involving white matter (thin arrow) and extending to grey–white-matter junctions (thick arrow). (C, D) CT and MRI changes in a patient with probable enterovirus encephalitis. In contrast to A and B, panel C demonstrates relative effacement of sulci (thin arrow), compared with normal sulcal spaces (thick arrow). Panel D is a T2-weighted inversion recovery (fluid-attenuated inversion recovery, FLAIR) MRI brain scan of the same patient, demonstrating areas of increased signal (arrow), reflecting increased water content in the oedematous brain.

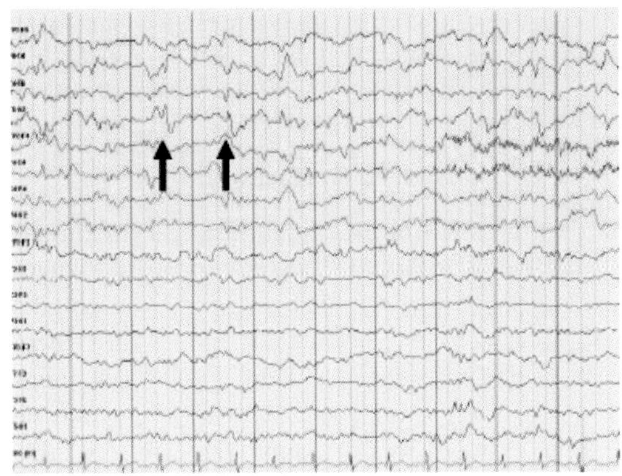

Fig. 41.2 EEG in HSV encephalitis may show non-specific slow waves. Periodic lateralizing epileptiform activities (PLEDs) are characteristic but they are not specific for HSE. This patient had right temporal PLEDs in the EEG (arrows).

PCR testing is useful for HSV-1, HSV-2, enteroviruses, VZV and cytomegalovirus.

Serology

Acute and convalescent serology may be useful for patients who fail to improve. Analysis of acute phase specimens can detect mumps and West Nile virus.

Brain biopsy

Brain biopsy is usually considered as a last resort where the aetiology remains unknown after all other investigations have been completed.

Management

Raised ICP requires the same supportive care as for bacterial meningitis.

There are no specific therapies for most CNS viral infections (with the exception of HSV). It is therefore essential to eliminate other treatable non-infectious causes of similar clinical disorders. These include tumours, autoimmune and neoplastic diseases and adverse effects of medications.

HSV-1 encephalitis can be treated with IV acyclovir. Failure to treat HSV in a timely fashion can significantly increase morbidity and mortality. Therefore unless HSV can be definitely excluded all patients with encephalitis should receive acyclovir (10 mg/kg 8-hourly). VZV can also respond to acyclovir therapy.

Prognosis

Encephalitis is difficult to diagnose. In one study of over 1500 patients with a clinical diagnosis of encephalitis a causative agent was only diagnosed in 16%. Those patients who presented with diffuse cerebral oedema or status epilepticus had a poor outcome. Those with localized seizures had a much better prognosis.

HSV is uniformly fatal without treatment. With high-dose acyclovir mortality can be reduced to 14% though over 20% of surviving patients will have epilepsy or neuropsychiatric disorders.

Key points

- Incidence of bacterial meningitis has decreased since the introduction of vaccines but continues to have high mortality and morbidity.
    - Classical presentation with fever, headache, neck stiffness and neurological signs may be variable or absent in some patients.
    - CSF samples remain the most important diagnostic tool but empirical antibiotic treatment can be started if there is delay in lumbar puncture. There is a potential risk of herniation with lumbar puncture in the presence of signs of raised intracranial pressure.
    - Steroid therapy should be instituted early and given before the first antibiotic dose.
    - Public health should be notified and contacts traced and treated.
- Encephalitis has remained difficult to diagnose and is associated with high mortality and morbidity.
    - MRI may be useful in diagnosis of encephalitis but CSF samples and viral serology are often needed to identify the organism.
    - Antimicrobial and antiviral treatment of patients with suspected meningitis and encephalitis should be discussed with microbiologist.

Further reading

- Steiner I, Budka H, Chaudhuri A *et al.* (2005) Viral encephalitis: a review of diagnostic methods and guidelines for management. *Eur. J. Neurol.* **12**(5): 331–43.
- Van de Beek D, de Gans J, Tuntel AR *et al.* (2006) Community-acquired bacterial meningitis in adults. *N. Engl. J. Med.* **354**: 44–53.

Traumatic brain injury

Randeep Mullhi and Sandeep Walia

Introduction

In the UK 1.4 million people annually attend hospital following a head injury. Every year, approximately 3500 patients are admitted to UK intensive care units with severe traumatic brain injury (TBI). The overall mortality of severe head injury is 23% with residual neurological deficit in 60% of survivors. Head injury often affects young individuals, particularly as a result of road traffic accidents. It represents a substantial economic burden in terms of ongoing rehabilitation. There has been a significant decline in mortality from severe TBI in adults over the last two decades, due to improvements in pre-hospital care as well as advances in neurocritical care.

The European Federation of Neurosurgeons has classified TBI into mild, moderate and severe based on the Glasgow Coma Score (Table 42.1).

Pathophysiology of traumatic brain injury

Primary and secondary brain injury

TBI has been divided into primary and secondary brain injury. Primary brain injury occurs at the time of impact. Secondary brain injury results from further physiological insults such as ischaemia and hypoxia to areas of the brain following the primary injury. The primary injury activates an autodestructive cascade of ionic, metabolic and immunological changes that render the brain more susceptible to the secondary physiological insults.

Pathology of primary brain injury

Intracranial lesions following TBI are classified into focal or diffuse injuries.

Focal injuries

These include extradural haematoma (EDH), subdural haematoma (SDH), cerebral contusions and intracerebral haematoma. These focal lesions expand with time resulting in potential delayed mass effect and clinical deterioration of the patient. Intracranial haematomas are the most important treatable cause of death and disability following TBI. Evacuation of a discrete haematoma is the primary goal of surgical treatment and life-saving surgery must be undertaken without delay.

Extradural haematoma

EDH occurs in about 1–2% of all head injuries and is due to a tear in a blood vessel between the dura and skull. Of these, 75% are caused by a middle meningeal artery tear in the temporoparietal area and 80% are associated with a skull fracture. Underlying brain injury is rare. CT scan demonstrates a biconvex opacity (Fig. 42.1). Almost 30% of EDHs present with rapid neurological deterioration following a lucid period after the initial injury. Prognosis is dependent on age and presentation. Overall mortality is between 10% and 30%.

Subdural haematoma

Subdural haematomas are much more common. They occur secondary to disruption of bridging veins between dura and arachnoid membrane. They are more common in the elderly, alcoholics and in patients with a coagulopathy. Severe underlying brain injury is common and the outcome is worse than that for EDH. If left untreated, subdural haematomas may become subacute or chronic. CT scan shows a crescenteric lesion (Fig. 42.2).

Core Topics in Critical Care Medicine, eds. Fang Gao Smith and Joyce Yeung. Published by Cambridge University Press.

Table 42.1 European Federation of Neurosurgeons (EFNS) definition of head injury severity

Classification	Admission Glasgow Coma Scale (GCS) and clinical characteristics
Mild	GCS 13–15
Category 0	GCS 15, no LOC, no PTA, no risk factors
Category 1	GCS 15, LOC <30 min, PTA <1 hour, no risk factors
Category 2	GCS 15 and risk factors present
Category 3	GCS 13–14, LOC <30 min, PTA <1 hour, with or without risk factors
Moderate	GCS 9–12
Severe	GCS ≤8
Critical	GCS 3–4, unreactive pupils and absent/ decorticate motor reactions (GCS motor scale 1 or 2)

LOC, loss of consciousness; PTA, post-traumatic amnesia.

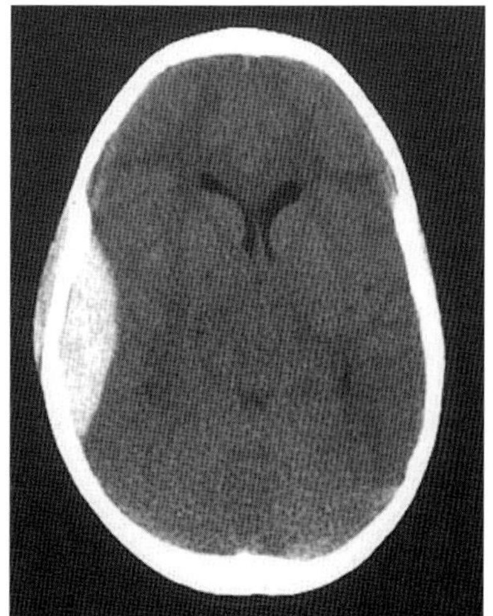

Fig. 42.1 Typical CT scan illustrating the biconvex opacity and midline shift seen in extradural haematoma (EDH).

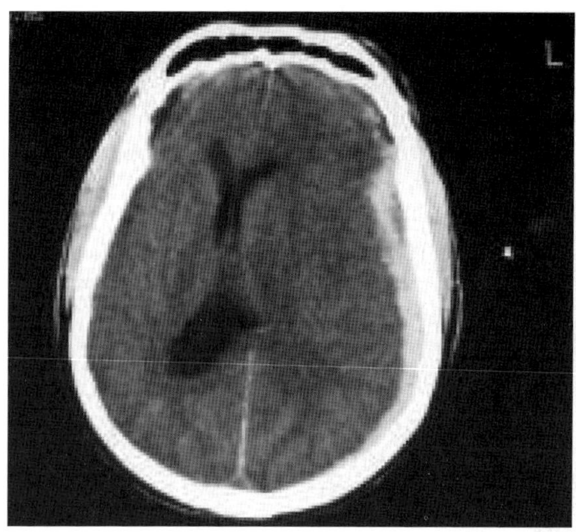

Fig. 42.2 Typical CT scan seen in subdural haematoma (SDH).

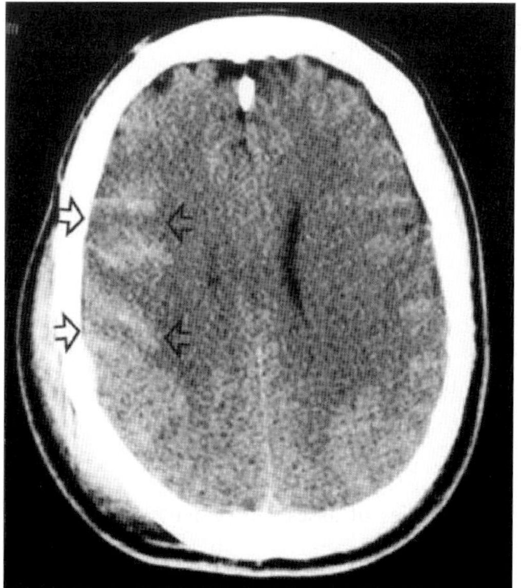

Fig. 42.3 CT scan showing cerebral contusions (arrows).

Cerebral contusions

These occur secondary to contact between brain and skull (Fig. 42.3). Coup injuries occur beneath the area of impact. Contre-coup injuries are remote from the area of impact and occur due to brain movement within the skull.

Diffuse injuries

These include diffuse axonal injury (DAI) and brain swelling. DAI is the result of acceleration and deceleration shear forces occurring at different rates across the brain. There is a non-focal pattern of injury. CT appearances vary from bright signals in brain matter to loss of grey/white differentiation (Fig. 42.4). Surgical treatment is difficult. DAI is the most significant cause of morbidity in patients in TBI.

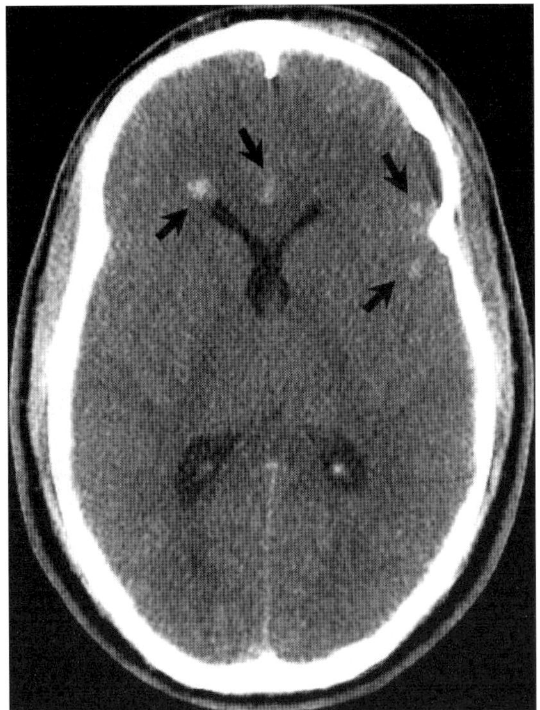

Fig. 42.4 CT scan showing small intracerebral haemorrhages in the junction between grey and white matter (arrows) seen typically in diffuse axonal injury (DAI).

Initial assessment and resuscitation

The major determinant of outcome from TBI is the severity of the irreversible primary insult. However, secondary injury resulting in cerebral ischaemia may be amenable to intervention. Thus early resuscitation and therapeutic intervention are essential to reduce the morbidity from TBI.

The principles of assessing patients with TBI are based on the ABC approach in common with all trauma victims. These were discussed in Chapter 41 and will be briefly outlined below.

Airway with cervical spine immobilization

Approximately 5% of patients with moderate and severe TBI will have cervical spine injury, commonly occurring between the level of the occiput and C3 vertebra. The risk of spinal injury increases with increasing severity of injury. Patients should have cervical spine immobilization with hard collar and sandbags until injury has been ruled out. Patency of the airway should be assessed and if signs of airway compromise are present, patients should have their airway secured by endotracheal intubation. Manual in-line stabilization should be used to maintain alignment of the cervical spine during intubation (see Chapter 43: Trauma and burns).

Breathing

Supplementary oxygen should be administered to patients with suspected TBI. Significant brain injury can lead to erratic patterns of breathing or apnoeic episodes. Patients should be monitored with pulse oximetry and arterial blood gas sampling to ensure that oxygenation is maintained.

Circulation

The patient's cardiovascular system should be assessed for the adequacy of perfusion and signs of shock. It is important to remember that patients with TBI are likely have to have suffered other injuries. Major extracranial injuries are found in 50% of patients with severe TBI and can lead to significant blood loss. Fluid resuscitation should be commenced if required.

Disability

Patients should be fully examined for neurological signs including level of consciousness with GCS or AVPU scale, pupil response and power, sensation and reflexes of limbs. Reassessment of the neurological system is needed regularly to look for signs of deterioration.

Exposure

Other signs of extracranial injury should be looked for. The patient should be log-rolled and their back examined for any signs of spinal injury.

Indications for CT scanning in head injury

CT scans are used to exclude lesions requiring urgent surgical intervention. Serial CT scans can be performed to monitor head injury progression. The National Institute for Clinical Excellence recently updated their recommendations for CT scanning after head injury (Fig. 42.5).

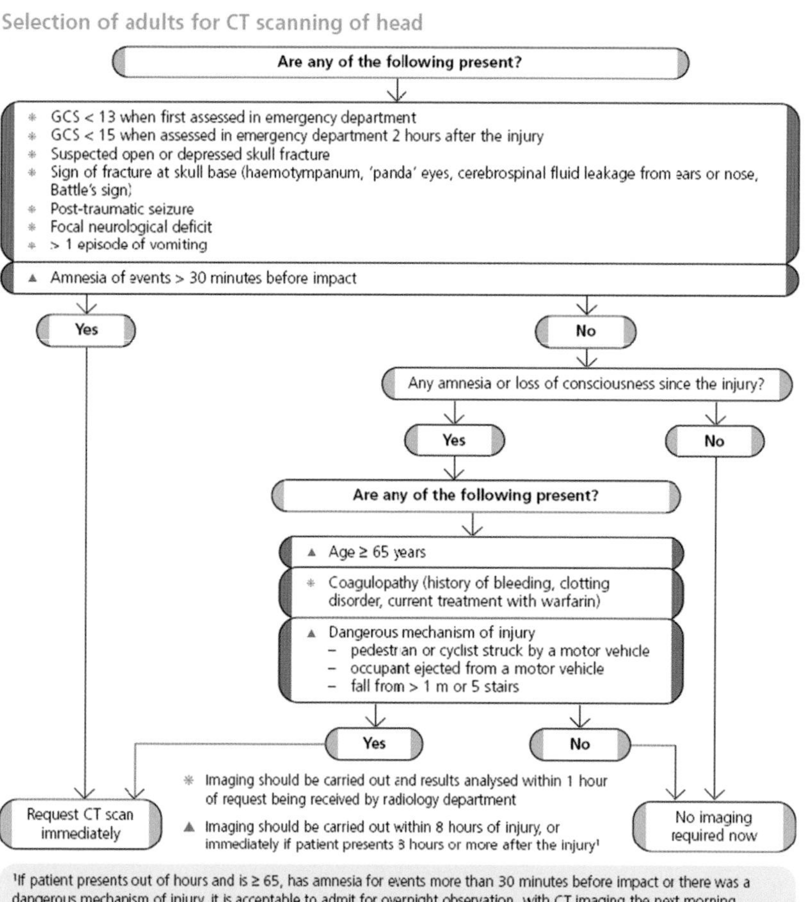

Fig. 42.5 Algorithm for selecting patients for CT scans. (From NICE Guideline no. 56 (2007) – see Further reading.)

Pathophysiology of intracranial pressure

Normal ICP is less than 10 mmHg when supine and breathing quietly. The ICP is determined by the volume of the intracranial contents: brain 1400 ml (85%), CSF 150 ml (10%) and cerebral blood volume (CBV) 100 ml (5%).

The brain is incompressible but CSF and CBV can change. The relationship between volume and pressure is shown in Fig. 42.6.

The rate of change of the intracranial volume is clinically important. In TBI, haematomas can cause a rapid increase in intracranial volume and intracranial pressure since normal intracranial compensation is overwhelmed. An increased ICP may cause distortion of cerebral structures and a reduction in cerebral blood flow, leading to cerebral ischaemia. Cerebral perfusion pressure (CPP) is estimated as the difference between mean arterial pressure and ICP (CPP = MAP – ICP). An elevated ICP, sufficient to compromise CPP, can lead to permanent brain damage, cerebral herniation and death.

Monitoring the injured brain

General monitoring allows maintenance of optimal systemic physiology but will not detect changes in the brain. Cerebral monitoring, on the other hand, allows measurement of CPP, cerebral blood flow (CBF) and assessment of oxygen delivery to the injured brain.

1. Intracranial pressure monitoring

Whilst there is no evidence base for ICP monitoring, it remains a useful adjunct for severe TBI management (Table 42.2). The Brain Trauma Foundation has recommended the use of ICP monitoring in all patients with severe TBI (GCS 3–8) and an abnormal CT scan

Table 42.2 Devices for monitoring intracranial pressure

Intracranial pressure monitor	Features
Intraventricular catheter	Gold standard Most accurate Allows CSF drainage High risk of infection
Intraparenchymal catheter	Cannot be recalibrated once inserted Examples are the Codman and Camino types
Subdural catheter	Prone to blocking Less risk of infection compared with intraventricular catheter
Epidural catheter	Least accurate

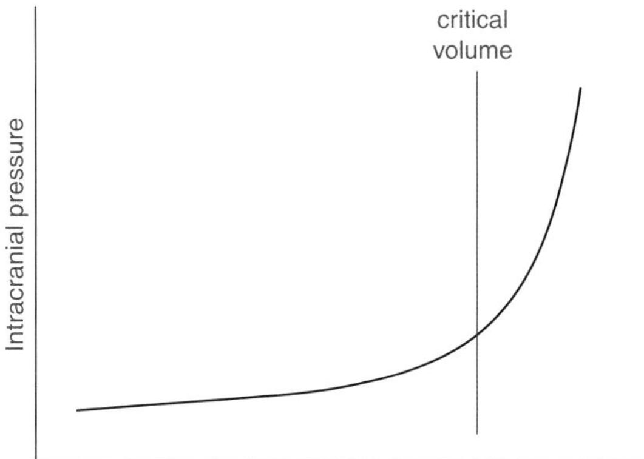

Fig. 42.6 Diagram illustrating the Monro–Kellie doctrine. An increase in mean arterial pressure (MAP) will improve cerebral perfusion, while an increase in intracranial pressure (ICP) will reduce blood delivery to the brain tissue and reduce perfusion. If cerebral perfusion pressure (CPP) falls below the threshold of 60 mmHg, aggressive efforts are instituted to either increase the MAP or reduce the ICP. ICP can only be decreased by reducing the volume within the cranial vault. Because the brain is contained within the non-compliant skull, as the volume within the brain begins to increase, so does ICP. At a critical volume there is no additional space and the pressure dramatically increases, leading to significant tissue ischaemia due to reduction in blood flow.

on admission. In those with severe TBI and a normal CT scan on admission, ICP monitoring is recommended if two or more of the following are present: age >40 years, motor posturing or systolic blood pressure <90 mmHg. Measurement of ICP via a ventricular catheter is regarded as the gold standard; however, other devices are also available (Fig. 42.7).

ICP monitoring allows calculation of CPP and determination of abnormal waveforms that occur due to phasic increases in ICP triggered by cerebral vasodilatation in response to a reduction in CPP.

Lundberg waves

- **A waves** – sustained pressure waves (60–80 mmHg) lasting 5–20 min (Fig. 42.8)
  - Represent cerebral vasodilatation due to decreased CPP
  - Urgent treatment needed
- **B waves** – high-frequency oscillations (<50 mmHg) every 30–120 s
  - Associated with normal breathing
- **C waves** – small oscillations (<20 mmHg)
  - Reflect changes in systemic arterial pressure
  - Considered normal.

2. Cerebral oxygenation

A fibreoptic catheter placed retrogradely via the internal jugular vein lies in the jugular bulb allowing sampling of venous blood draining from the brain. It gives a global assessment of the balance between cerebral oxygen supply and demand. Jugular desaturation ($SjVO_2 < 50\%$) is associated with increased mortality after TBI and worse outcome in survivors. However a normal value may give a false sense of security since regional ischaemia cannot be excluded.

Methods for measuring focal brain tissue oxygen tension include the use of invasive microprobes. Near-infrared spectroscopy is a non-invasive technique which measures the cerebral concentrations of oxygenated and deoxygenated haemoglobin by absorption of near-infrared light.

3. EEG and evoked potentials

These are used to assess activity and to gauge the level of sedation in barbiturate coma.

4. Brain tissue biochemistry

Cerebral microdialysis is a laboratory tool that can be used as a bedside monitor to provide analysis of brain tissue biochemistry. It has the potential to provide early warning of cerebral ischaemia.

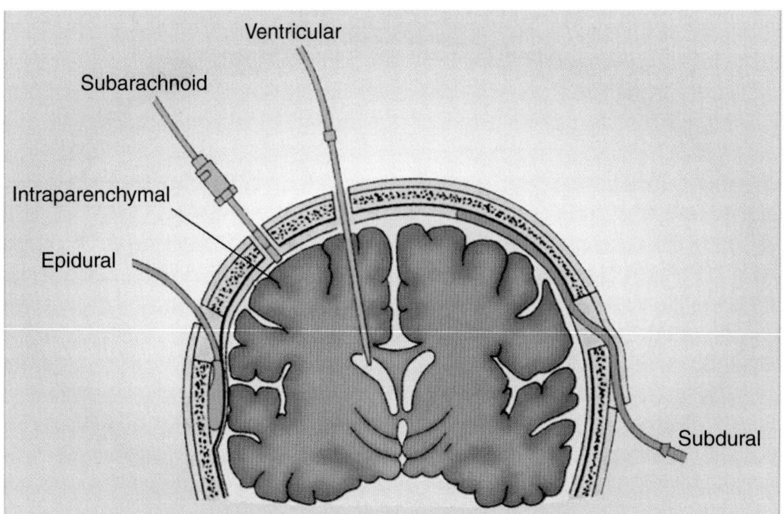

Fig. 42.7 Intracranial pressure monitoring devices: different placement of ICP catheters.

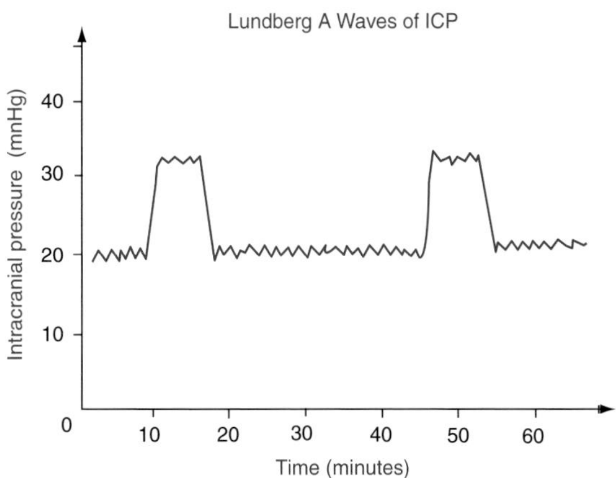

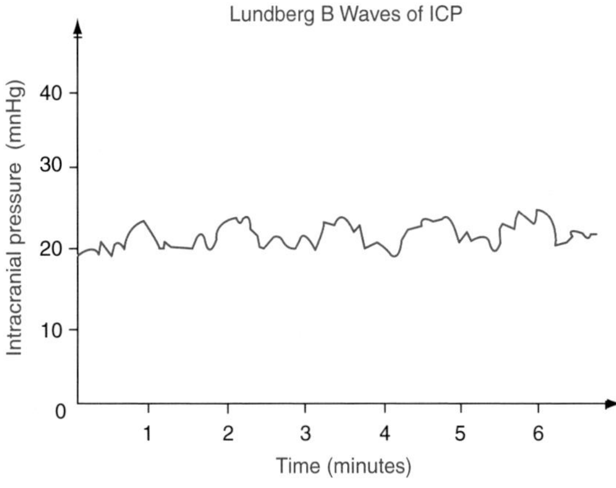

Fig. 42.8 Lundberg waves

5. Transcranial Doppler ultrasonography

This commonly involves measurement of blood flow velocity in the middle cerebral artery via the temporal bony window. It provides a non-invasive assessment of CPP but is not commonly used.

Intensive therapy management of traumatic brain injury

The main objective is to minimize secondary ischaemic brain injury by the maintenance of CPP and control of ICP.

General management

Secondary brain injury results from both systemic and intracranial causes. There is good evidence that protocolized management leads to improved outcome after TBI and may be further improved by treatment within a specialist neurocritical care unit.

Ventilation and sedation

Patients with TBI require mechanical ventilation to maintain PaO_2 >11 kPa and a $PaCO_2$ between 4.5 and 5.0 kPa. The use of minimal levels of PEEP to prevent rises in ICP has been challenged. It is now recognized that ventilation without PEEP often fails to correct hypoxaemia. Moreover, with adequate volume resuscitation, PEEP actually decreases ICP because of improved cerebral oxygenation. Permissive hypercapnoea should be avoided due to the cerebral vasodilatory effect that increases ICP. Hypoxia should be treated immediately to avoid the resulting increase in cerebral blood flow which leads to an increase in ICP.

Appropriate sedation must be provided to reduce the cerebral metabolic rate and to facilitate mechanical ventilation. A short-acting benzodiazepine such as midazolam is often used which is effective both as a sedative and as an anticonvulsant. Propofol is also commonly used for its superior cerebral metabolic suppressant effects, less interference with cerebral autoregulation, anti-inflammatory properties and a shorter half-life. It can however produce a precipitous fall in MAP which then leads to a reduction in CPP. Barbiturates such as thiopentone are used less frequently due to problems with immune suppression and increased risk of infection. They are now mostly reserved for controlling ICP when other methods have failed.

The mainstay of analgesia involves the use of opioid infusions which have minimal effects on cerebral haemodynamics.

Neuromuscular block can be used to minimize episodes of coughing and straining which may lead to an increase in ICP. Non-depolarizing muscle relaxants are used as boluses or infusion. Adequate sedation is important when muscle relaxants are used to reduce the possibility of awareness in a paralysed patient.

Cardiovascular support

Under normal conditions the brain autoregulates its blood flow between 50 and 150 mmHg. The injured brain is less able to do this and depends on systemic blood pressure to maintain blood flow. Hypotension (MAP <90 mmHg) must be avoided since it causes a reduction in cerebral blood flow and will ultimately result in cerebral ischaemia. Hypertension may conversely worsen vasogenic oedema with a detrimental effect on ICP. It is therefore imperative that a balance be attained by using values for CPP as a target to avoid cerebral ischaemia.

Euvolaemia is the primary resuscitative goal for patients with TBI. No resuscitation fluid has been shown to be superior and both crystalloids and colloids can be used. Isotonic crystalloids are widely available and 0.9% saline is scientifically justified although hyperchloraemic acidosis may result when large volumes are used. Glucose-containing solutions, on the other hand, must be avoided for two main reasons. Firstly, in the anaerobic brain, glucose is metabolized to lactate which worsens secondary injury. Secondly, the free water liberated following the metabolism of glucose can worsen cerebral oedema. If adequate maintenance of MAP cannot be achieved with fluids alone then a vasopressor such as norepinephrine should be introduced.

Nutritional support

Early nutritional support is essential with the enteral route preferred although no difference in outcome in severe TBI between enteral or parenteral nutrition has been demonstrated by clinical trials. Peptic ulcer prophylaxis is important as there is a 10% incidence of stress ulcers in severe TBI.

Glycaemic control

The stress response in TBI patients leads to hyperglycaemia. This exacerbates secondary ischaemic injury and worsens neurological outcome. It is unclear whether hyperglycaemia per se or lack of insulin affects outcome. However, clinical trials have failed to show improved outcomes following tight glycaemic control.

Thromboprophylaxis

Whilst there is no consensus of opinion as to when thromboprophylaxis should be commenced, it should be considered in all patients that are immobile, remembering that disseminated intravascular coagulation (DIC) may accompany severe TBI.

Specific management of traumatic brain injury

Conventional approaches to the management of TBI have centred around the reduction of a raised ICP to prevent secondary ischaemia. There has been a shift of emphasis from primary control of ICP to a multifaceted approach of maintenance of CPP and cerebral protection. Although the actual optimal level for CPP is contentious, there is consensus that it should be maintained between 50 and 70 mmHg. It is now thought that higher targets are often achieved only at the expense of significant complications. It is also now clear that an optimal CPP exists for individual patients and the use of multimodality monitoring may assist the clinician in selecting the optimal CPP target.

Management of intracranial hypertension

Position

Head-up tilt of 45° and a neutral position of the head and neck must be maintained to encourage venous drainage. Avoid tight ties around the neck which may cause venous congestion.

Hyperventilation

Hyperventilation is associated with adverse neurological outcome because regional ischaemia may be worsened by cerebral vasoconstriction. The desired range for $PaCO_2$ is between 4.5 and 5.0 kPa. Moderate hyperventilation may be indicated as rescue therapy in selected cases but should only be undertaken with cerebral oxygenation monitoring to ensure that hyperventilation itself does not cause cerebral ischaemia.

Osmotic therapy

Mannitol (0.5g/kg) effectively reduces ICP, and improves CBF and CPP in intracranial hypertension. Prolonged administration may lead to the movement of mannitol from the blood into brain tissue where it might paradoxically increase ICP. Mannitol should only be used as a bridge to more definitive treatment.

There are substantial data to support the use of hypertonic saline solutions as effective treatment of raised ICP. Their beneficial effects are likely to be multifactorial and include haemodynamic, vasoregulatory, immunological and neurochemical effects in addition to the more obvious osmotic effects. Further long-term functional outcome studies are needed to define the optimal osmolar load needed to lower elevated ICP.

Barbiturates

Barbiturates reduce ICP and have neuroprotective effects due to a reduction in cerebral metabolism and associated reduction in CBF, effects on vascular tone and free radical scavenging. However, the use of high-dose barbiturates for the control of raised ICP is highly contentious. Firstly, they are associated with significant hypotension. Secondly, the long half-life makes clinical assessment of patients difficult even after barbiturates are stopped. EEG monitoring should be used to titrate barbiturate therapy to ensure the minimum dose to achieve burst suppression and therefore minimize systemic complications. Despite the ability of barbiturates to reduce ICP, there is no good evidence demonstrating improvement in outcome.

Surgical methods

Drainage of CSF via an external ventricular drain is an effective means of reducing ICP. Another method for treating refractory intracranial hypertension is decompressive craniectomy, which is currently the subject of a multi-centre Randomized Evaluation of Surgery with Craniectomy for Uncontrollable Elevation of Intra-Cranial Pressure (RESCUE-ICP) study.

Therapeutic hypothermia

Although beneficial in animal models, the results of moderate hypothermia (33–35 °C) in human trials have been disappointing. This area is subject to ongoing research. What is certain is that hyperthermia should definitely be avoided. Brain temperature is higher than core temperature so this potential adverse effect may go unnoticed.

Steroids

The Corticosteroid Randomization After Significant Head Injury trial (CRASH) was terminated early because the risk of death from all causes within 2 weeks was higher in those receiving corticosteroids. There is therefore no place for steroids in the management of TBI.

Table 42.3 The Glasgow Outcome Scale

Score	Description
1	**Death**
2	**Persistent vegetative state** Patient exhibits no obvious cortical function
3	**Severe disability** Conscious but disabled: patient depends upon others for daily support due to mental or physical disability or both
4	**Moderate disability** Disabled but independent: patient is independent as far as daily life is concerned. The disabilities found include varying degrees of dysphasia, hemiparesis or ataxia as well as intellectual and memory deficits and personality changes
5	**Good recovery** Resumption of normal activities even though there may be minor neurological or psychological deficits

Source: After Jennett B, Bond M (1975) *Lancet* **i** (7905): 480–4.

Anticonvulsants

Anticonvulsant medication in the acute phase (first 7 days) after TBI does not reduce the incidence of post-traumatic seizures in the longer term and is therefore not recommended. Anti-epileptics should not be prescribed unless there is documented clinical or EEG evidence of seizures. Some neurosurgeons advocate the use of anti-epileptics in certain high-risk groups, such as those with depressed skull fractures, but these must be considered on an individual basis.

Outcome

Outcome after TBI is usually assessed using the Glasgow Outcome Scale 6 months after injury (Table 42.3). Early aggressive resuscitation is essential for optimizing outcome in TBI. It is also now apparent that genetic variation interacts with environmental factors to determine patients' outcomes. This opens up a whole new area of research into the management of TBI.

Key points

- Initial assessment and resuscitation of patients with TBI follows the same approach as all trauma patients.
- Primary brain injury often leads to a rise in intracranial cerebral pressure and a fall in cerebral perfusion pressure. In severe brain injury, ICP monitoring should be instituted to ensure adequate cerebral perfusion pressure.
- Specific management should aim to limit secondary brain injury.
- Management of raised ICP includes:
  - When ventilated, PO_2 should be maintained at 11 kPa and PCO_2 at 4.5 to 5 kPa to avoid cerebral vasoconstriction.
  - Sedation and paralysis is instituted to decrease cerebral metabolic rate and sudden increases in ICP.
  - Osmotic therapy with mannitol and hypertonic saline solution should only be used as a bridge until definitive surgery.
- Therapeutic hypothermia, steroids and anticonvulsants have no role in traumatic brain injury.

Further reading

- Brain Trauma Foundation (2007) Guidelines for the management of severe traumatic brain injury, 3rd edn. *J. Neurotrauma* **24** (Suppl. 1): S1–S106.
- Helmy A, Vizcaychipi M, Gupta A (2007) Traumatic brain injury: intensive care management. *Br. J. Anaesth.* **99**: 32– 42.
- National Institute for Clinical Excellence (2007) *Triage, Assessment, Investigation and Early Management of Head Injury in Infants, Children and Adults*, NICE Clinical Guideline no. 56. London: NICE.

Trauma and burns

Catherine Snelson

Trauma

Trauma remains a leading cause of morbidity and mortality worldwide, with an estimated 16 000 deaths due to injury in England and Wales in 2005. Death occurs in a trimodal distribution (Fig. 43.1). The first peak occurs immediately, with death due to catastrophic unsurvivable injuries such as rupture of the myocardium or major blood vessels or high cervical spine injury. The second peak occurs over minutes to hours, due to injuries causing hypoxia or haemorrhage. It is at this sta\ge, often termed the 'golden hour', where timely assessment and resuscitation can save lives. The Advanced Trauma Life Support Course (ATLS), co-ordinated by the American College of Surgeons, teaches basic principles to try and minimize these second-stage deaths. The third peak occurs days to weeks post injury, with patients dying of multi-organ failure or sepsis in the intensive care unit (ICU). In this chapter, we will mainly focus on management of the patient during the 'golden hour'.

Co-ordinated team care is essential for managing the multiple trauma victim. Regional trauma centres are now being established, but critical care doctors in all hospitals need to be aware of the principles of trauma resuscitation. The mechanism of the trauma gives clues as to the likely injuries sustained, so close attention should be paid to the handover given by the paramedic crews.

Primary assessment and treatment proceeds according to the standard ABCDE approach, with the added principles of cervical spine (C-spine) control and haemorrhage control (Table 43.2).

This is based on the concept that problems with the airway will kill before problems with breathing and circulation. Once this primary survey has been completed and immediate life-threatening conditions have been managed, then a secondary survey or top-to-toe examination is performed to pick up all other injuries and investigations performed as appropriate (Table 43.2).

It is not uncommon for this secondary survey to be completed several hours or days after admission when the patient is on the ICU.

Primary survey

Airway with cervical spine control

Assessment of airway patency occurs in the usual fashion beginning with opening the airway and looking for evidence of airway obstruction. There may also be direct injury to the maxillofacial area, larynx or trachea. During management of the airway, excessive movement of the cervical spine should be avoided, and the neck should be immobilized either with stabilization equipment with hard collar, sandbags and tape (Fig. 43.2) or manual in-line stabilization, in which an assistant holds the head and neck in the neutral position (Fig. 43.3). This limits the airway opening manoeuvres that can be performed to chin lift and jaw thrust, and can make oropharyngeal airways more difficult to insert. Nasopharyngeal airways should be avoided if there is a risk of basal skull fracture.

Establishing the definitive airway

Signs of airway obstruction, respiratory distress or inadequate airway protection due to reduced consciousness level mean that it is necessary to secure a definitive airway. Establishing a definitive airway in the trauma patient with a rapid sequence induction can be challenging. At least three assistants are needed: one person to maintain in-line stabilization of the cervical spine, one to provide cricoid pressure and

Core Topics in Critical Care Medicine, eds. Fang Gao Smith and Joyce Yeung. Published by Cambridge University Press.

Table 43.1 Principles of primary assessment and management of trauma.

Airway with cervical spine control
Breathing
Circulation with haemorrhage control
Disability
Exposure

Table 43.2 Secondary survey.

Head	Scalp or skull injuries
Maxillofacial	Eyes, pupils, facial bones and mouth
Neck	C-spine injury, laryngeal deformity, haematomas
Thorax	Thoracic wall injury, pneum/haemothorax, pulmonary contusions etc
Abdomen	Abdominal wall injury, intra/retroperitoneal injury
Pelvis	Perineal injuries, pelvic fractures, genitourinary tract injuries etc
Legs/arms	Soft tissue injury, fractures, dislocations, neurovascular defects
Spine	Vertebral injury with soft tissue swelling or steps, nerve injury

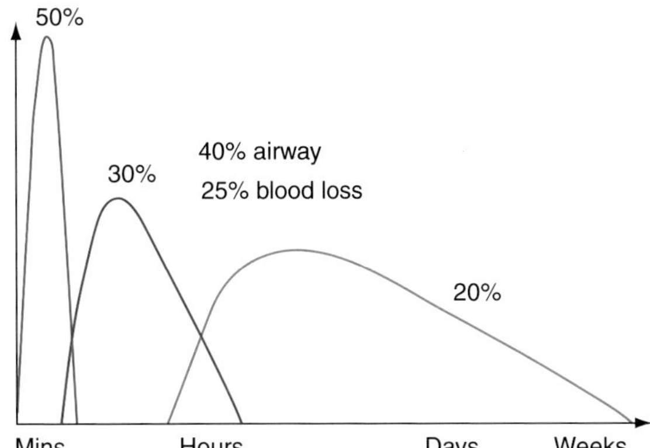

Fig. 43.1 Trimodal distribution of death from trauma. (With permission from Trunkey DD (1983) Trauma. *Sci. Am.* **249**: 20–7.)

hand airway equipment to the anaesthetist, and one person to administer drugs. The induction agent should be chosen carefully; thiopentone and propofol have to be used cautiously in the hypovolaemic patient due to the risk of cardiovascular collapse, ketamine may increase intracranial pressure (although further studies are ongoing) and etomidate is now widely recognized to cause adrenal suppression. Direct laryngoscopy with a Macintosh blade may be difficult due to the lack of neck movement. Adjuncts such as a bougie can be invaluable and difficult airway equipment such as an intubating laryngeal mask airway or an indirect laryngoscope such as Glidescope, McGrath or Airtraq, whereby visualization of the vocal cords is achieved indirectly through either an optical or a video system, should be made available. Even in the hands of the most skilled operator, it is occasionally impossible to intubate the trachea. The anaesthetist should keep in mind their failed intubation drill, and be prepared to perform a needle cricothyroidotomy if necessary (Table 43.3).

Breathing

In practice, assessment of the airway, breathing and circulation is often carried out simultaneously by different members of the trauma team. All trauma patients are administered high-flow oxygen and monitored by pulse oximetry. If respiratory distress is not relieved by clearing the airway, then search for other aetiologies by:

- Observation – look for asymmetrical chest movements, flail segments, open chest wounds, tracheal deviation and distended neck veins.
- Auscultation – listen for movement of air on both sides.
- Percussion – percuss for hyper-resonant or dull percussion notes (may be difficult in the noisy trauma room).

The major life-threatening thoracic injuries are shown in Table 43.4.

A tension pneumothorax is managed by immediate needle decompression in the mid-clavicular second intercostal space, followed by chest drain insertion. Pneumo- and haemothoraces are managed with thoracocentesis. Ensure that large-bore vascular access is in place prior to drainage of a haemothorax as cardiovascular collapse can ensue on decompression. Large open defects of the chest wall can suck in air resulting in an open pneumothorax. This can be managed initially by applying a sterile occlusive dressing that is taped on three sides, and then place a chest drain remote from the wound as soon as possible. Flail segments cause hypoxia through pain on breathing and underlying pulmonary contusion and the patient is likely to deteriorate before getting better. Patients with chest trauma should be monitored closely and given adequate analgesia. There should also be a low threshold for intubation and ventilation.

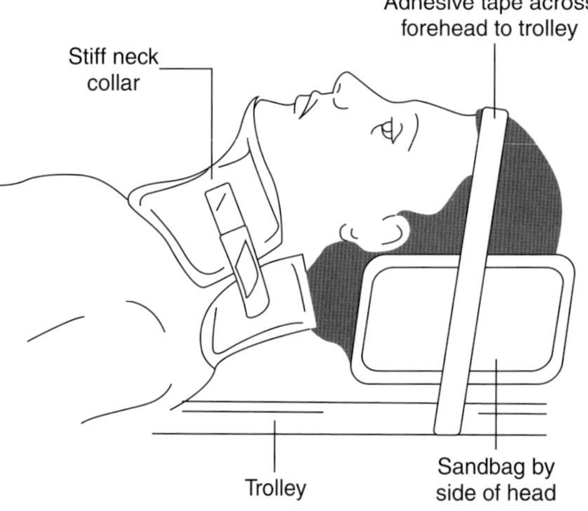

Fig. 43.2 Airway with cervical spine control. (With permission from *Update in Anaesthesia*, Issue 6 (1996), Article 2, The management of major trauma.)

Circulation with haemorrhage control

The causes of shock in trauma are shown in Table 43.5.

Shock in trauma is mostly caused by hypovolaemia secondary to haemorrhage. Cardiogenic shock due to tamponade can be difficult to detect clinically, but classically causes hypotension, distended neck veins and muffled heart sounds. Neurogenic shock results from disruption to the descending sympathetic pathways in the spinal cord. This causes loss of vasomotor tone and sympathetic innervation to the heart, thereby leading to hypotension and bradycardia. Septic shock on admission is rare, but may be present if transfer to hospital has been delayed or if the peritoneal cavity is contaminated with intestinal contents.

The most reliable clinical signs of hypovolaemic shock are cool peripheries and delayed capillary refill time. Tachycardia may not always be present (for example if the patient takes beta-blocking agents) and hypotension is a late sign. Base deficit and lactate measurements are sensitive markers to estimate and monitor the extent of bleeding and shock. Large-bore vascular access should be established; in cases where this is difficult, intra-osseous insertion devices for

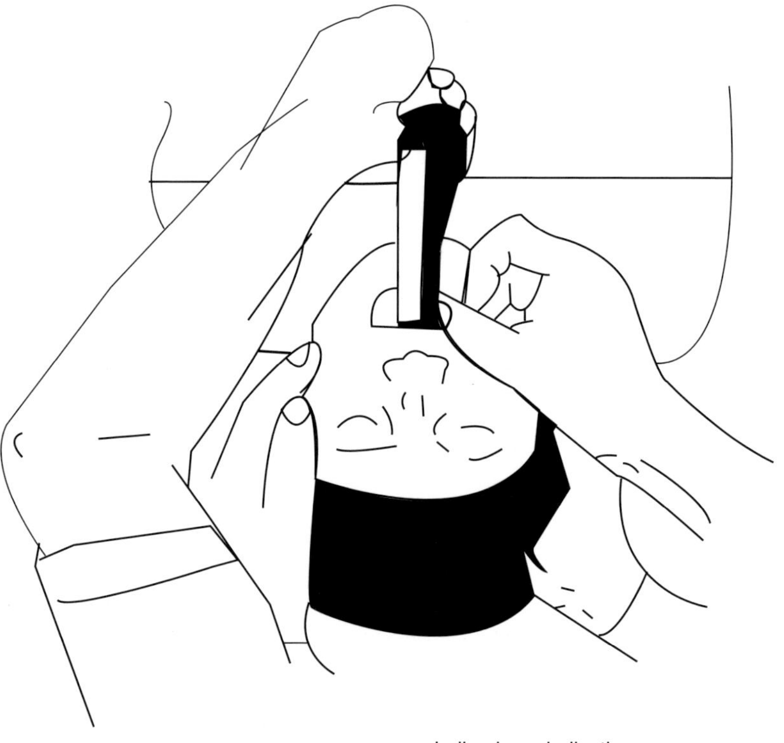

Fig. 43.3 Airway with cervical spine control. (With permission from *Update in Anaesthesia*, Issue 6 (1996), Article 2, The management of major trauma.)

Table 43.3 Establishing the definite airway.

Key points in airway management

- Maintain cervical spine immobilization
- Avoid nasopharyngeal airways if risk of basal skull fracture
- Consider use of bougies, indirect laryngoscopes or intubating LMAs to aid intubation of the trachea
- Always be prepared to call for help early and move on to failed intubation drill

Table 43.4 Immediately life-threatening thoracic injuries.

Tension pneumothorax	Shock, tracheal deviation away from side of injury, absent breath sounds, hyper-resonant percussion note
Pneumothorax	Reduced breath sounds, hyper-resonant percussion note, look for sucking open chest wound
Massive haemothorax	Shock, absent breath sounds, dull percussion note
Flail chest	Unco-ordinated respiratory movement, crepitus

Table 43.5 Causes of shock in trauma.

Hypovolaemia
Cardiogenic due to tamponade or myocardial dysfunction
Tension pneumothorax
Neurogenic
Septic

adults are gaining in popularity or femoral, subclavian or internal jugular access can be attempted. A thorough search should be made for the site of haemorrhage in the thorax, abdomen, pelvis and femurs, and the source should be controlled as soon as possible. Focussed assessment sonography in trauma (FAST) scans are now being used at the bedside in the trauma room to detect haemoperitoneum or pericardial tamponade. CT scan can provide more detailed imaging, but requires the patient to be haemodynamically stable for the transfer. Failure of haemorrhagic shock to respond to fluid and blood administration in the emergency department is an indication for immediate operative intervention. Unstable pelvic fractures causing major haemorrhage can be stabilized by wrapping a sheet round the pelvis as a sling or by using a pneumatic antishock garment, and embolization may be required.

Fluid resuscitation

Methods of fluid resuscitation in trauma remain controversial and a full discussion is beyond the scope of this chapter. In the early resuscitative phase prior to the control of bleeding, inadequate resuscitation increases mortality but restoration of full circulating volume prior to haemostasis may result in further haemorrhage. For penetrating trauma, 'permissive hypotension' is often advocated, where resuscitation is targeted to the ability to palpate the radial pulse or a systolic blood pressure of 80–100 mmHg as a bridge to surgical control of bleeding. There is no evidence for this in blunt trauma, and hypotension should be avoided if there is a risk of cerebral or spinal cord injury.

Choice of fluid continues to provoke much debate, and the available literature is confusing and difficult to interpret due to variations in study design. Trauma induces endothelial dysfunction with the consequent risk of interstitial oedema. Crystalloids are freely permeable to the vascular membrane and risk worsening this interstitial oedema, and normal (0.9%) saline induces a hyperchloraemic acidosis. Although colloids such as albumin, dextrans and hydroxyl-ethyl starch (HES) increase the plasma volume, they may also induce coagulation abnormalities and increase the risk of renal failure. The Saline versus Albumin Fluid Evaluation (SAFE) study compared 4% albumin with 0.9% saline in 6997 ICU patients; in the trauma sub-group that received albumin there was an increased incidence of intracerebral bleeding and a trend towards higher mortality ($P = 0.06$).

Currently, fluid resuscitation in trauma is generally performed according to local practice and personal preference. The ATLS manual recommends use of a crystalloid (Ringer's lactate) proceeding directly to blood products where necessary without the use of colloids. In the UK, a common practice is to use normal saline for traumatic brain injury, and in cases where surgical haemorrhage is controlled and significant head injury excluded to use Hartmann's solution for hydration and synthetic colloid to restore intravascular volume.

Coagulopathy

Trauma causes a coagulopathy through consumption, dilution and dysfunction of coagulation factors and platelets (Table 43.6). Coagulopathy, hypothermia and acidosis are often termed the 'lethal triad' of trauma as each factor exacerbates the others leading to life-threatening bleeding and exsanguination. Administration of red blood cells (RBCs) needs to be accompanied by correction of coagulation with fresh frozen plasma,

Table 43.6 Coagulopathy

Key points in control of circulation
• Shock is most likely to be due to haemorrhage and bleeding needs to be controlled as soon as possible
• Consider permissive hypotension in penetrating trauma without evidence of cerebral or spinal cord injury
• Look for sources of bleeding in the abdomen and exclude cardiac tamponade using FAST
• Only transfer to CT if you are confident the patient is sufficiently haemodynamically stable
• If the patient fails to respond to fluid administration consider other causes of shock or immediate surgery
• In head injuries use isotonic crystalloid as initial resuscitation fluid
• For massive transfusion consider 1:1 administration of packed cells to FFP
• Consider use of rVII if surgical approaches and administration of blood products fail to control bleeding

cryoprecipitate, platelets and calcium. Traditionally, this has been done according to results of laboratory investigations. However, recent evidence from the US military indicates that there is an association between mortality and the ratio of the number of units of plasma to the number of units of RBCs transfused. In many civilian trauma centres, a protocol using a 1:1 ratio of plasma to RBCs for massive transfusion is now being implemented, and scoring systems to predict patients at risk with massive transfusion are being evaluated.

Recombinant activated factor VII (rVII) binds to activated platelets at the site of injury and activates factors IX and X directly. Evidence indicates that its use may reduce RBC transfusion requirements and the incidence of acute respiratory distress syndrome (ARDS) in patients with blunt trauma. European guidelines suggest that the drug is considered if first-line treatment with a combination of blood products and surgical approaches fails to control bleeding. However, for rVII to be maximally effective, there must be sufficient levels of platelets and fibrinogen and an absence of severe hypothermia and acidosis.

Disability and exposure

A rapid neurological examination establishes the level of consciousness (see Fig. 40.2), pupillary size and reaction, and any spinal cord injury level.

A Glasgow Coma Score (GCS) of less than or equal to 8 is an indication for intubation for airway protection. Even with a higher GCS, if the patient is agitated and cannot be calmed, intubation may be required to allow appropriate investigation and management to proceed. Further management of head injuries is discussed in Chapter 42 (Traumatic brain injury). Remember that a decreased level of consciousness may also be due to decreased cerebral oxygenation and perfusion, and other problems such as hypoglycaemia, alcohol intoxication or drugs misuse. The patient should be completely exposed to allow a thorough examination without allowing hypothermia to develop, and it is at this stage where, if stable, the patient is usually log-rolled to allow examination of the back and vertebral column and removal of the spinal transport board.

Clearance of the cervical spine

Cervical spine injury can be excluded in a patient who is neurologically normal if there is no pain, tenderness or deformity along the spine and there are no distracting injuries. However, if all these criteria are not met then clearance is more problematic, and the risk of missing a significant injury in the comatose, polytrauma patient on the ICU has to be weighed against the morbidity and mortality of spinal precautions in terms of skin ulceration, pneumonias and sepsis. Most trauma centres are now performing CT scans of the neck, and the risk of missing an unstable cervical spine injury with modern scanners is less than 0.5%. MRI has a higher sensitivity for ligamentous instability, but has a low specificity. Most hospitals now have their own protocols for procedures in this situation. The Intensive Care Society suggests that the spine can be cleared on the basis of CT alone, and that it is not considered essential to routinely perform MRI to exclude ligamentous injury. An example of protocol is shown in Fig. 43.4.

Burns

Burns cause considerable morbidity and mortality. Although the initial assessment proceeds along the same principles as outlined above, it is vital that potential airway compromise is predicted and that the airway is protected early if at risk. The supraglottic airway is very susceptible to swelling and obstruction after exposure to heat, and this may develop after admission to the emergency department. In addition, smoke inhalation can severely compromise pulmonary function by causing inflammation, direct airway burns, bronchospasm, ciliary paralysis, reduced surfactant and acute lung injury. Evidence for possible airway obstruction and smoke inhalation includes:

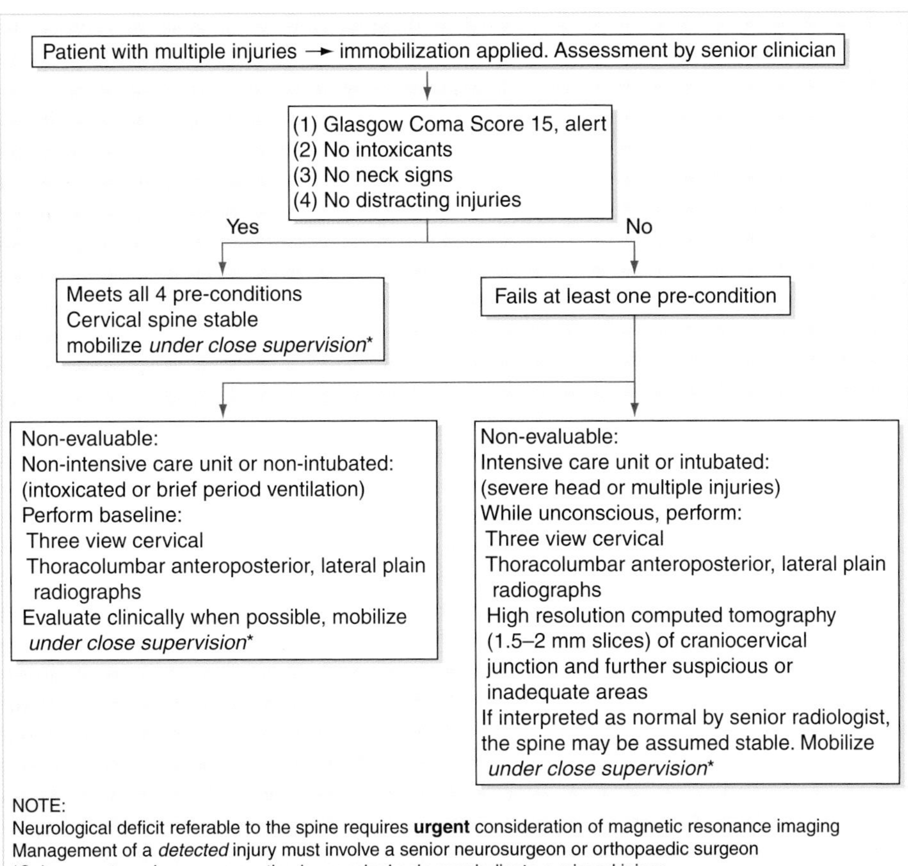

Patient with multiple injuries → immobilization applied. Assessment by senior clinician
(1) Glasgow Coma Score 15, alert
(2) No intoxicants
(3) No neck signs
(4) No distracting injuries
Yes
No
Meets all 4 pre-conditions
Cervical spine stable
mobilize under close supervision*
Fails at least one pre-condition
Non-evaluable:
Non-intensive care unit or non-intubated:
(intoxicated or brief period ventilation)
Perform baseline:
Three view cervical
Thoracolumbar anteroposterior, lateral plain radiographs
Evaluate clinically when possible, mobilize under close supervision*
Non-evaluable:
Intensive care unit or intubated:
(severe head or multiple injuries)
While unconscious, perform:
Three view cervical
Thoracolumbar anteroposterior, lateral plain radiographs
High resolution computed tomography (1.5–2 mm slices) of craniocervical junction and further suspicious or inadequate areas
If interpreted as normal by senior radiologist, the spine may be assumed stable. Mobilize under close supervision*
NOTE:
Neurological deficit referable to the spine requires urgent consideration of magnetic resonance imaging
Management of a detected injury must involve a senior neurosurgeon or orthopaedic surgeon
*Subsequent weakness, paraesthesia, or spinal pain may indicate a missed injury

Fig. 43.4 Example pathway for clearing the cervical spine in trauma patients. (Adapted with permission from Morris CG, McCoy W, Lavery GG (2004) Spinal immobilisation for unconscious patients with multiple injuries. *Br. Med. J.* **329**: 495–9.)

- Facial and/or neck burns
- Carbon deposits in the mouth or nose, or acute inflammation within the oropharynx
- Carbonaceous sputum
- Singeing of the eyebrows or nasal hairs
- Hoarse voice or stridor
- History of confinement within a burning area
- Hypoxaemia or increased carbon monoxide levels (>2%).

If one or more of these factors are present, then serious consideration should be given to securing the airway with a rapid sequence induction and orotracheal intubation. The endotracheal tube should be uncut to allow for swelling and facial oedema post intubation. There is no specific treatment for smoke inhalation injury other than ensuring adequate oxygenation and minimizing further iatrogenic lung injury. Carbon monoxide toxicity may cause falsely elevated pulse oximetry saturations and should be treated with 100% oxygen.

The 'rule of nines' is a useful way of assessing the extent of the burn (Fig. 43.5). The adult body is divided into areas that represent multiples of 9% of the total body surface area. In children, the head represents a larger proportion of the surface area and the legs a smaller proportion. Another method to assess smaller burns is for the patients' palmar surface of the hand to represent 1% of the body surface; this remains consistent at any age. The depth of the burn is important in evaluating severity. There are three types:

- First degree burns – characterized by erythema, pain and the absence of blisters
- Second degree burns (partial thickness) – painful erythema with associated swelling and blister formation

- Third degree (full thickness) – painless, leathery hard wound which fails to blanch on pressure; may be red or translucent, waxy and white.

Fluid resuscitation in burns can be difficult, and hypoperfusion caused by underfilling has to be balanced against the side effects of oedema caused by overfilling. There are many fluid regimes that have been suggested, but the one most commonly used is the Parkland formula (Table 43.7).

It should be remembered that any formula is a guide only, and it is important to assess the response clinically via vital signs and aiming for a urine output of 1 ml/kg per hour.

Full thickness burns will not stretch and if they are circumferential can cause neurovascular compromise in the limbs and ventilatory compromise in the chest. This can be prevented by division of the burnt tissue,

Table 43.7 Parkland formula for fluid resuscitation in burns.

Total fluid requirement in 24 hours = 4 ml × Total body surface area of burn (%) × body weight (kg)
Give 50% in first 8 hours and 50% in next 16 hours
Use crystalloid e.g. Hartmann's or Ringer's lactate
Starts at time of injury not time of admission to hospital

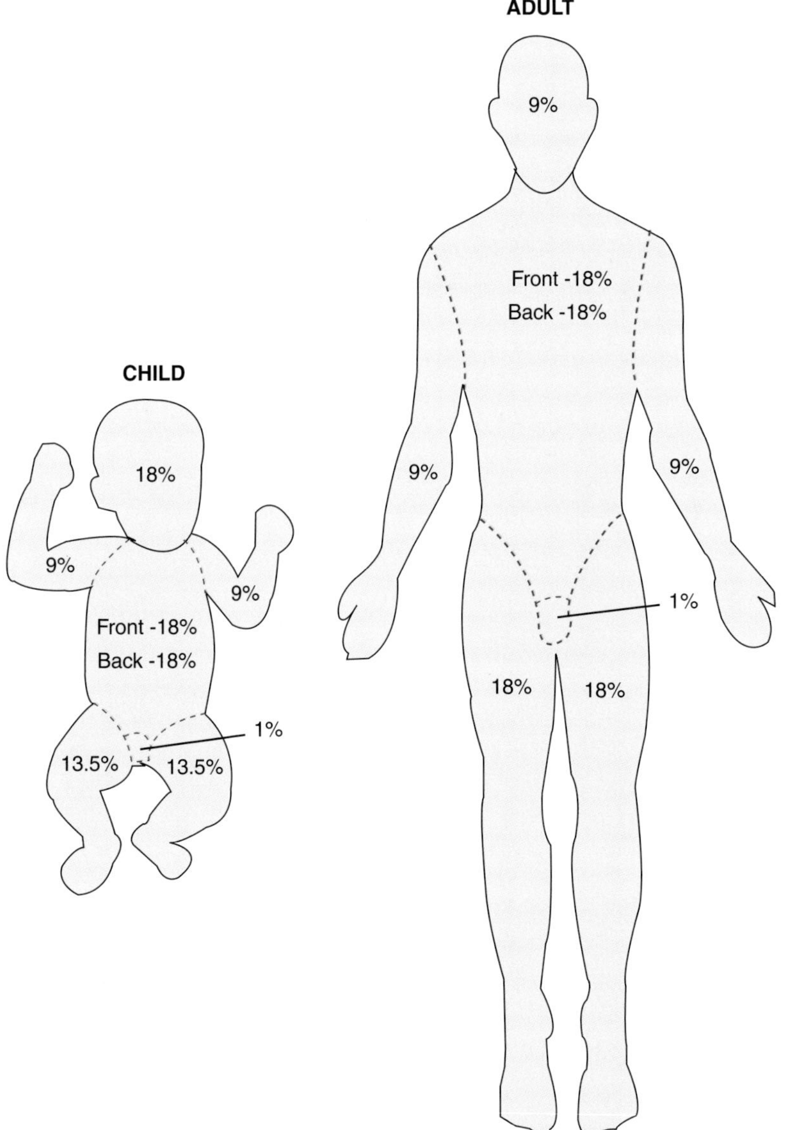

Fig. 43.5 Rules of nines.

termed escharotomy. This is best carried out in the specialist burns centre, but may need to be carried out in the local operating theatre if transfer is delayed. It is advisable to discuss all but the most minor burns with the local burns centre.

Key points

- Trauma is the leading cause of mortality and morbidity worldwide.
- Airway assessment of the trauma patient needs particular attention to the stabilization of the cervical spine.
- Difficult airway is more common in trauma patients and airway adjuncts should be made available.
- Shock in trauma is most commonly caused by hypovolaemia. Currently, there is no demonstrable survival benefit shown with the use of either crystalloids or colloids.
- Coagulopathy is common in trauma and the use of blood and clotting products should be considered early.
- In burns, airway compromise can happen quickly and airway should be secured early if problems are suspected.
- Burns injuries can lead to high loss of fluids and fluid requirement should be calculated and resuscitation started early.
- Management of all burns patients except the very minor ones should be discussed with the burns centre.

Further reading

- American College of Surgeons (2005) *Advanced Trauma Life Support for Doctors: Student Course Manual*, 7th edn. Chicago, IL: ACS.
- BMJ (2005) *ABC of Burns*. London: BMJ Publishing Group.
- Borgman MA, Spinella PC, Perkins JG *et al.* (2007) The ratio of blood products transfused affects mortality in patients receiving massive transfusions in a combat support hospital. *J. Trauma* **63**: 805–13.
- Intensive Care Society (2005) *Evaluation of Spinal Injuries in Unconscious Victims of Blunt Polytrauma: Guidance for Critical Care*. London: ICS. www.ics.ac.uk/icmprof/standards
- SAFE Study Investigators (2004) A comparison of albumin and saline for fluid resuscitation in the intensive care unit. *N. Engl. J. Med.* **350**: 2247–56.
- Spahn DR, Cerny V, Coats TJ *et al.* (2007) Management of bleeding following major trauma: a European guideline. *Crit. Care* **11**: R17.
- Vincent JL, Rossaint R, Riou B *et al.* (2006) Recommendations on the use of recombinant activated factor VII as an adjunctive treatment for massive bleeding: a European perspective. *Crit. Care* **10**: R120.

Eclampsia and pre-eclampsia

John Clift

Introduction

Pre-eclampsia is a multi-system disorder that is unique to pregnancy. It carries a significant morbidity and mortality to mother and baby alike. The incidence of pre-eclampsia in the UK is between 3% and 5% and for severe pre-eclampsia 0.5% of pregnancies. Eclampsia complicates 0.05% of pregnancies in the UK. In the Confidential Enquiries into Maternal and Child Health (CEMACH) report, *Why Mothers Die 2003–2005*, there were 18 deaths from eclampsia and pre-eclampsia. Ten died from intracranial haemorrhage, two from cerebral infarction, two from multi-organ failure that included acute respiratory distress syndrome (ARDS), one from massive liver infarction, and three from other causes.

It is important to realize that the management of pre-eclampsia and eclampsia should consist of a multi-disciplinary approach, involving obstetricians, midwives, anaesthetists, paediatricians and intensivists. There should be early engagement of intensive care specialists in the care of women with severe pre-eclampsia.

Definitions

Pre-eclampsia

This is defined as hypertension and proteinuria at greater than 20 weeks gestation.

Hypertension:

BP >140/90 mmHg on two or more occasions > 4 hours apart OR Diastolic BP >110 mmHg on one occasion

AND

Proteinuria >0.3 g protein in 24 hours OR

2+ or greater on urinalysis strip

Severe pre-eclampsia is defined as:

Systolic BP >170 mmHg OR Diastolic BP >110 mmHg
AND
Proteinuria

Pre-eclampsia may also be described as severe if there is evidence of other organ involvement such as:

- Severe headache, visual disturbances, papilloedema, clonus.
- Epigastric pain, liver tenderness, abnormal LFTs, vomiting.
- Platelets $<100 \times 10^6$/L, HELLP syndrome.

See Fig. 44.1 for the symptoms of pre-eclampsia.

Eclampsia

This is defined as convulsions, occurring after 20 weeks gestation, with no other underlying cause. The patient may or may not have signs or symptoms of pre-eclampsia.

Aetiology and pathogenesis

The pathophysiology is not fully known but is thought to result from incomplete trophoblastic invasion of the spiral arteries, resulting in narrowed spiral arteries and placental ischaemia (Fig. 44.2). The abnormal placenta releases one or more factors into the circulation, leading to endothelial damage and vasoconstriction, which account for the multi-system nature of the disease. The placental ischaemia causes the fetal complications.

Assessment

It is important that all patients are fully assessed due to the multi-system nature of the disease (see Fig. 44.1). It is best to consider the effects on each organ in turn.

Core Topics in Critical Care Medicine, eds. Fang Gao Smith and Joyce Yeung. Published by Cambridge University Press.

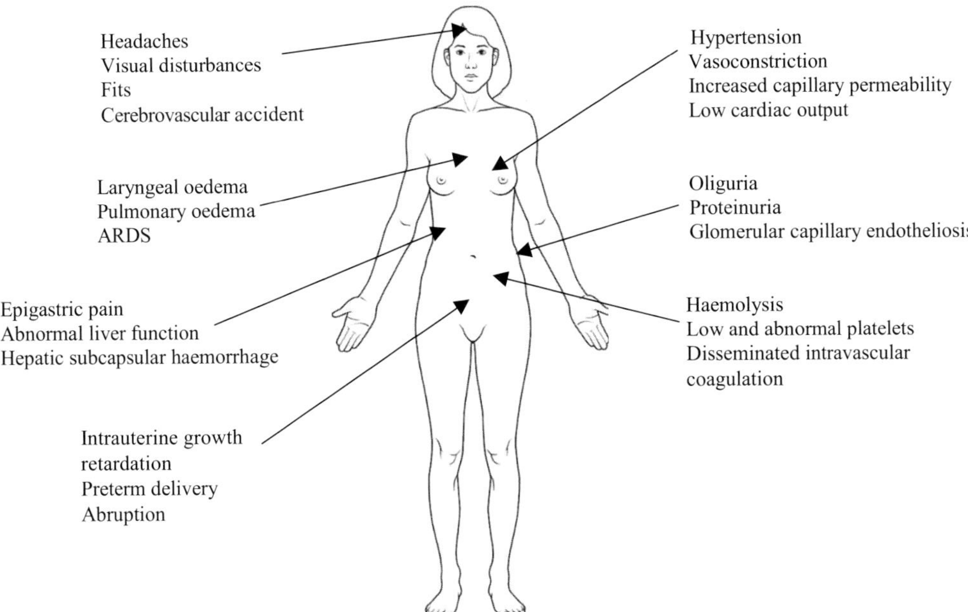

Fig. 44.1 Pre-eclampsia: a multi-system disorder.

Cardiovascular system

- Hypertension with increased sensitivity to angiotensin II, epinephrine and norepinephrine.
- Vasoconstriction and increased systemic vascular resistance.
- Low or normal cardiac output, with low volume pulse, cool peripheries and poor capillary return.
- Decreased circulating volume, which may result in profound hypotension if the patient is given vasodilator therapy.
- Decreased plasma protein, reduced plasma oncotic pressure and increased capillary permeability which together result in oedema in various organs.
- Pulmonary capillary wedge pressure (PCWP) is low or normal.
- Disparity between central venous pressure (CVP) and PCWP.
- Left ventricular failure.

Respiratory system

- Facial and laryngeal oedema.
- Acute lung injury/acute respiratory distress syndrome.
- Pulmonary oedema occurs in approximately 3% of patients, as a result of a reduced plasma oncotic pressure and increased capillary permeability; most cases occur after delivery.

Central nervous system

- Headaches.
- Visual disturbances.
- Hyperreflexia, clonus.
- Focal neurological deficit.
- Papilloedema.
- Cerebrovascular accident.
- Hypertensive encephalopathy.
- Cerebral oedema.
- Convulsions and coma, which may occur due to a combination of vasospasm, micro-infarcts and oedema.

Renal system

- Oliguria, which is relatively common.
- Reduction in glomerular filtration rate and renal perfusion leading to elevated renal function tests and plasma uric acid levels.
- Proteinuria.

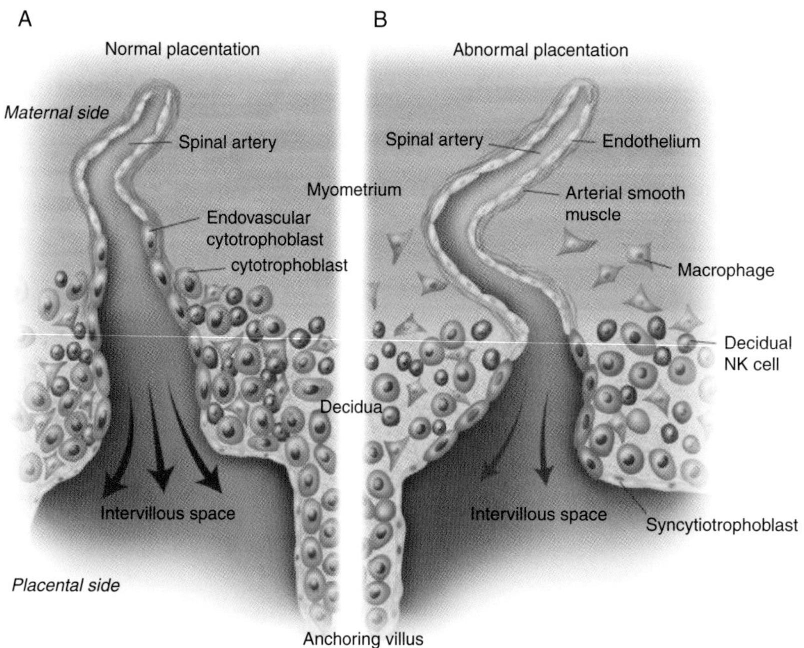

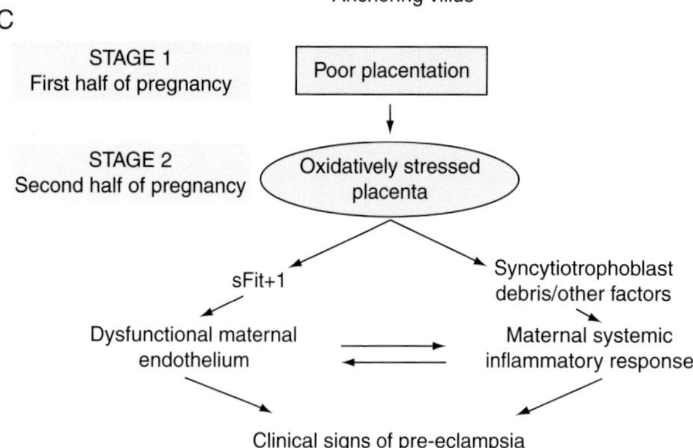

Fig. 44.2 Pathophysiology of pre-eclampsia. (A) Normal placentation where cytotrophoblasts (blue cells) invade the maternal decidua and adjacent spiral arteries. They penetrate the walls of the arteries and replace part of the maternal endothelium, stimulating remodelling of the arterial wall such that the smooth muscle is lost and the artery dilates. During normal pregnancy, NK cells and macrophages facilitate deep invasion of cytotrophoblasts into the myometrial segments and promote extensive spiral artery remodelling. (B) Abnormal placentation where invasion is restricted with impaired arterial remodelling. In the preclinical stage of pre-eclampsia, invasion is restricted (B) with impaired arterial remodelling.

- Temporary glomerular capillary endotheliosis, which if complicated by hypovolaemia may result in acute tubular necrosis.
- Rarely, acute renal failure.

Liver

- Epigastric pain and tenderness.
- Abnormal liver function tests.
- Liver dysfunction caused by periportal necrosis.
- Subcapsular haemorrhage.

Haematological system

- Haemolysis.
- Thrombocytopenia.
- Impaired platelet function.
- Disseminated intravascular coagulation.

Fetus

- Intrauterine growth retardation and increased perinatal mortality, due to placental insufficiency.
- Preterm delivery.
- Placental abruption.

Haemolysis, elevated liver enzymes and low platelets (HELLP) syndrome

This is characterized by:

- **H**aemolysis
- **E**levated **L**iver enzymes
- **L**ow **P**latelets

Management

Good management of pre-eclampsia is dependent on early diagnosis, careful assessment, monitoring and delivery of the baby at the optimum time. Important aspects of this management are:

- Control of blood pressure.
- Control and prevention of convulsions.
- Fluid balance.
- Planning the delivery.
- Postpartum care.
- Management of complications.

Control of blood pressure

The aim for controlling blood pressure is to reduce the incidence of maternal neurological complications: the end-point is a diastolic blood pressure <100 mmHg or systolic blood pressure <160 mmHg. This has been highlighted by the latest CEMACH report which indicated that the most significant failing in the clinical care received by mothers with pre-eclampsia was treatment of systolic hypertension, as this resulted in intracranial haemorrhage in several cases. Control of blood pressure may also have the advantage of prolonging the pregnancy. Antihypertensive treatment at lower blood pressures than above may be indicated in patients with heavy proteinuria or other symptoms or signs indicating severe disease.

Drugs used to control blood pressure acutely are:

- Oral labetalol 200 mg.
- IV labetalol 50 mg increments IV followed by an IV infusion 20–160 mg/hour.
- IV hydralazine 5 mg increments every 20 mins, followed by infusion 5–20 mg/hour.
- Oral nifedipine 10 mg, followed by 10–20 mg up to TDS.

Atenolol, angiotensin-converting enzyme inhibitors, angiotensin antagonists and diuretics should be avoided in pregnancy. Sublingual nifedipine should not be used as it may decrease placental perfusion thus causing fetal distress.

As there is often a decreased circulating volume, vasodilator administration may result in a sudden drop in blood pressure and placental perfusion, this must be corrected immediately. Small volumes of crystalloid IV can be given (250 ml) and boluses of a vasopressor, e.g. ephedrine 3–6 mg, will provide temporary support for the blood pressure and placental perfusion.

Magnesium IV will produce a transient reduction in blood pressure. In the labouring patient and post-caesarean delivery, epidural analgesia is effective at reducing maternal blood pressure.

Prevention of convulsions

Magnesium is the treatment of choice for preventing and controlling convulsions. Magnesium administration results in a 58% decrease in the risk of an eclamptic seizure. It should be given to women with severe pre-eclampsia and continued for 24 hours after the last delivery or 24 hours after the last seizure, whichever is longer.

A loading dose of 4 g IV should be given over 5–10 min followed by an infusion of 1 g/hour. A suggested regime is:

- Loading – 4 g made up to 40 ml at 240 ml/hour.
- Maintenance – 5 g made up to 50 ml at 10 ml/hour (1 g/hour).

There is no need to monitor plasma levels routinely but the patient should be regularly assessed for signs of magnesium toxicity, which include: urine output, respiratory rate, oxygen saturations and examination of maternal reflexes (see Table 44.1). Signs of toxicity include loss of deep tendon reflexes (patellar), respiratory depression and arrhythmias; if any of these are suspected the infusion should be halted immediately. As it is excreted in the urine, if the urine output is <20 ml/hour (over 4 hour period) the infusion should also be stopped.

If respiratory depression or arrhythmias are present due to suspected magnesium toxicity the

Table 44.1 Plasma levels of magnesium

	Plasma levels (mmol/l)
Therapeutic levels	2–4
ECG changes (wide QRS, prolonged PR)	3–5
Loss of tendon reflexes	>5
Heart block, CNS and respiratory depression	>7.5
Cardiac arrest	>12

infusion should be stopped, magnesium levels sent and 1 g IV calcium gluconate given over 10 mins.

Eclampsia

Eclamptic fits may occur in the antepartum (40%), intrapartum (20%) and postpartum (40%) periods. The patient may show the signs and symptoms of severe pre-eclampsia or the fit may precede these. The fits are usually generalized, short in duration and self-limiting. About 1–2% of women will have persistent neurological damage after an eclamptic fit.

The initial management is **A**irway, **B**reathing and **C**irculation with the patient being positioned in the left lateral position and IV access obtained. IV magnesium sulphate is given as stated previously (4 g bolus followed by 1 g/hour).

If the patient has recurrent seizures a further 2 g IV bolus of magnesium sulphate may be given or the rate increased from 1 to 2 g/hour. For further seizures IV diazepam may be used. If convulsions persist, thiopentone, intubation and ventilation in an intensive care setting will be necessary.

In the antepartum period a fit may cause a fetal bradycardia. The mother's health is the priority and her resuscitation will usually resuscitate the fetus.

Fluid balance

Pulmonary oedema is relatively common and has been associated with a significant morbidity and mortality. Radiological evidence of pulmonary oedema was found in 33% of pre-eclamptic patients and was most frequent between the 2nd and 3rd postpartum day, probably due to mobilization of extravascular fluid. On the other hand, although oliguria is common, acute renal failure is very rare. Therefore, the principle for fluid balance in the pre-eclamptic patient is to fluid restrict, with close monitoring of fluid balance, to facilitate the early identification of renal impairment.

Fluid restriction should consist of crystalloid infused at 1 ml/kg per hour continued until the patient develops a diuresis. Fluid management requires the patient to be catheterized, and there must be frequent clinical assessment and charting of fluid balance (input and output). There is no evidence that maintaining a specific urine output is important to prevent renal failure, and 20–30 ml/hour should be adequate; this should be averaged over a 4–6 hour period. If there is evidence of renal impairment a 500 ml crystalloid bolus may be given. The urea and electrolytes should be monitored regularly.

The use of central venous pressure (CVP) monitoring is controversial as there is poor correlation between the CVP and left-sided heart filling pressures. Diuretics are ineffective at preventing acute renal failure and should be reserved for pulmonary oedema. If pulmonary oedema does develop the management is fluid restriction, IV frusemide, oxygen and respiratory support if indicated.

Blood loss should be replaced with fluids and if significant there should be early recourse to invasive monitoring.

Planning the delivery

If the woman is >34 weeks gestation, once her condition has been stabilized delivery of the baby is recommended. The mode of delivery depends upon the likely success of a vaginal delivery. Although this is the preferred option, if success is not likely the baby should be delivered by caesarean section. Antihypertensive treatment should be continued throughout labour.

For a pregnancy of <34 weeks gestation, the mother should be stabilized and given corticosteroids, IM betamethasone 12 mg every 12 hours for 2 doses and allow 24 hours for maximum benefit. Steroids decrease the mortality of the neonate from respiratory distress syndrome (RDS). The delivery should be planned and organized so there is an on-site cot available in an appropriate neonatal unit.

The eclamptic patient should be fully resuscitated and stabilized prior to delivery; delivery is not an emergency. Appropriate blood tests should be done, magnesium started and blood pressure controlled prior to delivery. Once these have been done delivery should take place, usually by caesarean section.

Postpartum care

Some 40% of fits occur in the postpartum period and oliguria and pulmonary oedema are relatively common during this time, therefore the patient needs to be monitored very closely. Hourly monitoring of the following needs to take place:

- cardiovascular parameters
- respiratory parameters
- fluid balance
- signs and symptoms of magnesium toxicity.

Antihypertensive medication should be titrated against blood pressure, but not stopped abruptly. Hypertension and oliguria usually resolve in the first

48 hours. Magnesium should be continued for 24 hours post-delivery or 24 hours post-fit, whichever is longer.

These patients are at an increased risk of thromboembolism; therefore early mobilization, thromboembolic disease preventing (TED) stockings and low-molecular-weight heparin should be administered.

The patients are often young, awake and alert and care should be taken to optimize their psychological well-being. There should be the opportunity for early and frequent contact with the baby.

HELLP syndrome

HELLP syndrome complicates 0.3% of pregnancies and up to 20% of those with severe pre-eclampsia. It can occur in the postpartum period in 25% of cases. Its outcome is poor with a maternal mortality of up to 24% and perinatal mortality of 33%.

The syndrome is a consumptive coagulopathy that leads to the deposition of fibrin-like material in the liver. The clinical signs and symptoms include:

- Epigastric/right upper quadrant pain and tenderness.
- Jaundice.
- Nausea and vomiting.
- Hypertension.
- Proteinuria, oliguria, haematuria.

Laboratory investigations include:

- Abnormal liver function tests (↑AST, ↑ALT, ↑LDH, ↑bilirubin).
- Thrombocytopenia.
- Haemolytic anaemia.
- ↑ Serum haptoglobin.
- Hypoglycaemia.

Complications include: disseminated intravascular coagulation, placental abruption, acute renal failure, pulmonary oedema, and pleural effusions. Rarely intrahepatic haemorrhage, subcapsular haematoma and liver rupture may occur.

If HELLP occurs antenatally the treatment is resuscitation and prompt delivery, regardless of gestational age. Haematological abnormalities should be treated promptly and the advice of a haematologist should be sought at an early stage. Otherwise the treatment is similar to pre-eclampsia, with any complications being managed as they arise. Involvement of a liver unit is sometimes necessary.

Key points

- Pre-eclampsia is a multi-system disorder and it is important that patients are fully assessed for effects on their body systems.
- It is important to establish good control of patient's blood pressure to avoid neurological complications. Labetalol and hydralazine are popular agents.
- Magnesium is the treatment of choice to prevent and control convulsions and the patient should be monitored for signs of magnesium toxicity.
- Pulmonary oedema is common and fluid restriction is needed in pre-eclamptic patients. Oliguria, though common, rarely leads to acute renal failure.
- Once the patient's condition has stabilized, the delivery of the fetus should be planned.
- Monitoring of the patient should extend into the postpartum period as significant risks persist post delivery.

Further reading

- Altman D, Carroli G, Duley L *et al.* (2002) Do women with pre-eclampsia, and their babies, benefit from magnesium sulphate? The Magpie Trial: a randomised placebo-controlled trial. *Lancet* **359**(9321): 1877–90.
- Altman D, Carroli G, Duley L *et al.* (1995) Which anticonvulsant for women with eclampsia? Evidence from the Collaborative Eclampsia Trial. *Lancet* **345** (8963): 1455–63.
- Brodie H, Malinow AM (1998) Anaesthetic management of preeclampsia/eclampsia. *Int. J. Obstet. Anaesth.* **8**: 110–24.
- Confidential Enquiry into Maternal and Child Health (2007) *Why Mothers Die 2003–2005: The Seventh Report of the Confidential Enquiries into Maternal Deaths in the United Kingdom.* London: Royal College of Obstetricians and Gynaccologists Press.
- Da Silva E, Chimbira W (2007) Pre-eclampsia and hypertensive disorders of pregnancy. In *Obstetrics for Anaesthetists,* eds. Heazell A and Clift J. Cambridge: Cambridge University Press, pp. 70–87.
- Engelhardt T, MacLennan F M (1999) Fluid management in pre-eclampsia. *Int. J. Obstet. Anaesth.* **8**: 253–9.

- Mushambi MC, Halligan AW, Williamson K (1996). Recent developments in the pathophysiology and management of pre-eclampsia. *Br. J. Anaesth.* **76**: 133–48.
- Royal College of Obstetricians and Gynaecologists (2006) *The Management of Severe Pre-eclampsia/Eclampsia*, Guideline no. 10(A). London: RCOG Press.
- Tuffnell DJ, Jankowicz D, Lindow SW *et al.* (2005) Outcomes of severe pre-eclampsia/eclampsia in Yorkshire 1999–2003. *Br. J. Obstet. Gynaecol.* **112**: 875–80.

Obstetric emergencies in the ICU

John Clift and Elinor Powell

Introduction

Approximately 1% of maternity patients require ICU admission, the most common causes being obstetric haemorrhage and pre-eclampsia. Maternal mortality is between 3% and 33%, and neonatal mortality approximately 25%. The number of ICU admissions is likely to rise in future, as there are an increasing number of patients becoming pregnant with coexisting diseases, e.g. cardiovascular disease (both congenital and acquired), and a rise in obstetric haemorrhages.

The management of these patients is a particular challenge for several reasons:

- The presence of diseases that are specific to pregnancy e.g. pre-eclampsia and amniotic fluid embolus.
- The physiological changes of pregnancy should be taken into account during diagnosis and treatment (see below).
- There are two patients to consider (mother and baby), although optimal management of the mother should be the priority and will usually improve the fetal condition.
- Timing of delivery of the baby has to be considered.
- Emotional issues associated with mother, baby and family having to deal with serious illness in a young patient, during what should be a positive experience.

In the case of the critically ill obstetric patient, it is essential there is early involvement of senior obstetricians, anaesthetists and intensivists.

Maternal physiology

There are several good textbooks on maternal physiology (see Further reading) and a full description of the physiological changes occurring in pregnancy is beyond the scope of this book. This chapter highlights the changes that are relevant to modern-day critical care practice.

Cardiovascular system

There are increases in cardiac output, stroke volume and heart rate throughout pregnancy whilst the systemic vascular resistance decreases. The blood pressure falls until 20 weeks gestation and then rises towards, or slightly above, pre-pregnant levels at term (Fig. 45.1).

Supine hypotensive syndrome develops from mid-pregnancy and is due to the gravid uterus compressing the inferior vena cava, reducing venous return and hence cardiac output. This may result in placental hypoperfusion and maternal hypotension. The supine position should be avoided, using the left lateral position or left lateral tilt instead. This problem is exacerbated by multiple pregnancies or polyhydramnios.

The ECG may show left axis deviation and inversion of T waves in the lateral leads and lead III. There may also be a mild systolic flow murmur due to mitral regurgitation.

Patients with pre-existing cardiovascular disease are at risk of developing cardiac failure during pregnancy and post delivery. Care of these patients should involve a multi-disciplinary team approach with the involvement of anaesthetists, obstetricians, midwives, cardiologists and intensivists. After delivery these patients should be managed in a critical care environment.

Respiratory system

There is a reduction in the functional residual capacity (FRC) and an increase in maternal oxygen consumption which results in earlier desaturation when the

Core Topics in Critical Care Medicine, eds. Fang Gao Smith and Joyce Yeung. Published by Cambridge University Press.

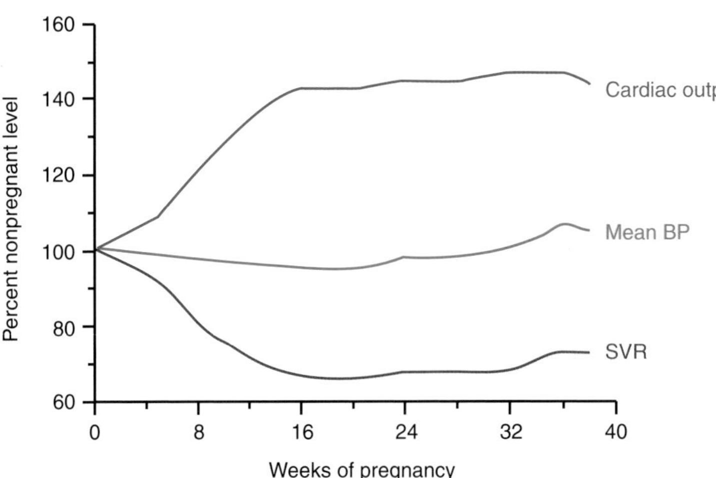

Fig. 45.1 Haemodynamic changes in pregnancy. Normal pregnancy is characterized by an increase in cardiac output, a reduction in systemic vascular resistance (SVR) and a modest decline in mean blood pressure.

patient is apnoeic, i.e. during an eclamptic seizure or prior to intubation (Fig. 45.2).

Progesterone produces an increase in both respiratory rate and tidal volume, therefore reducing the $PaCO_2$ to 4.1 kPa and a compensatory base excess decrease to −2 to −3.

Failed intubation is 7 to 8 times more common in the pregnant woman for various reasons including oedema of the upper airway (especially in the pre-eclamptic patient), engorged breasts, left lateral tilt and increased chest diameter. Pregnant patients are at risk from aspiration from 16 weeks (earlier if symptoms of reflux are present) due to the relaxation of the lower oesophageal sphincter by progesterone and the gravid uterus increasing the intragastric pressure. A rapid sequence induction, with cricoid pressure, is therefore always indicated.

Nasal intubation and nasal airways are best avoided due to capillary engorgement increasing the risk of nasal bleeding, bringing with it the potential for airway compromise.

Haematology

The circulating volume increases by 45% but the red cell mass by only 20%, thus resulting in a physiological anaemia of pregnancy (Fig. 45.3). The increased circulating volume may mask hypovolaemia, and delays the onset of its signs and symptoms until a relatively greater loss of blood has occurred.

The white cell count is increased during pregnancy, and may rise as high as 20×10^9/l in labour. All clotting factors are increased (except factors XI and XIII), as the patient is hypercoagulable to prevent bleeding at the time of delivery. This also means there is an increased risk of thromboembolic disease, and therefore all patients should be mobilized wherever possible. Patients with additional risk factors require thromboprophylaxis and/or thromboembolic disease preventing (TED) stockings. There is also an increased risk of sagittal vein thrombosis.

Biochemistry

There are reductions in plasma urea, creatinine and ionized calcium. Liver enzymes are slightly elevated, with a larger rise in alkaline phosphatase due to placental production.

Thromboembolism

Incidence

Pulmonary embolism is the leading direct cause of maternal death in the UK, with 33 deaths in the triennium 2003–2005, which is an incidence of 1.56 deaths per 100 000 maternities. Venous thromboembolism (VTE) is ten times more common in the pregnant, compared to the non-pregnant, woman. However, there are problems recognizing, diagnosing and treating patients with this condition.

Risk factors

Not only is pregnancy itself a significant risk but there are many additional risk factors (see Table 45.1), although it is difficult to quantify the degree of risk associated with each additional factor. VTE may occur

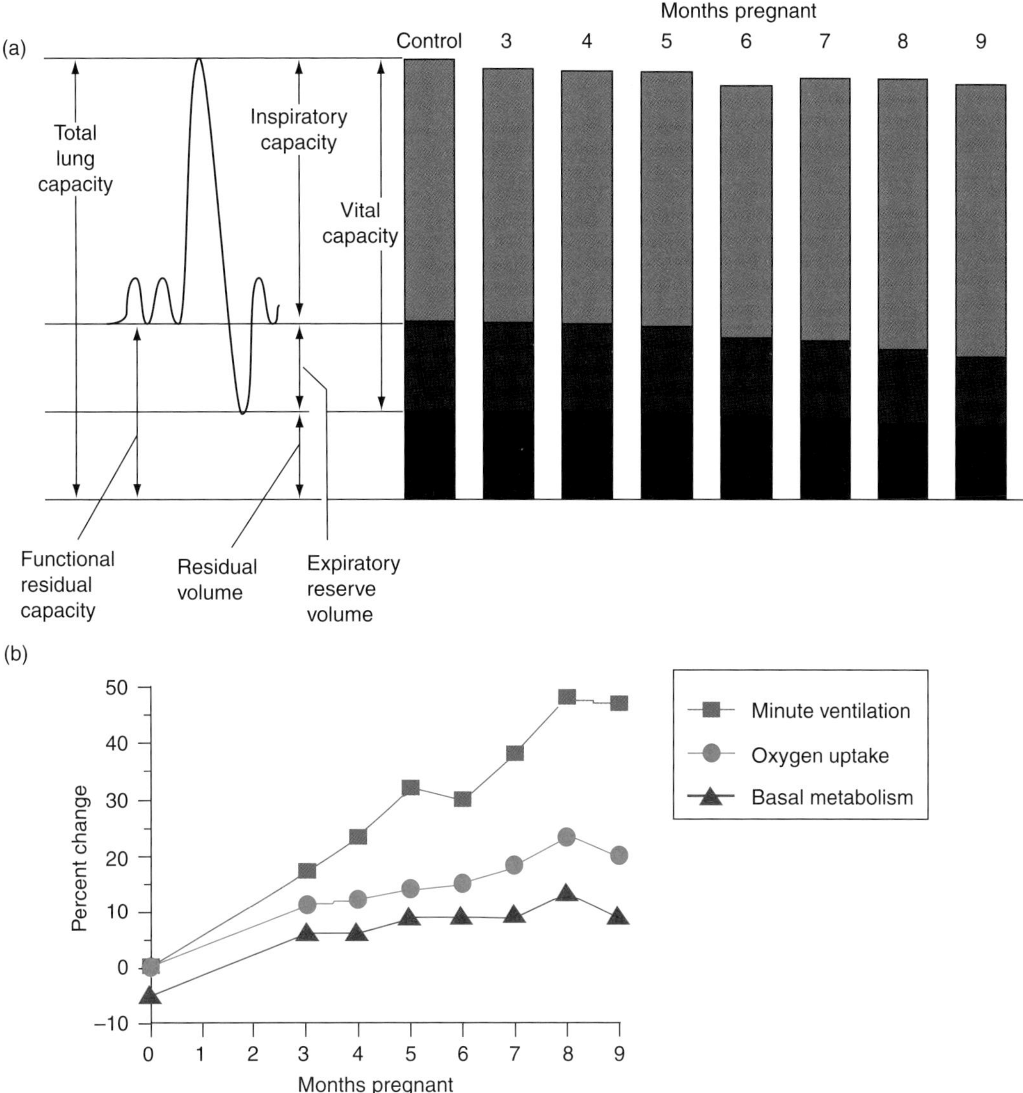

Fig. 45.2 These changes are associated with a 10-15 bpm increase in heart rate. (a) Serial measurements of lung volume components during pregnancy. Functional residual capacity decreases approximately 20% during the later half of pregnancy, due to a decrease in both expiratory reserve volume and residual volume. (b) Time course of percentage increase in minute ventilation, oxygen uptake and basal metabolism during pregnancy. (Adapted from Prowse CM, Gaenster EA (1965) *Anesthesiology* **26**: 381.)

at any time during pregnancy but is most common during the puerperium.

Investigations

Deep vein thrombosis

Many DVTs are asymptomatic but the classical signs and symptoms are:

- unilateral oedema in leg
- leg pain
- calf tenderness
- leg feels warm
- erythema and discoloration
- lower abdominal pain
- fever and raised white cell count.

Iliac vein thrombosis may produce lower back pain and swelling of the entire limb.

The commonest site for DVT is the femoral or iliac vein, with the left leg being more often involved.

Approximately 20% of DVTs will break off to form a pulmonary embolus (PE).

The following should be undertaken when DVT is suspected:

- Compression duplex ultrasound (Fig. 45.4) and Doppler (Fig. 45.5).
- Magnetic resonance venography or conventional contrast venography should be considered for suspected iliac vein thrombosis.

Pulmonary embolus

The origin of most PEs is the pelvic, subclavian and axillary veins. Fewer than 20% of patients present with dyspnoea, chest pain and haemoptysis. Other presentations include:

- chest wall tenderness
- wheeze
- tachycardia
- gallop rhythm or murmur
- fever
- cyanosis
- cardiovascular collapse or cardiac arrest.

The following should be undertaken when PE is suspected:

- Chest X-ray – normal in over 50% of women with proven PE. It may confirm other pulmonary disease and complications of a PE such as atelectasis, pleural effusion or regional oligaemia.

Table 45.1 Risk factors for venous thromboembolism in pregnancy and the puerperium

Pre-existing	New onset or transient
Previous VTE	Surgical procedure
Thrombophilias	Hyperemesis
Obesity (BMI >30 in early pregnancy)	Dehydration
Parity >4	Severe infection
Gross varicose veins	Immobility (>4 days)
Paraplegia	Pre-eclampsia
Sickle cell disease	Excessive blood loss
Inflammatory disorders	Long-haul travel
Cardiac disease	Prolonged labour
Nephrotic syndrome	Midcavity instrumental delivery
Myeloproliferative disorders	Immobility after delivery
Age >35	Ovarian hyperstimulation syndrome

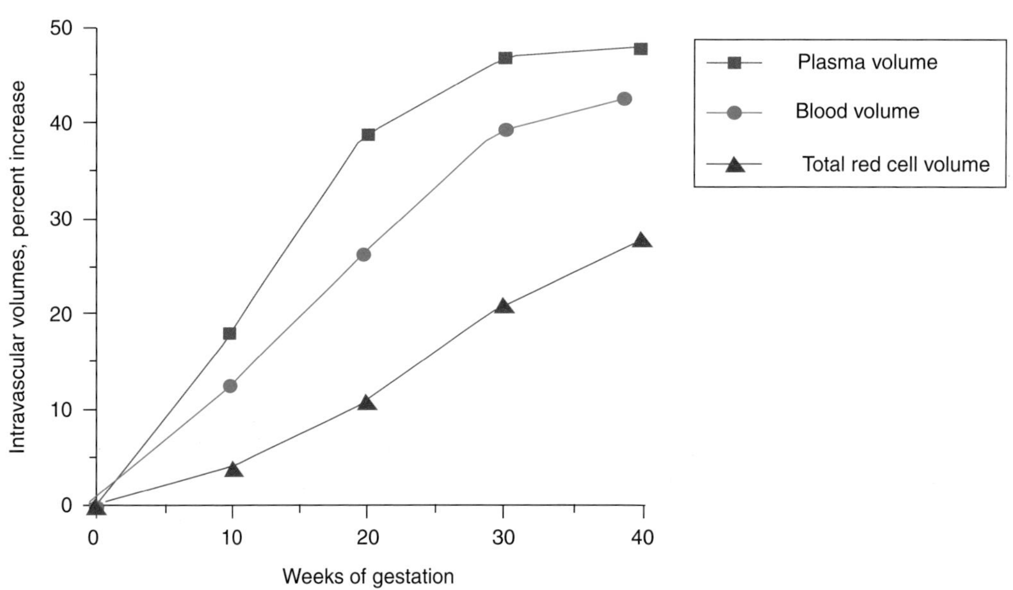

Fig. 45.3 Physiological anaemia of pregnancy. Plasma volume increases more than total red cell volume (50% vs. 25%), resulting in a 40% rise in blood volume and a dilutional fall in the haematocrit.

(a)
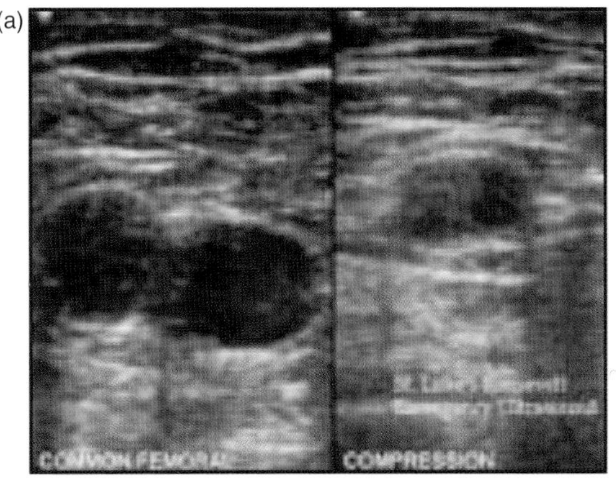

(b)
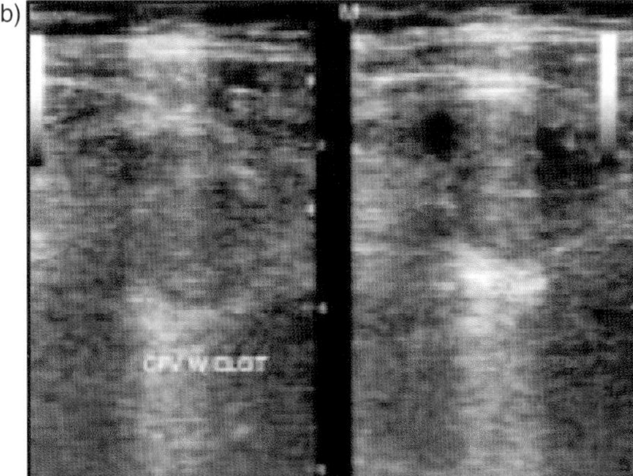

Fig. 45.4 Ultrasound images of (a) normal compressibility of the common femoral vein; (b) abnormal compressibility in deep vein thrombosis.

(a)
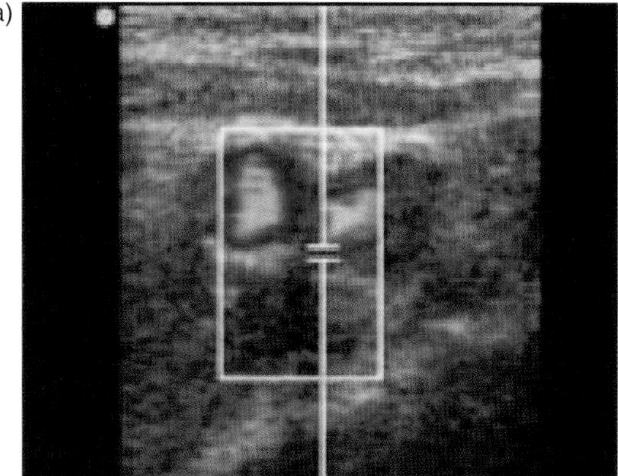

(b)
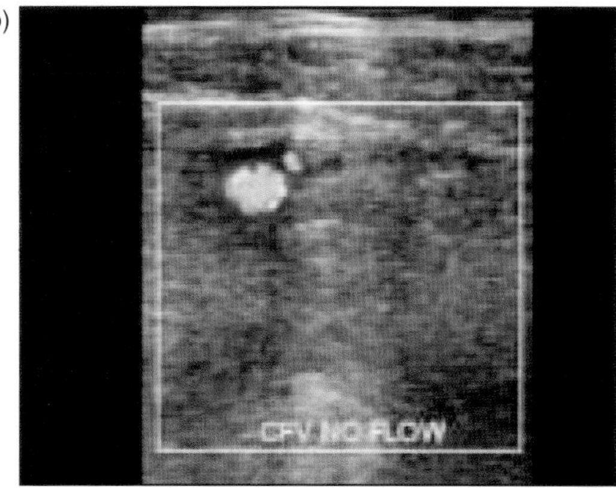

Fig. 45.5 Colour-flow Doppler images of (a) normal vessels; (b) deep vein thrombosis.

- Compression duplex ultrasound – a diagnosis of DVT will indirectly confirm a PE and the treatment is the same for both conditions.
- Computed tomography pulmonary angiogram (CTPA) (Fig. 45.6) or a ventilation–perfusion (V/Q) scan (Fig. 45.7) can be performed, if the above tests are negative. The ventilation component of the latter may be omitted in pregnancy to minimize the radiation to the fetus.

Management

Full anticoagulation should be commenced immediately if a VTE is suspected; this should be continued until the diagnosis is excluded by objective testing. The anticoagulant of choice is subcutaneous low-molecular-weight heparin and monitoring anti-Xa is not routinely required. If the VTE occurs in the antepartum period, discussions with the obstetricians, anaesthetists and haematologists are required to optimize anticoagulation and prevent bleeding during the peripartum period. Warfarin is teratogenic and should be avoided until after delivery. Anticoagulation should be continued for 6 weeks after delivery or for 3 months after the initial episode, whichever is longer.

Massive pulmonary embolus

The management of choice is intravenous unfractionated heparin, aiming for an activated partial thromboplastin time (APTT) ratio of 1.5–2.5. This is used because of its rapid onset and extensive experience in this situation. There may be problems with increasing resistance and requirements in later pregnancy; if this occurs the advice of a haematologist should be sought.

Where haemodynamic compromise is present initial treatment consists of supporting the **A**irway,

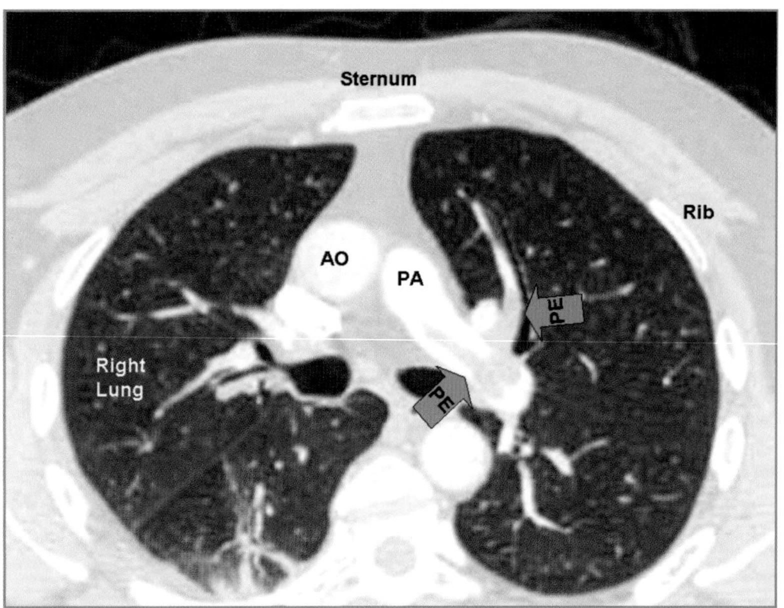

Fig. 45.6 Example of CTPA showing a large pulmonary embolus in the left branch of the pulmonary artery (PA). Pulmonary emboli are detected when the contrast fails to fill the entire artery, leaving voids that represent clots. This image shows a cross-section just above the heart where the PA and the aorta (AO) exit. The contrast has entered the PA making it bright white. A void in the left PA (arrow) and another void in a branch of the PA leading toward the sternum (arrow) indicate the presence of a large PE.

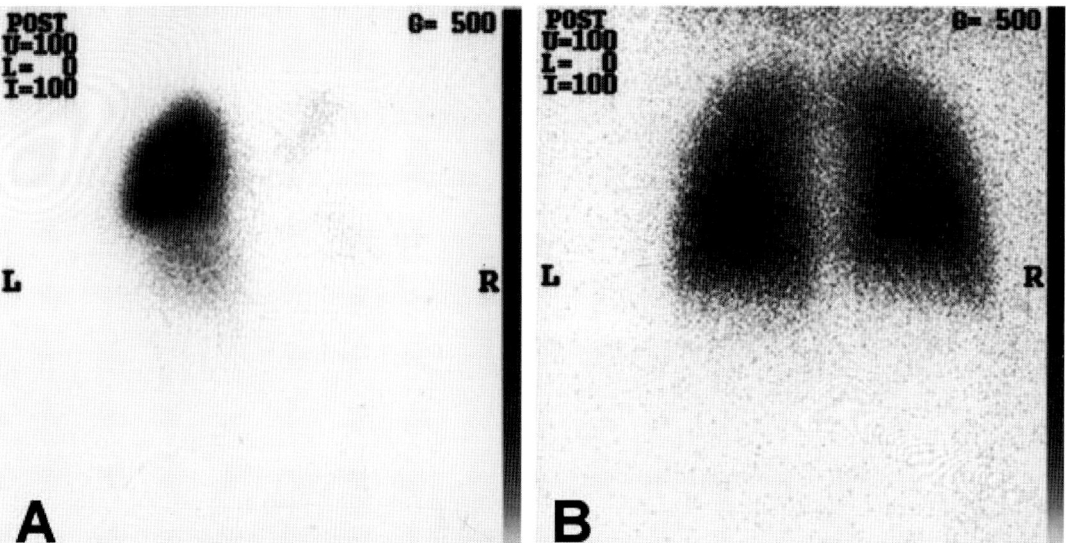

Fig. 45.7 V/Q scan showing normal ventilation to both lungs in (B) but no perfusion to right lung in (A).

Breathing and **C**irculation. Management should involve senior obstetricians, anaesthetists, intensivists and physicians. An urgent portable echocardiogram or CTPA should be arranged within the hour. Thrombolysis should then be considered as the next stage of treatment, although this has not been shown to improve long-term survival compared with heparin. No one thrombolytic agent has been shown to be superior. Once given, the patient should be commenced on intravenous heparin, whilst omitting the loading dose. The most common complication is bleeding around the puncture/catheter site.

Interior vena cava (IVC) filters have been used in pregnancy and the indications are:

- Anticoagulation is contraindicated.
- Patients who have further episodes of VTE whilst anticoagulated.

- Critically ill patients in whom another VTE is likely to be fatal.

These patients are at high risk of having complications from a long-term indwelling catheter and so a better option is to place a retrievable filter which can be removed after a short period.

Thoracotomy and surgical embolectomy should be considered in patients who are moribund or in whom thrombolysis is contraindicated. The incidence of fetal loss is 20–40% and therefore it should be restricted to women whose life is endangered.

If cardiac arrest has occurred the Adult Life Support Universal Algorithm should be used with the following modifications:

- Left lateral tilt.
- Consider perimortem caesarean section, to optimize resuscitation.

Amniotic fluid embolism

Definition

Amniotic fluid embolism (AFE) occurs when amniotic fluid, fetal cells, hair and debris enter the maternal circulation. It is a spectrum of disease that may range from subclinical to cardio-respiratory collapse and death.

Incidence

This is quoted between 1 in 8000 and 1 in 100 000 pregnancies. In the UK in the triennium 2000–2002, there were 20 cases of AFE reported to the register (see later); of these five died giving a mortality rate of 25%, although mortality has been quoted to be as high as 61%.

Pathophysiology

This is poorly understood but may be due to an anaphylactoid reaction and/or complement activation, rather than a direct embolic effect. However, it has been proposed that the condition should be renamed 'sudden obstetric collapse syndrome' due to the clinical nature of the diagnosis, the lack of evidence that amniotic fluid is harmful, low incidence of bronchospasm (to account for anaphylaxis) and the relatively common occurrence of seizures.

There are thought to be two phases:

- Phase 1 – amniotic fluid and cells enter the maternal circulation causing the release of chemical mediators, e.g. cytokines, surfactant, prostaglandins; these cause pulmonary artery spasm and hypertension. This results in:
    - right ventricular failure
    - hypoxia
    - hypotension
    - myocardial and capillary damage.

  This phase may last up to 30 minutes.
- Phase 2 – occurs in those who survive the initial insult and may result in:
    - left ventricular failure
    - acute respiratory distress syndrome
    - disseminated intravascular coagulation
    - massive haemorrhage
    - uterine atony.

Clinical presentation

The only risk factor is an increased incidence in multiparous patients. It is most likely to present in labour or shortly after, but can occur during caesarean section, abdominal trauma and abortions. It presents acutely and signs and symptoms may include:

- acute respiratory distress
- cough
- chest pain
- pulmonary oedema
- cyanosis
- cardiac arrest
- profound hypotension
- haemorrhage/coagulopathy
- seizures
- fetal distress.

Diagnosis

It is a diagnosis of exclusion but one that should be considered in all cases of maternal cardio-respiratory collapse or massive haemorrhage in the puerperium.

Most of the tests are non-specific and are looking to confirm the signs and symptoms in the clinical presentation; these include a full blood count, coagulation studies and arterial blood gases. An ECG may show rhythm abnormalities, a chest X-ray reveal pulmonary oedema and a V/Q scan may be abnormal. An echocardiogram should be done to assess ventricular function.

In the event of a patient dying, the diagnosis is confirmed by the presence of fetal squames or lanugo hair in the pulmonary vasculature at post-mortem.

Although this supports the diagnosis of amniotic fluid embolism, it is not specific to the condition.

Management

Women with symptoms suspicious of amniotic fluid embolism should be transferred to intensive care as soon as possible, to give them a better chance of survival, and the help of experienced obstetricians, anaesthetists, intensivists and haematologists should be sought.

Treatment is entirely supportive; resuscitation starting with **A**irway, **B**reathing and **C**irculation should be commenced immediately. The patients often require:

- Intubation, ventilation, high inspired oxygen and appropriate ventiatory strategies.
- Invasive monitoring, fluid resuscitation and inotropes.
- Clotting factors and platelets, recombinant factor VII should be considered when haemorrhage is difficult to control, after discussion with the haematologist.
- If in the antepartum period, the baby should be delivered as soon as possible. If cardiac arrest occurs the baby should be delivered within 5 minutes, to optimize maternal resuscitation.
- Drugs may be required to maintain uterine tone and continuous bleeding may necessitate surgery, including hysterectomy.

Amniotic Fluid Embolism Register

All suspected cases of AFE should be reported to the National Amniotic Fluid Embolism Register at UKOSS (United Kingdom Obstetric Surveillance System), website www.npeu.ox.ac.uk/UKOSS.

Obstetric haemorrhage

Introduction

There were 17 deaths in the 2000–2002 triennium which was increased compared to the previous 3 years. The increases occurred in postpartum haemorrhages, which are becoming more common, and could be explained by: an increase in age of childbirth, more women with complex medical disorders becoming pregnant, more multiple pregnancies and an increase in caesarean section rates. Women at high risk of bleeding should be delivered where there are facilities for blood transfusion and intensive care, and plans should be made for their management.

Obstetric haemorrhage may be divided into antepartum (APH) and postpartum (PPH) haemorrhage.

Antepartum haemorrhage, defined as vaginal bleeding after 24 weeks gestation, is caused by:

- Placental abruption – premature separation of placenta from uterine wall.
- Placenta praevia – the placenta covers the internal cervical os.
- Uterine scar dehiscence.
- Vasa praevia – bleeding from fetal blood vessels that are present in the fetal membranes.

Postpartum haemorrhage, defined as blood loss >500 ml in the first 24 hours following vaginal delivery, or >1000 ml following caesarean section, is caused by:

- Uterine atony – the uterus should contract after delivery closing the large blood vessels; failure to do so results in bleeding.
- Retained tissue – results in failure of the uterus to contract properly.
- Genital tract trauma.
- Ruptured uterus.
- Broad ligament haematoma.

Signs and symptoms

Pregnant patients may not show the signs of hypovolaemia until they have lost more blood, compared with non-pregnant women, because of their increased circulating blood volume and cardiac output. However, they may also show shock that is out of proportion to the observed blood loss due to concealed bleeding.

Clotting disorders may occur in pregnancy due to:

- Patients having anticoagulation therapy.
- Pregnancy-associated thrombocytopenia.
- Pre-eclampsia (DIC and thrombocytopenia).
- Sepsis.
- Intrauterine fetal death.
- Abruption.
- Amniotic fluid embolism.

Management

Resuscitation should concentrate on **A**irway, **B**reathing and **C**irculation and then a cause should be sought. An APH usually warrants delivery of the baby; the treatment for a PPH depends on the cause and will usually be done under the direction of the obstetrician. The mainstay of PPH treatment is uterotonic agents and surgery.

The consultant haematologist and staff in the blood bank should be informed at the earliest opportunity of every major APH and PPH. Resuscitation with appropriate blood and blood products should take place and recombinant factor VIIa should be considered for cases of PPH refractory to conventional treatment.

Ovarian hyperstimulation syndrome

Definition

Ovarian hyperstimulation syndrome (OHSS) is a systemic disease caused by vasoactive factors released by hyperstimulated ovaries, as a complication of assisted conception techniques.

There is an increase in vascular permeability which results in:

- Hypovolaemia and intravascular dehydration.
- Protein-rich fluid loss into the third spaces.

Factors that put patients at risk from OHSS include:

- Less than 30 years old.
- Polycystic kidneys.
- Use of gonadotrophin-releasing hormone agonists.
- Development of multiple follicles during treatment.
- Exposure to luteinizing hormone/human chorionic gonadotrophin
- Previous OHSS.

It can occur in up to 10% of patients undergoing in vitro fertilization (IVF) but the vast majority will have no or mild problems. However, a small number of patients will go on to develop a serious form of the disease which may be classified into severe and critical.

Severe disease

- Clinical ascites (occasionally hydrothorax).
- Oliguria.
- Enlarged ovaries >12 cm.
- Raised haematocrit >45%.
- Hypoproteinaemia.

Critical disease

- Raised white cell count.
- Tense ascites.
- Significant pleural and pericardial effusions.
- Oliguria/anuria.
- Hepatorenal failure.
- Acute respiratory distress syndrome.
- Cerebral infarction.
- Thromboembolic disease.

Patients who have signs or symptoms suggestive of critical disease are best managed on a critical care unit, with a multi-disciplinary approach, led by someone who is experienced in dealing with OHSS.

Management

It is important to monitor abdominal girth, weight and fluid balance. Increasing size and positive fluid balance are signs that the condition is deteriorating.

Pain is best treated with paracetamol and opiates; non-steroidal anti-inflammatory drugs (NSAIDs) are best avoided due to the risk of precipitating acute renal failure.

Fluid balance can be a major problem and invasive monitoring may be required, the main principle is to give the minimal amount of fluid to avoid renal failure, any more than this may result in ARDS or worsening of third space fluid loss. The amount of fluid required will vary, depending on the volume status of the patient when resuscitation is commenced. The patient may present in a state of cardiovascular collapse with a haematocrit >55%. Frusemide should not be given, unless there is evidence of pulmonary oedema.

Paracentesis should be considered in the following situations: persisting oliguria or worsening renal function despite adequate filling, severe discomfort, intra-abdominal pressures >20 mmHg or respiratory compromise due to the abdominal distension. Drainage should be done under ultrasound guidance to avoid puncture of ovarian cysts and bleeding. To avoid cardiovascular collapse, the rate of ascitic fluid removal should be controlled and intravenous fluid given. A catheter may be left in situ, to reaspirate if the fluid reaccumulates. Pleural and pericardial effusions may also require draining.

Prophylaxis against thromboembolic disease should be given, usually in the form of subcutaneous low-molecular-weight heparin and full-length TED stockings.

Ovarian torsion should be considered with worsening pain, ovarian enlargement and a rising white cell count; the treatment is surgery.

Outcome

The mortality rate from OHSS is very low. All deaths related to OHSS in the UK must be reported to the Confidential Enquiry into Maternal and Child Health (CEMACH).

Sepsis

The reported rate of septic shock in all obstetric patients is approximately 1 in 8000 and the mortality rate in these patients has been quoted at 12.5%. This is much lower than the non-obstetric patient and has been attributed to:

- Lower age group.
- Fewer coexisting diseases.
- The sepsis is often pelvic in origin and therefore more amenable to surgical treatment.

The pregnant female is more susceptible to sepsis due to:

- Reduced cell-mediated immunity.
- Raised corticosteroid levels.
- Pyelonephritis – due to smooth muscle relaxation of the renal tract and a reduction in renal concentrating ability (physiological changes of pregnancy).
- Chorioamnionitis and septic abortion – due to a decrease in pH and increase in glycogen in the vaginal epithelium.
- Pneumonia – diaphragm is elevated by the gravid uterus, reducing the FRC.

Gram-negative bacilli are the most common cause of sepsis (60–80%). Obstetric causes of infection must always be considered and sought. These include:

- intra-amniotic infection.
- postpartum endometritis.
- septic abortion.
- episiotomy infection.
- septic pelvic thrombophlebitis.
- mastitis.

Clinical features

The onset of life-threatening sepsis in the pregnant woman can be insidious, with rapid deterioration, and fever may not always be present.

The early cardiovascular changes of sepsis, tachycardia, raised cardiac output and peripheral vasodilatation can be difficult to detect as they mimic the physiological changes of pregnancy. The dependence of the blood pressure during pregnancy, on an increased cardiac output, makes cardiac function vulnerable and sepsis-induced myocardial dysfunction can lead to a rapid haemodynamic collapse in pregnancy.

The likelihood of acute lung injury in the pregnant patient is increased by the reduction in plasma osmotic pressure. Once ARDS has developed the mortality rate increases to more than 30%.

The increased levels of clotting factors in pregnancy may contribute to DIC and multiple organ dysfunction syndrome.

Management

The management of sepsis in the pregnant patient follows the same principles as for managing the non-obstetric patient and is based on the Surviving Sepsis Campaign guidelines (see Chapter 15: Sepsis):

- Initial resuscitation and goal-directed therapy.
- Source control to surgically remove infection.
- Antibiotics – initially broad-spectrum which are narrowed as the organisms and sensitivities become known.
- Thromboembolism prophylaxis.
- Stress ulcer prophylaxis.

In the patient with ARDS or pneumonia, careful consideration should be given to early delivery of the baby by caesarean section, as this will result in improved compliance and oxygenation.

Key points

- Pulmonary embolism is the leading direct cause of maternal death in UK and anticoagulation should be commenced immediately if this is suspected.
- Signs of hypovolaemia in significant obstetric haemorrhage may not be apparent until late due to altered maternal physiology. Haematologist and blood bank should be notified early about the possible need of blood products.

Further reading

- Clift J, Heazell A (2007). *Obstetrics for Anaesthetists.* Cambridge: Cambridge University Press.
- Confidential Enquiry into Maternal and Child Health (2007) *Why Mothers Die 2003–2005: The Seventh Report of the Confidential Enquiries into Maternal Deaths in the United Kingdom.* London: Royal College of Obstetricians and Gynaecologists Press.

- Davies S (2001) Amniotic fluid embolism: a review of the literature. *Can. J. Anaesth.* **48**: 88–98.
- Dedhia JD, Mushambi MC (2007) Amniotic fluid embolism. *Contin. Educ. Anaesth. Crit. Care Pain* **7**: 152–6.
- Farmer JC, Guntupalli KK, Baldisseri M, Gilstrap L (2005) Critical illness of pregnancy. *Crit. Care Med.* **33**: S247–397.
- Germain S, Wyncoll D, Nelson-Piercy C (2006) Management of the critically ill obstetric patient. *Curr. Obstet. Gynaecol.* **16**: 125–33.
- Heidemann BH, McClure JH (2003) Changes in maternal physiology during pregnancy. *Contin. Educ. Anaesth. Crit. Care Pain* **3**: 65–8.
- Karalapillai D, Popham P (2007) Recombinant factor VIIa in massive postpartum haemorrhage. *Int. J. Obstet. Anaesth.* **16**: 29–34.
- Royal College of Obstetricians and Gynaecologists (2001) *Thromboembolic Disease in Pregnancy and the Puerperium: Acute Management*, Guideline No. 28. London: RCOG Press.
- Royal College of Obstetricians and Gynaecologists (2006) *The Management of Ovarian Hyperstimulation Syndrome*, Guideline No. 5. London: RCOG Press.
- Wan S, Quinlan DJ, Agnelli G, Eikelboom JW (2004) Thrombolysis compared with heparin for the initial treatment of pulmonary embolism: a meta-analysis of the randomized controlled trials. *Circulation* **110**: 744–9.

Paediatric emergencies

Nageena Hussain and Joyce Yeung

Introduction

In England and Wales, 1 in 11 children is admitted to hospital each year, representing 16% of all hospital admissions. Intensive care clinicians will only be asked to assess a very small proportion of these children who are acutely unwell. For those of us who do not work regularly with children often a big fear is of being faced with a 'sick child'.

A full coverage of paediatric intensive care is beyond the scope of this book but this chapter will aim to provide a guide on how to deal with the sick child. There is an ample number of excellent textbooks dedicated to this topic (see Further reading).

Key differences between children and adults

Weight

Children are a diverse group of people and vary in weight, size, shape and intellectual ability. It is important to determine a child's weight accurately, as most drugs and fluids are given as dose per kilogram of body weight. The Broselow Tape uses the height (measured as length) to estimate weight and is relatively easy and quick method (Fig. 46.1). If the child's age is known then the weight can be estimated using this formula:

Weight (in kg) = 2 × (age in years + 4)

Anatomical differences

Airway

The paediatric airway can present a challenge:

- In children the head is large and neck is short, tending to cause neck flexion and airway narrowing.
- Face and mandible are small and there may be loose dentition.
- The tongue is relatively large and can obstruct the airway in an unconscious child and obscure the laryngoscopy view.
- Infants less than 6 months of age are obligate nasal breathers. The narrow nasal passages are easily blocked by secretions and cause airway compromise.
- Adenotonsillar hypertrophy is common and can cause obstruction when passing endotracheal tubes.
- Epiglottis is longer and projects more posteriorly and together with higher and more anterior larynx can make tracheal intubation trickier. Straight blade laryngoscope is useful in aligning the structures.
- The cricoid ring is the narrowest part of the trachea and it is important to use uncuffed endotracheal tubes in prepubertal children as pressure from cuffs can cause oedema.
- The trachea is short and carina is relatively symmetrical making tube displacement more likely. Foreign bodies can fall into the left as well as the right main bronchus.

Breathing

Both upper and lower airways are smaller and easily obstructed. As resistance of flow is inversely proportional to fourth power of the radius of the lumen, a smaller airway has large impact on airway resistance.

Children rely more on diaphragmatic breathing and can be prone to fatigue in respiratory distress.

Circulation

The circulating blood volume is 70–80 ml/kg and higher than in the adult, but the actual volume is small. A small amount of blood loss can be significant to the child.

Core Topics in Critical Care Medicine, eds. Fang Gao Smith and Joyce Yeung. Published by Cambridge University Press.

Table 46.1 Some physiological parameters in children

Age (years)	Heart rate (beats/ min)	Respiratory rate (breaths/ min)	Systolic BP (mmHg)
<1	110–160	30–40	70–90
1–2	100–150	25–35	80–95
2–5	95–140	25–30	80–90
5–12	80–120	20–25	90–110
>12	60–100	15–20	100–120

Source: Adapted from *Advanced Paediatric Life Support Manual*, 4th edn (2003).

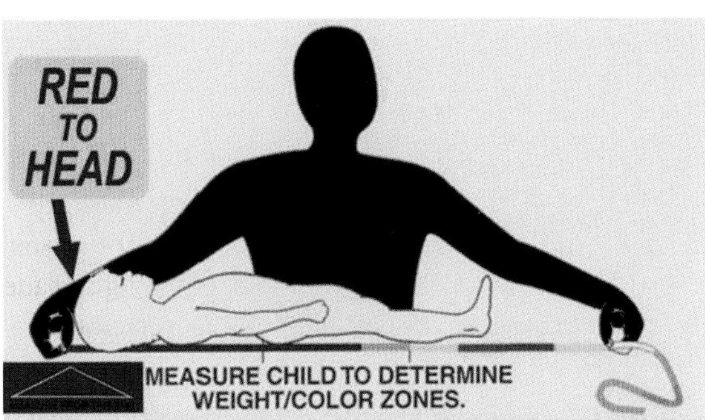

Fig. 46.1 Broselow Tape. (Courtesy of Armstrong Medical Industries Inc.)

Body surface area

Children have a higher body surface area to volume ratio, leading to a higher metabolic rate to cope with higher heat loss, and they are more susceptible to hypothermia.

Physiological differences

Some of the key parameters are summarized in Table 46.1.

Respiratory

Children have a higher respiratory rate to cope with a higher metabolic rate and oxygen consumption. The chest wall in children is more compliant and intrathoracic pressures are less negative and end expiratory lung volume can encroach on closing volume.

Cardiovascular

Infants have smaller heart and lower stroke volume resulting in a higher heart rate. Cardiac output is directly related to heart rate and stroke volume is relatively fixed; fluid loss is poorly tolerated. As the heart grows bigger and stroke volume increases, heart rate is lower in older children. Systemic vascular resistance rises from birth into adulthood resulting in higher blood pressure with age.

Recognizing the sick child

With the arrival of a sick child, there are also worried parents and distressed relatives. Healthcare staff can also be more emotional as the patient is a child but it is important to remember that basic principles should be applied to stabilize the child until more experienced help arrives.

Children cannot voice their complaints and do not present like adults. History can be vague or simply nothing more than 'not feeding', or 'not being their usual self'. Young children who become ill will stop their normal daily activities and become irritable, clingy and/or sleepier. Parents can provide an invaluable insight into the behaviour of their child and a detailed birth and developmental history should also be asked to identify any possible causes. Parents should be allowed to stay with the child if they want to and this can often help to pacify the child.

The seriously ill child can present with shock, respiratory distress, drowsiness, fitting or as a surgical emergency. Some common causes are listed in Table 46.2.

Approach to paediatric emergencies

Preparation

When asked to assess a sick child, or while waiting to receive a sick child, it is advisable to start with basic calculations in order to prepare for interventions needed for the child's airway, breathing and circulation to minimize mistakes. Drug doses can be calculated beforehand and can be diluted into 10 ml syringes (e.g. 10 mg per ml of suxamethonium) making it easier to give small doses (Table 46.3). Pre-drawn syringes of 0.9% saline to use as flushes can also be helpful.

Appropriate equipment needs to be available for different sizes of children. Most emergency departments and paediatric wards now have weight-specific

Table 46.2 Main modes of presentation of serious illness in children and their causes

Presentation	Causes	Conditions
Shock	Hypovolaemia	Dehydration, gastroenteritis Diabetic ketoacidosis Blood loss, trauma
	Maldistribution of fluid	Septicaemia, anaphylaxis
	Cardiogenic	Arrhythmias, heart failure
Respiratory distress	Upper airway obstruction	Croup, epiglottitis Foreign body, trauma
	Lower airway disorders	Asthma, bronchiolitis, pneumonia
Drowsy/fitting	Post ictal	Status epilepticus
	Infection	Meningitis/ encephalitis
	Metabolic	DKA, hypoglycaemia, electrolyte disturbances
	Head injury	Trauma, non-accidental injury
	Drug/ poisoning	
Surgical emergencies	Acute abdomen	Appendicitis, peritonitis

Table 46.3 Preparations and calculations of drugs for children

Important initial calculations
Weight – (age + 4) × 2 in kg
ET tube size – age/4 + 4 (ensure one size above and below is available)
ET tube at lips – age/2 + 12 cm
Fluids – 20 ml/kg in critically ill (Hartmann's solution or 0.9% saline)
Glucose – 5 ml/kg 10% dextrose
Energy for defibrillation – 4 J/kg
Adrenaline – 10 μg/kg
Atropine – 20 μg/kg
Additional calculations
ETT length at nose – age/2 + 15cm
LMA – size 1: up to 5 kg, size 1.5: 5–10 kg, size 2: 10–20 kg, size 2.5: 20–30 kg, size 3: 30–50 kg
Suxamethonium (intubating dose) – 2 μg/kg
Propofol (induction dose) – 5 mg/kg

sets available which contain all resuscitation equipment for a child of a particular size. Suitable airway equipment should also include face masks, Ambubags and paediatric anaesthetic circuits.

Parental support

Care of the sick child is stressful for all those concerned. Remember to consider the parents at this time and keep them as well informed as you can. It is kind to spare a member of staff if possible to be with them during the initial resuscitation phase, someone who can answer their questions, offer support and ensure they don't inadvertently hinder the medical team.

Cardio-respiratory arrest in children

Cardiac arrests in children are rarely due to primary cardiac disease but are usually secondary to hypoxia caused by respiratory pathology. This differs from adults where the cause of cardiac arrest is often cardiac. Respiratory arrests can occur secondary to neurological dysfunction caused by events such as convulsions. But whatever the cause, the child would have suffered a period of respiratory insufficiency, which will have caused hypoxia and metabolic acidosis. Cell damage and death takes place in sensitive organs such as brain, liver and kidneys before eventual myocardial damage results in cardiac arrests.

Outcome of cardiac arrest in children is invariably poor and neurological deficits are common in survivors. Early recognition of seriously ill children and prevention of cardiac arrests are the key to improved outcome in children.

In the event of a cardiac arrest, all advanced paediatric resuscitation is organized within one algorithm (Fig. 46.2) except in the newborn. From puberty the adult algorithm is used. For most up-to-date advanced paediatric life support, please refer to resuscitation guidelines issued by Advanced Paediatric Life Support Group.

The main differences when assessing and resuscitating the child compared to an adult are outlined below.

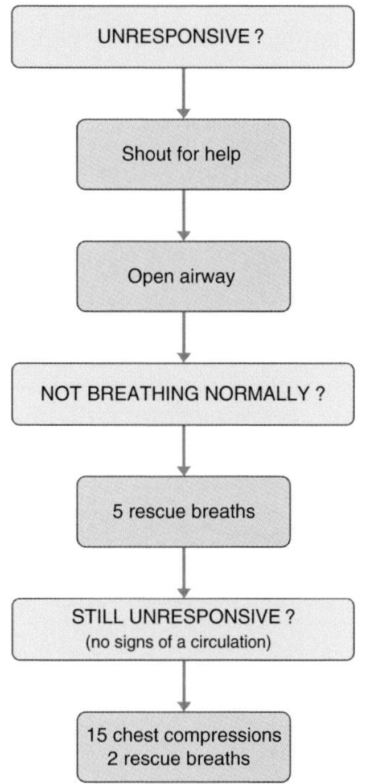

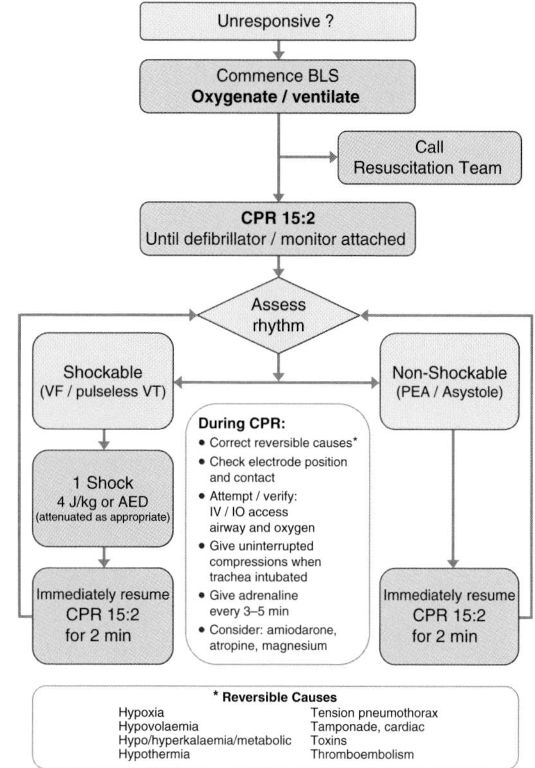

Fig. 46.2 Paediatric Basic Life Support and Advanced Life Support Algorithm.

Airway and breathing

- Start the assessment by a thorough clinical examination while looking for stridor, wheeze and signs of increased work of breathing, use of accessory muscles and sternal recession.
- If urgent intervention is needed, appropriate help from the anaesthetic consultant and an experienced ODP should be available.
- In airway obstruction, an inhalational induction in the operating theatre with the back-up of a senior ENT surgeon scrubbed up is the safest environment for endotracheal intubation in such children.
- Correct endotracheal placement should always be checked by auscultation, with capnography and chest radiograph.
- When placing the paediatric patient onto a ventilator, inadvertently high settings can cause barotraumas to the airway and this must be avoided. Pressure control ventilation is preferable, and the aim is for tidal volumes of 7–10 ml/kg initially.
- Once the patient is intubated and ventilated, ensure sedation is started promptly and a common combination is morphine and midazolam infusions.

Circulation

- When assessing central pulse, a different location is used in different age groups: brachial pulse in an infant, carotid pulse in those aged over 1 year.
- For external chest compressions, hands should be placed in the centre of the chest and depth should be one-third of chest diameter. In a large child, both hands are used; in a small child, just the heel of one hand; but in an infant, two thumbs with hands around the thorax will provide sufficient strength.
- Cardiovascular collapse in children can occur at lightning speed especially in sepsis or anaphylaxis. This can cause difficulties with gaining intravenous access and an intra-osseous needle is ideal in these situations (Fig. 46.3). Sites for insertion are the anterior surface of the tibia below the tibial

tuberosity or the distal femur proximal the lateral condyle. Once fluid resuscitation is under way, peripheral access can then often be easily placed. Some resuscitation drugs, and in particular adrenaline can be given via the endotracheal tube; with the increasing use of intra-osseous needles this if often unnecessary.

- Invasive central lines are best left for those experienced in siting them in children. However with the advent of ultrasound-guided line insertion central venous and arterial lines can be sited much more safely. The femoral CVC line is ideal in an emergency with less risk associated, but care must be taken to stay below the inguinal ligament in smaller children.
- Arterial lines are placed in the same locations as for adults but vessels vary in size and smaller arterial cannulae may be required.
- Fluid challenges of 20 ml/kg of crystalloid are used for resuscitation. Inotropes may need to be started in any child who does not respond to a third fluid challenge at this point seek advice from the local paediatric intensive care unit. Care must be taken with the doses and dilution of the drugs. Inotropes should ideally be given centrally but can be given peripherally if needed while waiting for central access.

DEFG – don't ever forget glucose

If blood glucose is <3 mmol then give 5 ml/kg of 10% dextrose to treat hypoglycaemia.

Common paediatric emergencies

Shock

Children are susceptible to fluid loss because they require higher fluid intake per kilogram of body weight than adults due to a higher surface area to volume ratio and higher basal metabolic rate (Table 46.3).

Clinical features

Children have good compensatory physiological mechanisms to maintain organ perfusion. In early, compensated shock, blood pressure is maintained by increased heart rate and respiratory rate. Blood flow is redistributed from venous reserve volume and diverted from non-essential organs. A fall in blood pressure is a late sign and the decompensation will lead to increasing lactic acidosis (Table 46.4).

Table 46.3 Fluid requirements in children

Body weight	Fluid requirement/ 24 hr	Volume/kg per hour
First 10 kg	100 ml/kg	4 ml/kg
Second 10 kg	50 ml/kg	2 ml/kg
Each subsequent kg	20 ml/kg	1 ml/kg

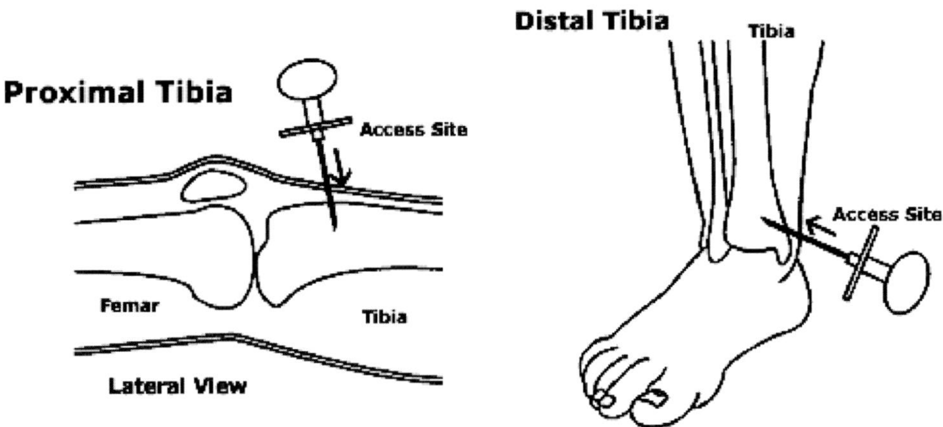

Fig. 46.3 Intra-osseous needle placement in children – proximal tibia and distal tibia.

Table 46.4 Signs of shock in children

Early (compensated)	Late (decompensated)
↑HR ↑RR	Kussmaul breathing
↓Skin turgor, sunken eyes and fontanelle	↓HR
CRT >2 s	Confusion
Pale, mottled skin	Oliguria
↓Urine output	↓BP

Management

Bolus of 20 ml/kg of 0.9% saline is recommended as first-line treatment of shock in children, with blood being used in trauma. If the child does not improve quickly after fluid bolus and there is worsening acidosis, a paediatric intensive care unit should be contacted and the child may need to be transferred. Patient should be intubated and mechanical ventilation started if in respiratory failure. Invasive blood pressure monitoring and inotropic support should be commenced to maintain organ perfusion.

Croup

Viral croup accounts for over 95% of laryngotracheal infections in children. The commonest causes include parainfluenza virus, metapneumovirus, respiratory syncytial virus and influenza. The peak incidence is in the second year of life but croup can occur from 6 months to 6 years of age. The infection causes mucosal inflammation and increased secretions affecting the upper airway. The oedema of the subglottic area can result in critical narrowing in the airway of a child.

Clinical features

The onset of symptoms is over a couple of days with preceding cold symptoms. A typical child will have a loud barking cough but there is no drooling of saliva and the child is able to drink. On examination, harsh, rasping stridor can be heard.

Management

When there is only minor airway obstruction, stridor and chest recession disappears when the child is at rest. Children with mild croup can be managed at home with parents monitoring their symptoms. Oral steroids (dexamethasone, prednisolone) and nebulized budesonide or adrenaline can reduce severity and duration of croup.

Pseudomembraneous croup (bacterial tracheitis)

This is a rare infection caused by *Staphylococcus aureus* or *Haemophilus influenzae*. Clinical features are similar to viral croup but the patient will also be septic with progressive airway obstruction. In 80% of children with bacterial tracheitis, severe respiratory distress occurs and these children should be intubated and given ventilatory support. Treatment is by intravenous antibiotics (combination of flucloxacillin and cefotaxime).

Acute epiglottitis

Incidence of epiglottitis has declined since the advent of HiB vaccines but cases still occur in vaccine failure and unimmunized children. Infection with HiB causes intense swelling of the epiglottis and causes airway obstruction. It is most common in 1–6 year olds but can also occur in infants and adults.

Clinical features

There is acute onset of illness with fever, lethargy, inspiratory stridor and respiratory distress. In contrast to croup, cough is minimal or absent. The typical child looks toxic and pale, and will sit immobile with saliva drooling, unable to swallow fluids or speak. The child must not be disturbed, for example to examine the throat or place an intravenous cannula, as this may provoke complete airway obstruction.

Management

Urgent arrangement should be made to intubate and secure the airway by senior anaesthetic staff with the back-up of intensive care and ENT surgeon. After securing the airway, blood cultures should be taken and intravenous antibiotics such as cefuroxime started. Extubation can usually take place after 24 hours but antibiotics should be continued for 3–5 days.

Bronchiolitis

Bronchiolitis is the commonest serious respiratory infection in infancy, occurring in 10% of all infants with 2–3% being admitted to hospital each year. The majority are under 1 year old and it is rare in children over 1 year old. In 80% of cases, RSV is the causative pathogen, with parainfluenza, influenza and adenoviruses causing the remaining cases.

Clinical features

Parents often complain of feeding difficulties and the child typically has coryzal symptoms preceding cough and increasing breathing difficulties. There may be fever, clear nasal discharge and wheezing. Recurrent apnoea is serious and can be potentially fatal especially in premature infants. Those at risk of developing respiratory failure are those with pre-existing chronic lung problems (e.g. cystic fibrosis), congenital heart disease and immune deficiency syndromes. Chest X-ray shows hyperinflation with flattening of diaphragm due to small airways obstruction and gas trapping.

Management

Management is supportive with supplementary humidified oxygen and close monitoring for apnoea. Nebulized bronchodilators have been used for symptomatic relief but their use does not reduce severity or duration of illness. Fluids maybe needed to be given nasogastrically or intravenously if there is feeding difficulties.

Status epilepticus

Status epilepticus is a seizure that lasts 30 min or longer, or when the patient does not recover consciousness in between successive seizures (see Chapter 39: Status epilepticus).

Management

After assessment of ABC, the priority is to terminate seizure. A typical protocol is shown in Fig. 46.4.

Non-accidental injury

All healthcare professionals have a responsibility to be alert to children who are endangered or abused. If child abuse is suspected, a consultant paediatrician with experience in dealing with child abuse should be alerted to conduct a further assessment of the child.

Presentation of physical abuse

- Head injuries – fractures, intracranial injury
- Fractures of long bones
  - Single fracture with multiple bruises
  - Multiple fractures in different stages of healing
  - Metaphyseal or epiphyseal injuries, often multiple
- Fractured ribs, spinal injuries
- Internal injuries, e.g. ruptured bowel
- Burns and scalds
- Cold injury – frostbite, hypothermia
- Poisoning
- Cuts and bruises – imprint of hands, sticks, belts can sometimes be seen.

Stabilizing the child for retrieval

In the UK, there is an excellent network of paediatric intensive care units (PICUs) which provide tertiary care of the critically ill child. They are an excellent source of advice and when a child is critically ill and requires transfer to a PICU, a retrieval team is normally sent to retrieve the child from the referring hospital. Effective preparation and planning is paramount to the safe transport of ill children.

The referral team should ensure good communication in organizing the transfer. The following should be discussed with receiving hospital. Advice can be obtained from receiving hospital and the retrieval team should be advised about the condition of the child. Parents should be informed about any plans at all times and reasons for transfer should be explained clearly. Joint management by the referring and receiving hospital should start immediately with the goal of managing the child effectively and safely until the retrieval team arrives. Whilst initial resuscitation responsibility lies with referring hospital, the retrieval team is responsible for bringing the necessary equipment and drugs.

All patients should have the following monitored prior to transfer:

- Heart rate and rhythm with ECG monitor.
- Oxygen saturation with pulse oximetry.
- Core and skin temperature with low-reading thermometer.
- Blood pressure with non-invasive monitor.
- Urine output with urinary catheter.
- Arterial pH and gases with arterial blood sample.
- CO_2 monitoring with capnography.
- Some patients will require invasive blood pressure and central venous pressure monitoring and/or intracranial pressure monitoring.

Airway and breathing

- Intubation should be maintained and monitored by capnography.

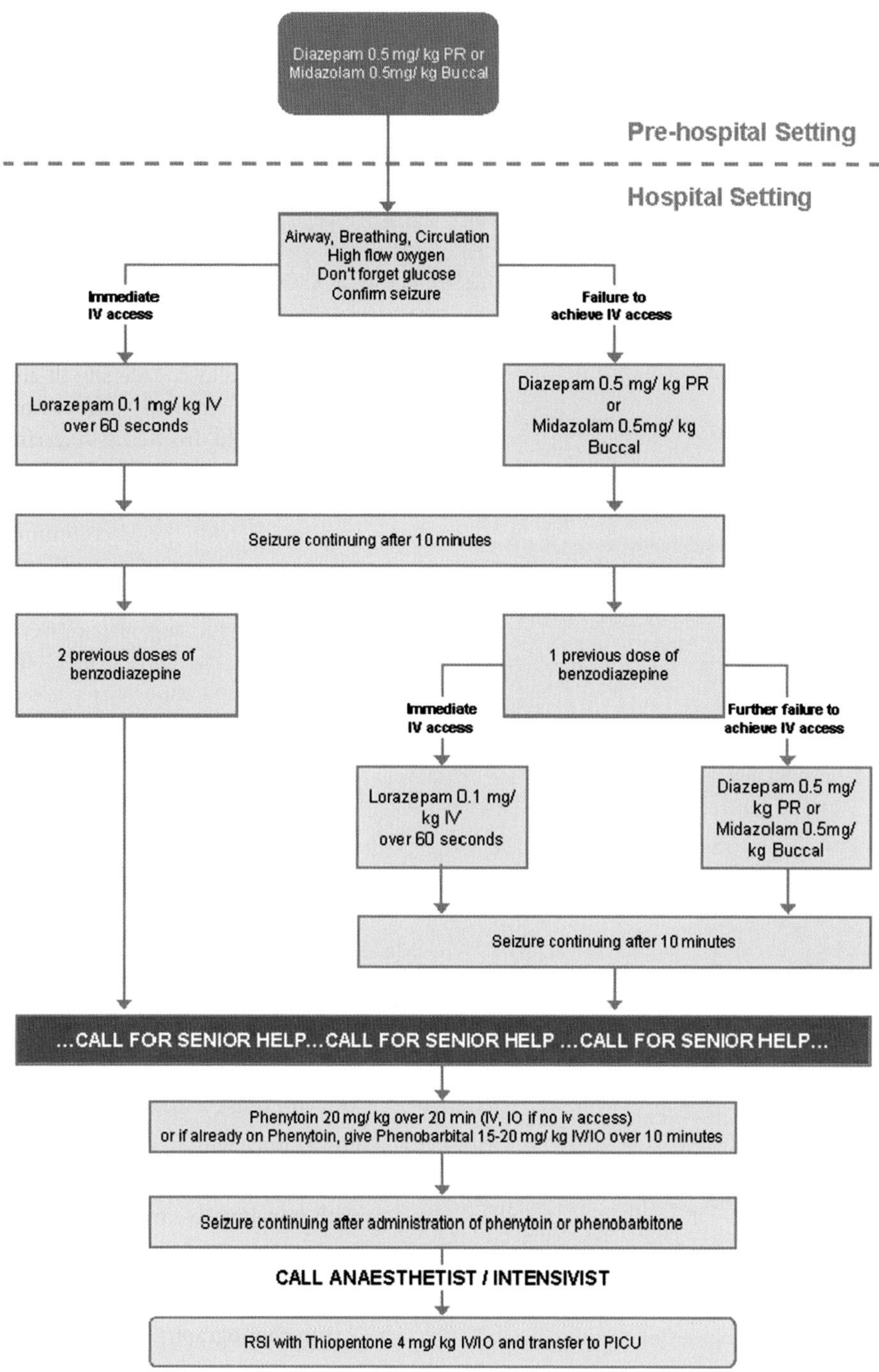

Fig. 46.4 Management protocol for children with status epilepticus. (Adapted from Chin RF *et al.* (2006) NLSTEPSS Collaborative Group. *Lancet* **368**, 222–9.)

- Endotracheal tube should be well secured with particular attention to length and position prior to transfer.
- Ventilation setting adjusted to keep PCO_2 <5.0 kPa and SaO_2 >95%.
- Suction must be available for the duration of transfer.
- Ample appropriate analgesic, sedative and muscle relaxant drugs should be available.
- Oxygen cylinders should be full and working.

Circulation

- If signs of poor perfusion are present, fluid boluses and inotropic support may need to be started to maintain normal arterial pH and oxygenation.
- Correct electrolyte disturbances and hypoglycaemia.
- Two good intravenous accesses are minimum.

Disability/exposure

- Blankets should be used to cover exposed areas and ambient temperature in transport vehicle should be warm.

Key points

- It is important to have senior help from anaesthesia, paediatrics and sometimes ENT in dealing with paediatric emergencies.
- Children are not small adults and have significant differences in their anatomy such as airway, and their cardiovascular and respiratory physiology.
- Outcome from cardiac arrests in children is poor and the emphasis should be on the recognition of the sick child and prevention of cardiac arrests.
- Preparation is the key to dealing with paediatric emergencies and drug dosages and equipment sizes should be calculated based on weight estimates prior to arrival of child whenever possible.
- Management of paediatric emergencies are mainly supportive with regular monitoring as the condition of a child can deteriorate quickly.
- No child should be transferred until they are stable. Close teamwork with the retrieval team will ensure a safe and smooth transfer.

Further reading

- Advanced Paediatric Life Support (2009) *UK Resuscitation Guidelines*. www.resus.org.uk
- Association of Paediatric Anaesthetists, Royal College of Anaesthetists and Royal College of Paediatrics and Child Health (2007) *Child Protection and the Anaesthetist: Safeguarding Children in the Operating Theatre*. London: RCOA, APA, RCPCH.
- Lissauer T, Clayden G (2007) *Illustrated Textbook of Paediatrics*, 3rd edn. London: Mosby Elsevier.

Section IV Chapter 47

Examinations

Core areas required for UK/European Diploma examinations

Zahid Khan

Introduction

The passing of a postgraduate examination in intensive care medicine (ICM) identifies the successful individual to all as someone who has been trained to a high standard in ICM. The knowledge required to thrive in clinical practice as well as examinations in ICM is broad based involving most hospital speciality areas. The candidate also needs to have thorough grounding in the basic sciences, clinical measurement and care of the critically ill including multiple organ support. Those gaining their training in the UK are increasingly sitting the Intercollegiate Diploma in Intensive Care Medicine (DICM) whilst others decide to sit the European Diploma in Intensive Care Medicine (EDIC) and some attempt to sit both examinations. The EDIC examination is increasing in popularity in Europe and internationally. Those who have completed their training in Australia or New Zealand may be eligible to sit the Joint Faculty of Intensive Care Medicine (JFICM) examination. In the US, a number of specialist societies run board examinations in ICM and in Ireland there is the Diploma of the Irish Board of Intensive Care Medicine (DIBICM).

Intercollegiate Diploma in Intensive Care Medicine

The DICM aims both to strengthen speciality status of intensive care and to improve the position of ICM doctors in the UK. The DICM institutes a body of knowledge, upholds high standards of training and acts as a prize for the most dedicated candidates.

Regulations

(1) The candidate must possess a postgraduate medical qualification in a primary speciality, e.g. MRCP, FRCS, FRCA or their equivalent.

(2) Candidates should be registered with the Intercollegiate Board of Training in Intensive Care Medicine (IBTICM) for training in ICM and have satisfactorily completed the intermediate training programme or another equivalent training programme acceptable to the IBTICM. Advice on appropriate experience and training available in each region can be obtained from the Regional Advisors in Intensive Care Medicine (RA) and Intercollegiate Board Tutors. The IBTICM administrative office provides guidance for overseas candidates.

(3) The application process is in two stages.

  (a) Firstly, a dissertation or high degree thesis summary is submitted; if this is approved then an application form for the examination is issued and the approval will stand for the next four sittings of the examination. The dissertation summary can be submitted at any time from September 2008 to the Board of Examiners. The Board will respond with their decision on the summary within 2 weeks.

  (b) Candidates must then submit hard copies of their dissertation and ten expanded case summaries.

(4) Diploma examiners can use their discretion to excuse the dissertation viva for those candidates with a higher degree in a subject relevant to ICM.

(5) The oral examination currently takes place annually in June but will become biannual with a November sitting from 2009.

Format of examination

There are three components to the examination: the dissertation, the oral examination and the expanded case summaries.

Core Topics in Critical Care Medicine, eds. Fang Gao Smith and Joyce Yeung. Published by Cambridge University Press.

The dissertation

The presentation of a 4,000 to 6,000 word dissertation on an ICM-related topic is an essential part of the examination. This commonly consists of a critical review of an intensive care related topic, an audit project or original intensive care research. Detailed guidance on how to prepare and layout the dissertation and the assessment criteria are available from the IBTICM. The RA will be able to offer counsel on the examination overall, the suitability of subjects for the dissertation and certify that appropriate training has been achieved. The submitted dissertation is reviewed by the two examiners who will conduct the oral examination. If the dissertation is found to be unsatisfactory then the candidate will not be invited to the remaining sections of the examination. It is advisable to work with local tutors familiar with examination to ensure that the dissertation is of an acceptable standard.

Oral examination

Those candidates deemed to have produced a satisfactory dissertation will be invited to attend the four-part oral examination. In all parts of the oral examination, one of the examiners will start the examination whilst the other takes notes and halfway through they will exchange roles. The examiners will each assess and mark the viva independently based on the candidate's performance and then jointly agree on a common mark.

(1) The first part of the examination is the viva based on the dissertation which consists of a discussion with two examiners for 45 minutes (this may be reduced to 30 minutes at the next sitting).

(2) The second oral examination is divided into two parts:

(a) First part is based on the ten expanded case summaries completed by trainees undertaking the IBTICM training programme. Candidates who are not in the IBTICM programme will need to produce ten case summaries for the use of entry to the examination. The case summaries should be about 1000 words long and contain no more than five references. They should consist of a selection of different cases from which a specific lesson about management has been learnt or a new modality has been used. Their format should be divided into the clinical problem, relevant management, discussion on the relevant literature and lessons learnt. Two different examiners will discuss the expanded case summaries with the candidate for 30 minutes. The discussion may focus on any aspect of the submitted case summaries including critical appraisal of the available literature, data interpretation and management.

(b) The second part tests the candidate's approach to clinical diagnosis, investigation and management of a given scenario. The candidate is given 10 minutes to read and formulate thoughts on a written clinical scenario. Two different examiners will then conduct a 30-minute oral examination with discussion around the clinical scenario followed by questions on up to three short cases. The short cases will include data commonly seen on intensive care units, e.g. electrocardiographs, X-rays and blood results and the candidates will be asked to discuss any findings.

(3) The third and fourth oral examinations will each last 30 minutes with two different sets of examiners. The questions for each will be structured and based on predetermined domains (see Table 47.1). All candidates will receive the same questions to ensure fairness and reliability of the examination.

The examination from 2009 will become modular with candidates being able to make an application in respect of dissertation alone (module 1) or combined with the expanded case summaries (module 2). Failure in module 1 or the combined modules will prohibit the candidate from the rest of the oral examinations. Success in module 1 will stand for the next four sittings of the examination.

The successful candidate will have submitted a satisfactory dissertation, satisfied the examiners in the viva and passed at least two of the subsequent three oral examinations.

European Diploma in Intensive Care Medicine

The EDIC examination is being taken in increasing numbers and is now widely accepted. It has grown from the 40 candidates who sat the examination in 1981 to 300-plus candidates who annually sit the examination today. The examination is also more accessible with additional venues such as Switzerland, Netherlands and Malaysia as well as during the European Society of

Table 47.1 Domains for structured oral examinations

Pathophysiology	**Ethics/management**
Cardiovascular	Patient rights/ withholding and withdrawing therapy
Respiratory	Scoring systems/ audit/ outcome prediction
Renal/ splanchnic/ liver	Design/ infection control
Neurological	Budgeting
Haematology	Progressive patient care/ outreach
Sepsis	Communication
Multiple organ failure	Brain death and organ donation
Hypothermia	
Obstetric emergencies	
Treatment	**Diagnosis**
Cardiovascular/ respiratory/ renal support	Imaging
CNS injury and disease	Laboratory
Pancreatitis	Electrophysiological
Liver failure	Organ function testing
Obstetric emergencies	
Hypothermia	
Sepsis	
Poisoning	
Sedation/ analgesia/ paralysis	
Nutritional support	
Equipment/clinical measurement	**Current trends/controversies**
Monitoring organ function	
Principles of measurement	
Equipment for organ support	
Monitoring: design, specification and ergonomics	

Intensive Care Medicines (ESICM) annual congress. The ESICM's education and training committee are responsible for the conduct of the EDIC examination. The principle objective of EDIC is to promote quality standards in education and intensive care medicine across Europe.

Regulations

(1) Candidates for the EDIC part 1 examination must be enrolled in a primary speciality training programme. The primary speciality can be anaesthesia, medicine, surgery, emergency medicine, paediatrics or intensive care medicine.

(2) The candidates must have satisfactorily completed 12 months of intensive care medicine experience and this may include no more than 6 months of complementary training. Complementary training involves training in acute medical care of patients in a speciality other than the candidate's primary speciality. Confirmatory evidence of satisfactory training must be submitted with the application for the EDIC examination.

(3) The candidate can progress to the EDIC part 2 examination if they have been successful in the EDIC part 1 examination and have completed 24 months of dedicated supervised full-time training in intensive care medicine. Complementary training can make up no more than 6 months of this training. Those who have completed training can sit the EDIC if they have a regular substantive commitment to intensive care medicine and must be able provide confirmatory evidence.

Format of examination

The EDIC examination is divided into two parts.

EDIC part 1 examination

Part 1 consists of a 3-hour examination with 100 multiple choice (MCQ) trunk questions each with 4–5 stems in English. The questions encompass all aspects of intensive care medicine including clinical practice, basic medical sciences, pathophysiology, diseases seen in ICM, complications, data interpretation, therapeutics, toxicology and ethics. The questions blueprint is seen in Table 47.2. The questions are divided equally into type A and type K:

- 50 type A questions have 5 options of which only one is correct.
- 50 type K questions have 4 options each of which requires an individual response of true or false.

There is no negative marking and the pass mark is set after each examination based on the mean value scored by the cohort and 0.6 standard deviation. In the 2007 sitting of the examination the pass mark was set at >56

Table 47.2 EDIC part 1 MCQ content blueprint

Blueprint topic	Combined number of questions
Cardiovascular	12
Respiratory	16
Neurocritical care	10
Gastrointestinal/ nutrition	8
Renal	4
Urology/ obstetrics	4
Endocrine/ metabolic	4
Bleeding/ coagulation	4
Oncology	4
Poisoning/ pharmacology	8
Severe infection/ sepsis	10
Surgery/trauma	6
Ethics/ law/ quality	4
ICM management	4
Transplantation	2
Total	**100**

points and 73% of the candidates were successful. Three attempts are allowed at the examination with 12-month intervals.

EDIC part 2 examination

The EDIC part 2 examination consists of a clinical and oral examination conducted in English or another language subject to availability of approved centre.

- The candidate will be asked to examine a major case for 30 minutes. The major case can be of a patient with a range of clinical problems, e.g. multiple organ failure, acute lung injury.
- Two or three short cases are discussed over 15 minutes, e.g. brainstem testing, examining cardiovascular system for signs or demonstrating equipment. The candidates will be assessed on their ability to elicit accurate comprehensive and relevant clinical information to form a differential diagnosis and to present this coherently. The candidates' approach to the patient, professionalism, compassion and due regard for patient dignity will also be assessed. The candidate must demonstrate consideration to other members of staff, local infection control and isolation procedures. The candidate will be observed examining more than one patient in the clinical setting by the examiners.
- The oral component of the examination will last 30 to 40 minutes and can be divided into two separate sessions. The oral examination may include clinical scenarios, ethical dilemmas, recent research and data interpretation including blood gases, biochemistry, imaging, electrocardiograms and equipment.

Part 2 of EDIC is usually sat within 24 months of passing the part 1 examination and no more than 4 years later. Two initial attempts are allowed to pass the examination followed by a 12-month interval before two further attempts are allowed. The candidates must obtain a pass mark in both components of the part 2 examination. The examiners may use their discretion to compensate a borderline fail in one component of the examination by an excellent pass in the other component. The EDIC is awarded after successful completion of part 2 of the examination provided base speciality specialist status has been achieved.

Examination preparation

Success in professional examinations requires a substantial investment of time. With conflicting demands of work and life, the candidate must allow sufficient time before sitting the examination and generally 6 to 12 months is recommended.

Meetings and conferences

Candidates preparing for examinations must avail themselves of all the educational opportunities at local, regional and national levels in ICM.

- Annual international congresses e.g. ESICM, Society of Critical Care Medicine (SCCM), each will normally have pre-congress educational courses as well as educational/continuing professional development sessions during the congress. The SCCM and American College of Chest Physicians run a Combined Critical Care Course to provide a multi-disciplinary review and preparation for the ICM Board examinations annually. The SCCM also provides a refresher course at its annual congress.
- In the UK, there are many specialist society ICM meetings, e.g. Intensive Care Society, some on

general topics and others on more specific topics that are held annually.

- The ESICM has a refresher course that takes place annually at its congress as preparation for the EDIC examination.

Literature

It is worth investing in one current standard textbook in intensive care medicine, e.g. *Oh's Intensive Care Manual*.

It is important for candidates to be aware of the current ICM literature, e.g. important papers related to ICM over the last 10 years in journals such as *New England Journal of Medicine, Critical Care Medicine* and *Intensive Care Medicine*. *Current Opinion in Critical Care* has detailed review articles on set topics in every bimonthly issue which are repeated annually. *Intensive Care Monitor* offers bimonthly reviews of the current literature with comments.

Electronic resources

- The ESICM primary educational resource and curriculum for the EDIC examination is its Patient-Centred Acute Care Training (PACT) distance learning programme. PACT consists of 44 modules which are available in hardcopy and electronically.
- ESICM's CoBaTriCE programme lists the core competencies required by those training in ICM. Candidates who have registered for the EDIC can get access to 35 MCQs recently used in EDIC examinations. Candidates can answer the questions online and get instant feedback on their performance; this offers invaluable experience on the difficulty and type of questions that will be encountered.

Useful websites

The internet offers a wealth of useful websites relating to ICM and all can be used to prepare for diploma examinations. A number are listed below:

- ESICM.org
- IBTICM.org
- SCCM Resident ICU
- The Evidence-Based Medicine Group of the Scottish Intensive Care Society
- Critical Care UK
- Emcrit.org

Key points

- Preparation for the diploma examinations requires a lot of time and effort to be successful.
- Preparation for diploma examinations will extend your ICM knowledge.
- Passing one of the diploma examinations marks you out as a holder of a credible qualification in ICM.

Further reading

- Dorman T, Angood PB, Angus DC (2004) Guidelines for critical care medicine training and continuing medical education. *Crit. Care Med.* **32**: 263–72.
- Fink M, Hayes M, Soni N (2003) *Classic Papers in Critical Care*. Chipping Norton, UK: Bladon Medical Publishing.
- Marini JJ, Wheeler AP (2006) *Critical Care Medicine: The Essentials*, 3rd edn. Philadelphia, PA: Lippincott Williams & Wilkins.
- Venkatesh B, Morgan TJ, Joyce CJ, Townsend SC (2003) *Data Interpretation in Critical Care Medicine*. Philadelphia, PA: Butterworth Heinemann.

Examples of mock MCQs and viva questions

Zahid Khan

Multiple choice questions

(1) Venous pressure increases in which of the following conditions:
- (A) Diabetic ketoacidosis
- (B) Medullary lesions
- (C) Obstructive airways disease
- (D) Opiate intoxication
- (E) Acute pulmonary embolus

(2) A 55-year-old farmer is admitted with suspected tetanus following an accident. Which of the following statements about tetanus is true:
- (A) Confers life-long immunity
- (B) Always causes muscular rigidity
- (C) Bacillus toxin may pass along sympathetic nerve fibres causing over-activity
- (D) Has approximately 50% mortality worldwide
- (E) Is caused by a gram-positive bacillus which will only grow in anaerobic conditions

(3) Specific antidotes exist for which of the following poisons:
- (A) Barbiturates
- (B) Phenol
- (C) Organophosphorus compounds
- (D) Aspirin
- (E) Cyanides

(4) A 45-year-old patient is being enterally fed via a nasogastric tube. Which of the following complications may occur:
- (A) Deficiency of fatty acids
- (B) Hyperglycaemia
- (C) Elevated circulating concentrations of potassium and phosphate
- (D) Constipation
- (E) Oesophagitis resulting from tube insertion

(5) A 65-year-old alcoholic patient is admitted with acute hepatic encephalopathy. Which of the following statements is true:
- (A) Protein should be withdrawn completely from his diet
- (B) EEG changes may be helpful in diagnosis
- (C) The presence of flapping tremor is diagnostic
- (D) Symptoms may be precipitated by dieresis
- (E) The degree of mental disturbance is closely related to the blood ammonia level

(6) A 50-year-old patient is admitted with acute pancreatitis. She may develop which of the following features:
- (A) Hypoxia
- (B) Tender lesions on her shins
- (C) Hyponatraemia
- (D) Hyperglycaemia
- (E) Obstructive jaundice

(7) A 60-year-old man presents to the emergency department with massive haemoptysis. Recognized causes include:
- (A) Pneumococcal lobar pneumonia
- (B) Cavitating tuberculosis
- (C) Acute pulmonary oedema
- (D) Goodpasture's syndrome
- (E) Carcinoma of the bronchus

(8) Non-cardiogenic pulmonary oedema is found with which of the following conditions:
- (A) Ketoacidosis
- (B) Head injury
- (C) Oxygen toxicity
- (D) Nitrofurantoin therapy
- (E) Paracetamol overdose

(9) A 52-year-old lady is admitted as an emergency with a thyrotoxic crisis. Which of the following does treatment include:
- (A) Administration of iodide

Core Topics in Critical Core Medicine, eds. Fang Gao Smith and Joyce Yeung. Published by Cambridge University Press.

(B) Immediate administration of propylthiouracil
(C) Administration of beta-blocker
(D) Keeping the patient warm
(E) High dose of dexamethasone

(10) A serum calcium of 3 mmol/l is compatible with which of the following conditions:
(A) Sarcoidosis
(B) Renal tubular acidosis
(C) Hyperthyroidism
(D) Myelomatosis
(E) Acute alcoholic pancreatitis

(11) The haemoglobin oxygen dissociation curve is moved to the right by:
(A) Anaemia
(B) Increasing age
(C) Passage through pulmonary capillaries
(D) Increasing body temperature
(E) Acidosis

(12) A patient is suspected to be digoxin toxic. Which of the following statements is true:
(A) The plasma digoxin level is a reliable guide to severity
(B) Corticosteroids may restore normal conduction if heart block is present
(C) Phenytoin may be helpful in the treatment of supraventricular arrhythmias
(D) Intravenous calcium gluconate may temporarily reverse the toxic effects
(E) The ECG characteristically shows widespread RST segment depression

(13) A patient is given a large overdose of gentamicin in error. Possible side-effects include:
(A) Ataxia
(B) Polyuric renal failure
(C) Neuromuscular block
(D) Tinnitus
(E) Bone marrow suppression

(14) A patient presents with an anaphylactic reaction to penicillin. Appropriate treatment includes:
(A) Intravenous chlorpheniramine
(B) Intravenous ranitidine
(C) Volume expansion with dextrans
(D) Subcutaneous adrenaline
(E) Intravenous hydrocortisone

(15) A patient presents with dyspnoea, abdominal pain and vomiting, and causes of the surgical emphysema found on examination include:
(A) Ruptured trachea
(B) Ruptured oesophagus
(C) Spontaneous pneumothorax
(D) Ruptured diaphragm
(E) Pulmonary embolism

(16) A patient is admitted with pulmonary fibrosis. This may be due to:
(A) Uraemia
(B) Pulmonary embolism
(C) Paraquat poisoning
(D) Rheumatoid arthritis
(E) Hypersensitivity

(17) Vitamin K can be used in the treatment of significant bleeding associated with:
(A) Factor XII deficiency
(B) Oral anticoagulant overdosage
(C) Heparin overdosage
(D) Scurvy
(E) Haemophilia

(18) Secondary causes of cardiomyopathy include which of the following:
(A) Prolonged artificial ventilation
(B) Alcoholism
(C) Dystrophia myotonic
(D) Porphyria
(E) Thyrotoxicosis

(19) An 18-year-old driver is admitted to the emergency department unconscious following an accident. Her blood pressure is 85/45 mmHg and pulse rate is 117 beats/min. She has fractured her right lower ribs but has no other obvious injury. Which of the following statements is true?
(A) Urgent laparotomy is indicated
(B) The tachycardia indicates that intracranial pressure is not raised
(C) She could be unconscious from hypotension
(D) Cyanosis may be caused by ARDS
(C) Tension pneumothorax is the most likely cause of the cardiovascular signs

(20) Which of the following are true of myasthenia gravis?
(A) Pyridostigmine is better than neostigmine because overdose does not cause a depolarization block
(B) Blood gases are a good guide to ventilator function
(C) Ophthalmoplegia alone is a presentation
(D) 15% will have a thymoma
(E) Disseminated lupus erythematosus is an association

(21) Alveolar hypoventilation is associated with which of the following:
- (A) Metabolic alkalosis
- (B) Emphysema
- (C) Pleural effusion
- (D) Asthma
- (E) Raised intracranial pressure

(22) Which of the following apply to the diagnosis of brainstem death:
- (A) Reflex movements of the legs may still occur
- (B) A peripheral nerve stimulator should be used to confirm the absence of neuromuscular blockade
- (C) Serial EEGs are required
- (D) The integrity of the fifth nerve is tested by caloric testing
- (E) The patient must not be breathing spontaneously

(23) A patient is admitted with a significant acute paracetamol overdose. Characteristic findings include:
- (A) Jaundice
- (B) Thrombocytopenia
- (C) Hyperventilation
- (D) Coma
- (E) Raised plasma alkaline phosphatase

(24) The following venous blood results – sodium 127 mmol/l, potassium 6 mmol/l, chloride 85 mmol/l, bicarbonate 18 mmol/l, urea 18 mmol/l – are compatible with which of the following conditions:
- (A) High small bowel obstruction with vomiting
- (B) Carcinoma of the lung with inappropriate ADH secretion
- (C) Renal failure
- (D) Hepatic failure
- (E) Adrenocortical insufficiency

(25) Which of the following are recognized complications of acquired immune deficiency syndrome:
- (A) Atypical mycobacterial infections
- (B) Cytomegalovirus pneumonia
- (C) Pulmonary veno-occlusive disease
- (D) Kaposi's sarcoma
- (E) Pneumocystis pneumonia

(26) Prolonged and excessive sedation and analgesia can cause which of the following:
- (A) Large gastric aspirates
- (B) Pneumonia
- (C) Pulmonary embolus
- (D) Bradycardia
- (E) Coma

(27) Which of the following statements regarding atrial flutter are true?
- (A) The radial pulse is usually regular or regular irregular
- (B) Carotid sinus massage usually slows the AV conduction
- (C) The heart is usually normal
- (D) Digoxin often converts the rhythm to atrial fibrillation
- (E) The atrial rate is usually 230 beats/min

(28) Critical illness polyneuropathy may lead to which of the following:
- (A) Problems after discharge from the critical care unit
- (B) Abnormal cardiac conduction
- (C) Hyperkalaemia with suxamethonium
- (D) Aspiration pneumonia
- (E) Abnormal neuromuscular transmission

(29) When considering mechanical ventilation in a patient with chronic obstructive pulmonary disease it is best to aim for:
- (A) Low frequency and low I : E ratio
- (B) Low frequency and low tidal volume
- (C) Hypercapnia and normal pH
- (D) Normocapnia and normal pH
- (E) Hypercapnia and acidosis

(30) A 70-year-old lady known to be hypertensive is admitted to the emergency department with acute severe chest pain radiating into her back. Her blood pressure is 180/100 mmHg. There is no evidence of a myocardial infarction. Which of the following interventions are indicated?
- (A) Administer intravenous hydralazine
- (B) Perform a transoesophageal echocardiogram
- (C) Give intravenous beta-blocker to reduce blood pressure slowly
- (D) Give a fibrinolytic agent
- (E) Insert an intra-arterial catheter to monitor blood pressure

Viva questions

(1) A 32-year-old female patient is admitted to the emergency department with rapid deep respirations. Clinical examination does not reveal

any other significant findings. The following results were obtained initially. Her pupils are fixed and dilated 24 hours later with fundoscopy revealing papilloedema. What are the biochemical abnormalities illustrated and what is the likely diagnosis?

pH 7.1

$PaCO_2$ 2.9 kPa

PaO_2 14 kPa

Sodium 131 mmol/l

Potassium 3 mmol/l

Glucose 14 mmol/l

Creatinine 70 μmol/l

Bicarbonate 16 mmol/l

Chloride 94 mmol/l

Measured serum osmolality 324 mosm/kg

Ionized calcium 1.2 mmol/l

Brain CT normal

CSF normal

(2) A 48-year-old man was admitted to the intensive care unit following the development of intra-abdominal sepsis from a perforated viscous. He is now recovering from multiple organ failure and has the following blood count and iron studies. What is the likely cause of his anaemia? In what setting is this anaemia normally seen and how can it be confirmed?

Hb 9.5 g/dl

WBC 10×10^9/l

Platelets 230×10^9/l

PCV 0.28

RBC 3.7×10^{12}/l

Mean corpuscular volume 81 fl

Mean corpuscular haemoglobin 23.6 pg

Mean corpuscular haemoglobin concentration 322 g/l

Serum iron 4 μmol/l

Serum ferritin 190 μg/l

Serum transferrin 1.1 g/l

Saturation 15%

(3) Outline the common risk factors for venous thromboembolism. When is anticoagulation contraindicated and what is the alternative?

(4) In the severely malnourished patient what are the major risk factors associated with rapid initiation of feeding?

(5) What is the cause of the haemodynamic deterioration in atrial fibrillation?
In which situations should verapamil never be given?

(6) What factors may contribute to the development of an ileus in the critical care unit?

(7) What are the causes of the endotracheal tube becoming dislodged? When is there increased risk of accidental extubation?

(8) What are the potential disadvantages of continuous renal replacement therapy?

(9) Discuss the causes of hyponatraemia following a transurethral prostatic resection and the associated risk factors.

(10) Discuss the use of low-dose dopamine in acute renal failure. Is dopamine renoprotective? How may it promote a dieresis?

(11) Discuss the different types of hypoxia and their causes.

(12) What are the common bacterial pathogens in hospital- and community-acquired pneumonia?

(13) How would you treat toxic shock syndrome?

(14) What are the advantages and disadvantages of using non-invasive positive pressure ventilation?

(15) What are the indications for and the common complications of central venous cannulation?

Answers to MCQs

(1) E, C
(2) B, C, E
(3) C, E
(4) A, B, E
(5) A, B, D
(6) A, B, D, E
(7) B, D, E
(8) A, B, C
(9) A, B, C
(10) A, C, D
(11) A, D, E
(12) E, C
(13) B, C, D
(14) A, D, E
(15) B, C
(16) A, B, C, D, E
(17) B

(18) C, D, E
(19) None
(20) C, D, E
(21) A, B, C, D, E
(22) A, B, E
(23) A, D, E
(24) E, C
(25) A, B, D, E
(26) A, B, C, D, E
(27) A, B, D
(28) A, C, D
(29) A, C
(30) E, C, B

Answers to viva questions

(1) The biochemical pathology is a metabolic acidosis with a high anion gap of 21. There is also a raised osmolar gap. The clinical picture and biochemistry combined with the normal CSF and CT scan suggest methanol ingestion.

(2) The likely cause of the anaemia is chronic disease. This is consistent with the mild microcytosis, normochromia, no reticulocyte response, low serum iron, low transferrin, low per cent saturation with normal ferritin. The anaemia of chronic disease is seen with neoplasia, infection and inflammation. It can be confirmed by lack of haemoglobin response to iron and bone marrow biopsy.

(3) The risk factors for venous thromboembolism include:

- Immobilization
- Trauma
- Recent surgery
- Obesity
- Smoking
- Congestive cardiac failure
- Old age
- Stroke
- Long-distance travel
- Pregnancy
- Oestrogen-containing contraceptive pill
- Family history of thrombosis.

If there is active bleeding, spinal cord injury, haemorrhagic stroke, ocular haemorrhage anticoagulation is contraindicated. A venacaval filter can be inserted.

(4) Refeeding syndrome can cause shifts of electrolytes resulting in severe hypokalaemia, hypophosphataemia and cardiac arrhythmias.

(5) Stroke volume is reduced because of the decrease in diastolic filling time with a rapid heart rate and the loss of the atrial systole. If the patient is on a beta-blocker or an accessory pathway is suspected then verapamil should never be used.

(6) A number of factors can contribute to the development of an ileus on the critical care unit. They include:

- Administration of opioids
- Critical illness polyneuropathy
- Hypokalaemia
- Residual neuromuscular blockade
- Pancreatitis
- Intra-abdominal hypertension
- Peritonitis
- Uraemia
- Hyperglycaemia
- Hypoalbuminaemia.

(7) The tracheal tube may become dislodged because of patient agitation, poor sedation, tracheal tube not placed in mid trachea or cut short, poor fixation, failure to support ventilation tubing appropriately. There is increased risk during physiotherapy, moving, proning patients or when there are not enough appropriately trained nursing staff.

(8) Continuous renal replacement therapy has a number of potential disadvantages; these include:

- Continuous anticoagulation
- Hypophosphataemia
- Loss of trace elements
- Difficulties in transferring patients for investigations
- Patient immobility.

(9) During transurethral resection of the prostate, large volumes of irrigation fluid containing glycine, sorbitol or mannitol are used. As much as 3 litres of this fluid can be absorbed into the circulation leading to a dilutional reduction in the plasma sodium concentration. The plasma sodium concentration may fall to as low as 100 mmol/l. The prolonged duration of surgery, excess height of irrigation

solution reservoir and large tissue resection are all risk factors. The history and the presence of an osmolar gap and hyponatraemia confirm the diagnosis.

(10) Dopamine is not renoprotective and the use of renal dose dopamine is no longer recommended. Dopamine can promote a diuresis by improving renal blood flow and glomerular filtration by elevating the blood pressure and cardiac output, it also modifies intrarenal haemodynamics via tubular dopamine receptors. The improvement in urine output must be balanced with the side effects such as arrhythmias and pituitary suppression.

(11) Hypoxia can be classified into four different types. These include:

- Circulatory hypoxia caused by a reduction in cardiac output, e.g. heart failure, severe hypovolaemia.
- Cytopathic hypoxia caused by a deficiency in cellular utilization of oxygen, e.g. sepsis, carbon monoxide and cyanide poisoning.
- Hypoxic hypoxia is a problem with saturating haemoglobin with oxygen, e.g. ARDS, pneumonia, carbon monoxide poisoning.
- Anaemic hypoxia results from a fall in haemoglobin, e.g. haemorrhage, bone marrow suppression.

(12) The usual pathogens involved with hospital-acquired pneumonia are *Pseudomonas aeruginosa*, *Klebsiella* spp. and *Acinetobacter* spp. *Haemophilus influenzae*, *Moraxella catarrhalis* and *Streptococcus pneumoniae* are found in community-acquired infection but can also be nosocomial.

(13) Source control would consist of wound drainage, removal of any foreign body associated with condition or wide excision if the cause is necrotizing fasciitis. Penicillin combined with clindamycin would be antibiotics of choice. Fluids and inotropes should be used to support the blood pressure. Immunoglobulins and hyperbaric oxygen may be used in severe cases although the evidence is lacking.

(14) The potential advantages of non-invasive positive pressure ventilation include:

Improved patient comfort with the reduced need for sedation

Reduced length of ICU, hospital stay and mortality

Airway reflexes preserved

Reduced airway trauma

Decreased incidence of nosocomial pneumonia

Potential disadvantages include:

Airway not protected

Gastric distention

Intubation delayed

Patient tolerance

Increased work for nursing staff

Difficulty in airway suction.

(15) The common indications for central venous cannulation include:

Measurement of central venous pressure

Administration of parenteral nutrition or irritating drugs

Haemodialysis

Large-bore venous access

Long-term venous access

Insertion of temporary pacing wire

Measurement of central venous oxygen saturations

Insertion of pulmonary artery catheter

Complications include:

Infection, thrombophlebitis, thrombosis

Pneumothorax, haemothorax, chylothorax

Haemorrhage

Air embolism

Cardiac arrhythmias

Local nerve, artery and vein damage.

Index